Fundamentals of Law for Health Informatics and Information Management

Second Edition, Revised Reprint

Melanie S. Brodnik, PhD, RHIA, FAHIMA;

Laurie A. Rinehart-Thompson, JD, RHIA, CHP, FAHIMA; and

Rebecca B. Reynolds, EdD, MHA, RHIA, FAHIMA

EDITORS

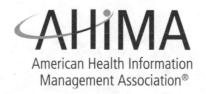

American Health Information
Management Association®

ISBN: 978-1-58426-073-8
AHIMA Product No.: AB241813

AHIMA Staff:
Angela K. Dinh, RHIA, CHPS, MHA, Technical Review, Second Edition
Julie A. Dooling, RHIA, Technical Review
Katherine E. Downing, MA, RHIA, CHPS, PMP, Technical Review
Katherine M. Greenock, MS, Production Development Editor
Jason O. Malley, Director, Creative Content Development
Diana M. Warner, RHIA, CHPS, MS, FAHIMA, Technical Review, Second Edition
Pamela Woolf, Managing Editor

For more information about AHIMA Press publications, including updates, visit http://www.ahima.org/publications/updates.aspx

American Health Information Management Association
233 North Michigan Avenue, 21st Floor
Chicago, Illinois 60601-5809

ahima.org

Brief Contents

Contents

CHAPTER 8   **The Legal Health Record: Maintenance, Content, Documentation,**

and Disposition 165

Laurie A. Rinehart-Thompson, JD, RHIA, CHP, FAHIMA,
Rebecca B. Reynolds, EdD, MHA, RHIA, FAHIMA, and
Keith Olenik, MA, RHIA, CHP

Keith Olenik, MA, RHIA, CHP, Melanie S. Brodnik, PhD, RHIA, FAHIMA,
Rebecca B. Reynolds, EdD, MHA, RHIA, FAHIMA, and
Laurie Rinehart-Thompson, JD, RHIA, CHP, FAHIMA

CHAPTER 13   **Required Reporting and Mandatory Disclosure Laws** 373
Elizabeth D. Bowman, MPA, RHIA

CHAPTER 16   **Medical Staff**. 461

Rebecca B. Reynolds, EdD, MHA, RHIA, FAHIMA, and
Melanie S. Brodnik, PhD, RHIA, FAHIMA

About the Editors and Authors

Melanie S. Brodnik, PhD, RHIA, FAHIMA, is an associate professor emeritus of the undergraduate program in health information management and systems, and coordinator of the graduate program in health informatics at Ohio State University. She has served on the AHIMA Board of Directors, was president of AHIMA in 2004, and is currently a commissioner of the board of directors of the Council on Accreditation of Health Informatics and Information Management Education (CAHIIM). Melanie received the AHIMA Literary Award in 1992, the Champion Award in 2006, and the Legacy Award in 2010; in 2006 she received the Ohio Health Information Management Distinguished Member Award. Melanie has championed the issues of patient privacy, confidentiality, and security throughout her career. She has taught legal courses at Ohio State University and was editor and column writer for *Topics in Health Information Management* for 20 years. She served on the editorial review board for AHIMA's *In Confidence Privacy and Confidentiality Newsletter* from 1996 to 2002 and currently serves on the editorial review board of *Perspectives in Health Information Management* and on the boards of several other professional journals. She has authored or coauthored many publications and has presented at numerous local, state, and national professional association meetings, workshops, and conventions. She received her associate degree in medical record technology from Fullerton Junior College, a bachelor's degree in health information management from Loma Linda University, a master's of science degree from the State University of New York at Buffalo, and her doctorate degree in educational research and evaluation from Ohio State University.

Laurie A. Rinehart-Thompson, JD, RHIA, CHP, FAHIMA, currently serves as the director of the undergraduate Health Information Management and Systems program and is an associate professor of clinical health and rehabilitation sciences at The Ohio State University. She earned her bachelor of science degree in medical record administration and her juris doctor degree from The Ohio State University. In addition to HIM education, her professional experiences span the behavioral health, home health, and acute care arenas. Laurie has served as an expert witness in civil litigation, testifying as to the privacy and confidentiality of health information. She has served on the AHIMA CHP Exam Construction, Advocacy & Policy, and Education Strategy committees and the AHIMA Privacy and Security Practice Council. She is currently a member of the AHIMA Professional Ethics Commiteee and serves on a Council on Excellence in Education subcommittee. She has served on the executive board of directors of the Ohio Health Information Management Association and is currently a project leader. A frequent speaker on the HIPAA Privacy Rule, she is the author of AHIMA's *Introduction to Health Information Privacy and Security*. She is also a contributing author to *Ethical Challenges in the Management of Health Information*, AHIMA's *Health Information*

Management Technology: An Applied Approach, AHIMA's *Documentation for Medical Practices*, and the *Journal of AHIMA*. She has also been published in *Perspectives in Health Information Management*. She received the Ohio Health Information Management Association's Distinguished Member Award and the AHIMA Legacy Award in 2010.

Rebecca B. Reynolds, EdD, MHA, RHIA, FAHIMA, is an associate professor and program director for the graduate program in health informatics and information management at the University of Tennessee Health Science Center (UTHSC) in Memphis. She has served on the AHIMA nominating committee and was chair of the 2010 AHIMA Education Strategy Committee. She is past president of the Tennessee Health Information Management Association and received its Outstanding New Professional Award in 1995 and Distinguished Member Award in 2004. She coordinated the HIPAA implementation program for the UTHSC system and provides HIPAA privacy and security training to all UTHSC students. She teaches the legal courses for both entry-level masters and post-professional graduate students and conducts legal workshops for attorneys, nurses, and other healthcare professionals. She served as a member of the Operations Committee of the Mid-South eHealth Alliance, which is a functioning health information exchange. She also serves on the Tennessee eHealth Network's Privacy and Security Work Group. She received her bachelor's degree in health information management from UTHSC and her master's degree in healthcare administration and doctorate in higher education administration from the University of Memphis. She received the AHIMA Legacy Award in 2010, and became a fellow of AHIMA in 2012.

Elizabeth Bowman, MPA, RHIA, has served as a professor in the Department of Health Informatics and Information Management at the University of Tennessee Health Science Center in Memphis for more than 35 years. She received a bachelor's degree from Millsaps College and a postbaccalaureate certificate from the Baptist Memorial Hospital School of Medical Record Administration. She also holds a master's degree in public administration with a concentration in healthcare administration from the University of Memphis. Bowman has served as chair of the AHIMA Assembly on Education and received the AHIMA Educator Award in 1999. She served as a commissioner and chair of the Commission on Accreditation for Health Informatics and Information Management Education, as well as chair of the AHIMA Professional Development Committee. She is a recipient of the Tennessee Health Information Management Association's Distinguished Member Award and the Chancellor's Distinguished Teaching Award, which recognizes excellence in teaching at the University of Tennessee Health Science Center. In 2009, Beth was awarded the Educator/Mentor Award from the Tennessee Health Information Management Association and the Outstanding Teacher Award from the University of Tennessee Alumni Association.

Sue Bowman, RHIA, CCS, is director of coding policy and compliance for AHIMA. She previously served as director of utilization review and data quality at St. Mary's Hospital in Centralia, IL; as a member of the board of directors of the Illinois Health Information Management Association (ILHIMA); and as chair of AHIMA's Society for Clinical Coding. She is the editor of the AHIMA publication *Health Information Management Compliance: Guidelines for Preventing Fraud and Abuse*. She has also participated in the development of the Office of Inspector General (OIG) compliance program guidance documents. Moreover, she has provided health information management consultative services to the OIG, the Federal Bureau of Investigation, and the Department of Justice on fraud and abuse and compliance issues. She has also provided an educational program to OIG officials on health record documentation and coding practices. Bowman has provided input on the development of the ICD-10-CM and ICD-10-PCS code sets and serves as secretariat on the World Health Organization's morbidity topical advisory group, which is contributing to the development of ICD-11. She holds a bachelor of science degree in medical record administration from Daemen College in Amherst, NY, and is currently enrolled in the master of jurisprudence in health law program at Loyola University Chicago School of Law. Sue has written numerous articles and provided a number of media interviews on fraud and abuse, compliance, and coding issues, in addition to giving a number of presentations on issues related to coding and compliance.

Jill Callahan Klaver, JD, RHIA, is principal of Health Risk Advantage, a Colorado-based risk management consulting firm that assists healthcare organizations in minimizing their risk of liability. Prior to this, she was senior vice president of public and industry leadership for AHIMA, where she helped plan and execute the association's policy and alliance agendas. Her leadership on health information management issues spans almost 30 years, and she is a frequent speaker on risk management, privacy, and electronic health information management topics. Her publications include numerous articles; chapter author of "Legal Issues in Health Information Management" in *Health Information: Management of a Strategic Resource* (Elsevier); author of *Privacy & Confidentiality of Health Information* (Jossey-Bass and AHA Press); and technical editor of *HIPAA by Example* (AHIMA). Jill served on AHIMA's Board of Directors from 2002 through 2007 and as the elected president in 2006. She was a member of the Confidentiality, Privacy, and Security Workgroup of the American Health Information Community (AHIC) of the US Department of Health and Human Services' Office of the National Coordinator for Health Information Technology. She has a law degree from Loyola University of Chicago, a master's in administration (health administration concentration) from Central Michigan University, and a bachelor of science degree in medical record administration from Ferris State University.

Keith Olenik, MA, RHIA, CHP, is principal of the Olenik Consulting Group in Chicago, IL, and a visiting professor for the University of Cincinnati Health Information Management Program. He also has worked as senior vice president of Consulting Services for Nauvalis Healthcare Solutions and as chief privacy officer at St. Luke's Health System in Kansas City, MO. Keith was a member of the AHIMA Board of Directors from 2004 to 2006, and chair of the AHIMA Foundation Board of Directors in 2009 and the AHIMA Certified in Healthcare Privacy Exam Construction Committee. He was president of the Missouri HIMA and has served on various state-level committees over the years. Keith is an active speaker on the topics of legal health records, electronic discovery, document imaging, project management, and various compliance topics at national and state meetings. He has a bachelor of science in health information management from the University of Kansas and a master of arts in health services management from Webster University.

Sebastian E. Proels, JD, MD, is the managing member of the law firm of Proels Winschel LLC, a litigation firm in Cleveland, OH. He has more than 20 years of combined experience in the physical sciences, medicine, and the law. He manages the firm's civil and criminal litigation, including its personal injury and tort practices. During the past 11 years, he has successfully prosecuted and defended thousands of civil cases at one of Ohio's largest litigation firms, including medical malpractice, personal injury, product liability, asbestos, toxic tort, wrongful death, insurance, commercial, and workers' compensation cases. Dr. Proels received his medical degree from the University of Chicago Pritzker School of Medicine and completed postgraduate permanent licensure requirements to practice medicine in the state of Illinois. He attended Case Western Reserve University School of Law on an academic scholarship. Since graduating from law school, he has devoted 100 percent of his professional time to the practice of trial law. Dr. Proels has diverse teaching experience that includes continuing legal education seminars for professional groups, including lawyers and paralegals, on a variety of legal and medical subject matters. He has published numerous articles and chapters in professional journals, trade journals, and university texts.

Marcia Y. Sharp, EdD, MBA, RHIA, is an assistant professor in the Department of Health Informatics and Information Management at the University of Tennessee Health Sciences Center. She has had an outstanding career in Health Information Management and in Human Resource Management, and has held various leadership positions in acute care hospitals and managed care organizations. She is an active member of the Memphis Health Information Management Association, serving as former treasurer and the Tennessee Health Information Management Association, serving as the Tennessee delegate to AHIMA House of Delegates, and former member of the Tennessee Nominating Committee. She is currently a member of the Editorial Review Panel for Perspectives on Health Information Management (PHIM). She has contributed chapters to several AHIMA publications, *Health Information Management Technology: An Applied Approach*, and *Fundamentals of Law for Health Informatics and Information Management*.

Preface

The use of health information technology, greater reliance on electronically stored information, and the federal government's promotion of electronic health records are all dramatically changing the way information is maintained in healthcare organizations. All healthcare professionals and employees with any relationship to patient information are challenged by the issues of confidentiality, privacy, security, and data integrity of this information. Subsequently, they are now charged with the responsibility of protecting its access, use, and disclosure. The complexities of managing health information are expanding as the industry faces increasing demands to share patient information and reduce healthcare costs while enhancing quality of care.

Traditionally, custodial responsibility for managing and safeguarding health information in either paper or electronic form rested with the health information management (HIM) department of a healthcare organization. With the increasing amount of electronic data and different health record formats, however, there are broader legal ramifications that extend beyond the traditional HIM department and encompass all departments and professionals who generate, access, use, and disclose patient information. Individuals who manage healthcare data and information in paper or electronic form and who control its collection, access, use, exchange, and protection are referred to as HIM professionals or health informatics professionals. However, healthcare administrators and healthcare providers such as doctors and nurses also have a role in understanding the legal aspects of healthcare and protecting the privacy, confidentiality, and security of health information.

This textbook was written to provide individuals responsible for managing and protecting health information and health records with the fundamentals of law surrounding the delivery of healthcare and the management and protection of health information.

Chapter 1, "Introduction to the Fundamentals of Law for Health Informatics and Information Management," introduces the complexity of healthcare law and legal issues surrounding the growing use of health information technology. It defines health information and health records as well as the concepts of privacy, confidentiality, and security. The issue of ownership of health records is introduced, followed by a discussion of custodial responsibility for health records and who functions in the role of custodian. It introduces the concept of ethics and professional codes of ethics as applied to the management and protection of health information.

Chapter 2, "The Legal System in the United States," provides the foundation for the role of law in the US healthcare system. It discusses the types and sources of law, government organization and its role in lawmaking, the court system, and resolution of disputes via mechanisms that exist outside the courtroom.

Chapter 3, "Civil Procedure," provides a working knowledge of the procedural aspects of the law. Healthcare professionals who respond to or attend legal proceedings must understand the issues related to malpractice, workers' compensation, subpoenas and court orders, and other legal matters routinely confronted by custodians of health information.

Chapter 4, "Evidence," introduces the concept of evidence, including the legal processes through which health records and information are requested and used as evidence during litigation. The health record as a business record made and kept in the usual course of business at or near the time of the event recorded is discussed. The chapter also emphasizes changes in evidentiary law as related to discovery of electronically stored information.

Chapter 5, "Tort Law," provides comprehensive coverage of tort law, which addresses the process for civil remedy to recover damages for wrongs involving personal or individual rights, rights to personal property, and rights to real property. Conduct that was entirely acceptable a century or even decades ago may now be totally unacceptable, giving rise to new causes of action. Examples include recovery of damages for discrimination, wrongful discharge from employment, strict product liability, negligent infliction of emotional harm, and wrongful use and disclosure of health information.

Chapter 6, "Corporations, Contracts, and Antitrust Legal Issues," describes the basic legal concepts that affect a healthcare organization as a business. It discusses the formation and types of corporations and the responsibilities of a corporate board. The general principles of contracts and antitrust are discussed along with issues related to vendor, physician-patient, and medical staff contracts.

Chapter 7, "Consent to Treatment," addresses one of the most valued rights in American society: the right to control one's own body, especially when it comes to medical decision making. This chapter discusses the right of an individual to consent or refuse consent to medical treatment. Because this right is not absolute and is governed by state and federal laws, individuals working in healthcare must be knowledgeable about the ethical and applicable legal principles of consent, the requirements for obtaining a legally defensible consent, and the potential liability resulting from treatment without proper consent.

Chapter 8, "The Legal Health Record: Maintenance, Content, Documentation, and Disposition," focuses on the laws and standards that dictate the maintenance of health records, essential documentation principles, the elements necessary for a legally defensible health record, and issues surrounding the retention and destruction of health records. The chapter also addresses the emerging concept of the legal health record. The chapter distinguishes between a legal health record and a designated record set, which is discussed in more detail in chapter 9.

Chapter 9, "The HIPAA Privacy Rule," addresses one of the most highly publicized laws to affect the healthcare industry in recent years, including changes brought about by HITECH and the subsequent January 2013 Final Rule. The HIPAA Privacy Rule is one of two key administrative simplification provisions of a federal law that governs the privacy and confidentiality of patient information. The chapter provides an in-depth discussion of the rule from its evolution to purpose to applicability to requirements. The chapter spells out the rules and the exceptions to the rules, which must be understood by those who manage the uses and disclosures of protected healthcare information.

Chapter 10, "The HIPAA Security Rule," deals with the second administrative simplification provision of HIPAA. This provision governs protected health information transmitted by or maintained in electronic media. Details of the security regulations are discussed in this chapter, including security safeguards and methods that prevent unauthorized access, alteration, deletion, and transmission of electronic health information.

Chapter 11, "Security Threats and Controls," discusses threats to the security of electronically protected health information in terms of access and system controls. Suggestions for preventing identity theft and medical identity theft are offered, along with issues to consider when transmitting information via fax, e-mail, the Internet, or other wireless devices. The importance of contingency or disaster recovery planning is also presented.

Chapter 12, "Access, Use, and Disclosure/Release of Health Information," discusses access to and protection of patient information, including highly sensitive information such as behavioral health, substance abuse, HIV/AIDS, genetic information, and adoption. Ownership and control of the health record and information therein are introduced along with practical situations regarding the use and disclosure of patient information with or without patient authorization. A discussion of the process for managing the release of patient information concludes the chapter.

Chapter 13, "Required Reporting and Mandatory Disclosure Laws," delves into the state and federal reporting laws that require certain healthcare entities or providers to report specific information to government and quasigovernment agencies in order to protect the health and safety of a community.

Reporting laws related to abuse and neglect of children and the elderly, communicable diseases, suspicious or unattended deaths, abortion, unusual events, registries, vital records, and more are discussed.

Chapter 14, "Risk Management and Quality Improvement," explores the concepts of risk management and quality improvement as they relate to the identification, analysis, evaluation, and elimination or reduction of possible risks to an institution's patients, visitors, and employees. It discusses the significance of advancing good medical outcomes and reducing costs while maintaining a high standard of quality care.

Chapter 15, "Corporate Compliance," provides an in-depth discussion of healthcare fraud and abuse issues that result in unnecessary costs and adverse patient outcomes. Compliance programs exist to ensure that healthcare organizations are meeting all pertinent laws, including the appropriate use of healthcare resources and proper billing for services rendered, in an effort to avoid investigations and resulting penalties for violations.

Chapter 16, "Medical Staff," addresses governing-body responsibility for medical staff organizations and the significance of medical staff bylaws that define the organizational structure of a healthcare organization's medical staff. The credentialing process, along with issues related to the granting of staff privileges and medical staff duties and responsibilities, is discussed, as is the legal concept of due process as it pertains to disciplinary and employment practices.

Chapter 17, "Workplace Law," focuses on employment laws related to the management of human resources. Labor laws related to discrimination, wages, and employee safety are discussed, in addition to issues related to unions and collective bargaining.

Appendixes include a glossary of terms and an online reference list. Throughout the chapters, boldface type is used to indicate the first substantial reference to a key term included in the glossary.

Acknowledgments

The editors would like to express appreciation to the many individuals who contributed to the writing, reviewing, and publication of this textbook. We are grateful for everyone's contributions and would particularly like to thank the AHIMA publications staff and book reviewers. We offer special recognition and gratitude to our chapter authors and coauthors Elizabeth Bowman, Sue Bowman, Jill Callahan Klaver, Keith Olenik, Sebastian Proels, Julie Roth, and Marcia Sharp. Without the collective contributions and expertise of these individuals, the publication of this textbook would not have been possible. We would also like to thank those who contributed to the first edition of the book, Joseph Brunetto, Denise Burke, Frances W. Lee, and Dianne Wilkinson. Special thanks go to Mary McCain, professor emeritus, University of Tennessee, Memphis, who served as one of the editors and coauthor for the book's first edition. Her dedication and hard work on the book's first edition is greatly appreciated. Finally, the editors wish to thank their families for their support and patience during the revision process of the book.

Foreword

To future health informatics and information management professionals:

Health informatics and information management (HIIM) professionals have many responsibilities, and none is more to the core of our profession than the protection of the information that has been entrusted to our guardianship. As HIIM professionals we must have an understanding of the various federal and state court systems and the associated health information legal processes therein, and we must ensure that the health information and systems with which we are entrusted are appropriately used and when needed said information disclosed. The HIIM professional must also have an in-depth knowledge of federal and state laws and regulations and accreditation standards governing who is entitled to have access to health information and under what circumstances.

The Health Insurance Portability and Accountability Act of 1996 (HIPAA) brought forth a new focus on the use and disclosure of health information. The HIPAA Privacy Rule is considered a "floor" as a national health information privacy standard; there are states that have rules that are more stringent and must be observed in those instances. The HIIM professional must be aware of the legislative rules within their respective state of employment. The HIIM professional focus on privacy and security increases when health information exchange is undertaken across state borders. The Health Information Technology for Economic and Clinical Health (HITECH) Act, enacted as part of the American Recovery and Reinvestment Act of 2009, was signed into law on February 17, 2009, to promote the adoption and meaningful use of health information technology. Subtitle D of the HITECH Act addresses the privacy and security concerns associated with the electronic transmission of health information, in part, through several provisions that strengthen the civil and criminal enforcement of the HIPAA rules. Healthcare organizations are also being forced into a compliance-critical condition by the HITECH Act, which expands the reach of HIPAA's data privacy and security requirements, as well as by a host of other industry standards and regulations. Today, healthcare organizations face increased liability and fines, as well as audits to demonstrate that electronic protected health information (ePHI) is adequately secured.

This textbook, Fundamentals of Law for Health Informatics and Information Management, 2nd edition, focuses on this body of knowledge from the HIIM professional's perspective. The contributors to this textbook expertly discuss the legal processes important to the HIIM professional, such as civil procedure, the medical record of evidence, and legal precedents. Also provided is guidance to the HIIM professional in responding to requests for uses and disclosures of health information and to assist in developing and maintaining systems to protect patient information. Additionally, the contributors discuss other legal aspects that the HIIM professional should be aware of, such as labor law, medical staff organization, risk management, quality improvement, and compliance.

HIIM professionals are the individuals entrusted to protect patient privacy and ensure appropriate security safeguards are in place. The future of true electronic health information that can be shared for the improvement in patient quality care depends on the public's trust in this role we provide to the healthcare industry.

Rita K. Bowen, MA, RHIA, CHPS, SSGB
Senior Vice President of HIM Best Practices and Privacy Officer
HealthPort Corporation

Chapter 1

Introduction to the Fundamentals of Law for Health Informatics and Information Management

Melanie S. Brodnik, PhD, RHIA, FAHIMA

Learning Objectives

- Discuss why protecting the privacy and confidentiality of health information is a challenge

- Describe the primary and secondary uses of health information

- Discuss the difference between a paper health record, a hybrid record, and an electronic health record

- Define and explain the theoretical concepts behind privacy, confidentiality, and security

- Discuss ownership of the health record and control over the use of information within the health record

- Discuss the role and responsibilities of the custodian of health records and who may serve in the role of custodian

- Describe the role of professional codes of ethics in protecting health information

Key Terms

American Health Information Management Association (AHIMA)

American Medical Association (AMA)

American Medical Informatics Association (AMIA)

American Recovery and Reinvestment Act of 2009 (ARRA)

American Society for Testing and Materials (ASTM)

Autonomy

Beneficence

Business record

Code of ethics (or code of ethical practice)

Confidentiality

Custodian of health records

Data security

Designated record set

Electronic health record

Electronic medical record

Ethics

Ethical principles

Health information

Health information exchange

Health information technology

Health Information Technology for Economic and Clinical Health Act (HITECH)

Health Insurance Portability and Accountability Act of 1996 (HIPAA)

Health record

Hybrid health record

Information governance

The Joint Commission

Justice

Law
Legal health record
Moral values
National Alliance for Health
    Information Technology
Nonmaleficence

Office of the National
    Coordinator for Health
    Information Technology
Ownership
Personal health record
Privileged communication

Privacy
Security
Steward
Stewardship
System security

Introduction

Law represents a set of governing rules designed to protect citizens living in a civilized society. Law establishes order, provides parameters for conduct, and defines the rights and obligations of the government and its citizens. It controls behavior that threatens public safety and sets penalties for disobedience. Law is divided into two types, public and private, which collectively define, regulate, and enforce rights and duties among people and businesses. Healthcare in the United States is a trillion-dollar industry that is complex and highly regulated by federal and state laws. It is also governed by various accrediting bodies' standards of practice. These laws and standards define how healthcare is delivered, financed, and reimbursed. They protect consumers and healthcare providers by requiring accountability for services rendered and the privacy, confidentiality, and security of **health information.**

Health information is often used as evidence in legal cases in which conflict arises and resolution is sought through the court system. Its primary use is for clinical care; however, secondary uses are numerous, such as public health reporting, population health studies, third-party reimbursement, and patient safety and quality improvement initiatives (Safran et al. 2007). During the past decade there has been unparalleled interest in decreasing healthcare costs and improving the quality and safety of healthcare through the use of **health information technology** (HIT). The main focus has been on moving from paper to **electronic health records** (EHRs) and **health information exchanges** (HIEs) that enable the sharing of information with multiple parties and across multiple boundaries to address healthcare cost, quality, access, and safety issues (President's Council of Advisors on Science and Technology 2010, v).

However, before seamless exchange of health information is common practice, differences in laws, standards, and program policies and procedures need to be addressed. Public and private collaborations have been working to eliminate legal barriers that prevent sharing of electronically stored health information as well as to identify practical solutions and implementation strategies that protect the privacy, confidentiality, and security of electronically stored and exchanged health information. For example, the federal government's Agency for Healthcare Research and Quality (AHRQ) funded the Health Information Privacy and Security Collaboration, which brought together 34 states to provide guidance in organization-level business practices, policies, and state laws that affect electronic exchange of health information. Several key reports have resulted from this collaboration, one of which is the *Health Information Security and Privacy Collaboration Toolkit* (AHRQ 2011).

Individuals responsible for protecting the privacy and security of health information within a healthcare organization are usually identified as health information management (HIM) or informatics professionals. They, along with healthcare providers and administrators, are challenged to understand the complexity of healthcare law and requirements to protect the privacy, confidentiality, and security of patient health information. In addition, they must accommodate changes to laws, standards, and programmatic policies and procedures that support the legal issues surrounding the delivery of healthcare and the growing use of electronically stored health information and health records.

This chapter sets the stage for this understanding by defining health information and health records. The concepts of privacy, confidentiality, and security are defined and discussed in terms of their significance for protecting health information. The issue of ownership of health records is introduced, followed by a discussion of custodial responsibility for health records and who functions in the role of custodian. The chapter concludes with a discussion of ethics as applied to the management and protection of health information.

Health Information and Health Records

Health information refers to the data generated and collected as a result of delivering care to a patient. It is collected from multiple sources and is used for a wide variety of purposes.

> [I]t is any information, whether oral or recorded in any form or medium, that: (1) Is created or received by a health care provider, health plan, public health authority, employer, life insurer, school or university, or health care clearinghouse; and (2) Relates to the past, present, or future physical or mental health or condition of an individual; the provision of health care to an individual; or the past, present, or future payment for the provision of health care to an individual (HIPAA 45 CFR 160.103).

What information is documented varies depending on several factors, including state or jurisdiction of healthcare provider, accrediting or licensing body requirements, type of healthcare provider (for example, hospital, clinic, physician practice, behavioral health center), and services rendered for the episode of care.

The information generated on a patient's episode of care comprises a patient's **health record** or record of care. A health record may also be known as a medical record, patient record, client record, inpatient record, outpatient record, or clinic record. The **American Health Information Management Association** (AHIMA) states that a health record "comprises individually identifiable data, in any medium, that are collected, processed, stored, displayed, and used by healthcare professionals" (AHIMA e-HIM Work Group 2010). It reveals the care rendered to the patient and the patient's healthcare status.

Health records are maintained in either paper or electronic formats or a combination of the two. The term **hybrid health record** refers to a record that consists of both paper and electronic records and media (for example, film, video, or imaging system) and uses both manual and electronic processes (AHIMA 2010). The record is usually composed of electronically stored information from numerous clinical information systems, such as laboratory, pharmacy, radiology, nursing, and other ancillary or administrative systems, along with paper documents. The data in the record may be handwritten, direct voice entry captured in a word-processing system, from provider wireless devices such as handheld personal computers, or any combination of these (Amatayakul 2013).

If the health record is completely electronic, it is called an EHR or **electronic medical record** (EMR). These terms are often used interchangeably but may be defined differently depending on the organization and how the record is designed or used. To help alleviate legal barriers and facilitate adoption of EHRs and HIEs, the **National Alliance for Health Information Technology** (NAHIT), sponsored by the **Office of the National Coordinator for Health Information Technology** (ONC), developed consensus-based definitions related to key HIT terms (NAHIT 2008). NAHIT's definitions for an EHR and EMR are as follows:

- **Electronic health record**—"an electronic record of health-related information on an individual that conforms to nationally recognized interoperability standards and that can be created, managed, and consulted by authorized clinicians and staff across more than one healthcare organization"

- **Electronic medical record**—"an electronic record of health-related information on an individual that can be created, gathered, managed and consulted by authorized clinicians and staff within one healthcare organization" (NAHIT 2008, 6)

The key difference in these definitions is that the EMR is considered an electronic record housed within an organization whereas an EHR is thought to contain data or information across more than one organization. However, as previously mentioned these terms are often used interchangeably. Healthcare consumers may also maintain a **personal health record** (PHR), which NAHIT defines as "an electronic record of health-related information on an individual that conforms to nationally recognized interoperability standards and that can be drawn from multiple sources while being managed, shared, and controlled by the individual" (NAHIT 2008, 6). Whether the health record is a paper record, a hybrid record, an EMR, or an EHR, it is the legal **business record** of an organization or healthcare provider. It is used for business, legal, and compliance purposes. For example, it serves as evidence in lawsuits or other legal actions. Information detailing the contents of a health record and including what constitutes a **legal health record** and **designated record set** are discussed in more detail in chapter 8.

Working within healthcare requires an understanding of the American legal system and the laws and standards that govern its delivery, financing, and reimbursement. Managing health data, information, and records also requires a clear understanding of laws and standards that protect the collection, access, use, exchange, and disclosure of health information and records. One of the most notable federal laws addressing privacy and security for "protected health information" (PHI) is the **Health Insurance Portability and Accountability Act of 1996** (HIPAA) (45 CFR 160, 164). HIPAA rules were originally enacted to protect patient information as a result of increasing use of information technology in healthcare. Specific HIPAA privacy rules went into effect in 2002, followed by security rules in 2003. Subsequently, in 2009, the **Health Information Technology for Economic and Clinical Health Act** (HITECH) (42 USC 17921) of the **American Recovery and Reinvestment Act of 2009** (ARRA) was passed to further promote the creation of a national healthcare infrastructure through adoption and meaningful use of EHR systems among healthcare providers and the sharing of health information through HIEs.

HITECH widens the scope of privacy and security protections under HIPAA to include companies previously untouched by HIPAA, provides for more enforcement of the rule, and increases potential legal liability for noncompliance (Callahan-Dennis 2010, 6). Many HITECH requirements were effective in 2010 with the remaining finalized in 2013. The Department of Health and Human Services (HHS) is charged with the promulgation of regulations to implement the HITECH legislation, which is discussed in more detail in chapters 9 and 10. HIPAA and HITECH are two of more than 50 federal laws and regulations addressing privacy, confidentiality, and security protections (Office of the National Coordinator for Health IT, Privacy & Security 2010).

Core to HIPAA, HITECH, and other federal and state laws related to the protection, access, use, and disclosure of health information, records, or both is an understanding of the concepts of privacy, confidentiality, and security.

Privacy, Confidentiality, and Security

Privacy and confidentiality have historically been key components of the patient-provider relationship. The information contained in a health record, regardless of its scope or format, can be some of the most private and sensitive information that exists about a person. In conjunction with a healthcare encounter, documentation is created to record the care that was provided, support medical decisions, and provide evidence of patient outcomes. Patients are encouraged to be truthful with their care providers regarding their mental and physical conditions because the truth is essential to the successful delivery of appropriate healthcare. Such truths, however, can place the patient in an extremely vulnerable position when intimate clinical and behavioral secrets are revealed or discovered as patient treatment is provided, test results are reported, and future options for care are discussed. Because of this, when a patient provides information and it is documented, there is an inherent trust that it will be kept private and protected from unauthorized access (Rinehart-Thompson and Harman 2006, 52–53).

The protection of individuals' health information is a central, defining obligation of healthcare providers, health information managers, and informatics professionals. In every area of law that relates to health information, the appropriate use and disclosure of that information must be a primary consideration. Although the protection of health information is discussed extensively later in the book, its significance warrants specific discussion in this introductory chapter. An understanding of the concepts of privacy, confidentiality, and security and the differences among the three concepts is important for the management of health information from a legal perspective.

Privacy

Privacy is an important social value that, described by jurists Samuel Warren and Louis Brandeis in 1890, means the right "to be let alone" (Rinehart-Thompson and Harman 2006, 53). It is an important aspect of one's freedom and one's legal right to be selective about what is revealed about oneself to others (Bankert and Amdur 2006, 143). One definition, which addresses the breadth of privacy, is provided by the **American Society for Testing and Materials** (ASTM) E 31 Health Informatics Subcommittee, which states:

> Privacy is a right of individuals to be let [*sic*] alone and to be protected against physical or psychological invasion or the misuse of their property. It includes freedom from intrusion or observation into one's private affairs, the right to maintain control over certain personal information, and the freedom to act without outside interference (ASTM Committee E31 on Healthcare Informatics Subcommittee E31.17 on Privacy, Confidentiality, and Access 2010, 4).

Although the US Constitution does not expressly grant the right of privacy, it does provide safeguards against government intrusion. Further, courts have interpreted the Constitution to give privacy rights with respect to religious beliefs (using the First Amendment as the basis), unreasonable searches (using the Fourth Amendment as the basis), marriage, and child-rearing. In addition, privacy rights have been further extended through such high-profile US Supreme Court cases such as *Griswold v. Connecticut* (contraception) and *Roe v. Wade* (abortion).

While a constitutional right of privacy related to one's own health information is nonexistent, privacy protection has been established through other means such as court decisions, accrediting body standards, individual state laws, and federal laws like HIPAA and the HITECH provisions of ARRA. For example, the predominant accrediting body and standards-setting organization in healthcare is **The Joint Commission**. The Joint Commission is an independent, not-for-profit organization that administers accreditation programs for hospitals and related health organizations. It defines privacy as an individual's "right to limit the disclosure of personal information" (The Joint Commission 2010, GL-26). Its standards require the maintenance of information privacy, confidentiality, and security and supports efforts to ensure the integrity of data, which is the assurance that the data has not been modified without authorization or corrupted, either maliciously or accidentally (The Joint Commission 2010).

Standards of professional practice are also defined by professional healthcare organizations that offer protection of privacy rights as a main component of professional codes of ethics as discussed in more detail later in this chapter.

Confidentiality

Privacy and confidentiality are often used interchangeably; however, there are important distinctions between the two terms. **Confidentiality** results from sharing private thoughts with someone else in confidence (Amatayakul 2009, 225). The ASTM E 31 Subcommittee on Health Informatics defines confidentiality as the "status accorded to data or information indicating that it is sensitive for some reason, and therefore it needs to be protected against theft, disclosure, or improper use, or both, and must be disseminated only to authorized individuals or organizations with a need to know" (ASTM 2010, 5).

Confidentiality, as recognized by law, stems from a relationship where information is shared between two parties such as attorney and client, clergy and parishioner, husband and wife, or physician and patient. The information or communication shared in these relationships is considered "privileged." What constitutes **privileged communication** is usually delineated by state law. Such laws in the case of healthcare providers may also further define what records of communication are privileged based on the healthcare provider's scope of practice (for example, physician, nurse, psychologist, licensed clinical social worker, or psychiatric nurse practitioner).

The concept of confidentiality of patient information resulting from a patient-provider relationship can be traced back to the fourth century BC. Hippocrates, considered the father of medicine, required Greek physicians to take the Hippocratic Oath. A modern translation of the Oath includes a tenet specific to protecting the confidentiality of information shared between patient and physician (MedicineNet 2011):

> I will respect the privacy of my patients, for their problems are not disclosed to me that the world may know. Most especially must I tread with care in matters of life and death. If it is given me to save a life, all thanks. But it may also be within my power to take a life; this awesome responsibility must be faced with great humbleness and awareness of my own frailty. Above all, I must not play at God.

Confidentiality obligates healthcare providers—both individuals and organizations—to protect patient information that is collected. When a patient reveals information to a physician or other provider of care, there is a presumption that this information will be considered confidential and protected as such (Rinehart-Thompson and Harman 2006). Healthcare organizations have the dubious task of balancing individual privacy rights and the use of confidential information to perform necessary clinical or business tasks (Herzig 2010). This includes the confidentiality of all information systems and verbal communication related to financial and business records, including employee information as well as clinical and service communication. As with privacy, The Joint Commission offers standards in support of confidentiality. It defines confidentiality as "protection of data or information from being made available or disclosed to an unauthorized person(s) or process(es)" (The Joint Commission 2010, GL-6).

Security

The concept of **security** is related to privacy and confidentiality in that it pertains to the physical and electronic protection of information that preserves these concepts (Harman 2010, 635). The Joint Commission definition of security reflects all administrative, physician, and technical safeguards to "prevent unauthorized access, use, disclosure, modification, or destruction of information or interference with system operations in an information system" (The Joint Commission 2010, GL-29). The ASTM E 31 Health Informatics Subcommittee (2010, 3) defines security from two perspectives, security related to data and security related to systems

- **Data security** is "the result of effective data protection measures; the sum of measures that safeguard data and computer programs from undesired occurrences and exposure to accidental or intentional access or disclosure to unauthorized persons, or a combination thereof; accidental or malicious alteration; unauthorized copying; or loss by theft or destruction by hardware failures, software deficiencies, operating mistakes; physical damage by fire, water, smoke, excessive temperature, electrical failure or sabotage; or a combination thereof. Data security exists when data are protected from accidental or intentional disclosure to unauthorized persons and from unauthorized or accidental alteration."

- **System security** is "the totality of safeguards including hardware, software, personnel policies, information practice policies, disaster preparedness, and oversight of these components. Security protects both the system and the information contained within from unauthorized access from without and from misuse from within. Security enables the entity or system to protect the confidential information it stores from unauthorized access, disclosure, or misuse, thereby protecting the privacy of the individuals who are the subjects of the stored information."

From a federal perspective, the US Code on Information Security (National Institute of Standards and Technology 2008, A-6) defines information security as follows:

> Protecting information and information systems from unauthorized access, use, disclosure, disruption, modification, or destruction in order to provide
>
> - Integrity, which means guarding against improper information modifications or destruction, and includes ensuring information non-repudiation and authenticity

- Confidentiality, which means preserving authorized restrictions on access and disclosure, including means for protecting personal privacy and propriety information

- Availability, which means ensuring timely and reliable access to and use of information

Harriet Pearson, chief privacy officer of IBM, affirmed the interdependence between privacy and security by identifying security as the way to implement an individual's expectation of privacy. "You can have outstanding security, yet violate people's perception of what their privacy ought to be. But you can't have privacy without having the right security measures in place. Privacy rests on a good security foundation always" (IBM Executive Interaction Channel 2007).

The interplay among the three concepts is important since they are supported through federal and state laws and accrediting body standards. In addition, a number of organizations have been working together on various initiatives that address privacy, confidentiality, and security concerns relative to EHRs and HIEs (AHIMA HIMSS HIE Privacy and Security Joint Work Group 2011).

Check Your Understanding 1.1

Instructions: Indicate whether the following statements are true or false (T or F).

1. A hybrid record is a record that is totally electronic.

2. An electronic health record can be managed across more than one healthcare organization.

3. Confidentiality refers to the right to be left alone.

4. HITECH widens the scope of privacy and security protections under HIPAA.

5. Privileged communication is a legal concept designed to protect the communication between two parties.

Custodian/Steward of Health Records

Ownership of the health record has traditionally been granted to the healthcare provider who generates the record. However, state and federal laws have long upheld the right of the patient to control the information within the record (Russell and Bowen 2012, 282). The HIPAA Privacy Rule (45 CFR 164.524–526) (see chapter 9) grants a patient the right to access, view, copy, or amend his or her record. Even though healthcare providers may own the physical health record—regardless of the media in which it is contained—such ownership does not permit providers to share or sell patient-identifiable medical information as they wish. This is an important issue as healthcare organizations expand their use of EHRs and HIEs. For example, the question of whether patients should consent to or authorize the disclosure of their information to HIEs is under debate by several government and private organizations (Office of the National Coordinator for Health IT, HIT Policy Committee, Privacy and Security Tiger Team 2010; AHIMA HIMSS HIE Privacy and Security Joint Work Group 2011).

Associated with ownership of health records is the legal concept of the **custodian of health records.** The custodian of health records is the individual who has been designated as having responsibility for the operational functions related to the development and maintenance of records (AHIMA e-HIM Work Group 2010). This includes the care, custody, control, and proper safekeeping and disclosure of health records whether stored in paper or electronic format for such persons or institutions that prepare and maintain records of healthcare. An official custodian is required by both federal and state rules of evidence that permit health records to be entered as business records in legal proceedings.

This is discussed further in chapter 4. The official custodian is authorized to certify (that is, verify that the record or information is what it purports to be), through affidavit or testimony, the normal business practices used to create and maintain the record (AHIMA e-HIM Work Group on the Legal Health Record 2005a, b). The custodian supervises the inspection and copying or duplication of records and can be called to testify as to the authenticity of the record.

In most healthcare organizations, the health information management (HIM) department is the location from which requesters of health information receive information. The director of the HIM department (or designee) is traditionally the legal custodian of health records. In organizations that have hybrid or electronic health records, the custodian may differ depending on who is responsible for and can explain the procedures for compiling and maintaining patient information and records. This individual must also be able to validate the integrity of the information requested. See chapter 12 for a more detailed discussion of the process for releasing health information upon request or by subpoena or court order.

With the increasing use of HIT, the role of data or information **steward** is emerging. Similar to the role of custodian, **stewardship** goes beyond the physical record to include "responsibilities for ensuring integrity (accuracy, completeness, timeliness) and security (protection of privacy as well as from tampering, loss or destruction) within the context of electronic information and records management" (Davidson 2010, 42). Stewardship is a component of **information governance** that refers to the "strategic management of enterprise electronic information including the standards, policies, and procedures for access, use, and control of that information" (Davidson 2010, 42). The role of health record steward requires "leadership, responsibility, and governance to ensure the consistent application of and compliance with organizational record-keeping policies across the distributed information systems that comprise the health record" (Dougherty and Washington 2010, 44). Whether one is identified as a custodian or steward, key to either role is knowledge of the legal aspects of information management.

Regardless of the record format, patient information is routinely requested and relevant as evidence in legal proceedings, whether that information is used to allege a physician's negligence, used to assert that an individual is legally incompetent, or used in a variety of other types of legal proceedings in which the patient's health and treatment are an issue. Individuals charged with the custodial responsibility of protecting health information act as a gatekeeper for the appropriate access, use, and disclosure of that information for legitimate purposes and especially in conjunction with federal and state laws as well as the court system for use in legal proceedings.

Relationship of Law and Ethics

Law and ethics are closely intertwined. Remember, law refers to a set of governing rules used to protect the public, whereas **ethics** refers to standards of behavior that develop as result of one's concept of right or wrong. Ethics functions with a set of rules—rules of conduct that stem from **moral values** formed through the influence of family, culture, religion, and society. Professional ethics are "applied ethics designed to bring about the ethical conduct of a profession" (Edge and Groves 2006, 59). Taken together, law and ethics enable the healthcare professional to offer compassionate, competent practice while avoiding legal issues surrounding the delivery, financing, and reimbursement of healthcare.

In healthcare, ethics often encompasses economic, medical, political, social, and legal dilemmas that require decision making prefaced by law and moral values. Dilemmas such as the right to refuse treatment, right to die, right to life, denial of treatment based on cost, treatment of vulnerable others, and quality-of-life issues challenge healthcare professionals to make sound judgments and good decisions or choices based on values that work in unison with laws and standards of practice (Pozgar 2013, 3). Several of these dilemmas and legal implications are discussed in later chapters of the book.

To facilitate decision making as related to right or wrong, four **ethical principles** exist to assist healthcare professionals in addressing healthcare-related dilemmas (Pozgar 2013, 24–30):

- **Autonomy**—recognizing the right of a person to make one's own decision

- **Beneficence**—doing good, promoting the health and welfare of others, demonstrating kindness, showing compassion, and helping others

- **Nonmaleficence**—doing no harm

- **Justice**—obligation to be fair in the distribution of benefits and risks

These principles provide healthcare professionals with a framework for decision making that at times may involve conflicting principles. Harman (2010, 308) illustrates how these principles can be applied if, for example, an HIM professional must decide whether to release patient information:

- Autonomy would require the HIM professional to ensure that the patient, and not a spouse or third party, makes the decision regarding access to his or her health information.

- Beneficence would require the HIM professional to ensure that the information is released only to individuals who need it to do something that will benefit the patient (payment for an insurance claim).

- Nonmaleficence would require the HIM professional to ensure that the information is not released to someone who does not have authorization to access it and who might harm the patient if access were permitted (newspaper seeking information about a famous person).

- Justice would require the HIM professional to apply the rules fairly and consistently for all and not to make special exceptions based on personal or organizational perspectives.

The ideal is to uphold laws while demonstrating the moral values and ethical principles defined by one's professional code of ethics. A **code of ethics** reflects the values and principles defined by a profession as acceptable behavior within a practice setting. It represents the guiding principles by which a profession governs the conduct of its members. Protecting the health and well-being of a patient and the privacy, confidentiality, and security of patient information are well established in codes of ethical practice for health occupations. These codes not only assist those who treat patients but also serve as a guide for those occupations that manage health information, records, or both. Since codes of ethics represent standards of ethical practice they are often used as a benchmark for what constitutes acceptable practice in malpractice, negligence, or other litigious situations. Codes of ethics are dynamic in that they change as societal and practice expectations change. A brief discussion of several prominent professions and their codes of ethics follows.

American Medical Association

Ethical principles related to privacy and confidentiality have been inherent in the practice of medicine since the fourth century BC, when the Hippocratic Oath was created and "appealed to the inner and finer instincts of the physician" (American Medical Association 2007). The **American Medical Association** (AMA), from its first established code of ethics in 1847 to its most recent update in 2001, has upheld the preservation of patient confidentiality through its *Code of Medical Ethics*. Principle IV of the code states: "A physician shall respect the rights of patients, colleagues, and other health professionals, and shall safeguard patient confidences and privacy within the constraints of the law" (AMA 2001). The AMA *Code of Medical Ethics* also offers *Opinion 5.07* on the confidentiality of computerized medical records. The opinion provides guidelines "to assist physicians and computer service organizations in maintaining the confidentiality of information in medical records when that information is stored in computerized data bases" (Virtual Mentor 2011).

American Health Information Management Association

The ethical principle of protecting patient privacy has been a cornerstone and an inherent core value and ethical obligation within the AHIMA *Code of Ethics* since the beginning of the HIM profession in 1928. The discipline of HIM focuses on the process and systems for managing health information and records required to deliver quality healthcare to the public. HIM professionals work in a variety of businesses and health-related settings. HIM professionals may be found throughout the organization and have oversight responsibility for upholding federal and state laws regarding practices related to documentation, reimbursement, quality of care, employee and overall privacy, confidentiality, and security of health information. They are cognizant of the policies, procedures, rules, and regulations that allow for the legitimate fulfillment of requests for access, use, release, or disclosure of health information. The AHIMA *Code of Ethics* contains 11 key principles as shown in figure 1.1. Each principle is further enhanced by interpretive guidelines that can be accessed on the AHIMA website referenced at the end of the chapter. Crawford (2011) offers several examples of how the AHIMA Code of Ethics provides guidance for examining ethical issues related to complex work situations such as pressure to upcode, underreporting delinquent records, and denying professional development.

There is a need to balance the appropriate and lawful use of health information with the protection of the patient's privacy. Although all healthcare providers must be vigilant about protecting patient privacy, the HIM professional is often the individual designated by an organization to address privacy issues; protect patient information from unauthorized, inappropriate, and unnecessary intrusion; and make day-to-day operational decisions about disclosures and release-of-information policies and procedures. Core to the profession's *Code of Ethics* are Tenets I, III, and IV that specifically address

Figure 1.1. AHIMA Code of Ethics

Preamble

The ethical obligations of the health information management (HIM) professional include the safeguarding of privacy and security of health information; disclosure of health information; development, use, and maintenance of health information systems and health information; and ensuring the accessibility and integrity of health information. Healthcare consumers are increasingly concerned about security and the potential loss of privacy and the inability to control how their personal health information is used and disclosed. Core health information issues include what information should be collected; how the information should be handled, who should have access to the information, under what conditions the information should be disclosed, how the information is retained and when it is no longer needed, and how is it disposed of in a confidential manner. All of the core health information issues are performed in compliance with state and federal regulations, and employer policies and procedures. Ethical obligations are central to the professional's responsibility, regardless of the employment site or the method of collection, storage, and security of health information. In addition, sensitive information (e.g., genetic, adoption, drug, alcohol, sexual, health, and behavioral information) requires special attention to prevent misuse. In the world of business and interactions with consumers, expertise in the protection of the information is required.

Ethical Principles: The following ethical principles are based on the core values of the American Health Information Management Association and apply to all health information management professionals.

Health information management professionals:

I. Advocate, uphold, and defend the individual's right to privacy and the doctrine of confidentiality in the use and disclosure of information.

II. Put service and the health and welfare of persons before self-interest and conduct themselves in the practice of the profession so as to bring honor to themselves, their peers, and to the health information management profession.

III. Preserve, protect, and secure personal health information in any form or medium and hold in the highest regard the contents of the records and other information of a confidential nature, taking into account the applicable statutes and regulations.

IV. Refuse to participate in or conceal unethical practices or procedures.

V. Advance health information management knowledge and practice through continuing education, research, publications, and presentations.

VI. Recruit and mentor students, peers, and colleagues to develop and strengthen professional workforce.

VII. Represent the profession accurately to the public.

VIII. Perform honorably health information management association responsibilities, either appointed or elected, and preserve the confidentiality of any privileged information made known in any official capacity.

IX. State truthfully and accurately their credentials, professional education, and experiences.

X. Facilitate interdisciplinary collaboration in situations supporting health information practice.

XI. Respect the inherent dignity and worth of every person.

protecting the privacy and confidentiality of health information and records. The interpretive guidelines for these principles are shown in figure 1.2.

Figure 1.2.   AHIMA Code of Ethics Interpretive Guides for protecting health information and records

I.   Advocate, uphold, and defend the individual's right to privacy and the doctrine of confidentiality in the use and disclosure of information.

Health information management professionals shall:

1.1.   Safeguard all confidential patient information to include, but not limited to, personal, health, financial, genetic, and outcome information.

1.2.   Engage in social and political action that supports the protection of privacy and confidentiality, and be aware of the impact of the political arena on the health information issues for the healthcare industry.

1.3.   Advocate for changes in policy and legislation to ensure protection of privacy and confidentiality, compliance, and other issues that surface as advocacy issues and facilitate informed participation by the public on these issues.

1.4.   Protect the confidentiality of all information obtained in the course of professional service. Disclose only information that is directly relevant or necessary to achieve the purpose of disclosure. Release information only with valid authorization from a patient or a person legally authorized to consent on behalf of a patient or as authorized by federal or state regulations. The minimum necessary standard is essential when releasing health information for disclosure activities.

1.5   Promote the obligation to respect privacy by respecting confidential information shared among colleagues, while responding to requests from the legal profession, the media, or other non-healthcare related individuals, during presentations or teaching and in situations that could cause harm to persons.

1.6   Respond promptly and appropriately to patient requests to exercise their privacy rights (e.g., access, amendments, restriction, confidential communication, etc.). Answer truthfully all patients' questions concerning their rights to review and annotate their personal biomedical data and seek to facilitate patients' legitimate right to exercise those rights.

III.   Preserve, protect, and secure personal health information in any form or medium and hold in the highest regard the contents of the records and other information of a confidential nature obtained in the official capacity, taking into account the applicable statutes and regulations.

Health information management professionals shall:

3.1.   Safeguard the privacy and security of patients' written and electronic records and other sensitive information. Take reasonable steps to ensure that health information is stored securely and that patients' data are not available to others who are not authorized to have access. Prevent inappropriate disclosure of individually identifiable information.

3.2.   Take precautions to ensure and maintain the confidentiality of information transmitted, transferred, or disposed of in the event of a termination, incapacitation, or death of a healthcare provider to other parties through the use of any media.

3.3.   Inform recipients of the limitations and risks associated with providing services via electronic media (such as computer, telephone, fax, radio, and television).

IV.   Refuse to participate in or conceal unethical practices or procedures and report such practices.

Health information management professionals **shall not**:

4.6.   Participate in, condone, or be associated with dishonesty, fraud and abuse, or deception. For example,

- Allowing patterns of retrospective documentation to avoid suspension or increase reimbursement
- Assigning codes without physician documentation
- Failing to report licensure status for a physician through the appropriate channels
- Recording inaccurate data for accreditation purposes
- Allowing inappropriate access to genetic, adoption, or behavioral health information
- Misusing sensitive information about a competitor
- Violating the privacy of individuals
- Coding when documentation does not justify the diagnoses or procedures that have been billed
- Coding an inappropriate level of service
- Miscoding to avoid conflict with others
- Engaging in negligent coding practices

Source: AHIMA 2011a.

Complementing the Code of Ethics Tenets I, III and IV, is the AHIMA published the *Consumer Health Information Bill of Rights* (AHIMA 2011b). AHIMA created the Bill for the purpose of educating healthcare consumers about the protections and safeguards related to their personal health information. The Bill validates every individual's right to lawful access of their personal health information; prevent unauthorized access; ensure accuracy; and expect appropriate remedy when these privileges are violated (AHIMA 2011b). While the document is designed for healthcare consumers, it also offers those responsible for managing health information additional knowledge for ethical decision making regarding the protection and release of health information.

American Medical Informatics Association (AMIA)

Another professional group that addresses the appropriate use and protection of health information is the **American Medical Informatics Association** (AMIA). This not-for-profit organization supports the transformation of healthcare through science, education, research, and practice in biomedical and health informatics (AMIA 2010). Members of AMIA are asked to uphold the organization's *Code of Professional Ethical Conduct,* which specifically addresses the use of patient information in its first ethical guideline (see figure 1.3) (AMIA 2011). The *Code* also offers ethical guidance as related to patients, employers, colleagues, society, research, and general performance.

In adhering to this principle, AMIA has recently tackled ethical issues surrounding vendor-user contracts as related to the proliferation of EHRs systems, associated devices, and health-related software applications (Goodman et al. 2011). An AMIA-appointed task force has provided recommendations related to contract language, education and ethics, user groups, best practices, marketing, and regulation and oversight of the industry. Of particular note are recommendations related to contract language (discussed in more detail in chapter 6) and ethics education and corporate compliance focusing on topics such as patient safety; workflow and workarounds; disclosure of system defects versus intellectual property; and privacy, confidentiality, and security challenges (Goodman et al. 2011, 79). The legal and ethical issues facing HIT vendors and customers require attention as the healthcare industry continues to rely on HIT to address healthcare cost, quality, access, and safety issues.

The AMA, AHIMA, and AMIA are just three of the many professional organizations whose members adhere to ethical principles related to practice and the protection of patient privacy, confidentiality,

Figure 1.3.   AMIA Principles of Professional Ethical Conduct Related to Protecting Health Information

---

I. Key ethical guidelines regarding patients, their families, their significant others, and their representatives (called here collectively "patients"):

   A. Patients have the right to know about the existence of electronic records containing personal biomedical data.

      1. Do not mislead patients about how these data are used, about the origin of these data, or about how and with whom these data are communicated;

      2. Answer truthfully patients' questions concerning their rights to review and annotate their own biomedical data, and seek to facilitate a subject's legitimate right to exercise those rights.

   B. Advocate and work to ensure that biomedical data are maintained in a safe, reliable, secure, and confidential environment that is consistent with applicable law, local policies, and accepted informatics processing standards.

   C. Never knowingly disclose biomedical data in a fashion that violates legal requirements or accepted local confidentiality practices.

      1. Likewise, even if it does not involve disclosure, never use patients' data outside the stated purposes, goals, or intents of the organization responsible for these data.

   D. Treat the data of all patients with equal care, respect, and fairness.

Source: American Medical Informatics Association 2011.

and security of health information. These principles, recognized by court decisions along with an understanding of healthcare law, impose a legal duty on healthcare professionals to conform to professional standards of practice and codes of ethics in delivering healthcare as well as protecting health information.

Check Your Understanding 1.2

Instructions: Indicate whether the following statements are true or false (T or F).

1. Ownership of a health record generated by a doctor on a patient belongs to the patient.

2. A custodian of records is responsible for certifying that a record is what it purports to be.

3. When a patient refuses treatment, he or she is exercising the ethical principle of beneficence.

4. In a malpractice case, a professional code of ethics may be used as a benchmark for what should be acceptable practice by a healthcare professional.

5. The ethical principle of nonmaleficence refers to making sure rules are fairly and consistently applied to all.

Summary

Healthcare in the United States is a trillion-dollar industry that is complex and highly regulated by federal and state laws. It is also governed by various accrediting bodies' standards of practice. These laws and standards dictate the processes and safeguards used to deliver quality care and protect the health information derived from that care. Health information has many uses, and it is stored in various formats from paper to electronic records systems. There is government support for increasing the use of HIT to decrease healthcare costs and improving the quality and safety of healthcare. With increase in HIT comes concern for protecting the privacy, confidentiality, and security of health information. Privacy means the right to be left alone, confidentiality refers to protecting private thoughts shared with another, and security pertains to the physical protection of information that preserves confidentiality. HIPAA and HITECH rules provide individuals responsible for the access, use, exchange, and disclosure of health information with guidance for protecting privacy, confidentiality, and security of health information. Additional guidance comes from one's professional code of ethics and general ethical principles, all of which are central to the legal issues and implications that govern the protection of health information and health records.

References

Agency for Healthcare Research and Quality. 2011. Health information privacy and security collaboration. http://healthit.ahrq.gov.

AHIMA. 2011a. Code of ethics. http://www.ahima.org.

AHIMA. 2011b. AHIMA Consumer Bill of Rights: A Model for Protecting Health Information Principles. http://www.ahima.org.

AHIMA e-HIM Work Group. 2010. Practice brief: Managing the transition from paper to EHRs. Web extra. Chicago: AHIMA.

AHIMA e-HIM Work Group on the Legal Health Record. 2005a. Update: Guidelines for defining the legal health record for disclosure purposes. *Journal of AHIMA.* 76(8):64A–G.

AHIMA e-HIM Work Group on the Legal Health Record. 2005b. The Legal Process and Electronic Health Records. *Journal of AHIMA* 76(9):96A–D.

AHIMA HIMSS HIE Privacy and Security Joint Work Group. 2011. The privacy and security gaps in health information exchanges. Chicago: AHIMA. http://www.ahima.org.

Amatayakul, M. 2013. *Electronic Health Records: A Practical Guide for Professionals and Organizations,* 5th ed revised reprint. Chicago: AHIMA.

Amatayakul, M. 2012. Electronic health records. In *Health Information Management: Concepts, Principles, and Practice,* 4th ed., edited by K. LaTour and S. Eichenwald-Maki, 229-269. Chicago: AHIMA.

American Medical Association. 2001. Code of medical ethics. http://www.ama-assn.org.

American Medical Association. 2007. E-history. http://www.ama-assn.org.

American Medical Informatics Association. 2010. Strategic Alignment Summary. http://www.amia.org.

American Medical Informatics Association. 2011. Code of professional ethical conduct. http://www.amia.org

American Society for Testing and Materials Committee E31 on Healthcare Informatics Subcommittee E31.17 on Privacy, Confidentiality, and Access. 2010. Standard guide for confidentiality, privacy, access, and data security principles for health information including computer-based patient records. Publication no. E1869-04(2010). Philadelphia: ASTM.

Bankert, E., and R. Amdur. 2006. *Institutional Review Board: Management and Function,* 2nd ed. Sudbury, MA: Jones and Bartlett.

Callahan-Dennis, J. 2010. *Privacy: The Impact of ARRA, HITECH and Other Policy Initiatives.* Chicago: AHIMA.

Crawford, M. 2011. Everyday ethics. *Journal of AHIMA* 82(4):30–33.

Davidson, L. 2010. From custodian to steward. *Journal of AHIMA* 81(5):42–43.

Dougherty, M., and L. Washington. 2010. Still seeking the legal EHR. *Journal of AHIMA* 81(2):42–45.

Edge, R., and J. Groves. 2006. *Ethics of Health Care: A Guide for Clinical Practice,* 3rd ed. New York: Thomson Delmar.

Goodman, K., Berner, E., Dente, M., Kaplan, B., Koppel, R., Rucker, D., Sands, D., and P. Winkelstein. 2011. Challenges in ethics, safety, best practices, and oversight regarding HIT vendors, their customers and patients: A report of an AMIA special task force. *Journal of AMIA* 18(77):77–81.

Harman, L. 2010. Ethical issues in health information management. In *Health Information Management Concepts, Principles, and Practice,* 3rd ed., edited by K. LaTour and S. Eichenwald-Maki, 307–326. Chicago: AHIMA.

Herzig, T. 2010. *Information Security in Healthcare Managing Risk.* Chicago: Health Information Management and Systems Society.

IBM Executive Interaction Channel. 2007. Privacy is good for business: An interview with Chief Privacy Officer Harriet Pearson. http://www.ibm.com

The Joint Commission. 2010. Glossary. *Comprehensive Accreditation Manual for Hospitals: The Official Handbook. CAMH* Refreshed Core January. http://www.jointcommission.org.

MedicineNet. 2011. Definition of Hippocratic Oath. http://www.medterms.com/

National Alliance for Health Information Technology. 2008 (April). Defining key health information technology terms. http://healthit.hhs.gov

National Institute of Standards and Technology. 2008. An introduction resource guide for implementing the Health Insurance Portability and Accountability Act (HIPAA) Security Rule. NIST Special Publication 800-66 Revision I. http://csrc.nist.gov

Office of the National Coordinator for Health IT, HIT Policy Committee, Privacy & Security Tiger Team. 2010 (August). Letter of Recommendation to Dr. David Blumenthal, MD, on patient consent and the electronic exchange of patient identifiable health information. http://healthit.hhs.gov

Office of the National Coordinator for Health IT, Privacy & Security. 2010 (February). Summary of Selected Federal Laws and Regulations Addressing Confidentiality, Privacy and Security. http://healthit.hhs.gov

Pozgar, G. 2013. *Legal and Ethical Issues for Health Professionals*, 3nd ed. Boston: Jones and Bartlett.

President's Council of Advisors on Science and Technology. 2010 (December). Report to the President realizing the full potential of health information technology to improve healthcare for Americans: The path forward. Executive Office of the President. http://www.whitehouse.gov.

Rinehart-Thompson, L., and L. Harman. 2006. Privacy and confidentiality. In *Ethical Challenges in the Management of Health Information*, 2nd ed., edited by Laurinda Harman. Sudbury, MA: Jones and Bartlett.

Russell, L., and R. Bowen. 2012. Legal issues in health information management. In *Health Information Management: Concepts, Principles, and Practice*, 4rd ed., edited by K. LaTour and S. Eichenwald-Maki, 271–305. Chicago: AHIMA.

Safran, C., M. Bloomrosen, E. Hammond, S. Labkoff, S. Markel-Fox, P. Tang, and D. Detmer. 2007 (January–February). Toward a national framework for the secondary use of health data: An American Medical Informatics Association white paper. *Journal of AMIA* 14(1):1–9.

Virtual Mentor. 2011 (March). The AMA code of medical ethics' opinion on computerized medical records. *AMA Journal of Ethics* 13(3):161–162. http://virtualmentor.ama-assn.org.

Cases, Statutes, and Regulations Cited

Griswold v. Connecticut, 381 US 479 (1965).

Roe v. Wade, 410 US 113 (1973).

45 CFR 160.103: Definitions, Privacy rule. 2002.

45 CFR 160, 164: Standards for privacy of individually identified health information. 2002.

45 CFR 164.524–526: Amendment of protected health information. 2007.

42 USC 17921: Health Information Technology for Economic and Clinical Health Act. 2009.

Chapter 2

The Legal System in the United States

Laurie A. Rinehart-Thompson, JD, RHIA, CHP, FAHIMA

Learning Objectives

- Explain the relevance of law to the health information and informatics professional and other health professionals

- Differentiate between public law and private law

- Name and give examples of the four sources of law

- Explain resolution in cases where laws conflict with one another

- Compare the branches of government and the role that each plays

- Describe the separation of powers in a democratic society

- Summarize the federal and state court systems and the appeals process in both

- Discuss the role of nonlegal accrediting bodies, such as The Joint Commission, and their authority relative to the legal system

- Discuss types of alternative dispute resolution available as options to the court system

Key Terms

Administrative agencies
Administrative agency tribunals
Administrative law
Alternative dispute resolution
Appellate courts
Arbitration
Brief
Case law
Circuit courts
Civil law
Code of Federal Regulations (CFR)
Common law
Conditions of Participation
Conflict of laws
Constitution

Constitutional law
Court of Claims
Criminal law
Department of Health and Human Services (HHS)
District courts
Diversity jurisdiction
Due process of law
Executive branch
General jurisdiction
Judicial branch
Judicial law
Jurisdiction
Legislative branch
Limited jurisdiction
Mediation
Opinion

Oral argument
Persuasive authority
Petition for *writ of certiorari*
Precedent
Private law
Public law
Res judicata
Separation of powers
Special jurisdiction
Stare decisis
State action
Statutory law
Subject matter jurisdiction
Supremacy Clause
Supreme Court
Trial courts
United States Code (USC)

Introduction

Law is a "body of rules of action or conduct prescribed by a controlling authority . . . having binding legal force . . . which must be obeyed and followed by citizens subject to sanctions or legal consequences . . . (it is) a solemn expression of the will of the supreme power of the State" (Garner 2004).

In order to enjoy the benefits of living in a civilized society, it is necessary that laws be created to establish order, provide the parameters within which we lead our lives, and define the rights and obligations of both the government and its citizens. Nonetheless, laws are often broken and—because of their manmade imperfections—subject to dispute. It is, therefore, necessary for a legal system to not only create laws but also enforce and interpret them.

Role of Law in the US Healthcare System

Health information and informatics professionals and other healthcare professionals are employed in a wide range of settings, ranging from acute care hospitals to insurers to vendor corporations. Regardless of the venue, the legal system guides business decisions and practices. From wrongful disclosures of patient information to contract issues and employment matters, the law will constantly touch the decisions that health information and informatics professionals and other health professionals make.

Public vs. Private Law

In the United States, law can be divided into two types: public and private. **Public law** involves the federal, state, or local government and its relationship to individuals and business organizations. Its purpose is to define, regulate, and enforce rights where any part of a government agency is a party (Showalter 2012, 4). The most familiar type of public law is **criminal law**, where the government is a party prosecuting an accused who has been charged with violating a criminal statute or regulation. Public law also encompasses regulatory activities, which can be criminal in nature or within the realm of **civil law** (that is, noncriminal law). In health care, public law encompasses regulations at the state and national levels. For example, the Medicare Conditions of Participation, which involve the government and its relationship with individuals providing health insurance for the elderly and other designated groups, is federal public law.

Private law, conversely, is concerned with the rules and principles that define rights and duties among people and among private businesses. The government is not a party. Instead, private law consists of actions by one or more individuals acting in a private capacity against other individuals also acting in a private capacity. The rights and obligations of individuals in private law are generally enforced through the judicial (court) system. For example, private law applies when a contract for the purchase of a house is written between two parties. Normally, private law encompasses issues related to contracts, property, and torts (injuries). In the medical context, private law often applies when there is a breach of contract or when a tort occurs through malpractice. There are four sources of public and private law: constitutions, statutes, administrative law, and judicial decisions. Table 2.1 shows the relationship of public and private law to civil and criminal law.

Table 2.1. Relationship of public and private law to civil and criminal law

	Civil Law	Criminal Law
Public Law	X	X
Private Law	X	

Note: Public law encompasses both civil and criminal actions, but private law encompasses only civil actions.

Sources of Law

No one source or type of law governs the actions of individuals and governmental entities. Rather, the laws governing our society come from four sources: constitutions (federal and state), statutes (federal, state, and local), administrative law (rules and regulations created by **administrative agencies**), and common law (court decisions).

Constitutions

Constitutional law is the body of law that deals with the amount and types of power and authority that governments are given.

The US **Constitution** defines and lays out the powers of the three branches of the federal government. The **legislative branch** (the House of Representatives and the Senate) creates statutory laws (statutes) such as Medicare and HIPAA. The **executive branch** (the president and staff, namely cabinet-level agencies) enforces the law. For example, the Centers for Medicare and Medicaid Services (CMS), which enforces Medicare laws, are contained within the US **Department of Health and Human Services** (HHS), a cabinet-level agency that reports to the president. The **judicial branch** (composed of courts) interprets laws passed by the US Congress and signed by the president (federal level) and those passed by state legislatures and signed by governors (state level).

In addition to defining the three branches of government, the Constitution includes 27 amendments. These include the Bill of Rights (the first 10 amendments) and 17 additional amendments. The purpose of these amendments is to place restrictions on the federal government so that the most fundamental legal rights of US citizens are not infringed upon. Through the Fourteenth Amendment, these restrictions are also applied to state governments. **Due process of law**, provided for by the Constitution, serves to protect individuals' legal rights (substantive due process) and the implementation of fair legal processes when a person's life, liberty, or property is in jeopardy (procedural due process).

Each state also has a constitution. The state constitution is the supreme law of each state but is subordinate to the US Constitution, the supreme law of the nation.

Private organizations sometimes take on characteristics of a public organization or have a significant connection to the government. They are then held to government standards (for example, due process). Activities by these organizations constitute **state action.**

Statutes

Statutes (**statutory law**) are enacted by a legislative body. The US Congress and state legislatures are legislative bodies, and the compendiums of statutes they create are generally referred to as codes. The **United States Code** is the compilation of all federal statutes. Commonly known healthcare laws, such as Medicare and the Health Insurance Portability and Accountability Act (HIPAA, discussed later in the text), are statutes because they were enacted by the US Congress. Statutes can also be enacted by local bodies, such as municipalities. These statutes may be referred to as ordinances. Table 2.2 lists all the titles within the US Code.

There are many health information and informatics issues that can be impacted through legislation, both at the federal and state levels. An increasingly critical role of individuals charged with the management of health information is to stay abreast of legislative activity and advocate for changes that will positively affect the future of the profession.

Administrative Law

Administrative law falls under the umbrella of public law. As already noted, the executive branch of government is responsible for enforcing laws enacted by the legislative branch. Frequently, the legislative body (Congress, federally, and state legislatures at the state level) gives various executive

Table 2.2.   Titles within the US Code

Title Number	Title Name
1	General Provisions
2	The Congress
3	The President
4	Flag and Seal, Seat of Government, and the States
5	Government Organization and Employees (with Appendix)
6	Domestic Security
7	Agriculture
8	Aliens and Nationality
9	Arbitration
10	Armed Forces
11	Bankruptcy (with Appendix)
12	Banks and Banking
13	Census
14	Coast Guard
15	Commerce and Trade
16	Conservation
17	Copyrights
18	Crimes and Criminal Procedure (with Appendix)
19	Customs Duties
20	Education
21	Food and Drugs
22	Foreign Relations and Intercourse
23	Highways
24	Hospitals and Asylums
25	Indians
26	Internal Revenue Code
27	Intoxicating Liquors
28	Judiciary and Judicial Procedure (with Appendix)
29	Labor
30	Mineral Lands and Mining
31	Money and Finance
32	National Guard
33	Navigation and Navigable Waters
34	Navy (Repealed)
35	Patents
36	Patriotic Societies and Observances
37	Pay and Allowances of the Uniformed Services
38	Veterans' Benefits
39	Postal Service
40	Public Buildings, Property, and Works
41	Public Contracts
42	The Public Health and Welfare
43	Public Lands
44	Public Printing and Documents
45	Railroads
46	Shipping
47	Telegraphs, Telephones, and Radiotelegraphs
48	Territories and Insular Possessions
49	Transportation
50	War and National Defense (with Appendix)

Source: US Government 2009.

Figure 2.1. President's cabinet

Executive agencies	Cabinet-rank agencies and individuals
• Department of Agriculture • Department of Commerce • Department of Defense • Department of Education • Department of Energy • Department of Health and Human Services • Department of Homeland Security • Department of Housing and Urban Development • Department of Justice • Department of Labor • Department of State • Department of the Interior • Department of the Treasury • Department of Transportation • Department of Veterans Affairs	• Council of Economic Advisers • Environmental Protection Agency • Office of Management and Budget • United States Ambassador to the United Nations • United States Trade Representative • Vice President of the United States • White House Chief of Staff

Source: The White House n.d.

and Medicaid funds, standards for providers receiving Medicare and Medicaid reimbursement (CMS); healthcare research (National Institutes of Health); and healthcare issues relating to specific populations, such as those represented by the Indian Health Service and the Administration on Aging. In particular, a high-profile regulation that has been finalized by CMS in recent years was the reconfiguration of the payment system to severity-adjusted diagnosis-related groups (DRGs) for Medicare beneficiaries. The complete list of agencies within the HHS is illustrated in the organizational chart in figure 2.2.

The HHS is also actively involved in combating healthcare fraud and abuse that occurs through fraudulent billing. As with other federal administrative agencies, one of the HHS offices is the Inspector General. In conjunction with the Department of Justice (another federal cabinet-level agency), the Inspector General for HHS investigates providers that are believed to be receiving Medicare and Medicaid funds fraudulently. The tenacious efforts of the government, while costly, have proven beneficial in ferreting out criminal activity and allowing the government to recoup dollars obtained illegally by healthcare providers.

State Regulation of Healthcare

Healthcare is an important policy objective for state governments as well as for the federal government. Issues and populations that are addressed and regulated at the state administrative level are disbursement of Medicaid dollars; funding and operation of facilities for state residents with mental illnesses, developmental disabilities, and substance abuse problems; public health issues, such as naturally occurring epidemics and bioterrorism threats; regulation of facilities that receive state reimbursement, including nursing homes, mental health facilities, and facilities for the developmentally disabled and those suffering from substance abuse; and regulation of healthcare professionals, such as physicians, nurses, and allied health professionals. With such a broad spectrum of responsibility and oversight, numerous statewide administrative agencies divide the responsibility for managing operational and policy issues.

Legislative Branch

The legislative branch of government enacts laws in the form of statutes. The federal legislative body, the US Congress, is a bicameral (two-chamber) model consisting of a Senate (with two senators representing each state) and a House of Representatives (with each state entitled to at least one representative, and the total number based on the population of each state). Numerous committees that operate within

Figure 2.2. Department of Health and Human Services organizational chart

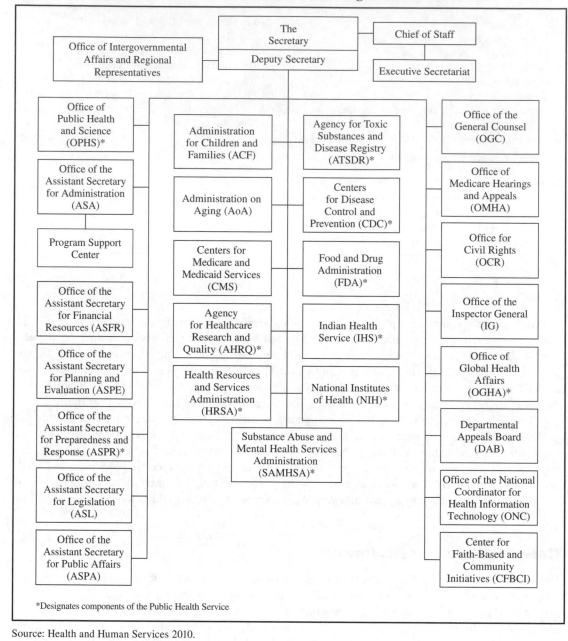

*Designates components of the Public Health Service

Source: Health and Human Services 2010.

both the Senate and the House initially create proposed legislation. When it has successfully moved through research and hearings, it must be passed by both chambers of Congress in identical form before it can be presented to the chief executive of that jurisdiction for approval. All state legislatures, except unicameral Nebraska, are bicameral (Pozgar 2011).

Judicial Branch

The third (judicial) branch of government interprets the law and adjudicates disputes, thus creating common law. Disputes may arise from personal controversies (for example, a contract dispute or medical malpractice action), constitutional challenges to existing laws (for example, a federal or state statute that allegedly violates one's constitutional rights), or conflicts between laws. Depending on the nature of the dispute and the jurisdiction, courts may apply the law of federal or state constitutions, statutes, regulations, or case law of that jurisdiction. Common law within a jurisdiction is constantly evolving based on newly litigated disputes and the resulting judicial decisions. Both state and federal courts apply the legal doctrine of *res judicata* ("a matter already judged") to limit excessive litigation. It prohibits subsequent lawsuits about the same matters and involving the same parties once a decision has been made by a court and all appeals have been exhausted.

Separation of Powers

Separation of powers among the three branches of the federal and state governments limits the authority of each and inhibits any one branch of government from becoming autocratic. A related concept is checks and balances, which allows each branch to monitor the activities of the other branches to balance, or limit, the power of each.

Check Your Understanding 2.2

Instructions: Indicate whether the following statements are true or false (T or F).

1. Jurisdiction is a territory of legal control.

2. The US Congress is a bicameral model.

3. Federally, ultimate executive branch power rests with the president.

4. Under the theory of separation of powers, each branch of government is given expanded powers.

5. Judicial disputes may arise from constitutional challenges to existing laws.

Judicial System

Legal disputes are traditionally resolved through the court systems. In the United States, they exist at both the federal and state levels. (As described below, certain requirements must be met for a case to be filed in the federal court system.) The 50 states, US territories, and the District of Columbia each have their own court systems. Although the court system is the most familiar method for the resolution of legal disputes, there is increasing reliance on redirecting cases that are potentially set for trial toward alternative dispute resolution methods, described below, to lessen the burden on typically overwhelmed court systems and to provide less costly alternatives for opposing parties to settle their differences.

State Court System

State court systems generally use the same three-tier system as the federal court system, which will be described later in this chapter. **Trial courts** are the lowest tier of state courts and are divided into two courts. Courts of **limited jurisdiction** hear cases that pertain to a particular subject matter (for example, landlord and tenant cases or juvenile cases); or that involve crimes of lesser severity (for example, misdemeanors) or civil matters of lesser dollar amounts. Courts of **general jurisdiction** hear more serious criminal cases (for example, felonies) or civil cases that involve large amounts of money. At the trial court level, the judge or jury decides the facts of the case based on the evidence presented. For example, the plaintiff will present evidence that supports allegations of the defendant's wrongdoing. Likewise, the defendant will present evidence that disproves or tends to disprove wrongdoing. Given the evidence, the judge or jury will decide what they believe the facts are in order to determine liability or guilt, or the lack thereof.

Many states have **appellate courts**. Appellate courts hear appeals on final judgments of the state trial courts. The state **supreme court** is the highest tier. It hears appeals from the appellate courts or from trial courts when the state does not have appellate courts. Cases presented before appellate courts in both the federal and state court systems are not reenactments of the trial. Legal documents (**briefs**) are prepared by each party's attorney(s), who then argue the merits of the case in an **oral argument** before a panel of appellate judges. Witnesses are not called and, generally, the facts of the case are not revisited. Appeals are designed to solely address legal errors or problems that are alleged to have occurred at the lower court. At all tiers, a court's written determination outlining the facts of the case and the legal theories followed to reach an outcome is the **opinion**.

Federal Court System

The federal court system is arranged much the same as each state court system, with a three-level hierarchy: trial court, appellate court, and Supreme Court. Final judgments of the trial court may be appealed to the appellate level, with appellate decisions appealed to the Supreme Court of the United States.

In the federal court system, trial courts (called **district courts**) exist throughout the United States. At least one district court exists in each state, with the number of courts totaling 94. Bankruptcy, an area of law exclusively under the jurisdiction of federal law, is a unit of the district court system with its own courts and judges. Federal appellate courts (called **circuit courts**) are distributed throughout the United States. Each court represents a specific number of the district courts. Figure 2.3 illustrates the distribution of the federal circuit courts 1 through 11 nationwide. The twelfth circuit court covers the District of Columbia and the thirteenth circuit (federal circuit) court has the authority to hear certain appeals nationally depending on the subject matter.

The United States Supreme Court is the court of final decision making. It hears appeals most commonly from the federal appellate (circuit) courts and occasionally from state supreme courts in matters involving federal statutes or the US Constitution. Because its jurisdiction is federal law and the US Constitution, most cases come from the lower tiers of the federal court system. Thousands of cases with requests for review are submitted annually to the United States Supreme Court by parties who have lost at the lower court level and are appealing. The Supreme Court exercises considerable discretion in determining which cases it will hear. The process by which a party submits a request for the Supreme Court to hear a case is called a **petition for *writ of certiorari***. The Supreme Court either denies cert (and declines to hear the case) or grants cert (and accepts the case for oral argument). As with appellate courts (including supreme courts) at the state level, the US circuit courts and the US Supreme Court do not conduct trials. Rather, they review written briefs submitted by the parties (or their legal counsel) and listen to oral arguments presented by each party, often interjecting questions during each side's argument.

Judges for all federal courts are nominated by the president and confirmed by the US Senate. Because federal judicial decision making shapes the political landscape of the nation into the future, the nomination and confirmation process can become highly charged.

Jurisdiction

Referred to earlier in the chapter as a territory of legal control, jurisdiction is the legal authority that a body possesses to make decisions. Whether a case may be brought in the federal court system is generally subject to whether it meets two jurisdictional limitations: **subject matter jurisdiction** and **diversity jurisdiction**.

Subject matter jurisdiction is based on the content or substantive area of the case being brought. Because the jurisdiction of the federal court system is generally limited to federal laws and the US

Figure 2.3. Geographic boundaries of US Courts of Appeals (Circuit Courts) and US District Courts

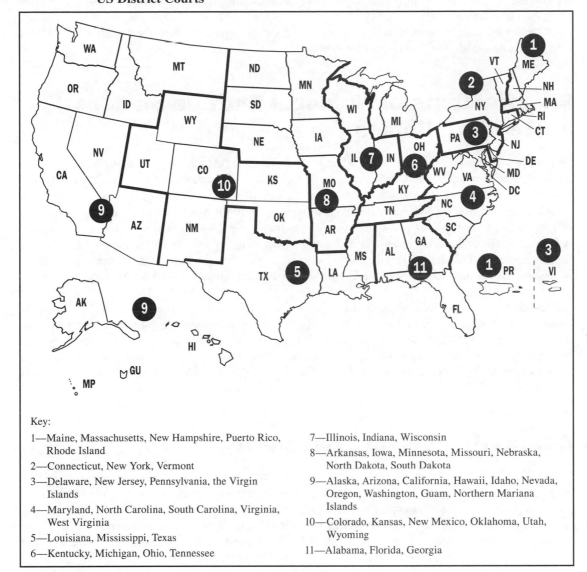

Key:

1—Maine, Massachusetts, New Hampshire, Puerto Rico, Rhode Island

2—Connecticut, New York, Vermont

3—Delaware, New Jersey, Pennsylvania, the Virgin Islands

4—Maryland, North Carolina, South Carolina, Virginia, West Virginia

5—Louisiana, Mississippi, Texas

6—Kentucky, Michigan, Ohio, Tennessee

7—Illinois, Indiana, Wisconsin

8—Arkansas, Iowa, Minnesota, Missouri, Nebraska, North Dakota, South Dakota

9—Alaska, Arizona, California, Hawaii, Idaho, Nevada, Oregon, Washington, Guam, Northern Mariana Islands

10—Colorado, Kansas, New Mexico, Oklahoma, Utah, Wyoming

11—Alabama, Florida, Georgia

Source: US Courts n.d.

Constitution, cases brought in federal court generally must relate to either federal law or the US Constitution. For example, lawsuits may be filed to challenge laws or governmental actions that limit free speech or freedom of religion. In the state court system, most trial courts are courts of general jurisdiction, meaning that they may hear all matters of state law except for those cases that must be heard in state courts of **special jurisdiction**, in which particular areas of the law have been carved out for resolution (for example, small claims, domestic relations, juvenile, and probate courts).

Diversity jurisdiction enables parties from different states to engage in a lawsuit in federal court, but federal statute limits the number of lawsuits brought this way by imposing two restrictions:

1. No plaintiff can be from the same state as any of the defendants.

2. The amount in controversy must be at least $75,000.

In a landmark US Supreme Court decision, *Erie Railroad Co. v. Tompkins,* 304 US 64 (1938), it was determined that, in diversity jurisdiction cases, the law of the state in which the lawsuit was filed would be applied by the court.

The federal court system, as well as many state court systems, has established a **Court of Claims** where lawsuits against the government are brought.

Requirements of Nonlegal Entities Such as Accrediting Bodies

Nonlegal entities, especially health care accrediting bodies, are often viewed as having a great deal of authority. However, they are voluntary and do not have the legal authority of laws created by statute, common law, constitutions, and regulations. Nonetheless, they often wield a great deal of power and exhibit a significant presence. Accreditation is often vital to the credibility of an organization and may be a prerequisite to provider reimbursement. For example, the Joint Commission and the American Osteopathic Association have been granted deeming authority by the US Department of Health and Human Services. This means that healthcare organizations accredited by either of these accrediting bodies will be deemed to have met the **Conditions of Participation** required for Medicare and Medicaid certification.

In addition to The Joint Commission and the American Osteopathic Association, other well-known accreditation organizations in the healthcare industry include the National Committee for Quality Assurance (NCQA) for managed care organizations and the Commission on Accreditation of Rehabilitation Facilities (CARF). Because the accreditation process imposes stringent standards and involves regular on-site surveys, continuous compliance is critical to a healthcare organization's ongoing success.

Alternative Dispute Resolution

Resolution of disputes through the judicial (court) system is a complex process that exacts a toll on financial resources, time, and emotions. While a considerable percentage of lawsuits filed eventually end in negotiation and settlement rather than proceeding to trial, many resources have already been expended by the time a case is settled. Therefore, the US legal system is a proponent of **alternative dispute resolution**, which provides means other than the court system to resolve lawsuits. The two primary types of alternative dispute resolution are **arbitration** and **mediation**.

In arbitration, a dispute is submitted to a third party or a panel of experts outside the judicial trial system. The process is the most effective when the parties to the dispute agree to have their differences heard and settled by an arbitrator or arbitration panel and agree that the settlement will be binding.

In mediation, a dispute is also submitted to a third party. However, the outcome of mediation occurs by agreement of the parties, not by a decision of the mediator. The role of the mediator is to facilitate agreement between the disputing parties.

Arbitration and mediation offer several advantages over the court system, including time and cost savings. These proceedings usually allow for more privacy than court proceedings do. Criminal misdemeanors may be handled through mediation. Smaller tort claims are often handled through arbitration. For example, a healthcare organization's wrongful disclosure of patient health information, particularly if it is not highly sensitive in nature, may be resolved by remedying the patient's injuries in an acceptable manner through arbitration or mediation rather than through a lawsuit.

Check Your Understanding 2.3

Instructions: Indicate whether the following statements are true or false (T or F).

1. Appellate courts hear appeals on final judgments of trial court decisions.

2. An opinion is the written argument of one of the parties in a lawsuit.

3. Courts of limited jurisdiction hear cases pertaining to a particular subject matter.

4. Diversity jurisdiction enables parties from different states to engage in a lawsuit in federal court.

5. In mediation, a third party makes a final decision about a dispute between parties.

Summary

Healthcare legal issues involve laws and the legal system at both the federal and state levels. Because a healthcare professional's involvement with the legal system can range from a medical malpractice lawsuit in a local state court to questions about compliance with a federal statute, such as the Medicare Conditions of Participation, it is important to be familiar with the various sources of law, where they can be located, and how disputes surrounding them might be resolved.

References

Code of Federal Regulations. http://www.gpoaccess.gov.

Department of Health and Human Services. 2010. Department of Health and Human Services organizational chart. http://www.hhs.gov.

Garner, B.A. 2004. *Black's Law Dictionary*. Abridged 8th ed. St. Paul, MN: West Group.

Pozgar, G.D. 2011. *Legal Aspects of Health Care Administration*. 11th ed. Sudbury, MA: Jones and Bartlett.

Showalter, J.S. 2012. *The Law of Healthcare Administration*. 6th ed. Chicago: Health Administration Press.

US Courts. n.d. Geographic boundaries of US Courts of Appeals (Circuit Courts) and US District Courts. http://www.uscourts.gov.

US Government. 2009. United States Code, 2006 edition. http://www.gpoaccess.gov.

White House. n.d. The cabinet. http://www.whitehouse.gov

Cases, Statutes, and Regulations Cited

Erie Railroad Co. v. Tompkins, 304 US 64 (1938).

Chapter 3

Civil Procedure

Laurie A. Rinehart-Thompson, JD, RHIA, CHP, FAHIMA

Learning Objectives

- Explain the role of civil procedure in the legal system
- Describe the parties to a lawsuit
- Describe the five methods of discovery
- Explain the difference between a court order and a subpoena
- Summarize the proper procedure for responding to a subpoena
- Describe each of the individuals involved in a trial
- Summarize the steps in a trial
- Explain the legal appeals process
- Explain the processes for the collection of judgment

Key Terms

Admissibility	Cross appeal	Interrogatories
Answer	Cross-claim	Joinder
Appeal	Default judgment	Judge
Appellant	Defendant	Judgment lien
Appellee	Deliberations	Judicial search warrant
Authentication	Deponent	Jury
Bailiff	Deposition	Jury instructions
Bench trial	Directed verdict	Lay witness
Burden of proof	Discoverability	Litigation
Civil procedure	Discovery	Mental examination
Class action	Dismissal	Motion to quash
Clerk of court	e-Discovery	Nominal damages
Closing argument	Equity	Opening statement
Compensatory damages	Expert witness	Parties
Complaint	Federal Rules of Civil	Peremptory challenge
Counterclaim	Procedure (FRCP)	Petitioner
Court order	Garnishment	Physical examination
Court reporter	In camera inspection	Plaintiff

Pleadings	Respondent	Summons
Pretrial conference	Service	Trial
Pro se	Settlement	Verdict
Procedural law	Subpoena	*Voir dire*
Production of documents	*Subpoena ad testificandum*	Writ of execution
Punitive damages	*Subpoena duces tecum*	
Requests for admissions	Substantive law	

Introduction

A working knowledge of the procedural aspects of the law is essential for any healthcare professional. For example, individuals who are responsible for the integrity of the health record, both inside and outside a healthcare organization, may be involved with procedurals such as responding to and/or attending civil or criminal legal proceedings relating to accidents, workers' compensation, malpractice, physical abuse, or other criminal activity. Responses to legal proceedings can involve functions such as responding to a subpoena or court order, described below; copying or preparing health records for legal proceedings; and appearing at either a deposition or trial to authenticate the health record and make it available to relevant parties. Therefore, the importance of familiarity with discovery methods and other legal procedures is emphasized in this chapter.

Definition of Civil Procedure

Substantive law, defines the rights and obligations that arise between two or more parties, such as torts (chapter 5) and contracts. However, of equal importance is **procedural law**; that is, the court's rules that guide a lawsuit from the time it begins through completion, whether it culminates in a **trial** or ends with a **settlement** or **dismissal**. Of further importance is the uniformity with which cases are handled. Procedural rules are the mechanisms used to guide substantive law in dispute resolution. Because most legal healthcare cases are civil rather than criminal in nature, they will fall within the rules and parameters of **civil procedure**. Those cases that are criminal in nature, conversely, will fall within the rules and parameters of criminal procedure.

In federal courts, **judges** presiding over civil cases at the trial level (that is, district courts) apply the **Federal Rules of Civil Procedure** (FRCP). Likewise, in federal criminal trials (again at the district court level), the Federal Rules of Criminal Procedure apply. Individual states follow their own state rules, which often are adaptations of the federal rules; further, even regions within a state court system follow their own sets of specific local rules (Cornell Law School 2006). Just as rules govern cases at the trial court level, the rules of appellate procedure govern procedures for appellate courts.

It is worth noting that plaintiff(s) may take legal action against the same defendant(s) both civilly and criminally. For example, a defendant who is charged criminally for assaulting a victim ("the government" vs. the defendant) can also be sued civilly by the victim in pursuit of monetary damages. The case caption then becomes the "victim/plaintiff" vs. the defendant. Damages will be discussed later in this chapter.

Parties to a Lawsuit

Parties are the individuals or organizations involved in a lawsuit. The party that initiates a lawsuit to enforce his or her rights and/or another's obligations is the **plaintiff**. The individual or organization that is the object of the lawsuit, and against whom a lawsuit is brought, is the **defendant**. There may be multiple plaintiffs and defendants, although a large number of people who have been similarly wronged may be categorized for certification (that is, approval and identification) as a class (Rule 23 of FRCP) and represented legally thereafter as a class. **Class action** lawsuits often proceed for groups of consumers to file lawsuits against a large and generally powerful entity for alleged wrongdoing.

Pretrial

From the time a lawsuit is filed until the date a trial is scheduled, a number of procedures will take place. This period of time is referred to as the pretrial phase of a lawsuit.

Commencement of a Lawsuit

Litigation refers to the legal proceedings that accompany a lawsuit. The first step in litigation is the commencement, or filing, of a lawsuit (also commonly referred to as a legal action) by a plaintiff or group of plaintiffs against one or more defendants. The filing is documented via a **complaint**. Courts vary in their jurisdictions (a concept discussed in chapter 2) and it is, therefore, incumbent upon the plaintiff's attorney or the plaintiff himself, if he or she is acting **pro se** through self-representation, to file the complaint in the appropriate court. Failure to do so will result in dismissal of the case and often re-filing of the case in the proper court.

Once a complaint is filed, a copy is served on the defendant along with a **summons**, which gives the defendant notice of the lawsuit and explains the defendant's procedural obligations. Through the summons and complaint, the defendant is informed of the nature of the case, including a listing of all causes of action (facts that give the plaintiff[s] the right to some type of remedy [Garner 2004]) and the amount of damages being sought. The defendant must respond to the complaint by filing an **answer** within the time frame specified by the court. Failure to answer may result in an automatic or **default judgment** by the court against the defendant. Usually, however, the defendant answers the complaint in one of several ways: by denying, admitting, or pleading ignorance to the allegations, or by bringing additional legal actions. Moreover, the defendant can ask the court to dismiss the plaintiff's complaint, but not without substantial reason.

The parties to a lawsuit are not solidified when the complaint is filed. Rather, a number of subsequent actions may ensue. A **counterclaim** is a claim by a defendant against a plaintiff. A **cross-claim** is a claim by one party against another party who is on the same side of the main litigation (Garner 2004). For example, two physicians may be named as codefendants by a plaintiff. One physician may then sue the other physician in a cross-claim, thus bringing a legal action against the other physician. **Joinder** is an action by a defendant to bring in (join) an outsider as a codefendant. For example, an orthopedic surgeon who is sued for negligence by a plaintiff patient who received a hip replacement may "join" the manufacturer of the hip replacement device, claiming that the manufacturer was negligent in its production of the device.

Under rules of civil procedure, **pleadings** refer to documents generated by parties involved in a lawsuit, including complaints and answers (Garner 2004). They are central to the litigation process. It is the responsibility of a government official, often a **clerk of court**, to officially maintain documents associated with legal actions filed in that court system.

An entire body of case law surrounds the legal process of **service** of a summons and complaint upon a defendant and what constitutes adequate notification of a lawsuit. Although service may be personal, by mail, or by publication, court requirements vary by jurisdiction, and proof of service may be required. Further, adequate time is required to allow the defendant(s) to sufficiently respond to a summons and complaint. Although at first glance this seems a mundane area of law, in actuality it has been the subject of a number of historic and lively lawsuits and court decisions. For example, service was disputed but found by the court to have occurred where a summons was placed on a defendant's car bumper after he was touched with the summons but refused to take it (*Nielsen v. Braland*, 1963). Likewise, a court found that service had been accomplished when a summons was placed under the windshield wiper of a defendant's car after the defendant refused to acknowledge it by remaining seated in the car with the windows rolled up while the summons was read to him (*Trujillo v. Trujillo*, 1945) (Casad, Fink, and Simon 1989).

Check Your Understanding 3.1

Instructions: Indicate whether the following statements are true or false (T or F).

1. Procedural law encompasses a court's rules that guide a lawsuit.

2. Class action lawsuits proceed for groups of consumers.

3. A cross-claim is a claim by a defendant against a plaintiff.

4. Joinder involves bringing an outsider into a lawsuit as a codefendant.

5. Notification of a lawsuit occurs through service of a summons or complaint.

Types of Discovery

Following the commencement of a lawsuit, the next pretrial stage is **discovery**. Discovery is both a process and a time period. It occurs during the period leading to trial and allows all parties (generally via their legal counsel) to use various strategies to discover or obtain information held by other parties and, subsequently, to assess the strengths and weaknesses in each party's case. Although discovery is time-consuming, information obtained as a result of the process can be invaluable in determining the course a case should take and whether negotiation and settlement is preferable to trying the case before a judge or jury. In fact, careful legal work during the discovery process may be significant toward winning a case through either trial or settlement. Although several discovery methods exist, those most pertinent to health information are the deposition and production of documents. These two methods of discovery, along with several others, are discussed below.

Discovery is also distinguishable from **discoverability**, which refers to limits on parties to discover pretrial information held by another. For example, state law may protect spousal or attorney-client communications from discoverability (that is, being accessed by other parties) during the discovery period of a lawsuit. Discoverability is also distinguishable from **admissibility**, which refers to evidence that is allowed to be admitted in a court of law and thus considered by the judge or jury in making a final determination about a case (Garner 2004). Admissibility, which will be discussed further in chapter 4, is an issue that is limited to the trial. Admissible evidence is often more restricted than discoverable evidence. Stated another way, more information is generally discoverable than is admissible. Information that has been obtained during the discovery period may or may not be admissible for consideration by a judge and jury during trial.

Deposition

A **deposition** is a formal proceeding by which the oral testimonies of individuals are obtained. Prior to a deposition, a subpoena (discussed in detail below) is issued, directing an individual (the **deponent**) to appear at an appointed time and place to testify under oath. Attorneys for both the plaintiff(s) and defendant(s) are present and the deponent's testimony is transcribed by a **court reporter**. Deposed individuals may be either parties to the lawsuit or independent witnesses. In any event, an attorney will be present to act on behalf of the deponent and to interject objections when legally impermissible questions are asked by an opposing attorney conducting a cross-examination. The accuracy of one's testimony at a deposition is important because the deposition is not only a discovery method; the transcript may be read into evidence at trial if the individual is unable to testify at trial or if opposing counsel wishes to use it to impeach or discredit a witness. Thus, consistency between the deposition and trial testimony is crucial to the credibility of a witness.

Testimony to Authenticate Health Records

Testimony is generally required to establish the authenticity or genuineness of a health record that is introduced as evidence. Such testimony is sought via a subpoena. (See appendix 3A for a sample subpoena.) **Authentication** is verification of the record's validity (that is, it is the record of the individual in question and it is what it purports to be) and, therefore, its reliability and truthfulness as evidence. As will be further discussed in chapter 4, rules of evidence generally permit health records to be used as evidence if it can be established that the records were made in the regular course of business (that is, they qualify as business records).

An individual who is called as a witness to testify as to the authenticity of a health record may expect the types of queries outlined in figure 3.1.

Authentication is the purpose of such testimony; however, at times attorneys may ask additional questions that may not be appropriate. It is inappropriate for an attorney to ask questions of a medical nature of an individual who is testifying for the purpose of establishing the authenticity of a health record. Examples of such inquiries include those that solicit personal opinion; seek the purpose of a medication or treatment regimen; or require interpretation of the health record. Other situations—such as asking the testifying individual to read entries that may be deemed illegible by others—are questionable and must be addressed on a case-by-case basis. If the individual is familiar with the practitioner's handwriting and is able to read the entries, guidance should be sought from the attorney acting on his or her behalf as to whether the attorney will object to the request and whether or not to proceed. If the individual is not comfortable with his or her ability to read the entries, however, this should be clearly stated and the request declined. It is acceptable to respond "I don't know" if the answer to a question is not known.

Interrogatories

A second discovery method, written **interrogatories**, provides a mechanism for questions to be presented to parties of the lawsuit and answered in writing during a more extensive time frame than that provided by a deposition. Because responses to written interrogatories may be prepared by a party's attorney or the attorney's legal staff instead of the party directly, these responses may provide less illuminating information than that provided directly by a party via a deposition. Nonetheless, the party must attest to the truthfulness and accuracy of the responses to written interrogatories.

Production of Documents

A third discovery method is particularly pertinent to health information because documentation is key evidence to legal actions in all industries, including healthcare. Requests for the **production of documents**, including health records, are initiated by a *subpoena duces tecum*, described below.

As the healthcare industry moves toward electronic health records (EHRs) and key evidence contained in other electronic documents such as e-mails, a new legal term has evolved: *e-Discovery*.

Figure 3.1. Types of witness queries

- Position/title
- Identification of the "custodian" of health records
- Length of employment as the "custodian" of health records, if applicable
- Whether the testifying individual currently has possession of the record(s) in question
- Confirmation of how and when the record was prepared
- Regarding health information from another facility that might be contained in the patient's record
  —This information was received in the normal course of business
  —The individual who is testifying cannot attest to recordkeeping practices of another facility

Source: Reynolds 2010.

The United States Supreme Court amended the FRCP to address the discovery of electronic records, creating a new paradigm with respect to the production of documents as a discovery method. The effective date for the new federal e-discovery rules was December 1, 2006. This issue will be discussed more extensively in chapter 4.

Physical or Mental Examination of a Party

When the physical or mental condition of a party is in question, the opposing party may request an independent **physical examination** or an independent **mental examination**, respectively, which is the fourth type of discovery. If the court determines that there is good cause for this request, such an examination will be ordered (Showalter 2012, 17). For example, a defendant may request that a physical examination be performed on the plaintiff in a personal injury lawsuit if the nature and extent of the injuries claimed are in question.

Requests for Admissions

The fifth discovery method is **requests for admissions**, which asks the opposing party to make certain admissions that will diminish the amount of time and money that would otherwise be spent proving those facts (Showalter 2012, 17). Although it is unlikely that an opposing party will admit to facts that would dramatically damage his or her case, this discovery device is nonetheless useful for eliciting facts that are not in dispute. For example, if asked to do so, a plaintiff may admit to the fact that he has been discharged from the course of medical treatment that he received as a result of the injuries allegedly suffered in the event that gave rise to the lawsuit. Admission of such a fact is more efficient than obtaining this information through a deposition or a subpoena for the production of health records.

Check Your Understanding 3.2

Instructions: Indicate whether the following statements are true or false (T or F).

1. Discovery allows parties in a lawsuit to use strategies to obtain information held by other parties.

2. Admissibility refers to evidence that parties can obtain during the pretrial period.

3. A deposition does not occur under oath.

4. Authentication is verification of a record's validity.

5. An independent mental examination may not be requested as a type of discovery.

Court Orders

A **court order** is a document issued by a judge that compels certain action, such as testimony or the production of documents such as health records. For example, a court order may command a hospital to disclose health records when the hospital, for whatever reason, refuses to disclose them pursuant to an authorization. Possessing greater legal force than a subpoena, valid court orders must be complied with, and failure to do so may result in a contempt-of-court citation with possible accompanying jail time. If there is any question as to which document has been received, legal counsel should determine whether the document is a court order or a subpoena. If a document requesting the production of health records is determined to be a court order, it must be complied with regardless of the presence or absence of patient authorization.

Subpoenas

A **subpoena** is a legal tool (rather than a method of discovery) used to compel one's appearance at a certain time and place to testify or produce documents or other tangible items either during discovery or at trial. A subpoena can be civil, criminal, or administrative in nature. It is generally issued by the clerk of court or by an attorney for one of the parties in the name of the court having jurisdiction over the case (a court order, conversely, is issued by a judge).

The subpoena is often confused with a court order because both are official in nature and may be issued to compel testimony or the production of documents. A subpoena is designated with a seal of the court and in the name of the presiding judge, which also appears on a court order, thus causing confusion between the two documents. A subpoena compels a timely response and requires proper service; failure to respond may result in a court order compelling attendance or a contempt of court citation. It is often served by law enforcement or sent via US mail and is not to be disregarded. Nonetheless, because it is issued by the court or an attorney and generally not by the judge presiding over the case, it does not have the same force and effect as a court order. In most cases where health records are requested, a subpoena must be accompanied by patient authorization to be valid. Patient authorization, however, is not always required. In light of the federal government's emphasis on reducing fraud and abuse in healthcare, the Office of the Inspector General (OIG) for the US Department of Health and Human Services has been given certain powers to compel both testimony and the production of documents without patient authorization as part of its investigations (5 USC 552a (App. 3 sec. (6)(a)(4)). The False Claims Act, discussed in chapter 15, and the Health Insurance Portability and Accountability Act (HIPAA) Privacy Rule, discussed in chapter 9, both include provisions for administrative subpoenas that can be enforced by the federal court system. Grand jury subpoenas, which are issued to obtain evidence for consideration by grand juries in criminal cases, also may not require an individual's authorization. Requirements will vary based on the jurisdiction.

There are two forms of subpoenas. A *subpoena ad testificandum* primarily seeks an individual's testimony. In a medical malpractice case, this type of subpoena is more likely to be directed toward physicians and other healthcare providers involved in the plaintiffs' care than toward health information management or informatics professionals. A custodian of health records would rarely expect to receive a subpoena that is primarily interested in his or her testimony. Rather, records custodians (who are often referred to legally as such) will likely find themselves served with a *subpoena duces tecum* (see appendix 3.A for a sample), which instructs the recipient to personally appear and produce documents and other records. Such subpoenas may direct the recipient to produce and bring originals or copies of health records, laboratory reports, x-rays, or other records to a deposition or to court.

States have different rules governing responses to subpoenas and the production of health records in litigation. State law and local court rules should be consulted to determine whether a specified amount of time is required between service of a subpoena and the requested appearance, to determine the acceptability of mailing health records in response to a subpoena, and to become familiar with other legal procedural requirements. Often, component state associations of the American Health Information Management Association (AHIMA) have legal handbooks that outline various conditions and the appropriate response to a *subpoena duces tecum*. Copies of records requested by this type of subpoena may often be substituted as long as appropriate steps have been taken to authenticate them. If copies may not be substituted and the original is ordered to remain with the court, the healthcare organization representative should confirm that the original record is in the custody of the court and obtain a receipt verifying this. Additionally, a copy of the health record should be retained at the healthcare facility in case the information is needed for patient care. For either form of subpoena, the individual who receives a subpoena should verify its validity.

Elements of a Valid Subpoena

A subpoena must be examined for validity before the recipient complies with it. For state cases, the required elements vary from state to state and are often present on a state-prescribed form.

Compliance with federal requirements is necessary for subpoenas issued in conjunction with federal cases. Elements of a valid subpoena commonly include the name of the court from which the subpoena was issued; the caption of the action (that is, names of plaintiff[s] and defendant[s]); assigned case docket number (to validate the case); date, time, and place of requested appearance; the information commanded, such as testimony or the specific documents sought in a *subpoena duces tecum* and the form in which that information (including electronic information) is to be produced; the name of the issuing attorney; the name of the recipient being directed to disclose the records; and the signature or stamp of the court/official or judge authorized to issue the subpoena (Reynolds 2010). The authorization of the person whose records are to be disclosed is nearly always required, although there are exceptions as described previously. If, in the case of a *subpoena duces tecum,* an authorization is required but does not accompany the subpoena, the subpoena should be declined and an authorization requested and received before the records are produced. If records requested per subpoena contain information that is specifically protected by state or federal law (for example, mental health or substance abuse information), the patient must specifically authorize the disclosure of those records. If requested records have been appropriately destroyed according to the facility's policies and in compliance with applicable laws, a certificate of destruction should be produced in lieu of the records.

Objections to Subpoenas

Certain protections are provided to persons who are subpoenaed. Like the specific requirements for subpoena content, these protections can vary based on the jurisdiction and type of subpoena. Subpoenas issued in federal civil cases include the following protections:

> The party issuing the subpoena must take reasonable steps to avoid imposing an undue burden or expense on the person subject to the subpoena.
>
> A person commanded to produce and permit inspection and copying of designated books, papers, documents, or tangible things, or inspection of premises need not appear in person at the place of production or inspection unless commanded to appear for a deposition, hearing or trial (FRCP 45(c)(2)(A) (2007)).

Although the recipient of a subpoena must respond to it in a timely manner to avoid a contempt of court action, the subpoena may warrant an objection. A person who is commanded to produce records for inspection or copying may, within 14 days of being served with the subpoena, provide a written objection to the party or attorney designated in the subpoena. Once written objections have been made, a court determines whether the subpoenaed information must be produced and issues an order accordingly.

Formal, written objections to subpoenas are often made in the form of a **motion to quash**. A motion to quash is a document filed with the court that asks the judge to nullify the subpoena for any number of reasons. Under FRCP 45(c)(3)(A) (2007), a court must quash or modify the subpoena if:

- The subpoena fails to provide adequate time for compliance

- A person who is not a party is required to travel over 100 miles to comply with the subpoena

- The subpoena requires the disclosure of privileged information that is not subject to any exception or waiver (privileges are discussed in detail later in the chapter)

- An undue burden is imposed on the person subject to the subpoena

State rules also allow parties to quash subpoenas. For example, in *Swartz v. Cartwright,* the administrator of the defendant's estate moved to quash the plaintiff's subpoena of a deceased physician's medical records on the grounds that the records were privileged. In finding that the physician's medical records were discoverable, the court stated,

> Here, given the deposition testimony of Dr. Voorhees's nurse, Gloria Gasnarez, who worked for Dr. Voorhees full-time from 1993 "until . . . 1997 or eight," that Dr. Voorhees demonstrated "more frequent hand shaking" in "the last year that [she] was there," and because the operation at issue occurred on March 14, 1997, the plaintiffs' request to examine Dr. Voorhees's medical records is "reasonably calculated to lead to the discovery of admissible evidence." Ms. Gasnarez's testimony suggests that Dr. Voorhees's physical condition may have effected [sic] his performance as a physician, and it is reasonable to suppose that his medical records would illuminate that issue.

However, the court limited the plaintiff's discovery of the deceased physician's medical records to dates ranging from approximately one year before the operation at issue in the case to approximately one year after that operation.

In *Fabich v. Montana Rail Link, Inc.,* the court denied the plaintiff's motion to quash on grounds of privilege because the plaintiff waived privilege by putting his own condition at issue by filing a claim for damages. However, the court provided that any specific records the plaintiff objected to producing to the defendant could instead be produced directly to the court. This is known as an **in camera inspection** and the judge personally reviews disputed records in his or her chambers and decides whether they are discoverable or admissible.

In addition to moving to quash on the basis of privilege, a party may move to quash a subpoena for medical records on the grounds that complying with the subpoena would be unduly burdensome. In *Smith v. Rossi,* the plaintiff moved to quash the defendant's subpoena of his medical records on the grounds that the subpoenas were oppressive and unreasonable. Specifically, the plaintiff claimed that the defendants had already received all of his medical records. However, because there was doubt as to whether the defendants had in fact received all records, the court denied the plaintiff's motion to quash and noted that such records were relevant to the defendant's defense in the case. Another example of an unduly burdensome subpoena that might be objected to is one that constitutes a "fishing expedition" for a broad range of documents that might not exist but, if they do, may benefit the requesting party's case (Servais 2008). The risk of these types of subpoenas increases with EHR systems that are capable of producing many types of data and metadata (data about data, which will be discussed in chapter 4). As discussed above, subpoenas may also be objected to based on the absence of patient authorization.

The HIPAA Privacy Rule, which is discussed in chapter 9, provides protections for records that have been subpoenaed from covered entities such as health plans, healthcare clearinghouses, and healthcare providers when patient authorization is not required. Specifically, records may be produced according to a subpoena only if:

- The covered entity has received satisfactory assurance from the party seeking the information that reasonable efforts have been made to ensure that the individual whose records have been subpoenaed has been given notice of the request.

- The covered entity has received satisfactory assurance from the party seeking the information that reasonable efforts have been made to secure a qualified protective order, limiting the use and disclosure of the protected information in the record (45 CFR 164.512(e)).

Further, court decisions may impose additional duties on providers to protect health information extending beyond statutory and regulatory protections. Individuals responsible for managing healthcare data and information must be aware of fiduciary duties to protect health information that may be imposed by such case law.

If a subpoena is invalid or otherwise unreasonable, an organization's legal counsel should be consulted regarding the legal mechanics of objecting to the subpoena according to court rules and in a manner that communicates with the party issuing the subpoena.

Duties in Responding to Subpoenas

While the law provides protections for persons who are subject to subpoenas, it also imposes certain duties relative to responding to subpoenas. The duties are specified by the applicable rules for civil procedure for the court in which the case is being heard. Generally, those responding to subpoenas must produce the records as they are kept in the usual course of business and claim any privileges that may be relevant.

Claiming Privileges

In addition to having the capability of identifying and producing records in accordance with the terms of a subpoena and applicable law, persons responding to a subpoena may also have a duty to claim a privilege on behalf of the individual whose records have been subpoenaed. As will be discussed in chapter 4, privileges protect certain information from being disclosed in court. Under the FRCP, if a records custodian withholds information based on a privilege, the custodian still must provide a description of the withheld information that is sufficient enough that the demanding party has enough information to contest the claim of privilege.

Preparation of Documents for a Subpoena Duces Tecum

Once the validity of a *subpoena duces tecum* has been verified, including the patient's authorization to release the requested records, appropriate measures must be taken prior to disclosure to ensure the completeness and integrity of the health record. Such careful preparation also applies when responding to court orders. The following steps should be taken.

1. Examine the health record for completeness and legibility.

2. Ensure the patient's name is present on every page.

3. Examine the record to determine if there is a basis for possible negligence action against the provider (and review with legal counsel, if necessary).

4. Remove material that is not requested in the subpoena (for example, correspondence).

5. Number the pages.

6. Prepare an index of the contents.

7. Photocopy the record and attempt to submit it in lieu of the original by authenticating the record and certifying the copy as an exact replica of the original record.

8. Personally deliver (never mail) original records and obtain a receipt if originals are delivered and left with the court.

9. Never leave original records with anyone other than a representative of the court (that is, opposing legal counsel is not entitled to original records).

As health records become increasingly electronic, issues such as document preparation and information integrity are paramount. The healthcare industry is now grappling with issues such as identifying the "legal" health record when information that was originally entered electronically is later printed to paper. The above document preparation guidelines—initially developed for still-existent paper health records—must also be viewed in light of the presence of both electronically imaged records and records created electronically at the point of care because records from all existing types of media must be produced in response to subpoenas and court orders. Currently, imaged and electronic records are often printed and added to paper records for legal process purposes, such as responding to subpoenas. However, as technology advances and electronic documents become more accepted in their native electronic form, both the legal system and those holding crucial evidence—such as records custodians providing health records created in a variety of formats—must adapt.

Check Your Understanding 3.3

Instructions: Indicate whether the following statements are true or false (T or F).

1. A subpoena is another name for a court order.

2. In most cases, a subpoena for health records must be accompanied by patient authorization.

3. Written objections to subpoenas may be made in a motion to quash.

4. A *subpoena duces tecum* primarily seeks an individual's testimony.

5. Material should always remain in a health record that has been subpoenaed, even if that material was not requested in the subpoena.

Warrants and Searches

Health records frequently are necessary as evidence in civil cases, such as medical malpractice actions; however, they can also play a significant role in criminal cases, such as healthcare fraud and abuse investigations (to be discussed in chapter 15). In criminal cases, obtaining evidence (including health records) often involves law enforcement actions such as warrants and searches. A **judicial search warrant** is a judge's written order authorizing a law enforcement officer to conduct a search of a specified place and to seize evidence (see FRCP 41).

Although the HIPAA Privacy Rule (42 USC sec. 1320), which will be discussed in chapter 9, requires an analysis of federal and state laws to balance an individual's privacy interests against governmental interests in preventing and stopping healthcare fraud and abuse, it generally does not prevent the disclosure of one's health information when it is provided to a government agency or law enforcement agency for the investigation of criminal or quasi-criminal activities. For example, a Pennsylvania court held that the confidentiality provisions of that state's Drug and Alcohol Abuse Act did not prevent the issuance and execution of a search warrant for patient health records maintained by an outpatient drug and alcohol clinic for a criminal investigation of the billing practices of that clinic (*In re Search Warrant App. No. 125-4,* 2004). In a well-publicized case involving the health records of Rush Limbaugh, *Limbaugh v. Florida,* a Florida court of appeals considered "whether the authority of the State to seize medical records in a criminal investigation by search warrant is limited by a patient's right of privacy." The court ruled that state statutory patient health record privacy protections relating to subpoenas are trumped by the State's authority to seize such otherwise protected records under a validly issued and executed search warrant.

Protections against unreasonable searches and seizures are provided by the Fourth Amendment of the Constitution (US Const. amend. IV), which provides that:

> The right of the people to be secure in their persons, houses, papers and effects, against unreasonable searches and seizures, shall not be violated, and no warrants shall issue, but upon probable cause, supported by oath or affirmation, and particularly describing the place to be searched, and the persons or things to be seized.

Although the vast majority of cases dealing with Fourth Amendment search and seizure considerations do so in the criminal context, the Fourth Amendment also applies to administrative and regulatory searches and seizures.

In addition to the federal right that is built into the Constitution, the constitutions and statutory schemes of individual states must be harmonized with federal principles and law.

A search that is conducted without obtaining a proper warrant is permissible under urgent circumstances or when conducted incident to an arrest. Warrantless searches are unique in that such searches proceed without the special statutory or legal protections built into most other types of searches. To pass constitutional muster, a warrantless search may be executed only in circumstances where an urgent need for a health record exists. Predictably, such circumstances are rare and limited.

Pretrial Conferences

From the time a lawsuit is filed and throughout the discovery period, when determined necessary by the parties and judge involved in a case, the parties and their attorneys will meet with the court to discuss the status of the case, the upcoming trial, and potential settlement negotiations. These meetings are **pretrial conferences.** Many times, a case is settled before it reaches trial. This saves time, money, and emotional hardship on the parties. A settlement may be reached between or among parties to a lawsuit with or without intervention from a third party.

Trial

If the parties fail to negotiate a settlement during the pretrial phase of a lawsuit, or if the case is not dismissed, it will proceed to trial.

Players in a Trial

The environment of a courtroom during trial is often very different from the overflowing courtrooms depicted by producers in action-packed TV legal dramas. There are, nonetheless, essential players involved in the trial itself.

The judge presides over the trial and the courtroom, making critical decisions regarding the admissibility of evidence, which will guide the outcome of a case. The judge makes decisions of law (for example, evidentiary decisions) and instructs the jury regarding the law of that jurisdiction. In a trial without a jury (**bench trial**), the judge also serves as the fact finder.

The **jury** is the fact-finding body that hears evidence given by the parties (if they testify) and other witnesses, observes evidence presented by both sides, and hears the opening statements and closing arguments of each side. Importantly, the jury decides facts based on the perceived credibility of the evidence, but does not decide law (for example, it does not determine which evidence shall be admitted and which shall not). Because opposing parties present conflicting evidence, it is the role of the jury to determine which evidence—in the form of testimony or physical evidence—is more believable and will be given greater weight in the jury's final decisions. The evidence that they choose to believe, therefore, becomes "fact" in the jurors' minds as they render their decision regarding the outcome of the case, such as liability or guilt. The number of jurors and alternates who are seated is determined by the FRCP for federal cases and by individual state rules of civil procedure for cases tried in state courts.

Parties in a trial include the plaintiff and defendant, accompanied by their respective attorneys, unless they are acting pro se. Both the plaintiff and defendant have the right to be present during the course of the trial.

Witnesses are individuals called by each of the parties to provide evidence supporting that party's case. A hostile or adverse witness is one who demonstrates such animosity or prejudice toward the party that called the witness to the stand that the witness can be declared hostile during the trial and subsequently cross-examined and treated as though he or she had been called by the opposing party (Garner 2004). Plaintiff(s) and defendant(s) may also become witnesses, taking the witness stand to testify.

The Fifth Amendment of the US Constitution protects a criminal defendant against self-incrimination, including the right not to testify. A prosecutor who brings to the jury's attention the fact that a criminal defendant declined to testify during a trial has compromised the defendant's Constitutional rights, and the statement may be grounds for a mistrial.

Generally, individuals called to the witness stand are **lay witnesses**, testifying based on their own observations of the situation(s). A second type of witness, an **expert witness**, is called to testify based on subject matter expertise rather than on personal observations (an expert witness generally was not present when the situation that prompted the lawsuit occurred). Individuals with considerable experience in HIM may be called as expert witnesses in cases involving the alleged wrongful disclosure of information, for example, and asked to proffer their opinions based on their experience and knowledge in the area.

The **bailiff**, assigned to a particular court, is responsible for maintaining order and decorum in the court as well as managing the schedule of the judge. Depending on state law, the bailiff may or may not be required to be a peace officer.

Although not a player in the trial and not present in the courtroom, the clerk of court is responsible for maintaining all court records, including pleadings that are generated as the case proceeds to trial. Often this is an elected position.

A court reporter is present during the entire course of a trial and is responsible for providing a verbatim transcript of the trial. The transcript provides key information when statements made during trial become a point of contention and, possibly, the basis for a successful appeal.

Check Your Understanding 3.4

Instructions: Indicate whether the following statements are true or false (T or F).

1. Cases are rarely settled before they reach trial.

2. Judicial search warrants are more likely to be used to obtain health records in criminal cases than in civil cases.

3. A pro se plaintiff is one who represents himself during litigation.

4. An expert witness is called to testify based on her own observations of the situation that prompted the lawsuit.

5. A bench trial is a trial without a jury.

Trial Procedures

Following the pretrial period, if the parties have been unable to negotiate a settlement, the case goes to trial. (See figures 3.2 and 3.3 for the sequence of civil and criminal trials, respectively.)

A jury is selected through a process called *voir dire* or, if a jury is waived, a judge hears the case (bench trial). The number of jurors assigned to a case will vary based on whether the case is civil or criminal and in what jurisdiction the case is being tried. Attorneys are given discretion to excuse potential jurors "for cause" (for example, a prosecutor may excuse an individual in a death penalty case if the individual states that he or she will not vote for the death penalty on moral or religious grounds). Further, attorneys are given a limited number of **peremptory challenges**, which allow jurors to be excused for unstated reasons. Attorneys may not use their peremptory challenges on prejudicial grounds that excuse jurors based on such protected classes as race, gender, religion, and ethnicity, although it is difficult to prove whether an attorney has done so. In the landmark US Supreme Court case of

Figure 3.2. Sequence of a civil trial

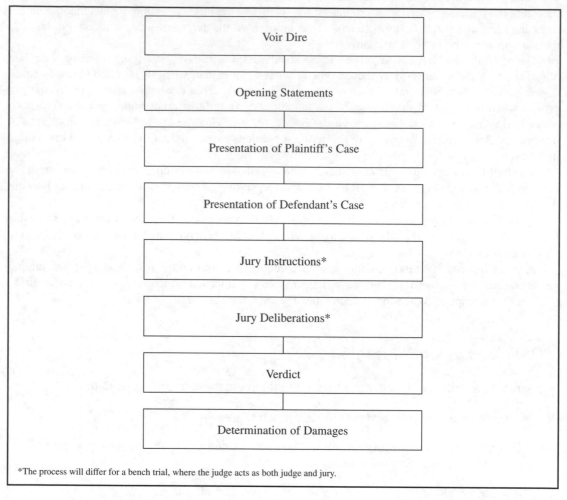

Voir Dire

Opening Statements

Presentation of Plaintiff's Case

Presentation of Defendant's Case

Jury Instructions*

Jury Deliberations*

Verdict

Determination of Damages

*The process will differ for a bench trial, where the judge acts as both judge and jury.

Batson v. Kentucky, the court held that using peremptory challenges to dismiss jurors solely on the basis of race was unconstitutional.

When the trial begins, each side gives an **opening statement** that outlines the evidence that will be heard. Evidence is then presented. The plaintiff's attorney is the first to call witnesses and present evidence. After the plaintiff's witness has been questioned by the plaintiff's attorney, the defense attorney has the opportunity to cross-examine him or her. After the plaintiff has rested his or her case, the defendant's attorney calls witnesses and presents evidence such as health records. After the defense witness has been questioned by the defendant's attorney, the plaintiff's attorney has the opportunity to cross-examine the witness. During the questioning of witnesses, objections are made by each side to prevent the admission of certain statements into evidence. Physical evidence such as exhibits or objects is submitted to the court as evidence to be considered by the fact finders. As each side rests its case, the attorneys for the opposing party may make a motion for a **directed verdict**, requesting the judge to determine that, at that point in time, the case is over and favorable to the requesting party. Although not generally granted by the judge, a directed verdict signifies that the plaintiff failed to present the minimal evidence necessary to prove his case (even without the opposition presenting its case) and could not win the case as a matter of law. After both sides have presented and rested their cases, each presents a **closing argument** urging the jury to find in its favor.

The **burden of proof** (that is, sufficiently proving or establishing the requisite degree of belief for each element of a case) usually belongs to the plaintiff (Garner 2004). In civil cases, the burden of proof

Figure 3.3. Sequence of a criminal trial

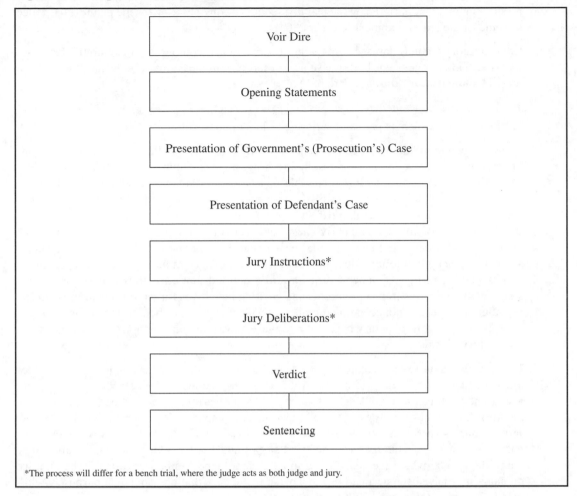

Voir Dire

Opening Statements

Presentation of Government's (Prosecution's) Case

Presentation of Defendant's Case

Jury Instructions*

Jury Deliberations*

Verdict

Sentencing

*The process will differ for a bench trial, where the judge acts as both judge and jury.

is the preponderance of the evidence standard, which requires the plaintiff to provide evidence proving it is "more likely than not" that each element of the case was met and that the defendant committed the alleged wrongdoing. This civil standard is lower than the burden of proof for criminal cases, whereby the prosecution must prove "beyond a reasonable doubt" that the defendant committed the act(s) alleged. A higher burden of proof is required for criminal cases because the stakes (jail or prison) are higher than the stakes in civil cases, which generally involve monetary damages.

The jury, having been given legal **jury instructions** by the judge, conducts **deliberations** secretly and renders a decision or **verdict**. In criminal cases, a unanimous vote is required to either convict or acquit a defendant. Any split in votes results in a hung jury. By contrast, civil cases often require only a certain majority in order to render a verdict of liability or no liability. This varies from state to state and is established by the FRCP in federal cases. A defendant is never declared innocent by the court, because a determination would indicate certainty that the defendant did not commit the act or acts alleged. Rather, "not guilty" or "not liable" verdicts indicate that the plaintiff or government did not present sufficient evidence to meet its burden of proof.

The final step in a trial where the defendant(s) have been judged liable by the jury or, in the case of a bench trial, the judge, is the determination of damages. (The criminal counterpart to this step is the sentencing phase.) The amount of damages, which was requested in the complaint, is determined by the jury. Types of damages are categorized as follows.

- **Nominal damages** are awarded simply to recognize wrongdoing by the defendant when there is no substantial injury suffered by the plaintiff requiring compensation, or the plaintiff has failed to demonstrate a dollar amount (Garner 2004).

- Compensatory (actual) damages are the most common and compensate the plaintiff for losses incurred. This category has been the subject of tort reform measures at both state and national levels. **Compensatory damages** are of two types:

  1. Economic, such as medical expenses and loss of wages
  2. Noneconomic, such as pain and suffering or loss of consortium

  Although economic damages can be readily verified through medical bills and calculations of days lost at work (and, as a result, lost wages), it is much more difficult—virtually impossible, in fact—to quantify intangible noneconomic damages. How does one attach a dollar value to a plaintiff's pain or disfigurement, or the diminished value of the quality of the relationship between the plaintiff and a spouse or other family member due to the event that led to the lawsuit? Quite clearly, these sums cannot be computed and, as a result, have created a significant challenge for the legal system. Plaintiffs and their attorneys, understandably, place high dollar values on noneconomic damages in an effort to recoup as much as possible. In turn, sympathetic juries award requested amounts, thus driving up professional malpractice insurance premiums and creating incentives for would-be plaintiffs to file lawsuits. As a result, noneconomic compensatory damages have been targeted by a variety of legislatures, with monetary caps put into place in various jurisdictions to stem the rising tide of jury awards.

- **Punitive damages** exceed compensatory damages and punish the defendant(s). Such damages are most likely to be requested and awarded where the actions of the defendant(s) were reckless, wanton, careless, fraudulent, or so egregious as to warrant excess action by the court. In an April 2006 high-profile case, the pharmaceutical company Merck was ordered by a New Jersey court to pay $9 million in punitive damages, in addition to $4.5 million in compensatory damages, to a 77-year-old man who suffered a heart attack after taking the anti-inflammatory painkiller Vioxx, which the court found to have contributed to his heart attack. The punitive damages may have been awarded due to a belief by the jury that the defendant purposely withheld information (Nordqvist 2006).

Testimony to Authenticate Health Records

As with depositions, discussed above, the custodian of health records or another designated individual may be called as a trial witness by one or more parties to testify as to the authenticity of a health record being sought as evidence. Testifying as to a record's authenticity refers to verification of the record's validity (in other words, that it is the record of the individual in question and it is what it purports to be) and is, therefore, reliable and truthful as evidence. Because individuals who document in a health record do not typically falsify their entries, the truthfulness of a health record is generally not questioned. As a result, the parties to litigation may agree (stipulate) as to a record's authenticity and allow it to be entered into evidence without requiring an individual to personally appear in court and testify. The parties may further agree to allow a photocopy of the record to be introduced into evidence instead of the original. This generally requires written certification that the photocopy being provided is an exact copy of the original. The dramatic increase in EHRs has introduced new challenges to the authentication process. Because the individual responsible for the management of health information may not be knowledgeable about the intricacies of an electronic system, the court may mandate a certificate of authorization from the software developer or testimony by the facility's chief information officer (CIO) or an individual from the information technology department to satisfy the court's authentication requirements (Servais 2008).

At trial, the types of queries that may be expected and the appropriateness of questions do not differ from queries at depositions. When the appropriateness of a question is doubtful, a legal objection may be made and the judge will make a ruling as to whether or not it is to be answered.

Post-trial

The completion of a trial does not mean that the case is over. The party or parties who are dissatisfied with the outcome will likely seek a different outcome by raising—through an appeal, discussed below—legal errors that purportedly occurred during the trial. In civil cases, once all legal arguments are exhausted and decisions rendered, a monetary amount may be required from the defendant(s) if the plaintiff(s) win(s) the case.

Appeals

After the court has rendered a verdict, the next stage in the litigation process is the **appeal**. A case may or may not be appealed to the next court in the tiered system for a review of alleged legal errors at the lower court. The party appealing a case is the **appellant**, who is thereafter also referred to as the **petitioner**. The party against whom a case is appealed is the **appellee**, who is thereafter also referred to as the **respondent**. There is not always a clear winner and loser at the conclusion of a trial. For example, a verdict may be rendered against the defendant, but the plaintiff may not believe that the amount of damages awarded was sufficient. In such cases, a **cross appeal** may occur, whereby the respondent, in addition to the petitioner who initially filed, files an appeal. In any event, appeals must be based on alleged errors or disputes of law, such as a judge admitting evidence contrary to the rules of evidence. Errors of fact, such as a jury believing an untruthful witness, cannot form the basis of a permissible appeal.

Collection of Judgment

The final stage of litigation, presuming a verdict of liability, is the collection of the judgment. Judgments may be in **equity**, such that the defendant is required to do or to refrain from doing something. However, more commonly, judgments are money awards and require collection. Because awarded damages may number in the millions of dollars, it may not be feasible for the defendant(s) to write a single check to satisfy the judgment. One method of collecting the award methodically and gradually is via **garnishment** of wages. Through this court-ordered method, a percentage of the defendant's wages are routinely set aside and paid to the plaintiff toward full satisfaction of the judgment. Another method, a court-ordered **writ of execution**, directs the appropriate law enforcement official to seize the defendant's real or personal property to satisfy the debt owed to the plaintiff. This may be accomplished by accessing the defendant's bank account or by holding a sale subsequent to seizure of the property. Likewise, a **judgment lien** may be placed on the defendant's property, encumbering it and preventing the debtor-defendant from taking any money from its sale until the judgment owed to the plaintiff has first been paid. Although the judgment lien method is dependent on the defendant selling the property and may not occur in time to benefit the plaintiff, it can nonetheless pose a surprise to a debtor-defendant who wishes to sell his or her property years after a judgment was rendered and, perhaps, all but forgotten.

Physicians and other healthcare professionals carry malpractice insurance as protection against lawsuits in which they are named as defendants and for which a settlement is reached or a court finds them liable. Depending on the terms of the malpractice insurance policy and the type of wrongdoing alleged, the defendant may or may not be covered. Some malpractice insurance policies may exclude wrongdoing that is found by the courts to be intentional. If a defendant is found liable or reaches a settlement on a legal matter that the policy covers, it will be the insurance company that pays the award to the plaintiff rather than the defendant. As a result, however, the defendant can expect that his or her malpractice insurance premiums will increase. If an individual is a defendant in multiple lawsuits, the malpractice insurer may discontinue coverage at some point, deeming the individual no longer insurable.

Check Your Understanding 3.5

Instructions: Indicate whether the following statements are true or false (T or F).

1. In civil cases, the burden of proof is "beyond a reasonable doubt."

2. Noneconomic compensatory damages have been targeted as a cause of rising professional malpractice insurance premiums.

3. The legal system does not allow photocopies of health records to be admitted into evidence.

4. The party that appeals a lower court's decision is the appellee.

5. Garnishment is a court-ordered collection of money damages that is awarded to the plaintiff through a set-aside of the defendant's wages.

Summary

Individuals responsible for the retention and integrity of health records are likely to be included in a lawsuit to provide critical evidence through production of health records. Therefore, it is important to understand the context around which a legal request for the health record occurs. This chapter discussed the structure of a lawsuit including the parties, discovery and other pretrial activities, trial procedures, and potential post-trial actions. The subpoena and court order should be differentiated to avoid the improper disclosure of information subsequent to legal process. Most information in this chapter was presented with an eye toward civil lawsuits because it is expected that these will be the most relevant to those responsible for health information. However, it is important to recognize that there are many similarities and corollaries in the context of criminal cases. It is important to be aware of these corollaries because health records do play a key evidentiary role in criminal cases as well.

References

Casad, R., H. Fink, and P. Simon. 1989. *Civil Procedure: Cases and Materials.* 2nd ed. Charlottesville, VA: The Michie Company.

Cornell Law School. 2006 (Sept. 27). Legal Information Institute. http://www.law.cornell.edu

Garner, B.A. 2004. *Black's Law Dictionary*, 8th ed. (abridged). St. Paul, MN: West.

Reynolds, R. 2010. *Tennessee Health Information Management Association Legal Handbook*, 11th ed. Winchester, TN: THIMA.

Nordqvist, C. 2006 (April 11). Merck to pay $9 million in punitive damages. *Medical News Today.* http://www.medicalnewstoday.com.

Servais, C. 2008. *The Legal Health Record.* Chicago: AHIMA.

Showalter, J.S. 2012. *The Law of Healthcare Administration.* 6th ed. Chicago: Health Administration Press.

Cases, Statutes, and Regulations Cited

Batson v. Kentucky, 476 US 79 (1986).

Fabich v. Montana Rail Link, Inc., MT Dist., 2005 ML 135.

In re Search Warrant App. No. 125-4, 852 A.2d 408 (PA Super.2004).

Limbaugh v. Florida, 887 So.2d 387 (2004).

Nielsen v. Braland, 264 MN 481, 119 N.W.2d 737 (1963).

Smith v. Rossi, 115 A.D. 2nd 899; NY App. Div. (1985).

Swartz v. Cartwright, 15 MS L. Rep. (2002).

Trujillo v. Trujillo, 71 CA App. 2nd 257, 162 P.2d 64 (1945).

45 CFR 164.512(e): HIPAA. 2006.

5 USC 552a (App. 3 sec.(6)(a)(4)): The Privacy Act of 1974.

42 USC 1320: HIPAA Privacy Rule. 1996.

FRCP 23: Class Action. 2007.

FRCP 45(c)(2)(A): Protection of persons subject to subpoena. 2007.

FRCP 45(c)(3)(A): Protection of persons subject to subpoena. 2007.

FRCP 41: Dismissal of Action. 2001.

US Const. Fourth Amendment: Search and Seizure.

US Const. Fifth Amendment: Rights of Person.

Appendix 3.A
Sample Subpoena Duces Tecum (Civil)

SUBPOENA DUCES TECUM (CIVIL) –
ATTORNEY ISSUED VA. CODE §§ 8.01-413, 16.1-89, 16.1-265;
Commonwealth of Virginia   Supreme Court Rules 1:4, 4:9

Case No.:..

....
HEARING DATE AND TIME

....Court

....
COURT ADDRESS

...................................**v./In re:**..........................

TO THE PERSON AUTHORIZED BY LAW TO SERVE THIS PROCESS:
You are commanded to summon

....
NAME

....
STREET ADDRESS

....
CITY   STATE   ZIP

TO the person summoned: You are commanded to make available the documents and tangible things designated and described below:

A certified copy of any and all records reflecting treatment received, including office visits, ER records,

diagnoses, histories and physicals, discharge summaries, consultations, operative reports, pathological reports,

x-ray reports and films, lab reports, echocardiogram reports and tapes, EKG reports and tracings, doctors' orders,

progress notes, nurses notes and any outpatient records concerning X, Date Of Birth, Social Security Number

at .... at ....
LOCATION   DATE AND TIME
to permit such party or someone acting in his or her behalf to inspect and copy, test or sample such tangible things in your possession, custody or control.

This Subpoena Duces Tecum is issued by the attorney for and on behalf of

....
PARTY NAME

....
NAME OF ATTORNEY   VIRGINIA STATE BAR NUMBER

....
OFFICE ADDRESS   TELEPHONE NUMBER OF ATTORNEY

....
OFFICE ADDRESS   FACSIMILE NUMBER OF ATTORNEY

....
DATE ISSUED   SIGNATURE OF ATTORNEY
Notice to Recipient: See page two for further information.

RETURN OF SERVICE (see page two of this form)

FORM DC-498   7/00
(MASTER, PAGE ONE OF TWO)

TO the person summoned:

If you are served with this subpoena less than 14 days prior to the date that compliance with this subpoena is required, you may object by notifying the party who issued the subpoena of your objection in writing and describing the basis of your objection in that writing.

TO the person authorized to serve this process: Upon execution, the return of this process shall be made to the clerk of court.

NAME: ....

ADDRESS: ....

....

☐ PERSONAL SERVICE   Tel. No. ....

Being unable to make personal service, a copy was delivered in the following manner:

☐ Delivered to family member (not temporary sojourner or guest) age 16 or older at usual place of abode of party named above after giving information of its purport. List name, age of recipient, and relation of recipient to party named above:

....

....

☐ Posted on front door or such other door as appear to be the main entrance of usual place of abode, address listed above. (Other authorized recipient not found.)

☐ not found   ...., Sheriff

.... by ...., Deputy Sheriff
DATE

CERTIFICATE OF COUNSEL

I, ... , counsel for .... , hereby certify

that a copy of the foregoing subpoena duces tecum was ....
                                                  DELIVERY METHOD

to .... , counsel of record for .... ,

on the .... day of .... , ...

_____
SIGNATURE OF ATTORNEY

FORM DC-498 7/00
(MASTER, PAGE TWO OF TWO)

Chapter 4
Evidence

Jill Callahan Klaver, JD, RHIA

Learning Objectives

- Explain the significance of health information as evidence

- Describe discoverability

- Explain electronic discovery (e-Discovery) and the associated changes to the Federal Rules of Civil Procedure

- Describe the significance of subpoenas to the litigation process

- Describe a legal hold

- Explain spoliation and the concern it raises in legal cases

- Describe admissibility

- Define and give examples of the three types of evidence

- Describe and apply the best evidence and hearsay rules

- Explain the principle of patient-provider privilege

- Discuss legal protections applied to incident reports and peer review records

Key Terms

Admissibility
Apology statutes
Authenticated evidence
Best evidence rule
Business records exception
Circumstantial evidence
Demonstrative evidence
Direct evidence
Discoverability
e-Discovery

Electronic health records
  (EHRs)
Electronically stored
  information (ESI)
Evidence
Federal Rules of Civil
  Procedure
Federal Rules of Evidence
Hearsay
I'm Sorry Laws

Incident reports
Legal hold
Metadata
Peer review
Physician–patient privilege
Relevant evidence
Spoliation
Subpoenas
Waiver of privilege
Weight of the evidence

Introduction

Patient information is routinely relevant in legal proceedings, whether that information is being used to allege a physician's negligence, to assert that an individual is incompetent, or to raise any number of other issues. Individuals charged with the responsibility of protecting health information must often act as the "gatekeeper" for the appropriate disclosure of that information in legal proceedings. In doing so, an understanding of state and federal privacy laws as well as the legal processes through which health records are actually requested and used as evidence during litigation is necessary. This chapter will discuss some of the key evidentiary rules that impact how health records are used as evidence.

Health Information as Evidence

Just as a variety of rules govern the trial process discussed in chapter 3, many additional federal and state rules specifically govern when and how evidence may be used during the trial process. **Evidence** is the means by which the facts of a case are proved or disproved (Garner 2004). It may be presented in the form of oral testimony, contained in written documents, or presented through pictures and objects. To manage how evidence is used during cases, both federal and state laws provide frameworks that govern the admission of evidence during litigation. Generally, if a case is presented in federal court because it involves a federal law (for example, the False Claims Act), or if the parties are from different states, the **Federal Rules of Evidence** (FRE) apply. If a case is tried in state court, then the rules of evidence for that particular state apply. State rules of evidence are often similar to the federal rules, although the degree of similarity varies from state to state.

Health information is an important kind of evidence that is relied upon in a variety of civil cases. If a plaintiff wishes to prove injury by the defendant in a personal injury case, health information will be used to establish the extent of the plaintiff's injuries. In a medical malpractice case, health information will be used to establish the standard of care that applied to the defendant's conduct and to establish whether the defendant's conduct caused the plaintiff's injuries. For example, in *Kohl v. Tirado,* the plaintiff alleged that his podiatrist had committed malpractice by failing to diagnose a fractured ankle and provide appropriate treatment. The health records kept by the podiatrist were instrumental in determining whether the podiatrist had in fact failed to diagnose the fracture and whether the podiatrist's overall treatment was reasonable. Similarly, if an injured worker wishes to claim benefits for a work-related injury, health information evidence will be used to prove the extent of the worker's injury. Individuals applying for federal disability benefits will use health information to establish that they qualify as disabled.

Courts will review health information evidence in cases involving custody, especially when the health of a child or custodial parent is at issue. In *In the Matter of J.B.,* the respondent appealed the trial court's order terminating her parental rights to her son. Specifically, the respondent argued that her mental health records should not have been admitted into evidence because they were protected from disclosure under a state statute. The appellate court disagreed, finding that the records were admissible under a statutory exception. (Admissibility will be discussed later in this chapter.) The court also noted that the contents of the records indicated that the respondent's mental health issues seriously impeded her ability to provide minimally acceptable parenting for her son. Health information evidence will also be used in cases where an individual's competence is at issue, such as in guardianship or commitment proceedings, which are discussed in more detail in chapter 7.

Health information evidence is central in criminal proceedings as well. Prosecutors use health information to prove injuries to victims in murder, manslaughter, criminal assault and battery, and abuse cases. Health information also may be used to establish a defendant's claim of self-defense in such cases. In *Connecticut v. Abney,* the defendant was convicted of manslaughter after she stabbed her ex-boyfriend. She claimed that the stabbing occurred in self-defense and sought to admit her own health records showing past treatment for injuries that she alleged were previously caused by her ex-boyfriend. Admission of health records would bolster the defendant's claim of self-defense by suggesting the defendant's state of mind at the time of the stabbing. The trial court excluded these records, but the appellate court disagreed, ruling that the records were relevant to her claim of self-defense.

Health information may also be used in white-collar crime cases, such as criminal fraud and abuse. For example, in *United States v. Syme*, health records were instrumental in the appellate court's finding that there was insufficient evidence to convict the defendant of intentionally billing Medicare for medically unnecessary ambulance services of a nursing home resident. The specific ambulance service at issue occurred on August 3, 1994. In determining that transporting the resident via ambulance was not medically necessary, the prosecutor's expert witness testified that he had reviewed the resident's nursing home records for January 20 and March 17, 1994. Those records showed that the resident was able to walk and sit up on her own, suggesting that absent an emergency, ambulance transportation would not be appropriate. However, the court found this evidence to be insufficient because other health records dated between March 17 and August 3, 1994, were not reviewed. The court determined that during those four months, the resident's condition could have deteriorated, thus making transportation via ambulance medically necessary.

Discoverability

Health information evidence presented at trial is usually obtained through the pretrial discovery process. **Discoverability** in general refers to the limitations on the ability of parties to discover pretrial information held by another. As discussed in chapter 3, discovery involves a pretrial exchange of information between the parties through depositions, interrogatories, requests for production of documents, physical and mental examinations of parties, and requests for admission. The idea behind the civil discovery process is that the parties should go to trial with as much knowledge about the facts of the case as possible. Information learned during discovery can also lead to settlements, avoiding the need for an expensive trial.

Whether a piece of information is discoverable depends on specific federal and state rules of evidence, statutes, and case law. As a general rule, to be discoverable, information must simply be related to the subject matter of the pending case. For example, if a plaintiff is claiming damages for a back injury as a result of a car accident, then information such as the plaintiff's medical bills and health records related to the accident obviously relate to the case. However, if the plaintiff had other injuries to his back before or after the car accident, records about those injuries would relate to the case as well because they could identify other sources of the plaintiff's claimed injuries.

Electronic Discovery (e-Discovery)

More than 90 percent of all information created today is done so electronically, and the healthcare industry is no exception to this trend. As a result, more and more evidence obtained through the discovery process and used in trials is found in an electronic format. Today, providers, insurers, and other health services entities routinely use electronic systems to document care, bill or reimburse for care, and arrange for ancillary services such as ordering pharmaceuticals or supplies (The Sedona Conference 2007). From a litigation standpoint, paper documents and electronic documents have important characteristics and differences that can change the discovery process. The Sedona Conference, a nonprofit research and educational institute dedicated to the advanced study of law and policy, outlines six key areas where electronic records differ from paper records as detailed in figure 4.1.

With increasing use of **electronically stored information** (ESI), which is information "created, manipulated, communicated, stored, and best used in digital form, and more widespread use of electronic records the concept of electronic discovery (e-discovery) has evolved" (AHIMA e-Discovery Task Force 2008). Just as paper documents significantly impact litigation, so do electronic documents. However, due to their differences, the processes by which each type of document is subject to discovery

Figure 4.1.   Six key areas where electronic records differ from paper records

1. **Volume and Duplicability:** With advances in information technology, at least 93% of information generated today is created using digital technology. Moreover, digital information is routinely and easily duplicated. Users can easily save files and disseminate them through e-mail. Most applications used to create electronic data and files have automatic backups, which help to protect against accidental loss of data.

2. **Persistence:** It is much more difficult to dispose of electronic documents than paper documents. Paper documents can be destroyed by shredding or some other form of physical destruction. However, as noted by the court in *Zubulake v. UBS Warburg LLC,* "The term 'deleted' is sticky in the context of electronic data. Deleting a file does not actually erase the data from the computer's storage devices. Rather, it simply finds the data's entry in the disk directory and changes it to a 'not used' status—thus permitting the computer to write over the 'deleted' data. Until the computer writes over the 'deleted' data, however, it may be recovered by searching the disk itself rather than the disk's directory. Accordingly, many files are recoverable long after they have been deleted even if neither the computer user nor the computer itself is aware of their existence."

3. **Dynamic Changeable Content:** Electronic information can be more easily modified than paper information. For example, correcting a spelling error on a document created using a typewriter involves physically "whiting out" the misspelled word and replacing it with the correctly spelled word. The same process is much easier in an electronic word processing application, and often only involves the use of an automatic spell checker. Further, simply accessing or moving electronic data can alter that data by changing file creation and modification dates.

4. **Metadata:** Electronic documents contain "metadata," which is "information about the document or file that is recorded by the computer to assist the computer and often the user in storing and retrieving the document or file at a later date." File designations, create/edit dates, authorship, and edit history are all examples of metadata. Where such issues are relevant or in dispute, metadata can be useful in authenticating documents or establishing exactly when documents were created. An electronic document's metadata may not be relevant in every case, especially when there is no dispute as to who authored a document or when a document was modified. However, in *Williams v. Sprint/United Mgmt. Co.,* the court held that "When a party is ordered to maintain documents as they are maintained in the ordinary course of business, the producing party should produce the electronic documents with their metadata intact."

5. **Environment-Dependence and Obsolescence:** Unlike paper documents, electronic data may not be readable once it is moved from its "environment." For example, if a file is transferred to a different computer, that computer must have the appropriate software loaded to open that file. If it does not, then the file may not open correctly or may not be readable at all. Further, with the continual advances and upgrades of information technology, many organizations routinely migrate to new or upgraded information systems. This can make it difficult to restore electronic data or files exactly as they were maintained in previous systems.

6. **Dispersion and Searchability:** Electronic documents are easily stored in multiple locations such as on computer hard drives, servers, or portable devices such as laptops, PDAs, cell phones, or jump drives. Searching electronic documents for specific pieces of information is often less cumbersome than conducting the same search on paper. For example, a "find" or "search" function in a word processing document can quickly find all occurrences of a certain word within electronic documents regardless of their size. To find all occurrences of the same word in a large paper document could take hours of manual labor.

Source: The Sedona Conference 2007.

differ depending on whether the document is paper or electronic. The AHIMA e-HIM Work Group on e-Discovery (2006) described **e-Discovery** as involving the

> . . . access, use, and preservation of information, data and records created or maintained in electronic media. It is more than rephrasing discovery requests to include electronic records and data, and it is more than printing e-mails. It includes obtaining new information, in new forms, in new places, from new sources and using it in a new manner. It includes the utilization of computer search capabilities, which creates enormous power to locate information in ways never before located. Electronic discovery also includes different approaches and disciplines:

- Computer forensics where scientific methods are employed to analyze sources of electronic data such as hard drives or servers to determine if evidence was accessed, destroyed or fabricated or to find computer generated evidence of which lay persons are unaware of such access logs or metadata;

- Searching, gathering, reviewing, analyzing, producing and using large amounts of relevant information, in "routine" litigation, i.e. the equivalent to searching warehouses, waste baskets, file cabinets, home offices, personal notes, etc., which is often performed or facilitated by outside service providers; and

- The focused search for ESI particularly relevant to the specific case such as cell phone records and e-mail or instant messaging of key participants. (AHIMA 2006, 68A)

Challenges that exist when an organization possesses ESI include locating all of an organization's relevant ESI when a discovery request is made and determining the procedures for identifying and disclosing relevant ESI (AHIMA e-Discovery Task Force 2008). **Metadata** is a result of ESI that is data about data—that resides outside the record that is normally released upon request. Metadata can provide valuable information to attorneys involved in litigation. For example, metadata can capture the time that documentation was created through an electronic time stamp, it can track when a document was created and by whom, when a document was accessed and by whom, and if any changes were made (Dimick 2007; Trites 2008). If, for example, metadata is obtained by opposing legal counsel during e-Discovery and shows that a patient encounter was documented prior to the encounter and by someone other than the patient's provider, this information can be damaging in a legal action (Trites 2008). It is now not uncommon in legal cases that an organization will be asked to produce ESI that includes any information found in **electronic health records** (EHRs) (computerized record of health information and associated processes), medical images, e-mail communications, medical bills, and other types of ESI for one or more patients and over a number of years of care. Thus, effectively managing ESI has become a particular daunting task as the volume of ESI continues to increase (Horn 2010).

To assist organizations and vendors who provide technology services and products designed to help organizations find and manage information required by the court, a group of interested parties (attorneys, vendors, and other stakeholders) developed the Electronic Discovery Reference Model (EDRM) to address the complexity of e-Discovery. The EDRM defines the process of e-discovery by using terminology that is meaningful to both healthcare providers and vendors. The model assists vendors in mapping their products and services to steps in the e-discovery process so that they can efficiently locate and prepare relevant electronic information (figure 4.2). One component of the EDRM, information management, will be further addressed through the Information Management Reference Model (IMRM), a project designed to develop common references for stakeholders including information technology, legal, business, and health information management professionals (Horn 2010).

Figure 4.2.   Electronic Discovery Reference Model

The EDRM diagram represents a **conceptual** view of the e-discovery process, not a literal, linear, or waterfall model. One may engage in some but not all of the steps outlined in the diagram, or one may elect to carry out the steps in a different order than shown here.

The diagram also portrays an **iterative** process. One might repeat the same step numerous times, honing in on a more precise set of results. One might also cycle back to earlier steps, refining one's approach as a better understanding of the data emerges or as the nature of the matter changes.

The diagram is intended as a basis for discussion and analysis, not as a prescription for the one and only right way to approach e-discovery.

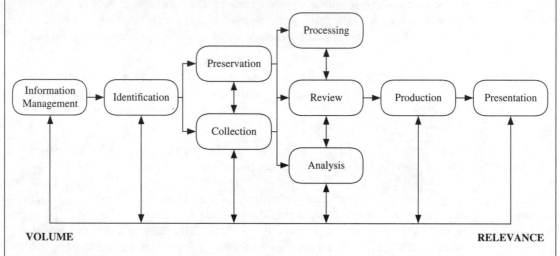

VOLUME   **RELEVANCE**

Information management: getting the organization's electronic house in order to mitigate risk and expenses should electronic discovery become an issue, from initial creation of electronically stored information through its final disposition

Identification: locating potential sources of electronically stored information and determining its scope, breadth, and depth

Preservation: ensuring that electronically stored information is protected against inappropriate alteration or destruction

Collection: gathering information for further use in the e-discovery process (e.g., processing and review)

Processing: reducing the volume of information and converting it, if necessary, to forms more suitable for review and analysis

Review: evaluating the information for relevance and privilege

Analysis: evaluating information for content and context, including key patterns, topics, people, and discussion

Production: delivering information to others in appropriate forms and using appropriate delivery mechanisms

Presentation: displaying the information before audiences (e.g., at depositions, hearings, and trials), especially in native and near-native forms, to attempt to persuade or elicit further information

Source: edrm.net 2009.

Check Your Understanding 4.1

Instructions: Indicate whether the following statements are true or false (T or F).

1. Health information is important as evidence in many types of civil and criminal cases.

2. In state court, a state's rules of evidence will determine whether a piece of information is discoverable.

3. Electronically stored information is now obtained more frequently through discovery than it was in the past. Electronic discovery includes computer forensics.

4. E-mail can generally not be sought as part of the electronic discovery process.

Amendments to the Federal Rules of Civil Procedure

In response to the increased use of electronic data in litigation, on April 12, 2006, the United States Supreme Court approved amendments to the **Federal Rules of Civil Procedure** (FRCP) (rules that govern civil cases at the trial level in federal court) to include requirements specifically tailored to the discovery of electronic data. The amendments, often referred to as e-Discovery rules, became effective December 1, 2006, and are found throughout the FRCP. These rules, which were subject to approval by both the US Supreme Court and the US Congress, apply to civil proceedings in federal courts. They encompass 11 different categories and 86 rule sets, which are summarized in table 4.1 (Baldwin-Stried 2006). The degree to which federal rules of civil procedure are used in state court proceedings varies from state to state. About half of all states have adopted these new rules already or have e-Discovery rules of their own in place. It is also important to note that a majority of the discovery rules, including references to e-Discovery, apply only to parties involved in a case—in other words, the plaintiff(s) and defendant(s). However, since the business records of nonparties are subject to subpoenas under Rule 45 of the FRCP, it is important for any organization that maintains ESI to be prepared to identify, protect, and produce that information.

The amended rules provide for early involvement of the court in managing e-Discovery and altering the process of when and how the courts make arrangements for the discovery of ESI with regard to scheduling, scope of discovery, preservation obligations, waiver of privilege, form of production, and the burden of deriving answers to interrogatories from electronically produced materials. Further, the amended rules modify what burdens may be applied via subpoena. The ramification of these new rules and their impact on the management of EHRs will be significant. They present a unique opportunity for collaboration among legal counsel, information technology, senior management, and individuals responsible for managing health information in developing policies and procedures that comply with new laws governing the management of electronic records. Some of the key amendments are discussed below with a more detailed discussion of the relevancy and practice considerations of the rule changes found in appendix 4.A (pp. 81–84).

Scheduling orders (Rule 16(b)), which outline key deadlines that apply to the case, may address the disclosure and discoverability of electronically stored information. They may also address agreements regarding how parties will handle privileged information that is inadvertently produced.

Initial disclosures (Rule 26(a)) are mandatory disclosures of certain basic information that must be provided before a formal discovery request and should include a copy or description and location of any electronically stored information that may be used to support parties' respective claims or

Table 4.1. Outline of the Federal Rules of Civil Procedure

Category	Category Description	Rules in Category	General Content in Category
I	Scope	1 and 2	Category I describes the purpose of the rules and their role in governing civil action in federal district courts.
II	Commencement of civil suits	3 to 6	Category II contains the rules that provide for the commencement of a civil suit, including the filing, summons, and service of process (legal notice).
III	Pleadings and motions	7 to 16	Category III provides for civil suit pleadings, motions, and defenses and counterclaims. The complaint is the plaintiff's pleading. The answer is the defendant's pleading.
IV	Parties	17 to 25	Category IV describes the capacities in which a party or parties can be sued. It maintains the provisions describing the mechanisms for the filing of countersuits, joinder claims, class action lawsuits, and other actions.
V	Discovery	26 to 37	Category V contains the rules governing discovery (e-Discovery included). In general, the discovery rules help ensure that neither party is subjected to surprises at trial. In many states discovery can occur only through formal request. In contrast, the FRCP requires parties to divulge certain information without a formal discovery request.
VI	Trial	38 to 53	Category VI provides for the plaintiff's right to a trial by jury or by the court. Additionally, this category contains the rules that describe how cases are assigned for trial, how actions are dismissed, and how subpoenas are handled. On December 1, 2006, FRCP 45 (subpoenas) was amended to conform with the e-Discovery rules.
VII	Judgment	54 to 63	Category VII maintains the provisions governing legal judgment and costs. "Judgment" is the decree and any other order from which an appeal lies. Category VII judgment rules maintain provisions for establishing new trials, amending judgments, and the enforcement of judgments.
VIII	Provisional and final remedies and special proceedings	64 to 71	Category VIII contains the series of rules that provide for the final provision or remedy of a case. The rules covered in this category include seizure of property, injunctions, offers of judgment, and execution of judgments.
IX	Special proceedings	72 to 76	Category IX contains the rules governing special civil action proceedings, such as condemnation of real and personal property, magistrate judges, and pretrial orders.
X	District courts and clerks	77 to 80	Category X provides direction concerning the business and operations of the district courts. The rules covered in this category include hours of operation, filing of pleadings and orders, trials and hearings, orders in chambers, procedures for books and records maintained by the clerk, the role of stenographers, and transcripts as evidence.
XI	General provisions	81 to 86	Category XI explains to which proceedings the rules apply (United States district courts vs. state courts) and provides direction on their general applicability, jurisdiction and venue, local rules applications, and judges directives.

Source: Baldwin-Stried 2006.

defenses. For example, if an EHR will be used as evidence in a case, the initial disclosure should describe that record and provide its location.

Reasonable access (Rule 26(b)(2)) allows for discovery of ESI to be limited if that information is not reasonably accessible because of undue burden or cost. What constitutes reasonably accessible can vary from case to case and court to court.

Discussion between two parties (Rule 26(f)) supports the requirement that very early on in the case, parties must confer with one another about a variety of issues, such as the nature of any claims and defenses, settlement possibilities, arrangements for initial disclosures, preservation of discoverable information, and the development of an overall discovery plan. Amendments to the rules now specifically require the parties to address "any issues relating to disclosure or discovery of electronically stored information, including the form or forms in which it should be produced." An understanding of an organization's document retention policies and the intricacies and capabilities of its information technology system is important to facilitating this process.

Interrogatories and Production of documents (Rules 33 and 34) now both contemplate the production of ESI. With respect to ESI, if a request does not specify the form for producing such information, the responding party must produce it in the form in which it is ordinarily maintained or in a form that is reasonably usable. Further, a party need not produce the same electronically stored information in more than one form.

Failure to make disclosures (Rule 37(f)) says a court may not impose sanctions on a party for failing to provide ESI lost as a result of the "routine, good-faith operation of an electronic information system." What constitutes good faith will vary from case to case and court to court. However, once there is reasonable notice of potential or actual litigation, an organization or party may need to suspend the routine destruction of electronic data that are potentially relevant to the litigation in order to satisfy the good faith standard.

Testing or sampling of documents (Rule 45) allows, in cases where large volumes of documents may contain relevant evidence, the testing or sampling of those documents to determine whether relevant evidence exists. The rules for subpoenas have been amended to allow for the testing and sampling of electronically stored information. As will be discussed in more detail below, the rules allow subpoenas to specify the form or forms in which subpoenaed information is to be produced.

Under the new rules, individuals responsible for the management of health information may need to be involved in the pretrial conference to discuss the scope of information being requested. Decisions will need to be made by the parties regarding what information needs to be preserved and the format in which it will be presented. These are new activities. In the past, paper records were simply retrieved and copied for discovery purposes. With ESI, discovery may involve information and data from source systems outside of those which are usually printed or viewed electronically, such as native file formats, computer files, erased files, e-mails, and others. It is important to be informed early in the discovery process if electronic information will be needed and to know the locations of all components of ESI in order to produce the information as requested. All information created in a health record—both electronic and paper—is potentially open to discovery unless otherwise directed by the court. Depending on how an organization has defined its business or legal record (discussed later in this text), a request for the "complete patient record" may encompass a wider range of information (including copies printed from an EHR system) than that which was typically considered to be part of the paper health record.

Other discovery process issues or concepts of importance relate to subpoenas and producing documents in the normal course of business, legal holds, spoliation, record retention and destruction polices, disaster recovery, and business continuity plans.

Subpoenas

Individuals responsible for the management of health information play an important role in the pretrial discovery process. Perhaps the most common way they participate in this process is by responding to subpoenas for health records. As described in chapter 3, a **subpoena** is a legal document that compels an individual to give testimony or commands the production, inspection, or copying of books, documents, ESI, or other tangible items. Subpoenas may be issued in both criminal and civil matters by both state and federal courts as well as administrative agencies.

Producing Records as Kept in the Usual Course of Business

Because documents produced in response to subpoenas are key evidence, appropriate responsiveness is essential. A person responding to a subpoena for documents must "produce them as they are kept in the usual course of business" or "organize and label them to correspond with the categories in the demand" (FRCP 45(d)(1)(A)). From a health information perspective, this requirement raises a number of important issues regarding the subpoena of health records. First, the facility must have a clear definition of what constitutes a health record that is kept in the usual course of business. For example, is e-mail or text message communication from a patient included in the record? What about x-ray films or any audio/video recordings made for patient care? If so, through what process are these items integrated into the record? Do staff members who release records have access to these items and a way to reproduce them?

As previously discussed, the FRCP now provides a framework for the discovery of electronic records. Under those rules, a subpoena may specify the form or forms in which ESI is to be produced (FRCP 45(a)). If no specification is made, then the records must be produced in the form(s) in which they are ordinarily maintained or in a form that is reasonably usable (FRCP 45(d)(1)(B)). However, the same rules provide some protection against producing ESI that is not reasonably accessible because of undue burden or cost (FRCP 45(d)(1)(D)). Further, the rules provide that ESI need not be produced in more than one form (FRCP 45(d)(1)(C)). Although the FRCP has created a framework for the discovery of electronic records, not all states have implemented similar frameworks. If a subpoena is issued for a case being tried under state law, then state rules establish the records custodian's duties in responding to that subpoena. Therefore, individuals responsible for the management of health information must be familiar with the subpoena requirements and discovery rules for their particular state. Further, the interpretation and application of both state and federal rules is influenced by judicial decisions, making an awareness of relevant judicial decisions equally important.

Once a facility has defined the content of records kept in the usual course of business, it must have a system to ensure that all records commanded by the subpoena have been produced. This can be especially challenging in settings where shadow records, hybrid records, or electronic records are used. A shadow record is a duplicate record kept for the convenience of the provider or facility (Burrington-Brown 2003). In theory, the shadow record should be an exact duplicate of the original health record and contain no documentation that is not in the original record. However, in practice, it is sometimes easy for staff to inadvertently file paperwork in a shadow chart instead of the original chart. When this happens, the original record becomes incomplete. As a result, the custodian of records risks representing that a true and complete copy of a patient's record has been produced in response to a subpoena when, in fact, this is not the case.

A hybrid record is one that is composed of both paper and electronic information. Release of information staff must know how to access both paper and electronic components of a hybrid record. It is important to remember that "the current hybrid records management encompasses EHRs as well as any and all information stored, created, or accessed within the organization, including e-mail, voice mail, text messages, metadata, back-up tapes, and legacy information systems" (Baldwin-Stried 2006). The same issues are important in facilities that have fully implemented EHRs.

Legal Hold

A **legal hold** (also known as a preservation order, preservation notice, or litigation hold) is issued by the court if there is concern that information may be destroyed in cases of current or anticipated litigation, audit, or government investigation. Individual circumstances of the litigation, investigation, or audit may determine the requirements for the legal hold.

The hold basically suspends the processing or destruction of paper or electronic records (AHIMA e-HIM Work Group on e-Discovery 2006). In a paper health record system, it is standard practice to physically "lock up" a record that is involved in litigation to protect the integrity of the documentation and evidence. If a legal hold is issued, then that is the process that is usually followed for paper documents. However, in an electronic environment an equivalent practice must be implemented. Organizational policies and procedures should encompass the process for communicating a hold to those responsible for all systems that contain relevant information so that no one system is purged in violation of the hold. The policies and procedures should also identify the individual or individuals who are responsible for implementing a legal hold, suspending destruction, and determining when the legal hold can be lifted (AHIMA e-HIM Work Group on e-Discovery 2006). This responsibility may fall to the custodian of records, who is usually an HIM professional.

Check Your Understanding 4.2

Instructions: Indicate whether the following statements are true or false (T or F).

1. The Federal Rules of Civil Procedure were amended in 2006 to address the discovery of electronic data.

2. Under the Federal Rules of Civil Procedure, court-imposed sanctions are not permitted if a party fails to provide electronically stored information lost as the result of a good-faith operation.

3. In general, documents must be produced in response to a subpoena as they are kept in the usual course of business.

4. A hybrid record is a fully electronic record.

5. A legal hold requires the preservation of both paper and electronic records.

Spoliation

Spoliation is "the intentional destruction, mutilation, alteration or concealment of evidence" relevant to a legal proceeding (AHIMA e-HIM Work Group on e-Discovery 2006). It is a legal concept applicable to both paper and electronic records. When evidence is destroyed that relates to a current or pending civil or criminal proceeding, it is reasonable to infer that the party had consciousness of guilt or another motive to avoid the evidence. In *Coleman Parent Holding Inc. v. Morgan Stanley & Co., Inc.,* the jury was instructed to find an adverse inference for the spoliation of evidence.

Spoliation of evidence has long been a concern of courts. The modern legal doctrine addressing spoliation of evidence began in 1959 (Eng 1999). It is this doctrine that drives the duty to preserve documents in the context of litigation. Various state and federal laws, such as the Sarbanes-Oxley Act, which enforces corporate accountability, broaden the reach of the spoliation doctrine from mere litigation matters to pending federal or state agency investigations.

Some jurisdictions have recognized a spoliation tort action, which allows the victim of destruction of evidence to file a separate tort action against the spoliator. This action, though, has been inconsistent in its application due to lack of clarity on whether the tort can be filed simultaneously with the civil action. In addition, some courts have required evidence of bad faith (that is, intentional destruction of evidence) for a plaintiff to successfully proceed. For example, *Phillips v. Covenant Clinic* involved a wrongful death action brought by the plaintiff after her father suffered cardiac arrest and died on his way from a physician clinic to a hospital for medical testing. The plaintiff sought discovery of her father's record from the physician clinic, and was informed that the record was missing. Witnesses for the clinic testified that the clinic record was delivered to the hospital and disappeared at some point thereafter. In a motion to the court, the defendants argued that the plaintiff failed to establish a causal relationship between the physicians' purported breach of the standard of care and her father's death. The plaintiff countered that the defendants' failure to produce the record entitled her to an inference that the missing medical record contained evidence unfavorable to the defendants. The court agreed that intentional destruction of or failure to produce relevant records supports an inference that the records would have been unfavorable to the party responsible for their destruction or nonproduction. However, the court went on to note that the inference can only be based on the intentional destruction of evidence, stating, "It is not warranted if the disappearance of the evidence is due to mere negligence, or if the evidence was destroyed during a routine procedure." Further, the court stated that the missing evidence must have been in control of the party who would ordinarily be responsible for its production. In granting summary judgment in favor of the defendants, the court found that no facts suggested that the clinic had intentionally destroyed the record. Without the inference provided by spoliation of evidence, the plaintiff was unable to establish the case. Other courts, further, have disallowed spoliation claims in conjunction with primary lawsuits alleging negligence rather than intentional wrongdoing.

Courts will allow the spoliator to rebut the inference of guilt through explanations that demonstrate a lack of bad faith. A good legal hold process, as outlined in the previous section, and sound policies on retention and destruction can prevent spoliation.

In 2003 and 2004, a series of legal cases (the *Zubulake* cases) related to e-Discovery and spoliation provided for the application of the Sedona Guidelines in the courtroom setting by Judge Shira Scheindlin of the federal district court for the Southern District of New York (The Sedona Conference 2007). Among the principles established were:

- "Electronic documents are no less subject to discovery than paper records, and this is true not only of electronic documents that are currently in use, but also of documents that may have been deleted and now reside only on backup disks" (*Zubulake v. UBS Warburg,* 217 FRD 309);

- There exists a "duty to preserve backup tapes" (*Zubulake v. UBS Warburg,* 220 FRD 212); and

- "When evidence is destroyed in bad faith, i.e., intentionally or willfully, that fact alone is sufficient to demonstrate relevance for purpose of sanction for spoliation of evidence; by contrast, when the destruction is negligent, relevance must be proven by the party seeking sanctions" (*Zubulake v. UBS Warburg,* 229 FRD 422).

Those principles were strengthened in a 2010 opinion by Judge Scheindlin, where failures among the defendants to produce documents were found to be negligent in some instances and grossly negligent in others, thus warranting the application of sanctions (*The Pension Committee of the University of Montreal Pension Plan, et al., v. Banc of America Securities, LLC, et al.,* 05 Civ. 9016 (SAS), opinion and order filed January 11, 2010).

With respect to the preservation of records as evidence, one court observed that the duty to preserve evidence applies both to the period of time preceding litigation when such litigation is anticipated as well as the time period of the litigation process itself (*Silvestri v. General Motors*).

Spoliation of electronic records should be prevented through the same standards as those used for paper records; however, there are some differences. Data that have been deleted whether appropriately or inappropriately from an electronic record can often be recovered using software tools. It is important that policies outline the proper steps for making changes to electronic documentation. Most importantly, procedures for making corrections must be followed to eliminate the inference that information was intentionally altered. EHR systems must have functionality that meets the organization's requirements for making corrections. Inaccurate entries are far more likely to result in a malpractice claim than spoliation is. Guidelines for ensuring documentation integrity to prevent liability are outlined in the next section.

Retention and Destruction of Health Information

Policies and procedures related to the retention and destruction of health information and records should offer some guidance and direction to a healthcare provider when addressing the discovery processes mentioned above. The AHIMA e-HIM Work Group on e-Discovery (2006) suggests that a healthcare provider must have knowledge of where its information is stored, how long it is kept, and when it may be destroyed, whether the information is in paper or electronic form. It goes on to suggest that health information management and information technology departments as well as other departments define the healthcare provider's legal health record and establish routine practices for retention and destruction. Guidelines should be developed that identify where information may be hidden, such as backup tapes, instant messages, voicemail, word processing drafts, and shadow records, as well as when parts or all of the legal record, audit trails, metadata, e-mails, and other business records should be destroyed. A healthcare provider must also ensure that any vendor or contractor possessing provider records is aware of the e-Discovery rules and has the ability to comply with the rules as required (AHIMA e-HIM Work Group on e-Discovery 2006).

Disaster Recovery and Business Continuity

As with retention and destruction guidelines, a healthcare provider must have plans that address how health information in either paper or electronic format will be preserved in the event of a natural or manmade disaster. The plan should provide for how the provider will return to normal operation as quickly as possible, with attention to prevention of loss and restoration of access to records including legal discovery within a reasonable time frame (AHIMA 2006).

Managing the Discovery Process

Managing the discovery process along with the new e-Discovery rules can be challenging. As the healthcare industry continues to transition from paper to electronic record systems, HIM professionals must, more than ever, be familiar with provider methods and formats used to retain, manage, store, and destroy paper and electronic records, as well as the production of records for litigation (Baldwin-Stried 2006). To assist in this process, AHIMA's e-HIM Work Group (2006) recommended that existing policies and procedures be reviewed and revised where necessary to include steps for responding to requests for information in electronic records. Figure 4.3 provides a list of these recommended steps.

Figure 4.3. Developing e-discovery policies and procedures

1. Develop a formal project charter to create and review the organization's procedures for providing evidence related to discovery for legal proceedings. Requirements for the project will include the allocation of resources to support the work of delivering a procedure document within a specified period of time. Members of this project team should include individuals with responsibility for:

   • Health Information Management

   • Privacy

   • Information Security

   • Risk Management

   • Information Technology

   • Patient Relations

   • Legal Counsel

   • Executive Management

2. Prepare an education session for the appointed team covering the Federal Rules of Civil Procedure with respect to e-Discovery including the findings from your research of state laws and AHIMA resources.

3. Locate existing policies and procedures for the definition of the legal health record, retention, destruction, and electronic record management. Review existing procedures for adequacy and identify gaps and issues that should be addressed in the new or revised policies and procedures.

4. Locate any existing procedures for providing material in response to subpoena, court order, or request from an attorney. Review existing procedures for adequacy and identify gaps and issues that should be addressed in the new or revised policies and procedures. Be sure to include information for the following three situations in the procedures:

   • Legal discovery process that does not involve your organization.

   • Discovery process in which your organization or a member of your staff is being sued. The procedure must provide for measures to protect the information from modification or destruction by the employees involved. This information must also be reviewed to ensure that privileged information is not being furnished.

   • Discovery process that involves your organization, specifically the health information management and/or information technology departments. Alternate custodians of the information must be assigned to ensure that measures to protect the information from modification or destruction by the employees involved are implemented. The information must also be reviewed to ensure that privileged information is not being furnished.

5. Prepare drafts of the policies and procedures for review by the team, senior management, and legal counsel if not already done as part of the team. Revise the drafts based on comments and submit for further review as needed until approved.

6. Develop a plan to purchase and install any software and hardware identified to support implementation of the policies and procedures.

7. Develop a comprehensive communication and education program to inform all members of the organization about the existence of the procedures including their responsibilities with respect to electronic discovery.

8. Publish the approved policies and procedures.

Source: AHIMA e-HIM Work Group on e-Discovery 2006.

Admissibility

Admissibility refers to evidence that is allowed to be admitted in a court of law. It is important to distinguish between discoverability and admissibility. Evidence that is discoverable during the pretrial process may not necessarily be admissible at trial. As a general rule, only **relevant evidence** is admissible at trial (FRE 402). Relevant evidence is evidence having a tendency to make the existence of any fact more probable or less probable than it would be without that evidence (FRE 401).

Even if evidence is relevant, it may still be excluded from a trial on a number of grounds. For example, if a piece of relevant evidence also happens to be unfairly prejudicial, confusing, or misleading, or if it is needlessly redundant, then the court must conduct a balancing test before allowing the piece of evidence to be admitted. The probative value of this evidence must substantially outweigh the dangers of unfair prejudice and/or undue delay associated with presenting that evidence (FRE 403). *Broek v. Park Nicollet Health Services* involved a wrongful death action brought by the plaintiff regarding the death of her husband. The plaintiff appealed the trial court's decision to admit certain health records of her husband, who had been diagnosed with a ventricular septal defect as a teenager. Specifically, the records noted that her husband experienced an episode of dizziness while playing basketball several months before his sudden cardiac arrest, but he had not sought any treatment at that time. In upholding the trial court's decision, the appellate court noted that evidence is not unfairly prejudicial merely because it is damaging to one party's case.

Even if evidence appears to be relevant, it must also be authenticated. As with health records, as introduced in chapter 3, the evidence itself must be shown to have a baseline authenticity or trustworthiness. As a general rule, **authenticated evidence** is present if there is "evidence sufficient to support a finding that the matter in question is what its proponent claims" (FRE 901(a)). Generally, this is established by a record custodian's affidavit that the record was:

- Documented in the normal course of business (following normal routines)

- Kept in the regular course of business

- Made at or near the time of the matter recorded

- Made by a person within the business with knowledge of the acts, events, conditions, opinions, or diagnoses appearing in it (AHIMA Work Group on Maintaining the Legal EHR 2005)

While the authentication requirements established by the FRE comport with paper records, establishing the authenticity of electronic records presents additional challenges for individuals responsible for the management and integrity of health information. Electronic documents can be easily modified and, depending on the system used, those modifications are not always apparent. Therefore, a records custodian or other witness may need to describe how an electronic system monitors or manages modifications or different versions of electronic documents in order to satisfy the court that the record should be admitted into evidence.

The accuracy and trustworthiness of electronic records are determined by:

- The type of computer used and its acceptance as standard and efficient equipment

- The record's method of operation

- The method and circumstances of preparation of the record (AHIMA Work Group on Maintaining the Legal EHR 2005)

Other indicators of the reliability and issues relating to preparation of electronic records are shown in figure 4.4.

Each state establishes its own rules for authenticating evidence similar to the rules outlined above. Individuals responsible for the management of health information must be aware that failure to follow applicable rules could lead to the exclusion of health records from evidence. For example, in *American Color Graphics v. Rayfield Foster,* the appellate court determined that health records were improperly admitted into evidence because they had not been properly authenticated. In that case, the plaintiff wished to demonstrate the extent of his claimed injuries by offering a variety of health records and reports into evidence. However, the doctors and psychologists who compiled the reports were not deposed and did not testify at trial. Under Alabama discovery rules, if copies of health records and

Figure 4.4. Indicators of the reliability of and issues related to preparation of electronic records

---

Reliability

- Validation of computer systems to ensure accuracy, reliability, consistent performance, and the ability to conclusively discern invalid or altered records;

- The ability to generate accurate copies of records in both human readable and electronic form;

- Protection of records to enable their accurate and ready retrieval throughout the records retention period;

- Use of hardware, software, records management procedures (including trusted third party storage of electronic records) and/or third party notarization and time certification, to ensure reliability as to the identity of the creator and the time of creation of an electronic record, and to ensure that the electronic record has not been altered since the time of creation;

- Limiting system access to authorized individuals, and use of authority checks to ensure only those individuals who have been so authorized can use the system, electronically sign a record, access the operation or device, alter a record, or perform the operation at hand;

- Use of appropriate controls over systems documentation including adequate controls over the distribution, access to, and use of documentation for system operation and maintenance; and established written policies which hold individuals accountable and liable for actions involving creation of electronic records, and where appropriate, the use of system audit trails that track creation, use, modification and disposition of electronic records.

Preparation

- The sources of information on which it is based

- The procedures for entering information into and retrieving information from the computer

- The controls and checks used as well as the tests made to ensure the accuracy and reliability of the record

- The information has not been altered

Sources: Adapted from Cavanaugh et al. 2000, AHIMA e-HIM Work Group on Maintaining the Legal EHR 2005.

bills are certified and sealed, they may be admitted "without further need for authenticating testimony" (*American Color Graphics v. Rayfield Foster*, 2001). To be properly certified, there must be a written attestation that

1. The record was made in the regular course of business.

2. It was the regular course of the business to make such a record at the time of the act (of medical treatment) or within a reasonable time thereafter.

Some of the reports offered into evidence contained the following certification by the treating physician: "I hereby certify that the attached is a true and correct copy of the health records kept on file in my office." With respect to these records, the court stated, "Because none of the language on any of these documents reference that these reports were compiled in the regular course of business and at a time consistent with the regular course of business, we conclude that their certifications fail and they were improperly admitted into evidence" (*American Color Graphics v. Rayfield Foster*, 2001).

Other reports offered contained this certification:

I hereby certify and affirm in writing that the attached is a true and complete copy of the records regarding treatment of [the plaintiff], which are kept in the office of [the physician], in my custody and control. I further certify that I am the legal custodian and keeper of the records. The attached records were made in the regular course of business and it was in the regular course of business for such records to be made at the time of the events, transactions, or occurrences to which they refer, or within a reasonable time thereafter.

The appellate court found that the certification language followed the requirements of Alabama law. However, because a notary public did not seal those records, the court still found that they had been improperly admitted (*American Color Graphics v. Rayfield Foster*, 2001).

Even if evidence has been properly authenticated under the rules for a particular jurisdiction, the evidence itself may not necessarily be error-free. For example, incorrect information may inadvertently be documented in a patient record, a provider may fail to document enough information in the record, or the record may contain conflicting information. In such cases, courts generally find that those errors or inconsistencies relate to the **weight of the evidence**, not its admissibility. In other words, the court may still admit the record into evidence, but the jury will then determine how much weight to give that record as they decide the factual issues of the case. If the jury determines that the record contains errors, they may find the record to be untrustworthy and, therefore, discount the information in the record.

Types of Evidence

Three major types of evidence exist: direct evidence, circumstantial evidence, and demonstrative evidence.

1. **Direct evidence** is "real, tangible or clear evidence of a fact, happening or thing that requires no thinking or consideration to prove its existence."

2. **Circumstantial (indirect) evidence** is "evidence in a trial which is not directly from an eyewitness or participant and requires some reasoning to prove a fact."

3. **Demonstrative (real) evidence** is actual objects, pictures, models, and other devices that are supposedly intended to clarify the facts for the judge and jury—how an accident occurred, actual damages, medical problems, or methods used in committing an alleged crime (Garner 2004).

Evidence, including health information evidence, can take a number of specific forms. Evidence is often in written form or "writing," such as medical reports and records. With the onset of new technologies such as EHRs, courts take a broad view of what constitutes writing. The general definition of writing includes "writings and recordings consisting of letters, words, or numbers, or their equivalent, which are set down by handwriting, typewriting, printing, photostatting, photographing, magnetic impulse, mechanical or electronic recording, or other form of data compilation" (FRE 1001(1)).

Evidence may also take the form of oral testimony. (See chapter 3 for information about expert witnesses.) Oral testimony is provided when a witness is deposed or questioned at a hearing or trial. Often, testimonial evidence and documentary evidence are combined. For example, a witness on the stand may refer to a document to refresh his or her recollection of an event, or the witness may be asked to read or explain the contents of writing to the court. Sometimes, documents may not be presented at all unless they are accompanied by witness testimony. *Fred's Stores of Tennessee v. Brown* involved a negligence claim brought by the parents of a 10-year-old girl who was injured after a bicycle assembled by Fred's broke as it was being ridden by the girl. At trial, authenticated health records were entered into evidence, but the physicians who created those records were never deposed and were never called to testify about the contents of those records. Although the court noted that presenting unexplained health records could cause the judge and jury to be confused, it noted, "The health records were introduced without objection at the beginning of trial. If Fred's believed that the testimony in the documents might require expert explanation, the time to make the objection was then. Therefore we find that the records could be used by the trial judge, subject to a reasonable layperson's limits on what may be gleaned from such records."

Evidence may also be presented through photographs. Generally, photographs include still photographs, x-ray films, videotapes, and motion pictures (FRE 1001(2)). As with writings, photographic evidence must be authenticated and trustworthy.

Evidentiary Rules

Rules of evidence, such as those relating to relevance and admissibility mentioned above, are governed by state and federal rules of evidence. These rules establish a comprehensive framework for the admissibility and use of evidence during trials. Some key evidentiary rules are discussed below.

Best Evidence Rule

Under the **best evidence rule**, to prove the contents of a writing, recording, or photograph, the original writing, recording, or photograph is required (FRE 1002). The rule serves mainly to protect against intentional perjury or simple faulty memory regarding the contents of writings, recordings, and photographs. Original means the writing or recording itself or a negative or any print of a photograph. With the healthcare industry's trend toward keeping EHRs instead of paper, the issue of what constitutes an original of an EHR is important. With respect to data stored in a computer or similar device, the best evidence rule states that a printout or other output readable by sight and shown to reflect the data accurately constitutes an original (FRE 1001(3)).

The best evidence rule also permits the use of duplicates in lieu of the original unless (FRE 1003):

- A genuine question is raised as to the authenticity of the original.

- Under the circumstances, it would be unfair to admit the duplicate in lieu of the original.

Therefore, authenticated copies of health records are often used at trial rather than the original patient health record. However, original health records or their duplicates are not always available—records may be lost, destroyed by accident or in accordance with records retention laws, stolen, and so on. In such cases, the best evidence rule provides that other evidence of the record's contents may be admissible if:

- All originals have been lost or have been destroyed (unless done so in bad faith).

- No original can be obtained by any available judicial process or procedure.

- At a time when an original was in possession of the opposing party, that party was put on notice, by the pleadings or otherwise, that the contents would be a subject of proof at the hearing, and that party does not produce the original at the hearing.

- The writing, recording, or photograph is not closely related to a controlling issue (FRE 1004).

Lipschitz v. Stein involved a malpractice claim brought by the plaintiff against his eye doctor. One basis of the claim was that the doctor negligently delayed diagnosis of postoperative eye problems because he did not see the plaintiff until 11:45 a.m., when the appointment was supposed to be at 9:00 a.m. According to the plaintiff, the delay in diagnosis and treatment caused permanent injury to the plaintiff's eye. Although the plaintiff testified that he arrived at the defendant's office at 9:00 a.m., a receptionist working for the defendant testified that the plaintiff did not arrive until 10:00 a.m. The receptionist based her testimony on a patient log, but the actual patient log itself was never entered into evidence. The appellate court ruled that the receptionist's testimony violated the best evidence rule because the best evidence of what was contained in the patient log was the patient log itself, not the receptionist's memory of what was contained in the log. Notably, the pretrial records of the case suggested that the log was not produced by the defendant because the receptionist had altered the times listed on the log. As a result, the appellate court awarded the plaintiff a new trial.

Hearsay

Hearsay is a written or oral statement made outside of court that is offered in court as evidence to prove "the truth of the matter asserted" (FRE 801(a)). For example, if a nurse in a malpractice case against Dr. Jones testifies, "Doctor Smith said that Doctor Jones committed malpractice," the nurse's statement would constitute hearsay. It is testimony about a statement that was made outside of court, and it was offered to prove the truth of Dr. Jones's negligence. This evidentiary concept is applicable to health information because much documentation in the health record is hearsay. As a general rule, hearsay is not admissible as evidence unless one of several hearsay exceptions applies (FRE 803).

Business Records Exception

Because health records consist of out-of-court statements that are often used in court to prove the truth of the claim, they technically constitute hearsay. However, a major exception to the prohibition against using hearsay as evidence is the **business records exception** (FRE 803(6)). Under this rule, a record (for example, a memorandum, report, record, or data compilation) in any form, of acts, events, conditions, opinions, or diagnoses is not hearsay if it meets the following requirements:

- It was made at or near the time by, or from information transmitted by, a person with knowledge.

- It was kept in the course of a regularly conducted business activity.

- It was the regular practice of that business activity to make the record.

Generally, the custodian of records testifies as to the three requirements mentioned above.ww

Other Exceptions

Other hearsay exceptions, in addition to the business records exception, involve health information. For example, statements made for purposes of medical diagnosis or treatment and describing medical history; or past or present symptoms, pain, or sensations; or the inception or general character of the cause or external source thereof insofar as reasonably pertinent to diagnosis or treatment are excepted from the hearsay rule (FRE 803(4)). Records or data compilations, in any form, of births, fetal deaths, deaths, or marriages, if the report thereof was made to a public office pursuant to requirements of law, are also excepted from the hearsay rule (FRE 803(9)).

American Color Graphics v. Rayfield Foster involved both the business records exception to the hearsay rule as well as the exception pertaining to statements made for purposes of medical diagnosis or treatment. The plaintiff in that case filed a workers' compensation claim against the defendant-employer. To demonstrate the extent of his injuries, the plaintiff sought to admit a detailed medical report by a physician who had examined him after he had filed his claim. However, the plaintiff did not call the physician to testify as a witness. The defendant argued that the report was inadmissible because it constituted hearsay—it was an out-of-court statement offered to prove the truth of the plaintiff's work-related injuries. At issue was whether the report met either the business records exception or the statements for purposes of medical diagnosis or treatment exception to the hearsay rule. The defendant argued that the report did not meet the business records exception because it was not kept in the regular course of business, but was prepared specifically in anticipation of litigation (that is, it was prepared specifically for use at trial). In finding that the report constituted hearsay and met neither of the two exceptions at issue, the court stated:

> We first note that according to the case action summary, Foster filed his case on April 8, 1999. Plaintiff's exhibit 2(A), the medical examination report of Dr. Allen, is dated June 28, 1999—almost three months after he first filed his complaint. See plaintiff's exhibit 2(A). Furthermore, in support of its motion *in limine,* ACG submitted to the trial court a copy of Foster's deposition, in which he admitted that although he visited Dr. Allen on a number of occasions after he had back surgery in 1997 and although he paid for his consultations through his wife's insurance, he was referred to Dr. Allen by his own attorney. Although Dr. Allen's report constitutes a statement "made for purposes of medical diagnosis or treatment and describing medical history, or past or present symptoms, pain, or sensations, or the inception or general character of the cause or external source thereof" and, according to its certification, constitutes a report of conditions, opinions, or diagnoses, made the day of the examination by Dr. Allen, certified by the custodian of records within one day thereafter, allegedly kept in the course of regularly conducted medical business, in the regular practice of medical evaluators to make such report, all as shown by the certification of the custodian of records and the sealing thereof by a notary public, we are not as convinced that the source of the information does not indicate a lack of trustworthiness in the sense that it has been prepared solely in anticipation of, and preparation for, litigation. . . . Given the fact that the date of Dr. Allen's evaluation and Foster's own testimony that it was his attorney who sent him to Dr. Allen for consultation, we cannot conclusively say that plaintiff's exhibit 2(A) was not prepared in anticipation and preparation for the lawsuit Foster filed against ACG. Thus, we conclude that Dr. Allen's medical report constitutes inadmissible hearsay; the trial court erred in admitting plaintiff's exhibit 2(A) into evidence.

Physician–Patient Privilege

Courts have long recognized that health records are private and "deserve the utmost constitutional protection" (*Mapes v. District Court,* 1991). The **physician–patient privilege** is a common tool for protecting that privacy in the context of litigation. While it varies from state to state and is not provided for by every state, the physician–patient privilege generally legally protects confidential communications between physicians and patients related to diagnosis and treatment from being disclosed during civil and some misdemeanor litigation. The rationale behind the privilege is that it encourages patients to fully disclose all relevant information to their physicians without fear of the information being made public during a trial. Originating with the Hippocratic Oath, the American Medical Association's Principles of Ethics continue the professional tradition of confidence between a physician and patient unless provided otherwise by law. Similar privileges exist and are recognized by law for relationships such as psychologist-client, attorney-client, and clergy-parishioner.

Generally speaking, the patient (or his/her legally authorized representative) is the holder of the privilege, and must assert that privilege in order to prevent his/her medical information from being disclosed in court. However, case law may impose a duty on a physician or hospital to claim the privilege on behalf of the patient. For example, in *Wesley Medical Center v. Clark,* the hospital sought to protect certain records from disclosure in court based on the physician-patient privilege. The Kansas Supreme Court recognized that the hospital did not meet the statutory definition of holder of the privilege; however, the court stated:

> While it is true that the physician, or in this case the hospital, is not the holder of the privilege that does not mean that a physician, absent statutory authority, may reveal, ex parte, information subject to the privilege without the knowledge and consent of the patient or holder of the privilege. Similar restraints apply to confidential records of hospitals and other treatment facilities unless otherwise provided by statute. Records in the possession of Wesley, which are subject to the physician-patient privilege under Kan. Stat. Ann. 60-427(b), would not ordinarily be discoverable without notice to and the consent of the holder of the privilege (*Wesley Medical Center v. Clark,* 1983).

In *Fierstein v. DePaul Health Center,* the plaintiff sued the defendant for breach of fiduciary duty for wrongful release of her health records. In that case, the plaintiff's ex-husband (through his attorney) issued a subpoena to DePaul Health Center. The subpoena ordered DePaul's custodian of records to appear at a deposition and to bring any and all records pertaining to a hospitalization of the plaintiff. The subpoena was accompanied by a letter stating that the records custodian would not need to appear at the deposition if the requested records were mailed to the ex-husband's attorney's office prior to the deposition. The records custodian testified that she telephoned the ex-husband's attorney's office and was told that the plaintiff's attorney had authorized the release of the records. The records custodian executed an affidavit and mailed the records to the ex-husband's attorney. The plaintiff subsequently sued DePaul for breach of fiduciary duty for wrongful release of her health records. She testified that she never authorized the release of her records or waived any privilege protecting the records. Further, the attorney's office testified that no one had ever represented that the plaintiff had authorized the release of her records.

After hearing the evidence, a jury awarded the plaintiff $10,000 in actual damages and $375,000 in punitive damages. The trial court reduced the punitive damage award to $25,000. The Missouri Court of Appeals (Eastern District) upheld the decision of the trial court, stating, "If a physician discloses any information, without first obtaining the patient's waiver, then the patient may maintain an action for damages in tort against the physician." (Waiver is discussed below; torts are discussed in chapter 5). A key factor in the court's decision was that the plaintiff was never given the opportunity to object to the release of her records. The Court of Appeals also upheld the trial court's decision to reduce the punitive damage award, finding that $25,000 in punitive damages was appropriate to deter the defendant from similar future conduct.

As noted earlier, the existence of privilege statutes varies from state to state. The scope of privilege also varies, although certain common principles apply. Information is not generally considered privileged when it is obtained by a physician in a social situation that is outside the treatment setting. Likewise, information that is subject to public observation (for example, the fact that an individual is bleeding) is not privileged. Information obtained during an employment or pre-employment physical exam is generally not privileged because it lacks a contractual physician–patient relationship. Other parameters that may be defined by state law include:

- Whether privilege survives the presence of a third party during a physician–patient communication

- The survival of privilege even when a third party is paying the patient's medical bill

- The survival of privilege even when a patient is unwilling to be treated (for example, emergency mental health treatment) or unable to give express consent (explained in chapter 7)

- What constitutes a physician–patient relationship

Check Your Understanding 4.4

Instructions: Indicate whether the following statements are true or false (T or F).

1. The best evidence rule prohibits the use of a duplicate record in lieu of the original.

2. Much documentation in the health record is hearsay.

3. The business records exception often enables health records to be admitted as evidence.

4. The physician–patient privilege is used to encourage full disclosure of relevant information by patients to their physicians.

5. It is the physician who holds the physician–patient privilege.

Waiver of Privilege

Like the hearsay rule discussed above, physician–patient privilege is riddled with exceptions. One of the most common exceptions involves **waiver of privilege**. Specifically, "when a party claims damages for physical or mental injury, he or she places the extent of that physical or mental injury at issue and waives his or her statutory right to confidentiality to the extent that it is necessary for a defendant to discover whether plaintiff's current medical or physical condition is the result of some other cause" (*Fabich v. Montana Rail Link, Inc.*, 2005). However, "This waiver is not unlimited, and the defendant may only discover records related to prior physical or mental conditions if they relate to currently claimed damages. The plaintiff's right to confidentiality is balanced against the defendant's right to defend itself in an informed manner. A defendant 'is not entitled to unnecessarily invade plaintiff's privacy by exploring totally unrelated or irrelevant matters'" (*Fabich v. Montana Rail Link, Inc.*, 2005). The waiver of privilege may apply to both health records and to testimony about a patient's condition and/or treatment.

Another exception to the physician–patient privilege involves using the results of blood alcohol tests at trials for driving while under the influence. An individual on trial for driving while under the influence of drugs or alcohol cannot claim the physician–patient privilege to prevent the results of drug and alcohol tests from being admitted as evidence. Likewise, in a proceeding to determine whether an individual's mental capacity is such that he or she needs to be committed, that individual cannot use the physician–patient privilege to prevent testimony and health records regarding mental capacity from being admitted into evidence.

Privilege between Patients and Other Providers

The concept of privilege extends beyond the physician–patient relationship to relationships between patients and other types of providers. Privileges exist between patients and their psychologists, therapists, counselors, social workers, optometrists, dentists, and so on. The scope of these privileges is defined by state statutes and regulations, but generally prohibits providers from disclosing treatment information without patient authorization unless specific circumstances exist. For example, state laws generally allow psychologists to reveal client information to appropriate authorities when there is reasonable belief that the client presents a clear and present danger to the health and safety of himself or herself, another individual, or the public at large. For example, see Kansas Administrative Regulation 102-1-10a(g). As with physician–patient privileges, patients or clients of nonphysician providers can waive their privilege rights. For example, under Kansas law, an individual waives the privilege between himself or herself and a licensed social worker by bringing charges against the licensed social worker. However, the waiver is valid only to the extent that the otherwise privileged information is relevant to the case (KSA 65-6315(a)(3)).

Apology Statutes

Related to privilege (which belongs to the patient) are **apology statutes** that protect communications made by providers to patients (and perhaps patients' relatives) from being admitted as evidence in court. When healthcare providers apologize for unanticipated outcomes following medical procedures or treatments, the apologies may be perceived as admissions of fault rather than merely as compassionate or sympathetic expressions. Informally referred to "**I'm Sorry Laws**," over thirty states have enacted these protective statutes that vary in scope. For example, Ohio and Georgia deem all statements or conduct that express apology or sympathy inadmissible as an admission of liability, and Colorado law specifically excludes statements of fault from admission. Vermont law excludes only oral apologies or statements of regret. California and Texas protect sympathetic statements made relative to an accident, but allow statements of fault to be admitted into evidence (AMA Advocacy Resource Center 2008). Although the intent of apology laws is to protect healthcare providers, defense counsel may prefer that apologies be admitted because juries often view compassionate defendants more favorably.

Protection of Related Medical Documentation

Not all documentation related to patient care is made solely in the health record. In some circumstances, usually when there has been a medical error or some other unexpected adverse event, additional documentation is made in incident reports and peer review records. As discussed below, incident reports and peer review records are part of facility processes designed to document, investigate, and learn from errors and other unexpected events. The law, to varying degrees among different states, generally protects these records from disclosure in court.

Incident Reports

Incident reports are the means through which occurrences that are inconsistent with a healthcare facility's routine patient care practices or operations are documented (Dunn 2003, 46, 49). For example, an incident report should be generated if a nurse administers an incorrect dosage of medication to a patient or if a visitor slips and falls on a freshly mopped hospital hallway. The purpose of an incident report is to document the facts of the incident so that an internal investigation of that incident may be conducted. The main goals of incident reporting are to:

- Describe the unexpected occurrence or incident

- Provide the foundation for an investigation of the occurrence or incident

- Provide information necessary for taking remedial or corrective action

- Provide data useful for identifying risks of future similar occurrences (Dunn 2003, 49)

Incident reports involving patient care are created not to treat the patient, but rather to provide a basis for investigating the incident. Specific requirements for incident reporting are addressed to varying degrees by individual states, often in their risk management statutes. Chapter 14 provides a thorough discussion of the legal requirements related to risk management programs.

From an evidentiary standpoint, incident reports should not be placed in a patient's health record, nor should the record refer to an incident report. This is because state law may protect incident reports from being admitted into evidence during legal proceedings. This rationale is based on the belief that protecting the documents from being used in legal proceedings against providers or organizations will encourage full and frank incident investigations. As a result, organizations can reduce the likelihood of similar incidents in the future. The state law protection or "privilege" of incident report documentation can be waived, however, if the health record contains or refers to the incident report.

After an incident has occurred, documentation in the health record should occur in the same manner as it is routinely completed for patient care. In other words, all the information relevant for a patient's treatment, such as a description of what occurred, the results of evaluation, and the treatment provided, should be documented by those providing care (Dunn 2003, 57). The health record generally should not refer to names (unless necessary for patient care), nor should it make excuses or cast blame for any incident (Dunn 2003, 57).

It is important to note that in individual cases, not all state law privileges or protections for incident report documentation actually prevent the records from being admitted into evidence. From a plaintiff's standpoint, incident reports or related documentation may be critical to proving a negligence claim. The plaintiff may therefore seek a court order or ruling that allows that documentation to not only be discovered but also be admitted into evidence. In such situations, the court will often weigh the rights of the plaintiff against the policy behind the incident reporting protection or privilege. If the court determines that the information contained in the incident report is necessary to the plaintiff's case, it may admit the incident report into evidence despite the existence of the privilege. Alternatively, the court may conclude that the documents at issue fall outside the scope of the privilege or that the defendant waived the privilege in some way (for instance, by referring to the incident report in the health record). Individuals who manage health information should be aware of incident reporting laws and court decisions that are applicable in their own states.

A recent case addressing the admission of incident reporting documentation into evidence is *Riverside Hosp., Inc. v. Johnson*. In that case, the plaintiff's wife was initially hospitalized for lymphoma but suffered a hip fracture during her hospital stay after leaving her bed without assistance. She died several months later as a result of lymphoma. The plaintiff sued on behalf of his wife's estate, alleging that Riverside failed to accurately assess his wife's risk of falling and then failed to implement appropriate measures to prevent her from falling. The jury returned a verdict against Riverside and one of its nurses in the amount of $1 million. The defendants believed that certain evidence was improperly admitted during trial and appealed the judgment. Specifically, the defendants argued that the trial court erred in allowing a quality care control report (QCCR) and a quality management services (QMS) database report, which were used to document factual information about the plaintiff's wife's fall (date, place, time, circumstances, severity, and so forth, of the fall). The defendants argued that the documents constituted incident reports and were therefore protected from being admitted into evidence under Virginia law. The court ruled that the documents fell outside the scope of the Virginia privilege law. According to the court, the documents were not "generated by a peer review or other quality care committee referred to in the statute" (*Riverside v. Johnson,* 2006). Nor were the documents created during a deliberative process involving the overall evaluation of patient safety conditions and the design of initiatives to improve the healthcare system. The court went on to state:

> Factual patient care incident information that does not contain or reflect any committee discussion or action by the committee reviewing the information is not the type of information that must 'necessarily be confidential' in order to allow participation in the peer or quality assurance review process.

The court concluded that the reports were health records of the hospital, made and kept in the normal course of operation of the hospital, and were therefore not protected by the Virginia privilege law from disclosure in court (*Riverside v. Johnson,* 2006).

Peer Review Records

Another type of documentation that is generated outside of the health record involves documentation of peer review activities. **Peer review** involves a broad range of activities undertaken by a peer review committee to ensure that a facility provides quality care and may include such activities as the review of quality and safety issues and determinations of medical staff credentials. Individual state law generally defines the specific scope of peer review activities. It may also provide statutory protection to peer review documentation from being disclosed in court or in preliminary proceedings. For example, in Kansas, hospital peer review activities include:

- Evaluating and improving the quality of healthcare services rendered by healthcare providers

- Determining that health services rendered were professionally indicated or were performed in compliance with the applicable standard of care

- Determining that the providers of professional health services in this area considered the cost of healthcare rendered reasonable

- Evaluating the providers' qualifications, competence, and performance or taking action in disciplinary matters

- Reducing morbidity or mortality

- Establishing and enforcing guidelines designed to keep healthcare costs within reasonable bounds

- Conducting research

- Determining whether a hospital's facilities are being properly utilized

- Supervising, disciplining, admitting, determining privileges for, or managing members of a hospital's medical staff

- Reviewing the professional qualifications or activities of healthcare providers

- Evaluating the quantity, quality, and timeliness of healthcare services rendered to patients in the facility

- Evaluating, reviewing, or improving methods, procedures, and treatments being utilized by inpatient and outpatient staff (KSA 65-4915 (d)).

As with incident reporting, it is common for plaintiffs to attempt to discover and admit peer review records into evidence during cases alleging negligence. As mentioned above, state law may provide a peer review privilege generally protecting these records from being used in litigation. The rationale behind the privilege is that providers will be more candid in admitting fault or identifying problems if they know that this information will not later be used against them in court. By encouraging complete candor, hospitals are better able to identify, respond to, and prevent acts falling below the acceptable standard of care.

However, whether the privilege will actually apply to keep records from being introduced as evidence depends on the facts of the particular case. For example, in *Adams v. St. Francis Regional Medical Center,* the plaintiffs brought a wrongful death suit against the defendants after their daughter died from a ruptured ectopic pregnancy at the defendant hospital. One issue in the case was the admissibility of several reports, including disciplinary reports of a nurse who treated the plaintiffs' daughter. The defendant objected to the admission of the reports based on peer review privilege.

The court recognized that, based on a literal reading of the Kansas peer review statute (detailed above), the disciplinary reports were protected from discovery. This, however, did not end the court's inquiry. According to the court, the privilege had to be weighed against the plaintiff's right to "due process and the judicial need for the fair administration of justice." The court concluded that, based on the facts of the case, the peer review privilege was outweighed by the plaintiffs' right to have access to all relevant facts to their case. The court specifically noted, "Forms and documents containing factual accounts and witnesses' names are not protected simply because they also contained the officers' or committee's conclusions or decision-making process." Instead, the court can simply order the redaction (removal) of the parts of the documents containing analysis but still grant plaintiffs access to portions of documents containing relevant facts.

It is again important for individuals responsible for managing health information to understand the scope of the peer review privilege law that applies in their states.

Check Your Understanding 4.5

Instructions: Indicate whether the following statements are true or false (T or F).

1. Incident reports are created for patient treatment purposes and should be a part of the health record.

2. State law may protect incident reports from being admitted into evidence.

3. Peer review involves activities undertaken to ensure the provision of quality care.

4. Plaintiffs commonly attempt to discover and admit peer review records into evidence during negligence cases against health care providers.

5. The physician-patient privilege may be waived when a party claims damages by the physician and puts his physical or mental condition at issue.

Summary

With the complexity of today's healthcare system and legal environment, it is essential that individuals responsible for the management of health information understand how patient information is used as evidence in legal proceedings. Individuals managing health information are accountable for appropriately maintaining and producing patient information for use in legal proceedings. This means that awareness of federal and state privacy, procedural, and evidentiary law and facilitation of organizational policies that foster compliance with those laws are imperative.

References

AHIMA e-Discovery Task Force. 2008. Litigation response planning and policies for e-Discovery. *Journal of AHIMA* 79(2):69–75.

AHIMA e-HIM Work Group on e-Discovery. 2006. Practice brief: The new electronic discovery Civil Rule. *Journal of AHIMA* 77(8):68A–H.

AHIMA e-HIM Work Group on Maintaining the Legal EHR. 2005. Practice brief: Maintaining a legally sound health record—Paper and electronic. *Journal of AHIMA* 76(10):64A–L.

American Medical Association Advocacy Resource Center. 2008. I'm Sorry Laws. Summary of State Laws. http://www.physicianspractice.com.

Baldwin-Stried, K. 2006. Practice brief: E-Discovery and HIM: How amendments to the Federal Rules of Civil Procedure will affect HIM professionals. *Journal of AHIMA* 77(9):58–60ff.

Burrington-Brown, J. 2003. On the line: Professional practice solutions. *Journal of AHIMA* 74(1):62.

Cavanaugh, F., W. Rishel, P. Spitzer, and J.P. Tomes, eds. 2000. *Comprehensive Guide to Electronic Health Records.* New York: Faulkner and Gray.

Dimick, C. 2007. E-discovery: Preparing for the coming rise in electronic discovery requests. *Journal of AHIMA* 78(5):24–29.

Dunn, D. 2003. Incident reports: Their purpose and scope. *AORN Journal* 78(1):46, 49.

EDRM (edrm.net). 2009. The electronic discovery reference model. http://edrm.net/.

Eng, K. 1999. Legal update: Spoliation of electronic evidence. *Boston University Journal of Science and Technology Law*. 5:L13.

Garner, B.A. 2004. *Black's Law Dictionary*, 8th ed., abridged. St. Paul, MN: West.

Horn, W.S. 2010. Easing e-Discovery: The electronic discovery reference model and the information management reference model. *Journal of AHIMA* 81(1):44–46.

The Sedona Conference. 2007 (June, 2nd ed). The Sedona Principles addressing electronic document production. http://www.thesedonaconference.com/.

Trites, P. 2008. Metadata you need: Determining what must be collected and retained. *Journal of AHIMA* 79(7):52–53, 60.

Cases, Statutes, and Regulations Cited

Adams v. St. Francis Regional Medical Center, 264 KS 144, 955 P.2d 1169 (1998).

American Color Graphics v. Rayfield Foster, AL Civ. App., 838 So.2d 374 (2001).

Broek v. Park Nicollet Health Services, MN App. Unpub. (2003).

Coleman Parent Holding Inc. v. Morgan Stanley & Co., FL Dist. Ct. App. 892, So. 2d 496 (2004).

Connecticut v. Abney, 88 CT App. 495; 869 A.2d 1263 (2005).

Fabich v. Montana Rail Link, Inc., MT Dist., 2005 ML 135.

Fierstein v. DePaul Health Center, MO Ct. App. E.D., 24 S.W.3d 220 (2000).

Fred's Stores of Tennessee v. Brown, MS App., 829 So. 2d 1261 (2002).

In the Matter of J.B., 172 NC App. 1; 616 S.E.2d 264 (2005).

Kohl v. Tirado, 256 GA App. 681, 569 S.E.2d 576 (2002).

Lipschitz v. Stein, NY App. Div., 10 A.D.3d 634, 781 NYS.2d 773 (2004).

Mapes v. District Court, 250 MT 524; 822 P.2d 91 (1991).

The Pension Committee of the University of Montreal Pension Plan, et al., v. Banc of America Securities, LLC, et al., SDNY, 05 Civ. 9016 (2010).

Phillips v. Covenant Clinic, 625 N.W.2d 714, Iowa (2001).

Riverside Hosp., Inc. v. Johnson, 272 VA 518, 636 S.E.2d 416 (2006).

Silvestri v. General Motors, 4th Cir., 271 F.3d 583, 591 (2001).

United States v. Syme, 3rd Cir., 276 F.3d 131 (2002).

Wesley Medical Center v. Clark, 234 KS 13, 669 P.2d 209, 220–221 (1983).

Williams v. Sprint/United Management Company. 230 F.R.D. 640 (D. Kan. 2005).

Zubulake v. UBS Warburg, SDNY, 217 FRD 309 (2003).

Zubulake v. UBS Warburg, 220 FRD 212 (2003).

Zubulake v. UBS Warburg, 229 FRD 422 (2004).

FRCP 45: Subpoena. 2007.

FRE 401: Definition "Relevant Evidence." 1975.

FRE 402: Relevant Evidence Generally Admissible; Irrelevant Evidence Inadmissable. 1975.

FRE 403: Exclusion of Relevant Evidence. 1975.

FRE 801: Definitions. 1975.

FRE 803: Hearsay Exceptions; Availability of Declarant Immaterial. 1975.

FRE 901: Requirement of Authentication or Identification. 1975.

FRE 1001: Definitions. 1975.

FRE 1002: Requirement of Original. 1975.

FRE 1003: Admissibility of Duplicates. 1975.

FRE 1004: Admissibility of Other Evidence of Contents. 1975.

Kansas Administrative Regulation 102-1-10a(g): Unprofessional conduct. Misrepresenting the services offered or provided. 2002.

Kan. Stat. Ann. 60-427(b): Privileged communications. Physician/patient. 2000.

Kan. Stat. Ann. 65-4915(d): Peer review officer or committee. 2000.

Kan. Stat. Ann. 65-6315(a)(3): Confidential information and communication exception. 2000.

Sarbanes-Oxley Act of 2002. Public Law 107-204, 116 Stat. 745.

Appendix 4.A

Changes to the FRCP Relevant to HIM

FRCP	Intent, Description of Rule	Relevance	Professional Practice Considerations
16	Pretrial conferences, scheduling, management	Describes the process attorneys will follow before litigation.	HIM professionals must be aware that the attorneys (parties) will meet and agree upon matters related to discovery before litigation. HIM and IT must work with the organization's attorney prior to a pretrial conference to discuss information and record availability.
16(b)	Early attention to electronic discovery issues	Presents a framework for the parties and the court to give early attention to issues relating to electronic discovery, including the frequently recurring problems of the preservation of evidence and the assertion of privilege and work-product protection. It inserts and creates a much stronger role for the judge in the discovery process.	HIM professionals will need to be aware that the rule gives the court discretion to enter an order adopting agreements the parties reach for asserting claims of privilege or protection as trial-preparation material after inadvertent production in discovery. Credibility is established at the beginning of the process; therefore, HIM and IT must communicate with their attorneys before a meeting with the judge. HIM professionals should work with legal and IT to ensure added privilege protections for HIV, mental health, substance abuse, and employee records. In addition, HIM must be prepared to answer or research questions pertaining to the organization's systems such as location, retention, and accessibility of electronic health information.
26	General provisions governing discovery, duty of disclosure	Describes legal obligation to maintain and disclose relevant records. An organization has roughly 90 days after the complaint is answered to make the initial disclosure.	Organizations and HIM professionals need to be aware of this obligation, which is the same as the duties surrounding maintenance of paper records.
26(a)	Early attention to electronic discovery, required disclosures, methods to discover additional matter	Describes responsibilities of parties in initial disclosure and clarifies the party's duty to include initial disclosures of electronically stored information for data compilations.	HIM and IT professionals must be aware that parties involved in litigation are required to meet ahead of time to review and discuss matters related to electronic discovery. Communication between HIM, IT, and legal should be conducted prior to the parties meeting.

(continued on next page)

FRCP	Intent, Description of Rule	Relevance	Professional Practice Considerations
26(b)(1)	Early attention to electronic discovery, required disclosures, relevance of information produced	Limits the scope of party-controlled discovery matters "relevant to the claim or defense of any party," allowing discovery into "the subject matter involved in the action." The content of the medical record will be an extremely important factor in e-Discovery.	HIM and IT must work carefully with legal and have communication channels established ahead of time. HIM professionals must know the specific documents being requested and their relevance to the claim. Take, for example, a party with a cause of action related to a broken arm in the ER. Records relating to an earlier OB delivery probably will not be relevant, despite a request that specifies "any/all records."
26(b)(2)	Information that is not reasonably accessible	Provides that a responding party need not provide electronically stored information that is inaccessible because of undue burden of cost. The responding party has the burden to show that the sources are not reasonably accessible. Even when such showing is made, a court can still order discovery of those materials for good cause shown and could specify conditions for that discovery, including a reallocation of the costs of the discovery.	"Reasonable" accessibility will be more of an issue for IT professionals and HIM professionals practicing in IT. Organizations will need to establish mechanisms to determine the true costs and burdens for producing data that they determine "not reasonably accessible." HIM and attorneys never want to be in a position of not knowing what is reasonably accessible. Organizations must be proactive and identify ahead of time what information is available and how it will be accessed.
26(b)(2)(C)	Information that is not reasonably accessible, balancing the costs, and potential benefits of discovery	Sets up factors for the judge to consider. Provides whether the responding party is required to search and produce information not reasonably accessible depending on whether the costs and burdens are justified.	HIM professionals may need to be apprised of whether a court order was issued requiring the organization to produce information not reasonably accessible in response to rule 26(b)(2)(C). HIM and IT may need to assist in preparing a summary evaluation supporting legal counsel's definition of "reasonably accessible." HIM and IT should already know what is relevant and what is not, and what is burdensome to produce and what is not. An organization must determine the costs of producing and the privacy concerns ahead of time.
26(b)(5)	Procedure for assertion of claims of privilege and work-product protection after inadvertent production	Established to present to the court claims that parties inadvertently produced information protected by attorney-client privilege or work-product doctrine. It provides that if a party discovers information inadvertently produced, protected, or privileged as work product, it must notify the receiving party and set forth in writing the basis by which the party believes the information is privileged.	This may become an issue for legal, risk management, HIM, or IT professionals if they produce electronic health records that are not requested or relevant to the request (for example, inadvertent production of electronically stored incident reports or peer review records). Also, provisions should be made regarding the inadvertent production of HIV, mental health, and substance abuse records.

FRCP	Intent, Description of Rule	Relevance	Professional Practice Considerations
26(f)	Early attention—discussion between parties, preserving discoverable information	Directs parties to discuss "any issues relating to preserving discoverable information."	HIM and IT professionals may need to be made aware of issues related to discovery of electronically stored information.
26(f)(3) and Form 35	Early attention—discussion between parties, issues relating to disclosure, discovery of electronically stored information, and forms of document production	Directs parties to discuss "any issues relating to disclosure or discovery of electronically stored information, including the form or forms in which it should be produced." Form 35 enables the parties to report to the court their proposed discovery plan and their proposals for disclosure or discovery of electronically stored information.	HIM professionals will need to be apprised of Form 35 and the parties' proposed discovery plan. HIM professionals will be responsible for producing those electronic documents agreed upon between the parties. Issues such as the formats in which the data are to be produced, how much, and what is relevant will need to be provided to HIM.
26(f)(4)	Early attention—discussion between parties, issues relating to privilege and work-product production	Provides for parties to ameliorate costs and delays of document production created by steps necessary to avoid waiving privilege or work-product production during discovery through agreements that allow for the assertion of privilege or work-product production after documents of electronically stored information are produced.	Organizations will need to establish specific policies and procedures outlining examples of what privileged and protected work products include. Legal, IT, and senior management will need to establish mechanisms to determine exact costs and burdens of producing electronically stored information. The policy should include provisions outlining how an organization will respond to requests for records subject to added protections such as HIV, mental health, and substance abuse records.
33	Interrogatories to parties	Provides for the procedure and process in which answers to interrogatories are provided and covers both business records and electronically stored information.	HIM and IT professionals may be required to attest to authenticity of electronically stored information produced in answer to an interrogatory. HIM professionals must therefore be deeply familiar with the operations of the EHR system, particularly the vital legal functionality.
33(d)	Interrogatories to parties, option to produce business records	Allows responding party to respond to an interrogatory by providing electronically stored information.	When HIM professionals provide answers to interrogatories by providing electronic documents, they are responsible for ensuring information can be located and identified by the interrogating party. They must also give the interrogating party a "reasonable opportunity to examine, audit or inspect" the information.
34	Production of documents, electronically stored information, and things and entry upon land for inspection and other purposes	Provides for discovery of the electronic health record and recognizes that on occasion the opportunity to perform testing of documents and electronically stored information.	Discovery of electronically stored information will require new collaborative processes between HIM and other professionals (for example, IT, legal) within the organization.

(continued on next page)

FRCP	Intent, Description of Rule	Relevance	Professional Practice Considerations
34(a)	Discovery of electronically stored information (stands on equal footing with discovery of paper documents)	Provides that electronically stored documents are equally as discoverable as paper documents and are normally required to be produced unless the request clearly indicates the party is seeking only traditional documents.	HIM professionals working in organizations with both paper and electronic records need to be aware of this rule and ensure polices and procedures are in place to access and produce electronically stored health records in response to a legal request (including a legal hold, preservation order, and subpoena). HIM professionals should implement EHR management processes that include periodic review of existing policies and procedures and technical capabilities in support of the discovery process.
34(b)	Production of documents, forms in which documents are to be produced	Provides that a party must produce documents that are kept in the usual course of business or must organize and label them to correspond with the categories in the discovery request. The production of electronically stored information is subject to comparable requirements to protect against inadvertent or deliberate production that raise unnecessary obstacles for the requesting party.	HIM and IT professionals need to be aware of requesting parties' requirements relative to document production. HIM and IT will need to establish organizational policies and procedures for retention, storage, and production of data, including native file format and metadata maintenance. Information that is retained for business reasons must include a plan for how it will be disclosed (in a reasonable format). If information is not needed for business purposes it should not be retained.
37	Failure to make disclosures in discovery, sanctions	Describes if, why, and what sanctions an organization will be subject to if it fails to produce agreed-upon documents.	Organizations as well as HIM and IT professionals must be aware of Federal Rules of Civil Procedure regarding sanctions for inability to produce (absent good faith activities) electronically stored information.
37(f)	Sanctions and safe harbors for certain types of loss of electronically stored information	Provides that absent exceptional circumstances, a court may not impose sanctions for failure to provide electronically stored information lost as a result of the routine good faith operation of an electronic system. Good faith may require that a party impose a litigation hold, that it complies with agreements it reaches between parties on preservation, and that it complies with any court orders entered addressing preservation.	Organizations with the input of legal counsel and HIM and IT professionals must establish policies and procedures regarding retention and destruction of electronically stored information, including metadata. Additionally, HIM professionals need to be aware of new requirements that will be placed upon them such as legal holds and preservation obligations. Procedures will need to be established defining who will be the designated recipient of a legal hold notice and who is notified. The efficacy of the HIM program will be an issue for the judge to consider. The better the HIM systems, the better protection for the organization. Include e-Discovery in periodic compliance reviews and activities to ensure ongoing monitoring and evaluation.

Source: AHIMA e-HIM Work Group on e-Discovery 2006.

Chapter 5

Tort Law

Sebastian E. Proels, MD, JD

Learning Objectives

- Explain the various types of torts

- Discuss strict liability

- Discuss causes of action for improper disclosure of health information

- Discuss defamation, invasion of privacy, breach of confidentiality, and infliction of emotional distress and defenses thereto

- Discuss liability of the health information professional

- Contrast healthcare provider and health information professional immunity issues

- Discuss relevant statutes of limitation

- Discuss criminal liability in healthcare

- Articulate issues related to medical malpractice insurance, the existence of an insurance crisis, and tort reform measures

Key Terms

Act of God
Affidavit of merit
Affirmative defense
Assault
Assumption of risk
Battery
Breach of confidentiality
Charitable immunity
Civil law
Collateral source payments
Common law
Comparative negligence
Compensatory damages
Contingency fee

Contract law
Contributory negligence
Corporate negligence
Criminal law
Criminal negligence
Damages
Defamation
Defendant
Emotional distress
False imprisonment
Felony
Fiduciary duty
General damages
Gross negligence

Health Insurance Portability and Accountability Act of 1996 (HIPAA)
Infliction of emotional distress
Intentional torts
Invasion of privacy
Joint and several liability
Judge-made law
Jurisdiction
Liability
Libel
Malfeasance
Medical malpractice

Medical malpractice insurance	Punitive damages	Structured settlement
Misdemeanor	*Res ipsa loquitur*	Sudden emergency doctrine
Misfeasance	Rescue doctrine	Tolled
Negligence	*Respondeat superior*	Tort
No-fault insurance	Slander	Tort law
Noneconomic damages	Special damages	Tort reform
Nonfeasance	Standard of care	Tortfeasor
Ordinary negligence	Statute of limitations	Trier of fact
Plaintiff	Statute of repose	Unavoidable accident
	Strict liability	

Introduction

More than any other area of the law, the law of torts reflects our cultural and social views as to what is acceptable and unacceptable conduct. The word "tort" is derived from the Latin *tortes* or "twisted." Tortious conduct is conduct that is crooked or twisted.

In today's legal terminology, a **tort** is a civil wrong for which the law will provide a remedy in the form of a lawsuit to recover damages. **Damages** in the form of monetary compensation are awarded by a court to an individual in a civil action who has been injured by another party. The law of torts is constantly evolving and expanding. Conduct that was entirely acceptable decades or a century ago may now be totally unacceptable, giving rise to new causes of action. Examples include recovery of damages for discrimination, wrongful discharge from employment, strict product liability, or the negligent infliction of emotional harm. **Liability** in general means a legal obligation or responsibility (amount owed) that one party in the lawsuit may have to another party in the lawsuit.

The law of torts can be divided into three broad subgroups: a wrong involving the person or individual rights, a wrong involving the rights to personal property, and a wrong involving the rights to real property. Tort law is to be distinguished from **criminal law,** which refers to a type of law in which the government is a party to prosecuting an accused charged with violating a criminal statute or regulation (by committing either a **felony** or a **misdemeanor,** which is a less severe crime than a felony). The commission of a crime is an offense against society or the public at large. The government, usually the state representing the people, prosecutes the defendant for violating a criminal statute. The objective is to protect the public interest and to punish wrongdoers, hopefully deterring them from committing similar offenses in the future. A criminal prosecution generally does not involve any compensation to the injured victim of the crime. Rather, the victim is the chief witness on behalf of the state. In contrast, a **tort law** or proceeding involves the right of an individual, corporation, or other legal entity to recover damages for a loss caused by the defendant (**tortfeasor**). As discussed in chapter 2, the one who brings the suit is the **plaintiff,** and the wrongdoer is the **defendant.** The private individual or corporation pursues the action against the defendant in a civil suit. The remedy varies depending on the type and nature of the tort, but in general, a tort victim seeks monetary compensation. If the plaintiff is successful in his or her lawsuit, he or she is awarded a judgment at trial (or through a settlement between the parties) for an amount of money to be collected from the defendant.

Certain actions are both criminal and tortious. For example, theft of an individual's property is a crime against the state that may subject the defendant to criminal prosecution and imprisonment. The same wrongful act may give rise to a civil action for a conversion, entitling an individual to recover money damages against the individual who committed the criminal act. In a criminal proceeding, the state is responsible for prosecution of the case, and the objective of the suit is to punish the wrongdoer. In a civil action, the plaintiff is responsible for pursuing legal action, and the objective is to recover money damages to compensate for the loss.

As noted earlier, the development and evolution of tort law over the years has followed the path of social reform and the development of public policy. We as a society and a culture decide the types of conduct that are considered acceptable or unacceptable. Thus, the law of torts reflects society's current views on issues such as morality, fairness, and reasonableness.

Types of Torts

The US concept of torts originated in the **common law** of England. In the early days of English law, the right to recover damages for a wrongful act depended on whether the king was willing to issue a writ, a formal written order issued by one with administrative or judicial jurisdiction over the case. **Jurisdiction** refers to the legal authority an entity possesses to make a legal decision. A limited number or forms of writs were prescribed. Unless the plaintiff could identify a writ that applied to his or her situation, no remedy was available. In general, two writs were available for tortious conduct: trespass and trespass on the case.

An action for trespass generally involved a breach of peace. A defendant who committed a trespass was imprisoned or fined. The civil remedy was in the form of direct and intentional interference with a person's protected interest. The protected interest could be personal (such as bodily harm) or related to a property interest (such as harm to a person's possessions). Trespass on the case evolved from trespass and was directed toward remedying conduct that was not necessarily intentional or directed toward the plaintiff's interest.

The US legal system of today generally distinguishes between **intentional torts,** which involve a deliberate or intentional act, and unintentional acts or negligence, in which the defendant does not necessarily intend to cause harm but harm is a foreseeable consequence of the defendant's conduct. A third type of tort, strict liability, will also be discussed in this chapter.

Intentional Torts

Battery, assault, false imprisonment, and intentional infliction of emotional distress are all examples of intentional torts. A medical abandonment claim may also be brought as an intentional tort for the alleged wrongful termination of a provider-patient relationship, but depending on the circumstances, it may be negligence or a breach of contract (Showalter 2012). Abandonment is discussed in more detail in chapter 6 as a breach of contract. Other torts, which may also be intentional, are relevant to health information. They include defamation, invasion of privacy, breach of confidentiality, and infliction of emotional distress and will be discussed in the section about causes of action for improper disclosure of health information.

Battery

Battery is intentional and nonconsensual contact with the plaintiff. Whether touching rises to the level of bodily harm depends on the circumstances and whether the touching occurred in a context that society views as acceptable. For battery to occur, the defendant must have performed some positive or affirmative act that resulted in an impermissible contact with the plaintiff. The defendant may be liable not only for contact that physically harms the plaintiff but also for relatively minor contacts that are offensive or insulting. Thus, spitting in the plaintiff's face or forcibly removing his or her hat may constitute battery. The law does not require that the defendant intended a certain result, but merely that the defendant intended a "touching." A defendant may be liable for battery where he or she intended only a joke or even a compliment, as when a woman is kissed without her consent or the defendant makes a misguided effort to offer assistance. In the medical context, performing a procedure on a patient without the patient's consent (and presuming no exception allowing it, such as a medical emergency) could give rise to a cause of action for battery. Patient consent is detailed in chapter 7.

A certain amount of personal contact is inevitable in society and must be accepted. Thus, consent is implied and there is no tort where contact is customary and reasonably necessary, such as a tap on the shoulder to attract attention, a friendly grasp of the arm, or casual jostling among other people (Prosser 1971).

The time, place, and circumstances of an act determine whether the touching is impermissible. A person is not expected to tolerate actions by a stranger that would be allowed by an intimate friend. However, unless the defendant has special reason to believe that the plaintiff is more or less sensitive, the test is what would be offensive to an ordinary person who is reasonable about the type of personal contact generally encountered in society. The intent required is only that the defendant intended to make contact. Given that, liability will depend on whether there is a privilege or whether the plaintiff has otherwise consented (Prosser 1971). Privilege is a special relationship recognized by the law that permits certain conduct that would be prohibited under other circumstances. For example, a parent may be privileged to touch or restrain a child in a manner that a stranger would not.

In some circumstances, the intent to commit a battery on one person may be transferred to a third person. If the defendant intended to commit a battery on one person but caused an unintended harmful contact to a different person, the latter may be entitled to recover damages as if the defendant intended to affect him or her. In this case, the intent is transferred to the victim.

Assault

The intentional tort of **assault** involves conduct that causes apprehension of a harmful or offensive contact instead of actual contact. Thus, no actual contact is necessary for an assault. The interest of the plaintiff is protection against a mental disturbance of his or her personal integrity.

An act that is likely to bring about an apprehension or fear of battery may constitute an assault. Thus, shaking a fist under another's nose, taking aim with a weapon, or even holding a weapon in a threatening position may constitute an assault. In these examples, the harm is the plaintiff's mental apprehension that he or she may be the victim of a battery or other impermissible contact. The mere fact that the plaintiff is subjected to such apprehension is enough to give rise to a cause of action for an assault, even without actual contact.

Mere words may allow a plaintiff to recover for an assault. Hostile words that arouse apprehension in the plaintiff, such as threatening words or behaviors, may lead to the plaintiff's apprehension and a right to recover for assault.

False Imprisonment

False imprisonment is the intentional confinement of a person against that person's will. The elements of this intentional tort are:

- Confinement of a person against his or her will

- Absence of a reasonable means of escape

- No legal authority on the part of the person acting to confine another

A cause of action for false imprisonment may occur when an individual is hospitalized against his or her will, although legal exceptions exist regarding individuals in need of mental health treatment who pose harm to themselves or others, and individuals with certain contagious diseases. A familiarity with relevant state laws is necessary to appropriately address this type of situation.

Intentional Infliction of Emotional Distress

Intentional **infliction of emotional distress** is a common law tort for intentional conduct that results in extreme emotional distress. The elements are:

- An intentional or reckless act (the defendant does not have to intend that emotional distress will occur; acting with reckless disregard is sufficient to meet this element)

- Extreme and outrageous conduct that is beyond the standards of civilized decency or is utterly intolerable in a civilized society

- The act of the defendant must have actually caused the emotional distress

- The emotional distress suffered by the plaintiff must be "severe"

A cause of action for the intentional infliction of emotional distress may occur when an individual engages in extreme and outrageous conduct that is so egregious as to cause another person severe emotional injury. Examples may include defamation with serious emotional and psychological consequences.

Emotional distress may include manifestations such as sleeplessness, anxiety, irritability, or the emotional inability to perform activities or go places that the plaintiff was capable of prior to the event for which a lawsuit has been filed. To prove emotional distress, the plaintiff must demonstrate that he or she has suffered from one or more manifestations that have negatively impacted his or her life.

Potential defenses to intentional torts, depending on the specific tort alleged, are consent by the plaintiff and necessity, including self-defense or defense of others.

Check Your Understanding 5.1

Instructions: Indicate whether the following statements are true or false (T or F).

1. A tort is a civil wrong.

2. Battery is an intentional tort that involves nonconsensual contact with the plaintiff.

3. Assault is an intentional tort that involves nonconsensual contact with the plaintiff.

4. The law provides exceptions to false imprisonment liability where involuntarily hospitalized patients pose harm to themselves or others.

5. Intentional infliction of emotional distress is a tort that results in extreme emotional distress to the plaintiff.

Negligence

The second type of tort, unintentional, is negligence. It is the basis for most medical malpractice lawsuits. **Medical malpractice** is an alleged wrongful act committed by a healthcare provider against a patient. **Negligence** involves failure to act in a way that a reasonably prudent person would act under the same circumstances, thus causing harm or injury to another (57A Am. Jur. 2d Negligence 7 [2004]). *Restatement of the Law (Second), Torts* (1965) defines negligent conduct as "conduct which falls below the standard established for the protection of others against unreasonable risk of harm." The law recognizes that when one person commits negligence and injures another, the injured person is entitled to compensation for his or her injuries. As contrasted with intentional torts, negligence results from unintentional conduct.

A negligent tort may result from a person acting or failing to act as an ordinarily careful and prudent person would act under similar circumstances (57A Am. Jur. 2d Negligence 5 [2004]). Negligence is careless conduct outside the generally accepted standard of care (57A Am. Jur. 2d Negligence 5 [2004]). **Standard of care** is what an individual is expected to do or not do in a particular situation (57A Am. Jur. 2d Negligence 132 [2004]). Standards of care are established by statute or ordinance, judicial decision, professional associations, or practice (57A Am. Jur. 2d Negligence 135 [2004]).

The standard of care in the healthcare professions is the exercise of reasonable care by healthcare professionals with similar training and experience in the same or similar communities (see 61 Am. Jur. 2d Physicians, Surgeons, and Other Healers 188 et seq. [2002]). Some courts define standards of care on a national level as opposed to a community level. In *Strickland v. Pinder* (2006), the court stated that for an expert's testimony to establish a national standard of care, the testimony should be supported by a published standard, certification process, current literature, or conference or discussion with other knowledgeable professionals. Without such support, the court held that the expert's testimony was merely personal opinion, insufficient to prove the applicable standard of care. The standard of care on a national level would generally be expected to be stricter or more rigorous than a community standard in a small, isolated, or less technologically sophisticated community. Further, as technology has enabled healthcare providers in remote locations to access more sophisticated medical resources for their patients, the community standard has become disfavored and has been replaced by prevailing national standards.

Negligence may occur where an individual has evaluated alternatives and their consequences and has exercised his or her best possible judgment. Therefore, a person can be found negligent when he or she fails to protect against a risk that he or she knew could happen. Furthermore, negligence can occur where it is known, or should have been known, that a particular behavior would place others in unreasonable danger.

Types of Negligence

Negligence may occur in the form of:

- Malpractice: Misconduct of a professional person, including a physician, nurse, attorney, or accountant

- **Criminal negligence:** Reckless disregard for another individual's safety or, stated differently, willful indifference to a harm that could result from an act

Negligence can also be categorized in other ways. For example, negligent torts can be categorized as (see 57A Am. Jur. 2d Negligence 13 [2004]):

- **Nonfeasance**: Failure to perform an act (including protecting another from harm) that a person is under a duty to do and that a person of ordinary prudence would have done under the same or similar circumstances.

- **Misfeasance**: Improper performance of an act that a person might lawfully do, or active misconduct that causes injury to another. Misfeasance exists if the defendant is responsible for making the plaintiff's position worse; that is, the defendant has created a risk. Conversely, nonfeasance is found if the defendant has failed to aid the plaintiff through beneficial intervention.

- **Malfeasance**: Similar to nonfeasance and misfeasance but characterized by the additional element of intentional conduct in that such conduct is intended to cause damage.

Degrees of Negligence

Negligence can be categorized by the degree of wrongdoing. **Ordinary negligence,** which is the failure to exercise ordinary care, is "the failure to exercise such care as . . . mankind ordinarily exercises under the same or similar circumstances" (57A Am. Jur. 2d Negligence 226 [2004]). **Gross negligence** is very great or excessive negligence that implies an extreme departure from the ordinary standard of care and shows a reckless disregard for the rights of others.

Elements of Negligence

To recover damages caused by negligence, the plaintiff must demonstrate that all four of the following elements of negligence are present (57A Am. Jur. 2d Negligence 78–143 [2004]):

- The defendant owed the plaintiff a duty of care. In a medical malpractice action, the plaintiff must demonstrate that a physician-patient, nurse-patient, therapist-patient, or other healthcare provider–patient relationship existed at the time of the alleged wrongful act.

- The defendant breached that duty of care. The plaintiff must demonstrate that the defendant failed to exercise reasonable care under the given circumstances.

- The plaintiff suffered an injury as a consequence of the defendant's breach. Injury includes physical and mental suffering (and may include invasion of the plaintiff's rights and privacy), monetary damages, and other damages.

- There is a causal connection between the defendant's breach and the plaintiff's injury. There are two types of causation in the law: cause-in-fact (actual) and proximate (legal) cause. Cause-in-fact is determined by the "but-for" test: but for the action, the result would not have happened. For example, but for running the red light, the collision would not have occurred. Proximate cause is different from cause-in-fact. It is an event that is sufficiently related to a legally recognizable injury so as to be held as the cause of that injury. In other words, it is an act that results in injury through a natural, direct, uninterrupted consequence and without which the injury would not have occurred. Proximate cause entails an analysis of foreseeability (that is, was it foreseeable that the defendant's actions would result in the plaintiff's injury?).

In some circumstances, a statute, ordinance, or judicial decision may define the standard of care to which a defendant must conform (*Restatement of the Law* 1965, 285; 57A Am. Jur. 2d Negligence 135 [2004]). However, when none exists to define what is reasonable in a particular situation, the **trier of fact** (judge or jury responsible for deciding factual issues) must determine what a reasonably prudent person would have done if faced with the circumstances that faced the defendant. Generally, a reasonably prudent person is a hypothetical person that a community believes exhibits ideal behavior in a particular situation and can differ from one situation to another (*Restatement of the Law* 1965, 283). Considering the above, the trier of fact defines what the behavior of the reasonably prudent person would have consisted of under particular circumstances. The trier of fact then compares that definition with the defendant's behavior. Negligence has not occurred if the defendant's behavior meets or exceeds the reasonably prudent person standard. However, if the defendant's conduct does not meet the reasonably prudent person standard, negligence has occurred. In the latter case, the trier of fact is then called on to determine whether (57A Am. Jur. 2d Negligence 124 [2004]):

- The defendant's negligent conduct resulted in injury to the plaintiff

- The injury that resulted from the failure to satisfy the reasonably prudent person standard could have been foreseen

Damages

The subject of damages in tort law is a continually evolving area of the law. A tort plaintiff may be entitled to several types of damages. Damages are intended to compensate a plaintiff for physical and monetary injuries. The principal types of damages can be divided into two broad categories: compensatory damages and punitive damages. **Compensatory damages** are further divided into general (noneconomic) and special (economic) damages. **General damages** naturally and necessarily flow from a tort and directly result from the tort. For example, pain and suffering are considered part of general damages. In contrast, **special damages** arrive out of the special character, condition, or circumstances of the event or person injured. Medical treatment costs and lost wages are the main types of special damages ordinarily at issue in a personal injury tort claim. **Punitive damages**, in contrast, are intended to punish and deter certain types of conduct, including tortious conduct. Punitive damages may not be awarded without a simultaneous award of compensatory damages.

Check Your Understanding 5.2

Instructions: Indicate whether the following statements are true or false (T or F).

1. Negligence is the second most common basis for medical malpractice lawsuits, following intentional torts.

2. The standard of care is what an individual is expected to do or not do in a particular situation.

3. Misfeasance is the failure to act per one's duty and according to ordinary prudence.

4. The two types of causation are actual and proximate.

5. Punitive damages punish the wrongdoer for tortious conduct that was committed.

Res ipsa loquitur

Generally, negligence is not inferred or presumed from an injury. The plaintiff usually has the burden of proof and must prove all elements of his or her case. The exception to this rule is the doctrine of *res ipsa loquitur* (the thing speaks for itself), where the facts or circumstances accompanying an injury may raise a presumption, or at least permit an inference, of negligence on the part of the defendant charged with negligence (57B Am. Jur. 2d Negligence 1163 [2004]). The defendant thus has the burden of proof to show that he or she was not negligent. This doctrine "derives from the understanding that some events ordinarily do not occur in the absence of negligence" (57B Am. Jur. 2d Negligence 1163 [2004]). A classic example of *res ipsa* application is in instances where a surgical team leaves surgical instruments in a patient's body after surgery, resulting in injury. Such events do not "ordinarily occur in the absence of negligence."

The three elements of the *res ipsa loquitur* doctrine are (57B Am. Jur. 2d Negligence 1164 [2004]):

- Injury of a kind that ordinarily does not occur in the absence of someone's negligence

- Injury caused by an agency or instrumentality within the exclusive control of the defendant

- Injury not due to any voluntary action or contribution on the part of the plaintiff

For example, in *Hake v. George Wiedemann Brewing Co.* (1970), the doctrine of *res ipsa loquitur* was applicable where a beer keg exclusively handled and controlled by the defendant rolled off an exterior second-story stairway platform, striking and injuring the plaintiff, who was walking underneath.

The doctrine may be applied in suits against hospitals to recover for injuries sustained by patients while receiving treatment or care in the hospital. However, courts have held that it is inapplicable when the patient's condition might be due to some other cause than the alleged injury or accident on the hospital premises, or when the evidence is insufficient to show that the injury complained of was caused by the instrumentality alleged. For example:

- In *Reese v. Bd. of Directors of Memorial Hosp. of Laramie Co.* (1998), a patient who alleged that she suffered a herniated disk because hospital employees failed to properly support her head and neck during oral surgery could not recover from the hospital on a *res ipsa loquitur* theory. While the plaintiff identified several acts by hospital employees that allegedly constituted negligence, the evidence permitted a reasonable inference that her injury could have stemmed from other causes, including turning wrong or sneezing.

- In *Hospital Authority of City of St. Marys v. Eason* (1966), the court did not apply the doctrine where a partially paralyzed hospital patient sustained injuries when his hospital bed caught fire after the patient's pipe was lit. The doctrine was inapplicable where the evidence failed to establish a presumption of negligence by the hospital according to the elements of *res ipsa loquitur.*

Several courts have warned that the *res ipsa loquitur* doctrine should be applied with caution and only under limited circumstances. In *Williams v. American Medical Systems* (2001), the plaintiff sued the manufacturer of a medical device implanted by the plaintiff's doctor. The court held that the *res ipsa loquitur* doctrine was not applicable where there was an intermediary cause that produced or could have produced the injury. Since the device was implanted by the plaintiff's doctor, it failed the *res ipsa loquitur* doctrine test because the device left the exclusive control of the manufacturer (defendant). The value of a *res ipsa loquitur* jury instruction to a plaintiff is that it permits the jury to infer negligence on an issue where the plaintiff may not have actual, discrete evidence or proof of negligence. Thus, mere control of an instrumentality permits an inference of negligence even though actual proof of negligence is lacking. Without the instruction, in certain circumstances it might be exceedingly difficult or impossible for a plaintiff to prove negligence.

Defenses to Negligence Claims

Defendants may raise a number of affirmative defenses in response to plaintiffs' negligence claims (Ernst 2007, 86). **Affirmative defenses** are those for which the defendant bears the burden of proving he or she is entitled to rely on them. Affirmative defenses to negligence claims are discussed below.

Contributory Negligence

The doctrine of **contributory negligence** bars a plaintiff from recovering damages from the defendant if the defendant is able to prove that the plaintiff's conduct contributed in part to the injury that the plaintiff suffered. "The gist of the doctrine of contributory negligence is that the person injured should not recover when it appears that the injury would have been avoided if the injured person had exercised reasonable care" (57B Am. Jur. 2d Negligence 798 [2004]). Contributory negligence has long been criticized because even if the defendant is 99 percent to blame for the plaintiff's injury and the plaintiff is only 1 percent to blame for his or her injury, the defendant would still be relieved from having to pay damages to the plaintiff. As a result, most states do not recognize this doctrine as an affirmative defense.

Comparative Negligence

Under the **comparative negligence** doctrine, a defendant demonstrates that the plaintiff's conduct contributed in part to the injury the plaintiff suffered. Unlike the doctrine of contributory negligence, in which the negligent plaintiff is completely barred from recovering damages, the doctrine of comparative negligence merely causes the plaintiff's recovery to be reduced by some amount based on his or her percentage of negligence. Using the example above, if the defendant is liable for 99 percent of the injury and the plaintiff is liable for 1 percent, the defendant must pay 99 percent of the damage award. This works from 51 percent on up in most jurisdictions, meaning that if the defendant is less than 50 percent negligent, the defendant pays nothing.

Comparative negligence can be further divided into pure and partial/modified types. Pure comparative negligence permits a plaintiff who is 90 percent to blame for an accident to recover 10 percent of his or her losses. Partial/modified comparative negligence allows a plaintiff to recover only if the plaintiff's negligence is "not greater than" or "not as great as" the defendant's negligence. For example, the plaintiff must be 50 percent or less at fault.

Assumption of Risk

Assumption of risk is an affirmative defense that bars a plaintiff from recovering on his or her negligence claim if the defendant proves that the plaintiff (57B Am. Jur. 2d Negligence 759 [2004]):

- Had actual knowledge of a danger

- Understood and appreciated the risks associated with the danger

- Voluntarily exposed himself or herself to those risks

In the medical context (for example, in defending a medical malpractice claim), a defendant would be more likely to rely on contributory or comparative negligence principles (such as a plaintiff's failure to follow up as ordered or failure to follow other important medical advice) than on assumption of risk. This is because the assumption of risk defense usually contemplates a voluntary exposure by way of an affirmative act. True voluntariness is generally lacking in a patient who seeks medical care, as opposed to an individual who chooses an activity such as skiing or snowboarding. In the latter examples, a defendant who is sued following a skiing or snowboarding accident may be able to demonstrate the plaintiff's voluntary exposure.

Rescue Doctrine

Some jurisdictions have adopted the rescue doctrine as a bar to the affirmative defenses of contributory negligence and assumption of risk. As the Alabama Supreme Court stated, "Neither contributory negligence nor assumption of risk is charged to him who comes to the rescue of others in peril without their fault, unless the act of the rescuer is manifestly rash and reckless to a man of ordinary prudence acting in emergency. In other words, unless the rescuer's own conduct in attempting the rescue is wanton, then the rescuer may recover from the negligent defendant" (*Dillard v. Pittway Corp.*, 1998; in which the court held that the plaintiff could sue the manufacturer of a smoke detector on the basis of harm the plaintiff suffered while attempting to rescue a family member from a burning house).

The **rescue doctrine** states that if a tortfeasor creates a circumstance that places a victim in danger, the tortfeasor is liable for the harm caused not only to the victim but also to any person injured in an effort to rescue the victim. This principle was demonstrated in *Wagner v. Int'l Railway* (1921), in which a railway company was held liable for injuries sustained by a rescuer who had fallen from a beam while searching for the body of his cousin, who had fallen from the train they were riding. The railway company argued unsuccessfully that it was not liable since the rescuer, while walking far out onto a beam, had time to consider the risk, thus breaking the sequence of the rescue. In a later case involving the rescue doctrine, Justice Cardozo wrote (*Lehman v. Haynam*, 1956):

> Danger invites rescue. . . . The wrongdoer may not have foreseen the coming of a deliverer. He is accountable as if he had. In contrast, the sudden (medical) emergency defense was established by the Supreme Court of Ohio in a 1956 case. The court said, "Where the driver of an automobile is suddenly stricken by a period of unconsciousness which he had no reason to anticipate and which renders it impossible for him to control the car he is driving, he is not chargeable with negligence as to such lack of control."

Sudden Emergency

According to *Herr v. Wheeler* (2006):

> The **sudden emergency doctrine** relieves a person of liability if, without prior negligence on his part, that person is confronted with a sudden emergency and acts as an ordinarily prudent person would act under the circumstances. (internal citations omitted)

Unavoidable Accident

Some jurisdictions recognize the "unavoidable accident" affirmative defense. An **unavoidable accident** is defined as an occurrence that could not have been foreseen or anticipated in the exercise of ordinary care and that results without the fault or negligence of either the defendant or the plaintiff. In *Uncapher v. Baltimore & O.R. Co.* (1933), the plaintiff sought damages against a railroad company for injuries resulting from a collision between the plaintiff's vehicle and the defendant's train. The court held that the plaintiff was unable to use unavoidable accident as an affirmative defense in a suit for damages against the railway company since the plaintiff admitted negligence when he failed to look both ways before crossing the railroad tracks.

Act of God

The term **Act of God** means "any irresistible disaster, such as earthquakes, unprecedented floods or the like, that is not human related. It may not be a reasonably foreseeable event. If the proper care and diligence on the part of a tortfeasor would have avoided the act, the act is not excusable" (Ernst 2007, 88). In an action where the defendant was held not liable for a car accident caused by fog, the court stated, ". . . if an 'Act of God' is so unusual and overwhelming as to do damage by its own power, without reference to and independently of any negligence by defendant, there is no liability" (*Smith v. McVicker*, 2004, citing *Andrews v. Ohio Dept. of Transp.*, 2002).

Theories of Hospital Negligence Liability

Hospitals have seen a growing exposure to negligence liability as they have assumed greater responsibility for monitoring the quality of care provided to patients and the medical staff who provide that care. Although hospitals were historically shielded from liability under the doctrine of **charitable immunity** due to their role as charitable organizations, this protection was gradually eliminated through state legislation and case law. *Darling v. Charleston Community Memorial Hospital* (1965), described in more detail in chapter 14, is a landmark case credited with significantly eroding charitable immunity protection. The courts have used two doctrines to establish liability: corporate negligence and *respondeat superior*.

Corporate Negligence (Primary Liability)

A hospital may be held primarily liable (that is, liable in its own right) under the **corporate negligence** doctrine. Under this doctrine, the hospital holds itself out as a provider of healthcare services and, therefore, also holds itself out as an entity subject to a lawsuit in an event of negligence.

Under the corporate negligence doctrine, a hospital owes its patients the following duties (see 40A Am. Jur. 2d Hospitals and Asylums 26 [2008]):

- The duty to use reasonable care to maintain safe and adequate facilities and equipment

- The duty to select and retain competent medical professionals

- The duty to oversee all persons who practice medicine within the hospital

- The duty to formulate, adopt, and enforce rules and policies that ensure quality care for all patients

As in any negligence action, a plaintiff seeking to establish liability under the corporate negligence doctrine must prove the following (40A Am. Jur. 2d Hospitals and Asylums 26 [2008]):

- The hospital deviated from the standard of care

- The hospital had actual or constructive notice of the defects or procedures that created the harm

- The hospital's act or omission was a substantial factor in bringing about the harm

Respondeat Superior (Secondary Liability) or Vicarious Liability

Generally, a hospital is liable to patients for the torts of its employees (including nurses and employed physicians) under the doctrine of ***respondeat superior*** (Latin for "let the master answer"), also referred to as vicarious liability. Under this doctrine the hospital holds itself out as responsible for the actions of its employees provided that these individuals were acting within the scope of their employment or within the hospital's direction at the time they conducted the tortious activity in question (40A Am. Jur. 2d Hospitals and Asylums 39 [2008]).

In the healthcare context, the legal status between physicians and the hospitals in which they practice must be considered. Most commonly, physicians are granted privileges to practice in a hospital. Such privileges make physicians independent contractors of the hospital rather than employees. A hospital is not held liable for the negligence of a physician with the status of independent contractor when the hospital (1) does not control the method or manner of the services the physician provides and (2) provides meaningful notice of an independent contractor status to the patient, acknowledged at the time of admission. A hospital is, however, liable for the torts of independent contractors in the following situations (see 40A Am. Jur. 2d Hospitals and Asylums 40, 41 [2008]):

- When the hospital contracts to provide medical services to a patient and has those services provided by an independent contractor

- When the hospital had reason to know that negligence would occur

- When the hospital holds out to the patient or the general public that the physicians associated with it are its employees, even if they are not. In this situation, liability would be premised on the legal doctrines of ostensible agency, apparent authority, or agency by estoppel

Some jurisdictions have enacted statutes that specifically provide that hospitals will not be held liable for negligent acts of healthcare professionals who are not agents or employees of the hospital. In *Fletcher v. South Peninsula Hosp.* (2003), the Alaska Supreme Court affirmed that a hospital was not liable for the negligent acts of an independent contractor surgeon since the plaintiffs went to see a specific doctor for care and the hospital repeatedly provided the plaintiffs with a disclaimer that stated that the surgeon was an independent contractor and not an employee or agent of the hospital. In *Lemuz By and Through Lemuz v. Fieser* (1997), the plaintiffs unsuccessfully challenged a Kansas statute that prohibited plaintiffs' independent liability/corporate negligence action against a hospital since the doctor at fault was not an employee or agent of the hospital.

Check Your Understanding 5.3

Instructions: Indicate whether the following statements are true or false (T or F).

1. Per the doctrine of *res ipsa loquitur*, an inference or presumption of the defendant's negligence is permitted.

2. Contributory negligence completely bars recovery by a plaintiff whose conduct contributed to the plaintiff's injury.

3. Assumption of risk is a viable defense by physicians in most medical malpractice cases.

4. Per the theory of corporate negligence, a hospital is liable for the torts of its employees.

5. Per the theory of *respondeat superior*, a hospital is liable in its own right to the patients it serves.

Strict Liability

Until the nineteenth century, an individual whose actions resulted in harm to another individual was, in most cases, held responsible for the harm simply because he or she had acted (74 Am. Jur. 2d Torts 12 [2001]). Under this theory of *strict* **liability** (liability without fault) a person is responsible for the damage and loss caused by his or her acts and omissions regardless of fault. In more recent times, liability without fault has become limited. Examples of strict liability may be found in cases where abnormally dangerous activities are carried on (such as the storage of explosives or the conducting of blasting operations) and in cases involving injuries caused by wild animals (see 74 Am. Jur. 2d Torts 13 [2001]; 31A Am. Jur. 2d Explosions and Explosives 94, 143 [2002]; 4 Am. Jur. 2d Animals 85 [2007]). In the former example, if a person were injured by an explosion in an explosives storage facility, regardless of whether there was fault by the defendant, the law would hold the facility strictly liable for injuries to persons because the storage of explosives is inherently an extremely hazardous activity.

According to 74 Am. Jur. 2d Torts 13 (2001), "The most common application of the doctrine of strict or absolute liability in tort has been in products liability cases." To prevail on a product's liability claim, the plaintiff need only prove an injury resulted while using the product in the proper manner. The plaintiff does not need to show that the defendant manufacturer, seller, or supplier acted negligently. To recover under the strict products liability theory, the plaintiff need only prove that the following four elements of strict liability exist (see 63 Am. Jur. 2d Products Liability 559 [1997]):

- The plaintiff sustained damages.

- The defendant was engaged in the business of manufacturing, assembling, selling, leasing, or distributing the product in question.

- The product was supplied by the defendant in a defective condition that rendered it unreasonably dangerous.

- The defective condition proximately caused the plaintiff's damages. A plaintiff must prove that a defective condition existed but need not prove that the defective condition occurred as a result of negligence. Thus, a plaintiff can establish a strict liability case simply by proving the existence of a defective condition without having to establish that the condition was caused by a negligent act.

Causes of Action for Improper Disclosure of Health Information

Civil causes of action encountered in healthcare settings are generally based either on negligence or on intentional torts (including previously discussed causes of action such as battery, assault, infliction of emotional distress, and false imprisonment). This section discusses causes of action that relate specifically to the improper disclosure of health information.

Basis for Liability

Conduct relating to improper disclosure of health information may lead to liability. In civil actions, it is necessary to distinguish negligence from intentional tort theory. As discussed previously, four elements must be present in a negligence action: duty, breach of duty, injury, and a causal relationship between the breach and the injury (figure 5.1).

The first element, duty, requires that a person conform to some identified standard of care. "The word 'duty' is used throughout the *Restatement* to denote the fact that the actor is required to conduct himself in a particular manner at the risk that if he does not do so he becomes subject to liability to

Figure 5.1.   The four necessary elements in a negligence action

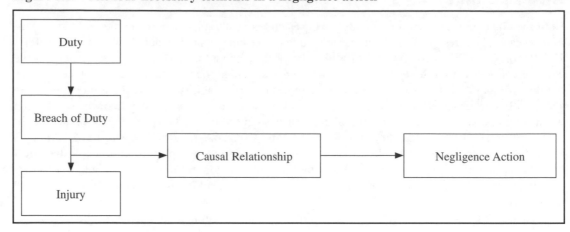

another to whom the duty is owed for any injury sustained by the other, of which that actor's conduct is a legal cause" (*Restatement of the Law* 1965, 4).

The second element, breach of duty, connotes a deviation from or breach of an applicable standard of care. The third element, injury, must be established to show that a person was harmed or injured. "The word 'injury' is used throughout the *Restatement* to denote the fact there has been an invasion of a legally protected interest. . . . It differs from the word 'harm' in this: 'harm' implies the existence of loss or detriment in fact, which may not necessarily be the invasion of a legally protected interest" (*Restatement of the Law* 1965, 7).

The fourth element, causation, must be established to show that a particular breach of duty caused the injury. It is worth emphasizing that, in addition to cause-in-fact causation, no lawsuit can succeed without proving the critical element of proximate cause. Proximate cause is defined as (1) a cause that is legally sufficient to result in liability; an act or omission that is considered in law to result in a consequence so that liability can be imposed on the actor; (2) a cause that directly produces an event and without which the event would not have occurred (Garner 2004). Thus, it is possible for someone to breach a duty but for that breach not to be the proximate cause of an injury. For example, a physician may have breached a standard of care but not proximately caused an injury. Under such circumstances, the breach and injury are coincidental and not sufficiently connected to result in legal liability. Without establishing the critical element of causation, no liability in tort may attach.

On the other hand, intentional tort law does not involve questions of negligence and what someone should have or should not have done. Intentional tort, as the name implies, is a separate and generally more serious cause of action that focuses on deliberate and unlawful conduct between parties that results in harm. The key feature of an intentional tort is the element of intent, which denotes "that the actor desires to cause consequences of his act, or that he believes that the consequences are substantially certain to result from it" (*Restatement of the Law* 1965, 8A). Intentional infliction of emotional distress and tortious interference with business relations are classic examples of intentional torts. Interestingly, tortious interference with business relations blurs the distinction between tort law and contract law. (Contract law will be discussed later in this chapter.) The most serious consequence for improper disclosure of health information is criminal liability, which is generally defined statutorily.

This section focuses on the more common causes of action that may be brought in connection with an improper disclosure of health information, including defamation (libel and slander), invasion of privacy, breach of confidentiality, and infliction of emotional distress.

Defamation

Defamation of character is a false communication about a person to someone else that harms the first person's reputation. The false communication may be either oral or written. If oral, the defamation is called **slander**; if written, it is called **libel.** To prove a cause of action for defamation, the plaintiff must show the following:

- The defendant made a false and defamatory statement about the plaintiff.

- The statement was not a privileged publication (that is, made appropriately and in good faith to persons with a legitimate reason to know) and was made to a third person.

- The conduct was an act of negligence or contained a higher degree of intent.

- Actual or presumed damages resulted.

Proof of special damages (such as economic losses) may be required to recover damages in a defamation case. Under certain circumstances, a plaintiff is not required to show proof of actual harm to his or her reputation, including when the defendant allegedly performs one of the following acts: accuses the plaintiff of a crime, accuses the plaintiff of carrying a loathsome disease, uses words that affect the plaintiff's professional or business activities, or calls a woman unchaste (Pozgar 2011). These types of attacks are inherently presumed to be damaging to a person's reputation, although an exception is granted to protect healthcare professionals against libel claims if they communicated information regarding loathsome diseases in compliance with laws requiring the reporting of communicable diseases.

There are two principal defenses available to defendants accused of defamation. First, a person accused of defamation is not liable if the statement made is true. That is, truth is a defense. Second, a defendant may use the defense of privilege. If the communication was made in good faith at an appropriate time and in an appropriate manner to persons who have a legitimate reason for receiving the communication (such as judicial proceedings or public safety), the defendant is not liable. The defense of privilege is grounded in the law's recognition that certain privileged communications take priority over statements that may allegedly be defamatory. In addition to the two principal defenses, authorization for the disclosure of information and lack of publication to a third party are also viable defenses.

Invasion of Privacy

A person's right to privacy is "the right to be left alone—the right to be free from unwarranted publicity and exposure to public view, as well as the right to live one's life without having one's name, picture, or private affairs made public against one's will" (Pozgar 2011). Under *Restatement of the Law, Torts* (1965, 652A), a person who invades the right of privacy of another is subject to liability for the resulting harm to the interests of the other. The right to privacy also includes the right to control personal information (Pozgar 2011).

To establish a claim for **invasion of privacy,** a plaintiff must establish the following elements:

- A duty to not invade the privacy of or disclose confidential medical information of a patient

- Breach of that duty

- Damages from the breach

While courts recognize that absolute privacy cannot be a practical reality in the healthcare setting, courts hold healthcare providers and personnel liable for negligent invasion of a patient's right of privacy. Courts are particularly sensitized to this right in instances where hospitalized patients cannot adequately protect their rights due to illness, altered states of mind, unconsciousness, or immobility.

In the healthcare setting, invasion of privacy can include disclosure of health information; the taking of photographs for medical, research, proprietary, or other purposes; and the presence of witnesses (for example, students) to a medical treatment or procedure. According to one author commenting on the invasion of privacy theory, "Most of the cases have alleged that the invasion consisted of publicizing a matter concerning the private life of another if the matter publicized is of a kind that would be highly offensive to a reasonable person and is not of legitimate concern to the public" (Moses 2000, 7; citing *Restatement of the Law* 1965, 652A, 652D).

Defenses to invasion of privacy claims include the patient's authorization or consent to the disclosure or other action that was taken; privilege, where legitimate interests are served by the disclosure or other action; and waiver, where the patient made public or otherwise placed his or her medical condition at issue.

Breach of Confidentiality (Fiduciary Duty)

A **fiduciary duty** is an obligation to act in the best interests of another party and is based on a special relationship of trust, confidence, and responsibility in certain obligations. Courts in various jurisdictions have concluded that a physician has a fiduciary duty to the patient to not disclose the patient's health and medical information. A patient may recover damages for violation of the fiduciary duty (Moses 2000, 526). To establish a claim for **breach of confidentiality,** a plaintiff must establish the following elements:

- Existence of a duty to not disclose health information

- A breach of the duty

- Damages

Breach of confidentiality and invasion of privacy have obvious similarities but are grounded in different principles. Invasion of privacy is grounded in principles of protecting privacy, whereas breach of confidentiality focuses on the special relationship—fiduciary in nature—between patients and healthcare providers.

Several cases have explored tortious conduct under the breach of confidentiality theory. For instance, in *Biddle v. Warren General Hospital* (1999), the Ohio Supreme Court held that "an independent tort exists for the unauthorized, unprivileged disclosure to a third party of nonpublic medical information that a physician or hospital has learned within a physician-patient relationship." In *Biddle*, a number of patients sued Warren General Hospital on learning that the hospital had entered an agreement with a law firm to screen patient intake forms to determine and pursue eligibility for Social Security reimbursements of medical expenses. Similarly, the Virginia Supreme Court in *Fairfax Hospital v. Curtis* (1997) concluded that a healthcare provider owes a duty of reasonable care to the patient to protect and preserve the confidentiality of patient information communicated to the provider in the course of treatment. A breach of that duty was held to be a tort. See also *Hammonds v. Aetna Casualty & Surety Co.* (1965), in which the court held that a physician has a fiduciary duty to the patient not to disclose the patient's medical information and that the patient may recover damages for violation of the fiduciary duty.

Whether particular conduct constitutes a breach of the duty to preserve confidential patient information depends on the specific facts of the disclosure. For instance, in *Estate of Berhinger v. Medical Center at Princeton* (1991), a New Jersey court held a hospital liable for failing to protect confidential information about one of its surgeons who was a patient at the hospital and happened to be HIV positive. Troubling facts in the case were that the medical records could be easily accessed and that no policy existed to limit access or prevent improper disclosures (see also *Martin v. Baehler*, 1993; breach of duty for failure to take reasonable precautions to safeguard records). In *Anderson v. Strong Memorial Hospital* (1988), a New York court recognized breach of fiduciary duty as a valid claim in a case where an identifiable picture of the silhouette of the plaintiff was published in connection with an article about an AIDS diagnosis.

Whether a particular action rises to the level of a breach of the fiduciary duty must be determined on a case-by-case basis. Courts will generally hold that even where a duty of nondisclosure exists, "confidentiality must yield to disclosure in the face of a countervailing public interest such as where the patient is a danger to himself or others" (where the welfare of minor children is involved) (Moses 2007; citing *Ace v. State of New York*, 1990; citing *Rea v. Pardo*, 1987).

Defenses to breach of confidentiality claims include the patient's authorization or consent to the disclosure; privilege, where legitimate interests are served by the disclosure; and waiver, where the patient made public or otherwise placed his or her medical condition at issue.

Infliction of Emotional Distress

Causes of action for the negligent or intentional infliction of emotional distress may be brought when a person whose medical information has been improperly disclosed can establish that the improper disclosure caused emotional harm or injury under applicable tort law. To recover under these causes of action, the injured person must establish that in making a nonprivileged disclosure, the defendant negligently, recklessly, or intentionally engaged in "extreme and outrageous conduct" that caused severe emotional distress (*Restatement of the Law* 1965, 46). (See also *Johnson PPA v. Atlantic Health Services*, 2000, in which the court granted a motion to strike a count of complaint alleging intentional infliction of emotional distress due to failure to establish outrageous conduct in connection with claimed improper disclosure of medical information; *Sanders v. Specter*, 1996).

Negligent infliction of emotional distress is generally considered to be a subcategory of negligence, which is recognized in some jurisdictions (Moses 2000, 529). Under *Restatement of the Law, Torts* (1965), a person who unintentionally causes emotional distress to another person is liable for causing injury to the other person if he:

- Should have realized that his conduct involved an unreasonable risk of causing the distress [and]

- From the facts known, should have realized that the distress might result in illness or bodily harm (*Restatement of the Law* 1965, 313; Moses 2000, 529)

A person whose medical information has been improperly disclosed may also be able to allege that the disclosure amounted to an intentional infliction of emotional distress. To recover, a plaintiff must show that, in making the disclosure, the defendant intentionally or recklessly engaged in "extreme and outrageous conduct" that caused severe emotional distress (*Restatement of the Law* 1965, 46; *Johnson PPA v. Atlantic Health Services, P.C.*, 2000).

An authorization from a patient that permits the disclosure of that individual's medical information may protect a defendant from liability in a claim for infliction of emotional distress.

Negligence for Improper Disclosure

Improper disclosure of an individual's health records may in some states be analyzed through a simple negligence inquiry, which was described earlier in this chapter under "Types of Torts." The elements of a cause of action for negligence are (*Restatement of the Law* 1965, 281, 282; Moses 2000, 530):

- The existence of a duty (protecting against unintentional invasion)

- Breach of duty (conduct falling below a standard of care for protecting against unreasonable risk of harm)

- Harm or injury

- Breach of a duty must be a legal and proximate cause of the harm or injury

In some states, malpractice statutes may support lawsuits that relate to improper disclosure of personal health information (Moses 2000, 530; citing *Berger v. Sonneland*, 2000). In *Berger*, the court recognized the validity of a malpractice claim that alleged unauthorized disclosure of confidential health information.

Liability of the Individuals Responsible for Protecting Health Information

The **Health Insurance Portability and Accountability Act of 1996 (HIPAA)** and state and federal privacy laws also impose liability for the improper use or disclosure of health information. Under HIPAA, civil and criminal liability may result from the improper use or disclosure of health information and for violating other HIPAA provisions. As revised under the Health Information Technology for Economic and Clinical Health Act (HITECH), the minimum civil monetary penalty for a HIPAA violation is $100 per violation, with a $1.5 million fine per calendar year for identical violations (AHIMA 2013). A discussion of criminal violations of HIPAA occurs later in this chapter. Chapter 9, "The HIPAA Privacy Rule," and chapter 10, "The HIPAA Security Rule," discuss HIPAA in greater detail. On the other hand, damages for tort claims discussed above are generally not controlled by statute. Instead, they are litigated under common law principles before a jury.

Individuals responsible for protecting health information should explore the need for professional liability insurance because they, in addition to their organization, may be named individually as defendants for the wrongful disclosure of patient information on the basis of one or more of the theories discussed in this chapter.

Immunity from Liability

In addition to the various tort defenses previously described, immunity is a defense to tort liability that is extended to a particular group of persons or entities. There are two important aspects of an immunity defense. First, the defense of immunity does not deny the existence of the alleged tort but merely denies any resulting liability. Second, immunity extends to only a limited group of people or entities. Immunity occurs because of the status or position of the defendant, not because of the facts of the case. The decision to extend immunity to a particular group of persons or entities is based on public policy. Therefore, others outside the group who engage in substantially similar conduct may be held liable for a tort.

Historically, immunity barred tort actions against governments, public officers, and charities and also barred litigation between spouses as well as parents and children. Today, the most important of these immunities is the immunity granted to governmental entities. Many of the other grounds for immunity have been eliminated. For example, immunity of charitable organizations as well as immunity between spouses no longer exists in most, if not all, states.

Governmental immunity, which is also referred to as sovereign immunity, originated from the common law idea that "the King can do no wrong." Certainly, under modern standards, this is flawed. Nevertheless, this defense continued as both the federal government and individual state governments were held to have immunity, absent consent, from tort liability. Additionally, the Eleventh Amendment to the United States Constitution prohibits a person or entity from suing a state in federal court.

Over time, courts and legislatures have adopted certain exceptions to governmental immunity. For example, in 1946 Congress adopted the Federal Tort Claims Act, which generally permits tort claims against the federal government for its negligence. However, the act does not extend governmental liability to intentional torts. Additionally, immunity exists where the government acts with due care in carrying out a statute or regulation and for acts or omissions within the discretionary function of a federal agency or employee.

All states now consent to lawsuits under certain circumstances, and most states have statutes that govern the tort liability of state and local governmental entities and employees. These statutes typically establish a general governmental immunity but provide for certain exceptions for particular types of activities. Some examples of exceptions include acts or omissions where the governmental agency is acting in a proprietary or private capacity and acts or omissions outside the scope of a governmental employee's job duties.

Another type of immunity from liability is related to state Good Samaritan statutes that provide legal immunity for ordinary negligence committed by persons who assist others in medical emergencies. The purpose of these statutes is to encourage individuals to provide good-faith emergency assistance, without fear of liability, in settings where lifesaving technology is not available. Such statutes vary from state to state, with some granting immunity only to specified healthcare professionals and others granting immunity to "any person." Because Good Samaritan laws eliminate otherwise applicable common law rights of victims to secure redress for their injuries, these statutes raise a number of constitutional questions.

Check Your Understanding 5.4

Instructions: Indicate whether the following statements are true or false (T or F).

1. The doctrine of strict liability is most common in product liability cases.

2. Libel is written defamation.

3. Fiduciary duty is the obligation to act in the best interests of another party.

4. To successfully claim breach of confidentiality, a plaintiff must establish that the defendant had a duty not to disclose the information.

5. Good Samaritan statutes encourage good-faith emergency assistance by providing immunity if ordinary negligence is committed by those who assist in medical emergencies.

Statutes of Limitations

As its name implies, a **statute of limitations** is a statutory enactment that places time limits on certain claims. For example, if a person is injured by the negligence of another, a statute of limitations will require an action to be brought against that person within a certain time period. The purpose of a statute of limitations is, first, to allow an injured person a reasonable amount of time in which to bring an action for recovery, and second, to allow claims to be resolved while evidence is reasonably available and fresh. As the US Supreme Court in *Order of Railroad Telegraphers v. Railway Express Agency* (1944) explained, a statute of limitations is "designed to promote justice by preventing surprises through the revival of claims that have been allowed to slumber until evidence has been lost, memories have faded, and witnesses have disappeared."

Generally, there are three steps involved in an application of a statute of limitations. First, one must identify the appropriate statutory period of limitations. Next, one must determine when that particular statutory period commenced or began to run. Finally, one must determine whether some condition or event suspended or postponed the operation of the statute of limitations.

Unlike the defense of immunity, a statute of limitations defense often varies depending on the type of tort claim asserted. For instance, intentional tort claims are usually subject to a different statutory limitations period than negligence claims. Additionally, although medical malpractice may be viewed as a form of negligence, many states have adopted special limitations periods for medical malpractice claims. Also, when a statute creates a cause of action, such as with claims for wrongful death, that particular statute will often contain its own limitations period.

The statutory period varies depending on the type of tort claim and from state to state. Each state has created a comprehensive set of legislatively imposed periods of limitation related to torts. Thus, a malpractice claim arising in Ohio may have a different period of limitations than a similar malpractice claim arising in Florida.

Finally, although a particular statute of limitations provides a certain time frame in which to bring an action, in some situations the parties involved may have contractually agreed on a different period of limitations. Unless such a contractual period is specifically disallowed by statute or public policy or is otherwise unreasonable, courts will usually enforce the agreement. For example, in *Thompson v. Ulysses Cruises, Inc.* (1993), a passenger on a cruise ship was injured when she slipped and fell. The court enforced a one-year limitations period contained on the five-page ticket that the passenger received.

Once the appropriate statute of limitations has been identified, one must next determine when the statutory period commenced or began to run. In some cases, the statute of limitations will provide specific guidance as to when the period begins to run. For example, a statute of limitations may provide that the period begins to run "from the date of the act or omission complained of" or "when the damage is sustained and is ascertainable." On the other hand, a statute of limitations is often vague as to when the period should begin to run. For instance, the statute may state that the period begins to run when the action "accrues." In such instances, judicial decisions provide guidance as to when the statutory period should begin to run.

If a statute of limitations does not specifically identify when the period begins to run and the claim involves a single act or omission causing injury, the general rule is that the period begins to run when the act or omission causing injury is complete. Thus, if one commits an assault on another, the statutory period of limitations for an intentional tort begins to run at the time of the assault. On the other hand, if the injury is one that accrues over time, such as by exposure to a toxic chemical, the statute generally will not begin to run until the last exposure. However, as with most rules, there are certain exceptions to the general rules regarding the running of a statute of limitations.

A statutory period of limitations may be **tolled** (postponed, suspended, or extended) for many reasons; primary reasons include the following:

- Inability to discover the injury
- Death of the injured individual
- Disability of the injured individual
- Wrongdoing by the individual or entity causing the injury

The Discovery Rule

The discovery rule provides that, if the nature of an injury is inherently undiscoverable, a person exercising reasonable diligence will not be barred by the statute of limitations from bringing a lawsuit. An injury is inherently undiscoverable if it is unlikely to be discovered within the specified period of limitations. For example, assume that during a surgery, a doctor inadvertently leaves a surgical sponge inside the patient. While the patient may experience some symptoms, he or she may have no reason to suspect that those symptoms are the result of negligent conduct. By the time the patient discovers the connection between the symptoms and the surgery, the statute of limitations may have expired. Thus, the discovery rule will toll the statute of limitations until the patient knows, or in the exercise of reasonable diligence should have known, of the injury.

Death of the Injured Individual

When a person is injured by a tort and later dies, the statute of limitations will be affected. For example, a cause of action may occur before the death of the injured person and the time for commencement of an action has not expired, but the person did not sue prior to death. In most cases, the statute of limitations will be tolled for a period of time to allow an executor or administrator to be appointed and to bring an action. This, however, is different from a claim for wrongful death, which is a distinct claim with a separate statute of limitations.

Disability of the Injured Individual

If the injured individual is legally under a disability (such as minors and mentally impaired individuals), the statute of limitations is usually tolled until the disability has been removed. For example, if one commits a tort against a minor child, the statute of limitations will not begin to run until the child becomes an adult under the law of the state.

Wrongdoing

Finally, a statute of limitations may be tolled due to the actions of the tortfeasor-defendant. For example, if the tortfeasor attempts to conceal wrongdoing, the statute of limitations will be tolled. Additionally, a tortfeasor may be prevented from asserting a statute of limitations defense. For example, presume that two people are involved in a car accident. The person responsible for the accident promises to settle any and all claims. In the meantime, however, the statute of limitations expires. A court may prevent the wrongdoer-defendant from asserting a statute of limitations defense due to the promises made to the other person. Finally, a defendant can also waive a statute of limitations defense if it is not specifically asserted against the opposing party. For example, an injured person initiates a lawsuit by filing a complaint and sets forth a number of claims. If the defendant fails to assert the statute of limitations defense in answering the complaint, the defense is deemed to have been waived.

Statute of Repose

Many states, in the course of enacting **tort reform** measures, retain existing statutes of limitations for malpractice cases (for example, one year in Ohio) and personal injury cases (for example, two years in Ohio) but then add new provisions, subject to certain exceptions, that provide a maximum amount of time within which to discover and file a claim. Such maximum or absolute limitations are called **statutes of repose.** For example, Ohio's Senate Bill 281 contained a statute of repose provision that limits the discovery and filing of claims to four years under most circumstances. (See Ohio Revised Code 2305.113.) Important exceptions to the five-year statute of repose include foreign objects (for example, a surgical instrument). Furthermore, certain classes of individuals, such as minors and persons of unsound mind, are subject to existing provisions of Ohio law that toll, or extend time limitations for bringing claims. Thus, the statute of repose does not apply to and does not run against individuals who are minors until they reach the age of majority.

Torts and Contracts

The focus of this chapter is torts, the causes of actions (that is, claims) that may be brought under tort principles, and defenses to tort claims. Another body of law often found in the healthcare context is contract law. **Contract law** is the body of **civil law** relating to agreements between parties, most often in the context of business or commercial relationships. Whereas the law of tort focuses on negligence or intentional wrongs committed by one party against another, the law of contract focuses on agreements between parties and the enforcement of such agreements. One critical difference between tort and contract law is that, by definition, negligence does not factor into the analysis and resolution of contract disputes. Contract law will be discussed in detail in chapter 6.

Criminal Liability in Healthcare

Wrongful acts committed in the healthcare environment generally lead to civil liability. However, wrongdoing in this arena can also constitute a criminal violation. One context in which criminal penalties may result is violation of the HIPAA Privacy Rule. Criminal violations of HIPAA privacy provisions are subject to penalties set forth in the United States Code at 42 USC 1320d-6(a). The key inquiry in a criminal violation is whether it was committed knowingly, which means either purposefully committing the act or acting in willful disregard of the existence of a statutory provision or scheme. Maximum penalties for criminal violations are set forth in 42 USC. 1320d-6(b). The imposition of penalties relating to federal crimes is subject to the Federal Sentencing Guidelines, which require the judge to consider the offense level and the defendant's criminal history in sentencing the defendant. Criminal penalties for privacy violations include the following:

- A fine of not more than $50,000, imprisonment for not more than one year, or both

- If the violation is committed under false pretense, the fine is not more than $100,000, imprisonment is for not more than five years, or both

- If the violation is committed with the intent to sell, transfer, or use personal health information for commercial advantage, personal gain, or malicious harm, the fine is not more than $250,000, imprisonment is for not more than 10 years, or both

In what is generally considered to be the first HIPAA privacy criminal prosecution, *U.S. v. Gibson* (2004), a covered entity employee was charged with illegal disclosure of a patient's personal health information to fraudulently obtain and use credit cards in the patient's name. Pursuant to the foregoing penalties, because the improper disclosure was for personal gain, the defendant was potentially subject to a fine of up to $250,000 and incarceration for up to 10 years. The defendant entered a plea bargain with the government, which included a recommendation for 10 to 16 months in prison and full restitution to the patient and credit card companies. In November 2004, District Judge Ricardo Martinez sentenced the defendant to 16 months in prison with three years of supervised release and more than $9,000 in restitution.

This case illustrates a further significant procedural and substantive legal point. The entity prosecuted by the government in this case was not a HIPAA-covered entity (which will be described in chapter 9) but an employee of a covered entity. This suggests that the government interprets HIPAA provisions to apply personally to members of a covered entity's (such as a hospital's) workforce. There is currently no legal consensus as to whether HIPAA provisions apply to persons individually or only to entities that are covered entities, and **judge-made law** (common law) continues to develop on this point.

Criminal liability for wrongdoing in the healthcare context may result in other circumstances, just as criminal liability may result in the business and other societal settings. For example, criminal liability issues may arise in antitrust, conspiracy, personal injury, health and safety, and fraud. Fraud, specifically fraudulent healthcare billing, has been aggressively pursued by the federal government. Led by the Office of Inspector General (OIG) for the Department of Health and Human Services, healthcare providers have been and continue to be aggressively investigated and prosecuted for receiving payments through fraudulent activity. This will be discussed further in chapter 15.

Medical Malpractice Issues

The question of whether a medical malpractice crisis exists in the US healthcare system is a highly debated, heavily studied, and exceptionally contentious issue among healthcare providers, physicians, attorneys, the insurance industry, and state and national legislatures. Volumes have been written on this issue, and views vary as widely as the sources from which they spring. This section summarizes and analyzes research and other findings relating to three interconnected issues: insurance and the overall rising cost of medical malpractice insurance, the argument for and against the existence of an insurance "crisis" in certain states, and various state tort reform measures enacted to address general healthcare systems, medical malpractice, litigation, and malpractice insurance concerns.

The Rising Cost of Medical Malpractice Insurance

Physicians must generally retain **medical malpractice insurance** to protect themselves from claims of medical negligence or other tortious injury arising out of care provided to patients (Danzon et al. 2004).

It is generally agreed that in recent years, physician malpractice insurance premiums have risen depending on the physician's area of practice and geographical location. Particularly steep premium increases have occurred in specialties such as obstetrics and gynecology, emergency medicine, and neurosurgery (Danzon et al. 2004). The reported median premium increase for internists, general surgeons, and obstetricians/gynecologists rose from 0–2 percent in 1996–1997 to 17–18 percent in 2003, reaching nearly 60 percent in some states in 2001–2002 (Danzon et al. 2004). These types of statistics have led to several states being labeled "crisis" states, meaning medical malpractice insurance premiums have risen dramatically in a relatively short amount of time (figure 5.2). In some instances, such increases are cited as the cause of physicians leaving their practice or moving away from their geographical area (Ranji et al. 2005).

Although it is clear that malpractice liability insurance premiums have increased in recent years, there are different opinions as to the cause of the increases, and evidence exists on both sides of the debate. On the one hand, some contend that physician insurance premiums seem to reach new heights annually. Also on this side of the argument are legislators who support legislative responses to a perceived crisis. Some have blamed trial attorneys for pursuing "junk" or "frivolous" lawsuits at the expense of increasing industry costs, although the cost of lawsuits is only a small percentage of America's annual healthcare costs (figures between 2 percent and 7 percent are often cited) (Center for Justice and Democracy 2002). Other common complaints tied to rising costs include the lack of availability and the affordability of medical malpractice insurance coverage, which are attributed to the rise in claims frequency and severity. Also cited is that fewer malpractice insurers are active in the market now, limiting competition on premiums. For example, St. Paul Insurance, previously the largest malpractice insurance carrier in the United States, discontinued underwriting policies in 2001. In addition, MIXX, PHICO, and Frontier Insurance Group each left the market in 2002 (Anawis 2003).

Another factor thought to play a role in the current crisis is the "downturn in the economy, which is reflected in lower stock values and bond interest rates, affecting insurers' investment returns" (Studdert et al. 2004). Some critics cite reduced insurance coverage, arbitrary policy cancellations, threats by insurers to abandon markets, and the mismanagement of the medical malpractice insurance industry as sharing in the blame for current problems (Center for Justice and Democracy 2002).

Despite the substantial number of individuals who believe the medical malpractice insurance industry is in crisis, critics point out that medical malpractice crises occurred in the 1970s and the 1980s and led to waves of tort reform measures—proof that today's malpractice landscape is not new (Medical Liability Monitor 2010). Many proponents suggest that the rise in medical malpractice premium expenses reflects a repeating and historically self-correcting cycle that the insurance industry routinely experiences (Kereiakes and Willerson 2004).

A number of other factors have been mentioned as possible catalysts for the current cost of medical malpractice insurance. These factors lead to the conclusion that the industry is not experiencing a crisis. Some allege that insurance premiums have escalated because of irresponsible underpricing of liability insurance products (Kereiakes and Willerson 2004). Others observe that insufficient data exist to determine what is driving up the cost of medical malpractice coverage, but speculate that underwriting losses triggered by jury awards and claims may be to blame (LeBlang 2006). In addition, inflation, subsequent changes in the insurance market competition, stock market returns, and interest rates have each been blamed for forcing the insurance premiums in an upward direction (LeBlang 2006). Figure 5.3

Figure 5.2. Medical liability "crisis" states

1. Arkansas	8. Mississippi	15. Oregon
2. Connecticut	9. Missouri	16. Pennsylvania
3. Florida	10. Nevada	17. Rhode Island
4. Georgia	11. New Jersey	18. Tennessee
5. Illinois	12. New York	19. Washington
6. Kentucky	13. North Carolina	20. West Virginia
7. Massachusetts	14. Ohio	21. Wyoming

Source: AMA 2007.

Figure 5.3.   The correlation between medical malpractice premiums and awards to plaintiffs, 1975–2005

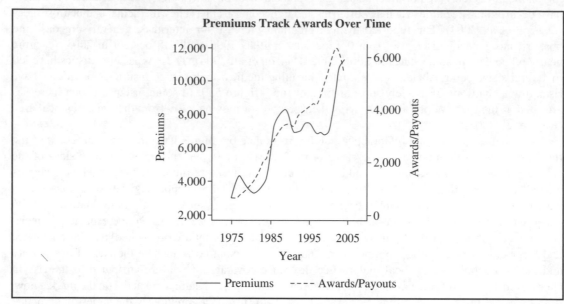

Source: Adapted from Tabarrok and Agan 2006.

shows the correlation between medical malpractice premiums and awards to plaintiffs (Tabarrok and Agan 2006).

Both proponents and opponents of the position that the healthcare system is experiencing a medical malpractice crisis have at least some compelling evidence to support their views. Whether one stands for or against the idea that the industry is in crisis, certain facts remain: Physician premiums have increased over the last several years, and the cost of healthcare continues to rise at rates above simple inflation (LeBlang 2006). Although critics are unlikely to arrive at a consensus, actuarial, demographic, and other statistical investigations will continue to analyze the causes, effects, and significance of medical malpractice costs. Another set of theorists believes that while there was a recent crisis in the medical malpractice industry, the crisis has since subsided (Doroshow and Hunter 2006). Others have reported that medical practice premiums and claims (inflation adjusted) are at the lowest they have been in 30 years, with an overall drop in claims of 45 percent since 2000 (Hunter et al. 2009).

Physician Medical Malpractice Insurance Crisis in Identified States

Due to the variety of ways in which states plan and respond to medical malpractice issues, the existence and extent of a medical malpractice insurance crisis varies from state to state (Excellus 2011). Predictably, the rates of malpractice insurance premiums vary among the states based on geographic region and medical practice. According to a 2010 study conducted by the Medical Liability Monitor, Florida, Illinois, and Michigan were among the states with the highest medical malpractice rates for general internists (Florida being the highest, with a rate of $48,245 per year). With a premium of $192,982 per year in Florida and $143,445 per year in Michigan, both states were also among those with the highest premiums for general surgeons (Medical Liability Monitor 2010). The same was true with regard to rates for obstetricians/gynecologists: Florida's 2010 annual rate was $201,808, second to New York's annual rate of $204,864. (See figures 5.4, 5.5, and 5.6.)

According to the American Medical Association's (AMA) 2007 medical liability, 21 states experienced a "full-blown medical liability crisis," up from 12 in 2002 (LeBlang 2006). (See figure 5.7.)

Figure 5.4. States with highest and lowest malpractice rates for internists, 2010

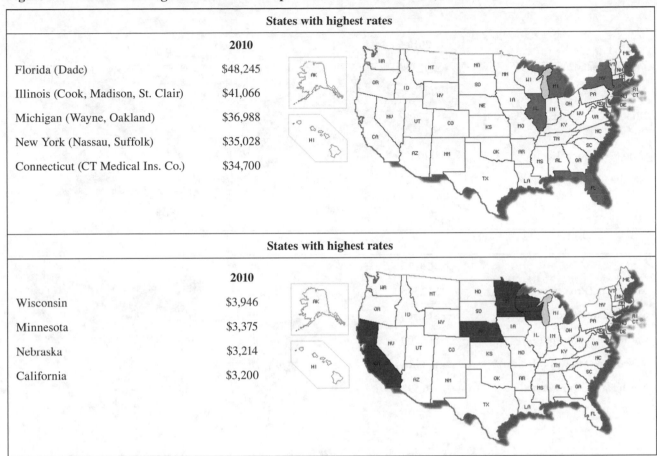

States with highest rates	
	2010
Florida (Dade)	$48,245
Illinois (Cook, Madison, St. Clair)	$41,066
Michigan (Wayne, Oakland)	$36,988
New York (Nassau, Suffolk)	$35,028
Connecticut (CT Medical Ins. Co.)	$34,700

States with highest rates	
	2010
Wisconsin	$3,946
Minnesota	$3,375
Nebraska	$3,214
California	$3,200

Source: Medical Liability Monitor 2010, as cited in Excellus 2011. Ranking is by state, based on the highest rate reported in each state for each specialty.

Among the states listed are Florida, Illinois, New York, and Ohio (LeBlang 2006). The AMA contends that these crisis states have certain common features: patients continue to lose access to care and obstetricians, rural family physicians no longer deliver babies, and high-risk specialists no longer provide trauma care or perform complicated surgical procedures (AMA 2007).

Other statistics from the AMA (2007) regarding "crisis" states include:

- In 2002, New York was considered a "Red Alert" state by the American College of Obstetricians and Gynecologists, which found that 67 percent of OB/GYNs have been forced to restrict their practice, retire, or relocate to another state.

- From 2001 to 2002, Ohio physicians faced medical liability insurance increases ranging from 28 to 60 percent.

- In 2004, the last two neurosurgeons in southern Illinois left because of medical liability insurance premiums of nearly $300,000 a year.

- FPIC, a leading medical liability insurance carrier in Florida, said during 1975 there were 380 lawsuits for medical negligence allegations resulting in $10.8 million in jury awards, costing $1.5 million to defend. In 2000, there were 880 lawsuits resulting in awards of $219 million, costing $36 million to defend.

Figure 5.5.   States with highest and lowest malpractice rates for general surgeons, 2010

States with highest rates		
	2010	
Florida (Dade)	$192,982	
Michigan (Wayne)	$143,445	
Illinois (Cook, Jackson, Madison, St. Clair, Will)	$127,083	
Ohio (Cuyahoga, Lorain)	$120,135	
Nevada (Clark)	$118,125	
States with lowest rates		
	2010	
Minnesota (ProAssurance)	$11,306	
South Dakota (ProAssurance)	$12,569	
California (CAP-MPT)	$13,200	
Wisconsin (Midwest Medical)	$13,813	
North Dakota (ProMutual)	$16,592	

Source: Medical Liability Monitor 2010, as cited in Excellus 2011. Ranking is by state, based on the highest rate reported in each state for each specialty. The Cooperative of American Physicians (CAP) is a physician-owned and -governed organization comprised of doctors practicing in the State of California. Membership in CAP gives physicians the opportunity to purchase medical professional liability coverage through the Mutual Protection Trust (MPT).

Despite the sobering account provided by the AMA statistics, editorials reported that certain states may experience relief in the near future. *Crain's Cleveland Business* reported that the market appeared to be slowly stabilizing after several years of insurance premium increases in Ohio (Mortland 2006). This prediction proved to be correct, as future editorials showed that net premiums written for the industry dropped every year from 2006 through 2009 (Medical Liability Monitor 2010). The Medical Liability Monitor (2010) commented that "rates for 2010 indicate a market that remains 'soft' or perhaps 'flat', with 67 percent of all rates holding at last year's levels." Each of the crisis states mentioned above has enacted some form of legislative tort reform (discussed below). California, having seen improvement in its malpractice and insurance crisis after legislative enactments in 1975, may continue to successfully stabilize its malpractice insurance costs through tort reform means.

Types of Tort Reform Measures

In response to medical malpractice insurance expenditures plagued by costly litigation and mounting judgment awards, state and local legislatures have initiated measures to lessen the industry's strain. Various states have instituted tort reform measures to control claims, causes of action, and judicial remedies to control malpractice costs.

Tort reform encompasses the variety of measures intended by legislatures to overhaul the justice system. With regard to medical malpractice, such reforms are intended to diminish the number of

Figure 5.6.   States with highest and lowest malpractice rates for OB/GYN, 2010

States with highest rates

	2010
New York (Dade)	$204,864
Florida (Miami, Dade)	$201,808
Illinois	$177,441
Connecticut	$170,389
Nevada	$168,750

States with lowest rates

	2010
California (CAP-MPT)	$13,400
Minnesota (ProMutual)	$16,449
Wisconsin (Midwest Medical)	$18,154
South Dakota (ProAssurance)	$21,073
North Dakota (ProMutual)	$22,486

Source: Medical Liability Monitor 2010, as cited in Excellus 2011. Ranking is by state, based on the highest rate reported in each state for each specialty. The Cooperative of American Physicians (CAP) is a physician-owned and -governed organization comprised of doctors practicing in the State of California. Membership in CAP gives physicians the opportunity to purchase medical professional liability coverage through the Mutual Protection Trust (MPT).

Figure 5.7.   AMA's "crisis map"

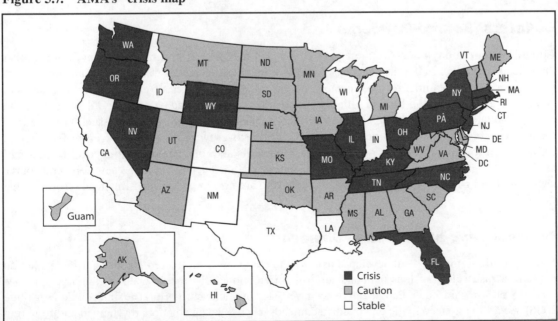

Source: AMA 2012.

lawsuits and large jury verdicts, stabilize the market, and ultimately reduce premiums for physicians. Several types of tort reform measures have been promulgated. For instance, several states have targeted specific tort reform issues by enacting laws that limit joint and several liability, consider collateral source payments, and place caps on noneconomic and punitive damages (NAMIC 2004). Additionally, Ohio has made systematic efforts to control tort litigation and medical malpractice costs through aggressive legislative efforts, resulting in various legislation including H.B. 292 (OH Rev. Code 2307.91-98 2004), which requires the establishment of minimum medical requirements before certain tort actions can be pursued.

California is often cited for its progressive tort reform measures under the 1975 Medical Injury Compensation Reform Act (MICRA), the legislative response to California's 1970s insurance crisis. Often considered a model for medical malpractice reform in other states, it limits attorney fees and awards for pain and suffering to $250,000. It is credited with reducing the amount of damages that doctors and their insurers are ordered to pay in medical malpractice lawsuits—30 percent in the opinion of some critics (Insurance Information Institute 2006). Other measures include shortening the statute of limitations period in which a lawsuit may be filed, limiting attorneys' contingency fees, allowing structured settlements in lieu of windfalls for plaintiffs, and establishing no-fault systems (Showalter 2012).

Nationally, federal tort reform measures have been proposed. However, because torts are generally a matter of state law and federal tort reform faces potential constitutional challenges, efforts to control tort damage award payments have generally been left to the individual states.

Joint and Several Liability

Joint and several liability allows each defendant in a legal action to be held responsible for the entire amount of damages that a plaintiff is awarded, regardless of the defendant's degree of fault (Insurance Information Institute 2006). The rule of joint and several liability has sometimes been referred to as the "deep pocket" rule because of the perception that plaintiffs are inclined to sue multiple defendants in order to find the most financially lucrative target. For example, under this theory, financially lucrative Defendant A may be required to pay 100 percent of the damages, even though it is only 60 percent responsible, because the nonfinancially lucrative Defendant B is unable to pay its 40 percent share. Tort reform measures replace the rule of joint and several liability with one of proportionate liability, which means that a tortfeasor is liable only for its share or proportion of the injury it caused. States that have enacted some form of joint and several liability reform legislation include California, Florida, Illinois, New York, Ohio, and Pennsylvania (Insurance Information Institute 2006).

Collateral Source Payments

Collateral source payments are those payments a plaintiff in a tort case receives from a source other than the defendant(s). Under the general collateral source rule, defendants were prohibited from presenting evidence that a plaintiff received compensation for his or her injuries from any other source. As of 2004, 24 states—including Florida, Illinois, New York, and Ohio—had passed laws allowing courts to consider collateral source payments. One example of a collateral source payment issue in the medical malpractice context is where an injured plaintiff might recover twice if he or she received $100,000 in medical care for his or her injury under Medicare benefits and then attempted to recover the costs of medical care against the person who caused the injury. The intended effect of the new collateral source laws is to diminish the damages awarded by juries who are now aware of other financial resources that the plaintiff has.

Noneconomic and Punitive Damages

Noneconomic damages were developed as a way to compensate an injured plaintiff for losses that do not have a cash value, such as pain and suffering or emotional distress. In contrast, punitive damages serve to punish and deter defendants who have acted maliciously (Insurance Information Institute 2006). Awarding noneconomic and punitive damages tends to be an emotionally charged and troubling process for juries, and the amounts given to injured plaintiffs often far exceed the actual damage award. As a result, 23 states have enacted noneconomic damage legislative reform as of 2004, with statutory limitations ranging from $250,000 to $1,000,000 (Insurance Information Institute 2006). In addition, as of 2004, 19 states have enacted punitive damage reform legislation requiring a stricter standard of proof and/or a higher degree of fault before punitive damages may be awarded. In addition to these general tort reform measures, New Jersey has implemented a Medical Malpractice Insurance Premium Assistance Fund that distributes funds to doctors in specialties with the highest medical malpractice insurance premiums. About 1,200 neurosurgeons, obstetricians, and radiologists who practice in the state will each receive about $11,000 (Insurance Information Institute 2006).

Affidavit of Merit

As a measure to deter excessive or frivolous litigation, some jurisdictions require that an **affidavit of merit** accompany a complaint. In the state of Ohio, any complaint that contains a medical claim, dental claim, optometric claim, or chiropractic claim must include an affidavit of merit by an expert witness relative to each defendant in the complaint for whom expert testimony is necessary to establish liability. The affidavit of merit must include all of the following, pursuant to Ohio Civ. R. 10(D)(2)(a):

- A statement that the affiant has reviewed all medical records reasonably available to the plaintiff concerning the allegations in the complaint

- A statement that the affiant is familiar with the applicable standard of care

- The opinion of the affiant that the standard of care was breached by one or more of the defendants to the action and that the breach caused injury to the plaintiff

The purpose of filing this affidavit is to establish the sufficiency of the complaint and to serve as a pretrial screening device. In Ohio, if an affidavit of merit is not filed with the complaint, the complaint may be dismissed without prejudice.

Limits on Attorney Contingency Fees

A **contingency fee** is a lawyer's fee paid on the basis of the percentage of the money awarded to the client. This fee is commonly one-third of the total recovery. As opposed to charging the client an hourly fee, a contingency fee structure allows plaintiffs who otherwise could not afford a lawyer to seek redress in court without any financial investment. The contingent fee system is unique to the US legal system and has been heavily criticized since it allows lawyers to take riskier cases and encourages them to make excessive demands and seek cases that may be settled quickly with minimal time invested. Many states have taken reform measures to curb the abuse of contingency fee arrangements by enacting statutes to limit the contingent fees in medical liability cases to certain percentages or provide that a court must review or approve the amount of such fees.

Structured Settlements

In personal injury or tort settlements, parties may agree to a **structured settlement** arrangement in which the claim is paid in installments rather than in one lump sum. Often the defendant will purchase one or more annuities to guarantee the future payments. Structured settlements were first developed in Canada and the United States and are now generally available in Australia and England as well. There is no set form for a structured settlement arrangement. While some uniformity exists, each country has its own definitions, rules, and standards for structured settlements. In the United States a structured settlement can significantly reduce taxes from the settlement and may even be tax-free. To help curb abuses by companies willing to purchase a structured settlement for a significantly discounted lump-sum payment, many states have enacted legislation to limit the sale of structured settlements.

No-Fault Systems

Broadly defined, **no-fault insurance** describes any type of insurance contract under which insureds are indemnified for losses by their own insurance company, regardless of fault in the incident generating losses. This is very similar to first-party coverage. However, the term "no-fault" is most commonly used in the context of state/provincial automobile insurance laws in the United States, Canada, and Australia, in which a policyholder (and his or her passengers) are not only reimbursed by the policyholder's own insurance company without proof of fault but also restricted in the right to seek recovery through the civil-justice system for losses caused by other parties. Thus, in states that have adopted no-fault systems, minor accident and injury claims are generally resolved without litigation. However, in instances of catastrophic injuries or damages, no-fault states still permit an individual to bring claims where basic no-fault principles would not adequately protect or compensate the injured party.

Check Your Understanding 5.5

Instructions: Indicate whether the following statements are true or false (T or F).

1. A statute of limitations places time limits on certain claims.

2. A tolled statute of limitations is one that has been delayed or suspended.

3. Wrongful acts committed in the healthcare environment can lead only to civil liability.

4. Diminishing returns on insurers' investments is believed to be a contributing factor to the medical malpractice insurance crisis.

5. Collateral source payments are payments received by the plaintiff from sources other than the defendant.

Summary

This chapter focused on tort law and the various causes of action that may be encountered in the health-care and health information settings. The author explained tort law's unique role in safeguarding the rights of individuals and other legal entities. Individuals responsible for the health information of others need to be familiar with negligence, intentional torts, strict liability, and contract principles, and the various causes of actions or claims that may be brought in the health information context. Specifically, this chapter reviewed a number of bases of liability, including defamation, invasion of privacy, breach of confidentiality, infliction of emotional distress, medical malpractice, and criminal conduct. Each of the causes of action has very specific elements that must be proved before a damages award may be made for claimed injuries. While HIPAA and HITECH revisions are discussed at length in chapters 9 and 10, it is clear that this legislation has broad and far-reaching implications in tort and criminal processes. Some of those implications were discussed in this chapter. Also important are the various defenses a defendant may bring. Because of the breadth and scope of legal issues faced by healthcare professionals, it is likely that in-house counsel or outside legal counsel would be involved in a number of active legal matters involving a particular healthcare provider. Obviously, the scope and implications of tort law are vast, yet a practical understanding of tort law, its various components, and how it applies in health information practice is crucial.

This chapter also focused on issues relating to medical malpractice insurance and tort reform measures. While the existence and extent of a medical malpractice crisis is the subject of heated debate, it is clear that healthcare costs and medical malpractice insurance costs have steadily climbed over the last decades. States have addressed these issues in myriad ways, some more successfully than others. This chapter discussed historical aspects and tort reform issues and initiatives in select states, with an eye toward the future.

References

4 Am. Jur. 2d Animals 85 (2007).

31A Am. Jur. 2d Explosions and Explosives 94, 143 (2002).

40A Am. Jur. 2d Hospitals and Asylums 26 (2008).

57A Am. Jur. 2d Negligence 5, 7, 13, 124, 132, 135, 78-143 (2004).

57B Am. Jur. 2d Negligence 798, 1163, 1164 (2004).

61 Am. Jur. 2d Physicians, Surgeons, and Other Healers 188 et seq. (2002).

63 Am. Jur. 2d Products Liability 559 (1997).

74 Am. Jur. 2d Torts 12 (2001).

American Health Information Management Association. 2013. Analysis of Modifications to the HIPAA Privacy, Security, Enforcement, and Breach Notification Rules Under the Health Information Technology for Economic and Clinical Health Act and the Genetic Information Nondiscrimination Act; Other Modifications to the HIPAA Rules. http://www.ahima.org

American Medical Association. 2007. Press Release: Medical liability crisis map. http://ama-assn.org

American Medical Association. 2012. Medical liability reform now. http://www.ama-assn.org.

Anawis, M.A. 2003. Tort reform 2003: Innovative practice applications. *DePaul Journal of Healthcare Law* 6(2):309–310.

Center for Justice and Democracy. 2002 (Sept. 25). A short guide to understanding today's medical malpractice insurance crisis.

Danzon, P.M., A.J. Epstein, and S.J. Johnson. 2004. *Brookings-Wharton Papers on Financial Services: The Crisis in Medical Malpractice Insurance*. Washington, DC: Brookings Institution.

Doroshow, J., and J.R. Hunter. 2006. Insurance crisis officially over: Medical malpractice rates have been stable for a year. Americans for Insurance Reform. http://www.insurance-reform.org.

Ernst, C. 2007. *Baldwin's Ohio Practice Series Tort Law*, Sections 5:40, 5:45. Eagan, MN: Thomson West.

Excellus. 2011. The facts about New York State medical malpractice coverage premiums: 2010–2011. https://www.excellusbcbs.com.

Garner, B.A. 2004. *Black's Law Dictionary*, abridged 8th ed. St. Paul, MN: West Group.

Hunter, J.R., G. Cassell-Stiga, and J. Doroshow, J. 2009. True risk: Medical liability, malpractice insurance and health care. Americans for Insurance Reform. http://www.insurance-reform.org.

Insurance Information Institute. 2006. Medical malpractice. http://www.iii.org.

Kereiakes, D.J., and J.T. Willerson. 2004. Health care on trial: America's medical malpractice crisis. *Circulation* 109(24):2939–2941. http://www.circ.ahajournals.org.

LeBlang, T.R. 2006. The medical malpractice crisis—Is there a solution? *Journal of Legal Medicine* 27(1):1–16.

Medical Liability Monitor. 2010 (October). Vol. 35, No 10. http://medicalliabilitymonitor.com.

Mortland, S. 2006. Docs find relief at last: Tort reform helps apply brakes to steep malpractice insurance hikes. *Crain's Cleveland Business* 27(37).

Moses, R.J. 2000 (November). *Privacy Actions and HIPAA: Using the Health Insurance Portability and Accountability Act to Protect Patient Privacy*. Practicing Law Institute (PLI Order NO B0-00RFW).

National Association of Mutual Insurance Companies (NAMIC). 2004. An overview of state legislative efforts to improve the legal system. http://www.namic.org.

Pozgar, G.D. 2011. *Legal Aspects of Health Care Administration*. 11th ed. Sudbury, MA: Jones and Bartlett.

Prosser, W.L. 1971. *Handbook of the Law of Torts*, 4th ed. St. Paul, MN: West.

Ranji, U., C. Gutiérrez, and A. Salganicoff. 2005. *Background Brief: Medical Malpractice Policy*. Menlo Park, CA: The Kaiser Family Foundation. http://www.kaiseredu.org.

Restatement of the Law (Second), Torts. 1965. Philadelphia, PA: American Law Institute.

Showalter, J.S. 2012. *The Law of Healthcare Administration*, 6th ed. Chicago, IL: Health Administration Press.

Studdert, D.M., M.M. Mello, and T.A. Brennan. 2004. Health policy report: Medical malpractice. *New England Journal of Medicine* 350(3):283–292.

Tabarrok, A., and A. Agan. 2006. Medical malpractice awards, insurance, and negligence: Which are related? *Civil Justice Report* 10. http://www.manhattan-institute.org.

Cases, Statutes, and Regulations Cited

Ace v. State of New York, 146 Misc.2d 954, 553 N.Y.S. 2d, 605 (1990).

Anderson v. Strong Memorial Hospital, 140 Misc.2d 770, 531 N.Y.S. 2d, 735 (1988).

Andrews v. Ohio Dept. of Transp, Court of Claims No. 2002-05336-AD (2002).

Berger v. Sonneland, 101 WN. App. 141, 1 P.3d 1187 (2000).

Biddle v. Warren General Hospital, 86 Ohio St. 3d 395 (1999).

Darling v. Charleston Community Memorial Hospital, 33 Ill.2d 326, 211 N.E. 2d, 253, 14 A.L.R. 3d 860 (IL Sept. 29, 1965).

Dillard v. Pittway Corp., 719 So.2d 188, 193 (Ala. 1998).

Estate of Berhinger v. Medical Center at Princeton, 249 N.J. Super. 597, 592 A2d 1251 (N.J. Super. L. 1991).

Fairfax Hospital v. Curtis, 249 VA 531; 457 S.E.2d 66 (1997).

Fletcher v. South Peninsula Hosp., 71 P.3d 833 (Alaska 2003).

Hake v. George Wiedemann Brewing Co., 23 Ohio St. 2d 65 (1970).

Hammonds v. Aetna Casualty & Surety Co., 243 F. Supp. 793 (N.D. Ohio 1965).

Herr v. Wheeler, 634 S.E.2d 317, 320 (Va. 2006).

Hospital Authority of City of St. Marys v. Eason, 222 Ga. 536 (1966).

Johnson PPA v. Atlantic Health Services, P.C., 2000 WL 1228275 (Conn. Super. Aug. 21, 2000).

Lehman v. Haynam, 164 Ohio St. 595 (1956).

Lemuz By and Through Lemuz v. Fieser, 933 P.2d 134 (Kansas 1997).

Martin v. Baehler, 1993 WL 258843 (Del. Super. 1993).

Order of Railroad Telegraphers v. Railway Express Agency, 321 U.S. 342 (1944).

Rea v. Pardo, 132 A.D.2d 442, 522 N.Y.S. 2d 393 (1987).

Reese v. Bd. of Directors of Memorial Hosp. of Laramie Co., 955 P.2d 425 (Wyo. 1998).

Sanders v. Spector, 673 So.2d 1176 (La. App. 1996).

Smith v. McVicker, 5th App. No. 2003AP120092, 2004-Ohio-4217 (Ohio 2004).

Strickland v. Pinder, 899 A.2d 770 (D.C. Ct. App. 2006).

Thompson v. Ulysses Cruises, Inc., 812 F. Supp. 900 (S.D. Ind. 1993).

Uncapher v. Baltimore & O.R. Co., 127 Ohio St. 351, at syllabus (1933).

U.S. v. Gibson, No. CR04-0374RSM, 2004 WL 2237585 (W.D. Wash. August 19, 2004).

Wagner v. Int'l Railway, 232 N.Y. 176 (1921).

Williams v. American Medical Systems, 248 Ga. App. 682, 684 (2001).

28 USC 1346(b), 2671-2680: Federal Tort Claims Act. 1946.

42 USC 1320d-5: General penalty. 1996.

42 USC 1320d-6(a): Wrongful disclosure of individually identifiable health information: Offense. 1996.

42 USC 1320d-6(b): Wrongful disclosure of individually identifiable health information: Defense. 1996.

Ohio Civ. R. 10(D)(2)(a).

OH Rev. Code 2305.113: Medical malpractice actions. 2006.

OH Rev. Code 2307.91-98: Asbestos Claims. 2004.

Chapter 6

Corporations, Contracts, and Antitrust Legal Issues

Jill Callahan Klaver, JD, RHIA

Learning Objectives

- Describe the most important benefits of forming as a corporation

- Analyze the key differences between a for-profit and not-for-profit corporation

- Articulate the key responsibilities of the governing board of a typical healthcare organization

- Describe the basic elements of a valid contract

- Discuss potential defenses against allegations of nonperformance (breach) of a contract

- Describe the purposes of a hold harmless/indemnification clause

- Articulate concerns associated with health information technology contracts

- Describe the physician–patient relationship as a contract

- Distinguish the parameters of three major federal antitrust statutes

- Explain contract and antitrust issues associated with the medical staff

Key Terms

Acceptance
Adhesion contract
Arbitration
Boilerplate
Breach of contract
Bylaws
Clayton Act
Compensatory damages
Consideration
Contract
Corporation
Due diligence
Duty of loyalty

Duty of responsibility
Economic credentialing
Exculpatory contract
Federal Trade
   Commission Act
Fiduciary duty
For-profit corporation
Hold harmless/
   indemnification clause
Horizontal restraint of trade
Injunction
Joint ventures
Learned intermediary

Noncompete agreement
Not-for-profit corporation
Offer
Partnership
Per se antitrust violation
Piercing the corporate veil
Rule of reason analysis
Sherman Act
Sole proprietorship
Specific performance
Ultra vires act
Vertical restraint of trade
Warranties

Introduction

On an ongoing basis, healthcare organizations must make business decisions that have legal implications. One decision is the legal form that an organization will take. Although small organizations assume legal forms such as partnerships and sole proprietorships, healthcare organizations commonly take the form of corporations. This chapter will discuss the structure and legal status of a corporation, as well as the myriad legal obligations associated with it. Regardless of the form that a healthcare organization takes, individuals within the organization have some level of contracting authority. From a provider standpoint, the physician–patient relationship itself is a contract. From a business standpoint, the authority to enter into contracts is most often held by healthcare administrators, managers, and department directors. Although contracts are diverse and created to carry out an organization's business purposes, prevalent today are health information technology (HIT) contracts, which have proliferated in response to the federal government's incentive program to adopt the electronic health record (EHR). In addition to contracting authority, decisions made by individuals in healthcare organizations may have potential antitrust or compliance implications. The goal of this chapter is to describe some basic, yet significant, legal concepts that affect the healthcare organization as a business and that may have implications for health information management (HIM) and informatics-related functions.

Healthcare Corporations

Most healthcare organizations are formed as **corporations**. A corporation is an artificial "being" created under the authority of a state statute (a business corporation act). These state laws permit groups of persons (or even individuals in some states) to incorporate an enterprise for any lawful purpose. The purposes of the corporation and the limits of its authority are stated in the articles of incorporation, filed with the state. Articles of incorporation function like a constitution for the corporation. The Internal Revenue Service (IRS) has certain requirements for the articles, as do various states. Typically, however, the IRS requirements include:

- Name and address of the corporation

- Name and address of the registered agent for the corporation (person or entity authorized to accept legal documents on behalf of the corporation)

- Overall purpose of the corporation (which is often written very broadly to permit flexibility in the future, for example, "to engage in any lawful purpose")

- Whether the corporation is organized as for-profit or not-for-profit (which are discussed later in this chapter)

- Whether the corporation will engage in political or legislative activity (since these activities are barred in not-for-profits organized under IRS code section 501c(3))

- How the corporation will distribute its assets upon dissolution

Healthcare organizations may take various legal forms, such as a **partnership** (for example, two or more physicians who agree to practice together) or even a **sole proprietorship** (a simpler legal form with a single owner who elects not to insulate his or her personal assets through the use of a corporation or other legal form). In a partnership, two or more parties, such as two physicians, agree to share the risks and the rewards of the enterprise. In a general partnership, the general partners usually share the profits or losses equally, and they are personally responsible for any liabilities or debts of the partnership. Decisions are made through consensus and agreement of the partners. But partnerships may also be classified as limited partnerships, in order to limit the potential liabilities attributable to some of the investors or limited partners. Limited partners have greater liability protection but also limited powers. They generally do not participate in the day-to-day management of the business.

Joint ventures are another form of partnership. They are created for a very specific purpose and are designed to have a limited lifespan. Joint ventures are sometimes seen when two separate healthcare corporations come together to provide a shared service, such as a dialysis center or a radiation therapy center. Healthcare organizations can also be sole proprietorships, such as where a single physician owns and operates a physician practice. In this structure, the physician is fully responsible for the debts and liabilities of the organization but is entitled to all the profits.

Advantages of a Corporation

So why do most healthcare organizations or practices form as a corporation? The main advantage of a corporation is that it is a legal entity or "person" under the law. As such, it is separate from the owners or incorporators. This generally shields the owners from personal liability for the debts of the corporation, although the corporation itself can both sue and be sued. And unlike a sole proprietorship or a limited partnership, a corporation can continue to exist despite the death of an owner. In for-profit corporations, owners can generally transfer their interests (shares) to others, without having to obtain permission to do so. Corporations can be either privately or publicly held. A publicly held corporation sells ownership shares to the public, while a privately held corporation is privately owned. In privately held corporations, the stock shares are not offered for sale to the general public. Private companies generally have relatively few shareholders, as compared to the thousands of shareholders that publicly traded companies have. The fact that publicly held corporations are beholden to many shareholders-owners can affect control of the corporation and its decision making options, since there are potentially far more owners to whom the key executives are accountable.

A corporation is taxed as an individual entity separate from the owners, meaning that the owners are taxed only on the income they actually receive from the corporation, and not all of the corporation's profits. Corporate income tax rates are generally lower than personal income tax rates. The limited liability for owners and investors also makes it easier for the corporation to attract investors.

But the liability protections offered by a corporation to its owners are not absolute. If a corporation is used for certain nefarious purposes, such as fraud or crime, those protections can be pierced and the owners may be liable for those bad acts. This concept is described as "**piercing the corporate veil**," and for a court to do this, three elements must be present:

- Complete domination of the corporation by its owners

- Such control was used to commit fraud or perpetrate a wrong, violate a statutory or other duty, or commit a dishonest or unjust act

- Corporate control was the proximate cause of the injury that is the subject of the suit (Fletcher 1983)

If the court finds these three elements, the protections of the corporation will be pierced and the owners can be found directly liable for the bad actions that are the subject of the suit.

For-Profit and Not-for-Profit Corporations

Healthcare organizations can be formed as for-profit or not-for-profit corporations. A **for-profit corporation** is allowed to distribute its income to the shareholders, directors, officers, and other individuals for their private gain. A **not-for-profit corporation** may not distribute its income for the private gain of individuals. A not-for-profit can certainly make money, but it must use that income for the purposes of the corporation. It is allowed to pay reasonable salaries to its members, directors, and employees. Making a profit is not the primary purpose of not-for-profit corporations. They usually have very specific social or beneficial purposes set forth in their charter. As a result of both their not-for-profit status and their beneficial purpose, they typically receive preferred treatment under tax laws as long as their actions adhere to their approved charter.

A charitable corporation is one form of a not-for-profit corporation—and perhaps the most common form that US hospitals adopt as their purpose—but it is not the only form. If formed for a charitable or benevolent purpose, charitable corporations are completely exempt from a variety of federal and state taxes. Because tax exemption is such a significant benefit, certain requirements must be met to qualify for it. Not only must the charitable corporation be organized and operated for a charitable purpose, but its net earnings must not benefit a private individual or corporation, which would, in effect, amount to an impermissible "profit." Instead, the charitable corporation must benefit the public or the community (this is referred to as the "community benefit standard," adopted in 1969 by the IRS). For the healthcare organization to be tax exempt it must meet at least five specific criteria set forth by the IRS as noted by Peregrine (2009) in figure 6.1.

In recent years, the charitable-purpose element of not-for-profit hospitals, which allows for tax-exempt status, has been challenged in part based on aggressive and inflated billing practices, particularly against the uninsured, who have no insurers to bargain on their behalf. Challenges can also be based on the amount of charity care provided. The Illinois Supreme Court, for example, in *Provena Covenant Medical Center v. Department of Revenue* (2000), decided that the tax-exempt status of a not-for-profit hospital should be revoked because the amount of charity care provided by the hospital was too low to justify tax exemption.

State corporation acts determine the qualifications a corporation must meet in order to maintain its not-for-profit status, and these vary somewhat from state to state. State corporation laws also vary in the duties and responsibilities assigned to the members of the corporation or governing body, but the detailed responsibilities of the corporation's governing body (often called board of trustees or board of directors) can be found in the corporate bylaws.

Figure 6.1. Factors used to determine whether a hopital meets the community benefit standard

- Whether the hospital maintains a governing body that includes community leaders (and not just hospital staff and physicians and other insiders)
- Whether the hospital has an open medical staff that permits all qualified physicians to practice there
- Whether the hospital has a full-time emergency department that is open to all, regardless of their ability to pay
- Whether the hospital provides nonemergency care to all persons able to pay (including through Medicare and Medicaid programs)
- Whether the hospital uses its surplus money to improve the quality of care, expand its facilities, and improve its medical education and training programs
- Whether, in the absence of some or all of the five factors above, there are other favorable factors that demonstrate benefit to the community
- Whether the hospital serves a broad cross-section of its community through charitable care or research

Source: Adapted from Peregrine (2009).

Responsibilities of the Governing Board

Bylaws refer to the internal rules of an organization or company. They describe the powers granted to the governing body, as well as their duties. Bylaws generally cannot be modified by the governing body unless the members or shareholders grant them that authority. In healthcare organizations, governing bodies are generally responsible for developing a strategic plan for the organization, setting broad policy, appointing medical staff members and delineating their clinical privileges, hiring and guiding the chief executive officer, and overseeing the overall performance of the organization (its clinical performance as well as overall administrative and financial performance). Governing body members may also have fundraising responsibilities in some organizations. The role is one of fiduciary oversight, not as an agent or employee of the corporation. They are generally not personally liable for the actions of corporation employees; however, they can be held responsible for failing to carry out their fiduciary duties properly. Fiduciary duty is further described below.

The bylaws often describe the actual makeup of the governing body, such as numbers, types of members (number of community members versus hospital administrators or medical staff members, which, as noted above, is a key factor in meeting the community benefit standard), terms of service, qualifications, duties of governing body officers, number of meetings and methods of calling for meetings and making decisions, whether governing body members are compensated, and so on. It is in a healthcare organization's best interests to select governing body members who can lend their expertise (for example, successful leaders in other industries and consumer members who represent the patient population being served).

The bylaws may provide for certain committees within the governing body. Often, committees made up of subsets of the full governing body are used to facilitate the completion of work between full meetings. Generally, these committees cannot operate and make decisions autonomously; rather, they make recommendations to the full governing body. The full body can then either accept or reject the recommendations. Some of the most commonly seen governing body committees in healthcare organizations include finance, building and grounds, human resources, corporate compliance, professional staff relations, and the executive committee. The executive committee is a key committee because it is often empowered to act on behalf of the full board in between official meetings, except where the bylaws have reserved specific decision-making authority to the full board.

Fiduciary Duty

As noted above, final decision-making authority generally rests with the full governing body. Individual trustees or board members cannot absolve themselves of their responsibility for decisions by arguing that they were not part of that committee and therefore are not responsible for that decision. They are responsible for all governing body decisions. They have a **fiduciary duty** to the corporation and its members and shareholders, and in the case of a not-for-profit corporation, they may have a duty to the community at large. Commentators often describe these duties as a duty of loyalty and a duty of responsibility (Showalter 2012).

The **duty of loyalty** means that board members must put the interests of the corporation ahead of their own personal interests. This does not bar a board member from ever benefiting from the corporation, such as by supplying certain services to the corporation—but the governing body must use great care to ensure that such arrangements are fair, fully disclosed, and the result of competitive bidding where possible. This is the reason behind conflict-of-interest policies in most corporations—such policies guard against practices that would call into question a board member's loyalty.

The **duty of responsibility** means that board members must act with due care in exercising their duties. They must attend meetings regularly, ensure that they understand the decisions under consideration, and perform **due diligence** (meaning they must exercise a legally acceptable level of care) in hiring key staff or appointing medical staff and in overseeing the performance of the corporation.

This does not mean that board members must not rely on the reports and assessments provided by the senior administrative staff, but they need to be active in asking appropriate questions and be willing to seek professional, independent advice when they suspect a problem.

An example may help clarify the difference. ABC Hospital's governing body selected a new chief executive officer who ultimately proved to be engaging in billing fraud. Was its selection a breach of its fiduciary duties? The answer depends on whether the decision was made with due care, in a responsible manner. If the governing body conducted an appropriate search for the position, checked relevant references and the candidate's background, and did not have undisclosed conflicts of interest in hiring the new CEO, it probably would not be liable for a breach of its fiduciary responsibilities. On the other hand, if ABC Hospital's governing body failed to conduct an appropriate candidate search and instead hired the friend of one of the board members on his recommendation alone, failing to check references and therefore never discovering evidence of past criminal activity by this candidate, the board members could be open to potential liability.

As long as board members fulfill their duties of loyalty and responsibility, they are generally protected from personal liability for their decisions. Corporate bylaws often indemnify the board members from personal liability for board decisions as well as some statutes. For example, the State of Tennessee has several statutes that provide protection to the board. The Tennessee Code for Nonprofit Corporations (T.C.A. 48-58-502) provides the authority to indemnify a board member of a corporation when the individual acts in the best interest and in good faith on behalf of the corporation. This means that if a board member faces a personal suit arising out of his or her board decisions, the corporation will pay for the associated expenses. However, the code also limits the immunity of members of the board for breach of their fiduciary duty (T.C.A. 48-58-601). Many corporations purchase insurance (directors' and officers' insurance) to protect their governing body and key officers from personal liability. But insurance will not protect board members from liability for gross negligence, intentional acts, or crimes.

Any decision by the governing body (or by corporation executives) that goes beyond the express or implied powers of the corporation is considered to be an ***ultra vires* act**, meaning "beyond the power of the corporation." *Ultra vires* acts are usually void and can be challenged. Governing body members (and corporation executives) can be held personally liable for any financial losses suffered by the corporation as an outcome of an *ultra vires* act that was taken with knowledge that the action was beyond their power or that was made in bad faith. The content of the minutes of the governing body can be extremely important in determining whether board members have satisfied their duties of loyalty and responsibility.

Restructuring an Organization

Governing body members may be called on to make decisions about the restructuring of an organization that occurs in the form of a merger, an acquisition, or a consolidation. While these types of restructuring are not uncommon in the healthcare arena due to organizations' needs to maintain financial stability or enhance marketability through a broader range of services, they are major undertakings that cannot be pursued without considering all the legal restrictions and ramifications, such as state corporation law and antitrust laws (discussed more fully later in this chapter). Mergers involve the absorption of one corporation by another where, theoretically, both corporations are similar in size and are in agreement. As an example, Riverview Hospital and Hilltop Hospital decide to merge. Riverview Hospital no longer exists as a separate entity but is now part of Hilltop Hospital. Acquisitions result in a similar consequence (that is, one company is subsumed by another), but they are often a takeover of a smaller organization by a larger organization. Consolidations involve the creation of a new corporation made up of two or more organizations that previously existed but then were dissolved (Showalter 2012). For example, Riverview Hospital consolidates with Hilltop Hospital. Both hospitals cease to exist, with a newly formed corporation—Rivertop Hospital—coming into existence.

Although individual department directors and managers may not be directly involved in the formation of the corporation or in governing bodies, they are sometimes called on to work on teams considering new joint ventures, or they may present information to the governing body. By understanding the overall corporate structure of the organization, and by appreciating the responsibilities of governing body members, they can help anticipate potential problems, questions, and the need for providing complete and accurate information for use in decision making.

Check Your Understanding 6.1

Instructions: Indicate whether the following statements are true or false (T or F).

1. The owners of a corporation are generally shielded from personal liability for the debts of the corporation, although the corporation itself can sue and be sued.

2. "Piercing the corporate veil" enables the owners of a corporation to be shielded from liability for wrongdoing committed through the corporation.

3. Fiduciary duty includes the duty of loyalty and the duty of responsibility.

4. A not-for-profit corporation is prohibited from making money.

5. A healthcare organization may not form as a partnership.

General Principles of Contracts

Healthcare administrators, directors, and managers often have the authority to enter into **contracts**. Corporations may also enter into contracts, and the articles of incorporation may specify who has the authority to approve contracts on behalf of the corporation, such as the chief executive officer. Contracts to purchase items or services are among the most common examples of contracts for which health information management and informatics professionals may be responsible (Rhodes and Hughes 2003). Sometimes an individual's contracting authority is limited by a dollar amount, with contracts involving greater sums requiring a higher level of approval. But because executing contracts is often part of one's job description, it is important to understand at least the basic principles of contracts. Many healthcare organizations use in-house counsel or outside legal counsel to advise on contractual matters, and it is also common to see corporate compliance officers and risk managers involved in reviewing potential contracts as well.

Elements of a Contract

As noted in chapter 5, a contract is a legally enforceable oral or written agreement. To be legally enforceable, it must comply with any applicable state and federal statutes and regulations, and it must meet the following conditions:

- It must describe an agreement between two or more persons or entities

- The agreement must include:

  — a valid **offer** (a communicated promise by one of the parties to do [or not do] something if the other party agrees to do [or not do] something)

  — **acceptance** of the offer (reflecting a meeting of the minds on terms that are sufficiently definite and complete)

  — **consideration** (what each party will receive from the other party in return for performing the obligations described in the contract)

Oral contracts, while valid if they meet these criteria, can be difficult to prove. Each party may claim a different recollection of the agreement. That is why requiring written contracts for important or high-value contracts is a wise practice.

In addition, the parties to the contract must be competent; that is, they must have the legal and mental capacity to contract (Pozgar 2011). Contracts can be either express (actually written or spoken) or implied. For example, if a patient makes an appointment to seek care at her physician's office, that act implies her offer—that if the office grants her that appointment, she will pay for the services she seeks. The physician's office confirming the appointment implies its acceptance of her offer.

Breach of Contract

Once a contract is effective, violations of one or more of its terms can result in a lawsuit alleging **breach of contract**. To prevail, the plaintiff seeking to prove the breach of contract must show that a valid contract was executed, the plaintiff met the requirements of the contract, the defendant failed to meet the requirements, and as a result, the plaintiff suffered an economic loss. This demonstrates why clear and complete contract terms are so important. If there was no true meeting of the minds, the contract would be considered invalid. Clear contract terms can help avoid nonperformance of both parties, by leaving no room for misinterpretations of the contract's terms.

Defenses for Nonperformance of a Contract

Not every instance of nonperformance will result in a finding of breach of contract. Defenses that can be raised for nonperformance include:

- Fraud—if the nonperforming party has been misled on a material fact or term of the contract and has been harmed by the misrepresentation, a breach of contract lawsuit will fail

- Mistake of fact—if both parties to the contract have relied on the mistake

- Duress—if unlawful threats or pressure was used to force a party to execute the contract

- Illegality—if the contract was for illegal purposes or against public policy (see below for additional information)

- Impossibility—if the contract required acts that were impossible to perform

Additional contracts that may fall under illegality nonperformance include exculpatory contracts and adhesion contracts. **Exculpatory contracts** contain clauses that seek to excuse a party in advance from any potential liability. For example, if a hospital admission consent form required the patient to waive in advance his or her right to sue the hospital in the event of a poor outcome, courts would generally void this clause or severely restrict its application because such agreements do not serve the public good. Another type of contract or clause that may be found against public policy are **adhesion contracts**, which, because the bargaining power between the parties is so unequal, essentially force the weaker party to agree to unfavorable terms because it cannot do without the stronger party's services. As an example, if a hospital were the only available medical facility within hundreds of miles, and it forced patients to sign an agreement to pay in full for all services before leaving the premises, such a provision would likely be struck down due to the unequal bargaining power of the parties.

It is important to keep in mind, however, that for a breach of contract lawsuit to go forward, it must be initiated within the statute of limitations (time period) for enforcing contract rights.

Remedies

If a breach of contract is found, the court's goal is to make the injured party whole. There are several potential remedies for breaches of contracts:

- Money damages (**compensatory damages**)—these damages attempt to return to the injured party the money it would have had, in the absence of the breach. But note that the injured party has a duty to mitigate, or reduce, the damages caused by the breach; it cannot simply do nothing so that the damages continue to increase.

- **Specific performance**—in some situations, an order requiring the breaching party to honor its contractual obligations is more desirable to the injured party than money damages. As a result, the court may order the breaching party to fulfill its obligations under the contract. This is often done via **injunction**, where the court orders a party to stop doing something (or in the case of a mandatory injunction, to do something) in order to prevent irreparable harm to the other party.

- **Arbitration**—it is increasingly common for contracts to call for arbitration of disputes as an alternative to lawsuits. In arbitration, a neutral party is agreed upon by the parties, hears the facts, and resolves the dispute. Arbitration may be binding or nonbinding on the parties—in other words, the contract may specify that the arbitrator's decision must be honored by the parties, or it may simply make the arbitrator's decision advisory in nature, with the option to proceed to lawsuit if an agreement cannot be reached.

Contract Provisions

Certain clauses are often found in contracts to help insulate and protect the parties from economic harm. Two of the most common provisions are hold harmless/indemnification clauses and warranties.

Hold Harmless/Indemnification Clauses

The purpose of **hold harmless/indemnification clauses** is to either transfer or assume liability. For example, the indemnitor (party assuming liability) may agree to hold the other party harmless against claims arising from the indemnitor's own actions or failures to act. This means that if actions (or inactions) result in harm to the other party, the indemnitor will seek to make that party whole, often through some sort of compensation. Or, the parties may agree to hold each other harmless for each other's actions/inactions. These clauses can be useful in clarifying each party's obligations under the contract, but if not understood and carefully executed, they can greatly expand one's potential liability under the contract (for example, by making one party potentially liable to indemnify the other party).

One often sees these clauses in contracts between healthcare organizations and vendors that provide products such as EHR systems or a special piece of equipment for diagnostic purposes. For example, the contract might read, "Hospital agrees to indemnify, defend, and hold harmless the Vendor and its officers, directors, agents, and employees from and against any and all demands, claims, and damages to persons or property, losses and liabilities, including reasonable attorney's fees, arising out of or caused by Hospital's negligence or willful misconduct."

Clauses of this nature can have a substantial impact on potential liability; thus, they should be reviewed closely by legal counsel.

Warranties

All contracts include representations or **warranties** of some sort, which are statements of facts existing at the time the contract is made. These statements are made by one party to induce the other party to enter into the contract. Typically, these statements relate to the quality of goods or services purchased or leased. For example, a software company may warrant that its product will perform as described in its technical manuals for a period of x years. If within that period the software fails to perform as described in the manual, the software company agrees to fix the problem or replace the software.

Warranties can be "express," as in the above example, where a statement is actually made from the seller to the buyer to promise performance or describe goods or services. Warranties may also be "implied" by law. For example, the Uniform Commercial Code section 2-314 states in part: "(1) Unless excluded or modified . . . a warranty that the goods shall be merchantable is implied in a contract for their sale if the seller is a merchant with respect to goods of that kind." And for the goods to be considered merchantable, they must be "fit for the ordinary purposes for which such goods are used." Section 2-315 describes an implied warranty of "fitness for a particular purpose," meaning that when the seller has reason to know any particular purpose for which the goods are required, and the buyer is relying on the seller's skill or judgment to furnish suitable goods, there is an implied warranty that the goods being sold will be fit for such purpose—as long as the buyer's reliance on that skill or judgment is reasonable.

Warranties may also be disclaimed by the seller by doing so in the contract. This is just one of many reasons why persons involved in negotiating contracts should seek assistance from counsel to understand the potential impact of the terms they are considering.

Health Information Technology Contracts

HIT contracts have been the subject of substantial concern as healthcare organizations adopt EHRs and other information technologies. Some commentators have noted that the terms within contracts for HIT are inadequate to protect purchasers or lessors from liability—even from problems directly attributable to the software or hardware. Healthcare organizations sometimes sign purchase/lease contracts without adequate review or negotiation of terms, accepting the **boilerplate**, or standard, vendor-written terms, which highly favor the HIT vendor. Koppel and Kreda (2009) reported serious liability concerns resulting from contractual terms that shift liability to the system users—even when the users are following vendor instructions for use. The vendors rely on the doctrine of "learned intermediaries" and on warranties prohibiting claims against their own products' fitness. **Learned intermediary** is a defense doctrine that "companies have a duty to warn physicians directly about potential adverse effects caused by their products, while physicians must serve as 'learned intermediaries' who interpret this information and advise patients appropriately" (Gemperli 2000). The doctrine is mainly used as a defense for pharmaceutical companies and medical device manufacturers.

What places the purchaser and subsequent user of an HIT product in an even more difficult position is that information sharing about HIT defects has been difficult in the past. Silverstein et al. (2007) noted that websites addressing HIT failures are very rare. More recently, however, American Health Information Management Association (AHIMA) and American Medical Informatics Association (AMIA) published a book on lessons learned from failed HIT implementation activities (Leviss 2009). Additional contract difficulties and HIT failures are further noted on a website maintained by Silverstein (1999–2010) in cooperation with AMIA's clinical information systems working group. To further address these concerns, the AMIA Board of Directors appointed a task force to provide recommendations ranging from stakeholder responsibilities and defect reporting to meaningful use standards and unintended consequences of HIT in an effort to help resolve issues related to vendor-user contracts and subsequent interactions (Goodman et al. 2010).

Concern regarding HIT contracts points to the need for careful review of contracts by someone familiar with contract law and, ideally, HIT issues. As mentioned in the AMIA task force report, there are many issues that could affect HIT purchasers and HIT vendors that both parties need to address. Healthcare providers who rely on HIT must pay close attention to these issues as greater reliance on HIT becomes the standard for information sharing and communication in healthcare.

Physician–Patient Relationship as a Contract

Courts have found that the physician–patient relationship itself is a form of contract. The physician agrees to provide services in exchange for payment. This contract can either be express (for example, a patient signs a consent to have the physician treat him and agrees to pay the bill) or implied (an unconscious patient is brought into the urgicenter, and the physician treats him). This contract imposes certain duties on the physician to treat the patient. However, physicians are not obligated to treat those with whom they have not established this contract. In other words, they do not have to treat those with whom they have not established a physician–patient relationship. A physician attending a party has no obligation to respond to or treat someone because that person has talked about his or her symptoms with the physician. Also, a physician offering informal consultation to a colleague about a patient the colleague is treating has no contractual obligation to the patient who is the subject of that informal consultation. However, if the consultation were a more formal one (for example, the consultant examined the patient, a specimen, or a tissue sample), and the physician was billing for those services, courts would find that a contractual relationship exists.

Physician warranties to a patient about the certainty of a particular outcome can also give rise to claims of breach of warranty contract. If, for example, the physician says to the patient, "You should have this surgery. And don't worry, I promise you will be pain-free a week after the knee replacement," and the patient relies on that promise and therefore has the surgery, the existence of pain beyond a week after the surgery would be grounds for a breach of contract lawsuit.

The existence of a physician–patient relationship as a form of contract is not everlasting. The relationship can be terminated by action of either party, such as when the patient ceases treatment or dies, when the parties mutually agree to end the relationship, when the patient dismisses or "fires" the physician, or when the physician dismisses the patient from his or her care. The physician must exercise care in terminating a physician–patient relationship to avoid claims based on abandonment of care. If, for example, a physician terminates the patient from his or her practice abruptly, without giving the patient time to secure another source of care, this can be considered abandonment. But if the physician notifies the patient in writing, gives him or her adequate time to secure other care and agrees to see the patient in the meantime, and cooperates in sharing relevant information with the new care provider once selected by the patient, the physician can likely avoid claims of abandonment.

Reasons vary for termination of physician–patient relationships. Some patients simply do not like the physician they have selected and therefore elect to leave the practice. Some physicians choose to terminate relationships with patients who repeatedly refuse to follow their medical advice or who are verbally abusive to the practice staff. Abandonment cases do make it clear, however, that once a physician–patient relationship has been established, a clear, careful stepwise approach to terminating the relationship will make abandonment claims more defensible.

Check Your Understanding 6.2

Instructions: Indicate whether the following statements are true or false (T or F).

1. A "hold harmless" clause may provide for compensation by one individual to another.

2. A breach of contract judgment always requires monetary compensation.

3. An acceptance of an offer reflects a meeting of the minds regarding the contract terms.

4. To be valid, a contract must be in writing.

5. Mistake of fact is a potential defense for nonperformance of a contract.

General Principles of Antitrust Law

To understand how antitrust laws affect healthcare organizations and their medical staffs, it is important to have a basic understanding of three federal antitrust statutes: the Sherman Act, the Clayton Act, and the Federal Trade Commission Act. These statutes seek to protect the public against trusts and monopolies that are so large they have the power to control a market, and thereby restrict free trade and freedom of choice. If, for example, a single healthcare organization controlled all healthcare services in a single market, the consumer would be at the mercy of the pricing and practices of the monopoly, simply because the monopoly controlled the market. This can result in inflated prices, and even in poor quality, because there essentially is no competition.

The Sherman Act

The general purpose of the **Sherman Act** (15 USC 1 et seq), which has been in effect since 1890, is to prevent restraints of trade among the states (or with foreign countries). It does so in Section 1 of the act by declaring that "every contract . . . or conspiracy, in restraint of trade or commerce among the several states, or with foreign nations, is . . . illegal." Section 2 of the act seeks to prevent monopolies in a market. Restraints of trade can be classified as either horizontal or vertical. In a **vertical restraint of trade**, two or more entities at different levels in a distribution chain act together to restrain trade (for example, a manufacturer of hospital supplies collaborates with a wholesaler to keep prices artificially high). In a **horizontal restraint of trade**, competitors agree to fix prices, divide the market (for example, "I will serve residents on the west side of town only; you serve them on the east side"), or try to exclude others from competing in the same market. Section 1 of the act applies to joint actions (two or more parties), while Section 2 can apply to a single organization. For example, if a healthcare organization attempts to create a monopoly, even if the actions it takes are solely its own and not in concert with any other organization, it can be found in violation of the Sherman Act.

The Clayton Act

Because the language of the Sherman Act was very broad, and therefore was being used in unintended ways (notably union-busting), Congress passed the **Clayton Act** (15 USC 12 et seq) 24 years later, in 1914. The Clayton Act exempted union activities from antitrust laws, but it also prohibited, among other things, discriminatory pricing practices (where different purchasers are given different prices for commodities of like grade and quality, where the effect of that pricing practice is to lessen competition—but note that there are many important exceptions to this prohibition), tying arrangements (exclusive dealing contracts where the selling party requires the buyer to not use or deal in the goods or commodities of a competitor, where the effect lessens competition), and mergers and acquisitions that reduce competition.

The Federal Trade Commission Act

The **Federal Trade Commission (FTC) Act** (15 USC 41-58), also passed in 1914, gave the FTC broad powers to act against organizations engaging in unfair methods of competition, or unfair or deceptive acts that affect commerce (including advertising). Practices that could apply to healthcare organizations include:

- Failing to reveal material facts about a product
- Making false claims and misrepresentations
- Offering misleading prices
- Disparaging a competitor's product by making misleading or untrue assertions
- Presenting advertising that is intended to attract a customer who will then be switched to a higher-priced product (Showalter 2012)

Rule of Reason and Per Se Violations

Not all restraints of trade are actual antitrust violations. For example, by virtue of having a superior product or services, an organization may lawfully dominate a local market. If antitrust challenges are raised for activities that are *not* automatically considered to be antitrust violations (automatic violations are called **per se antitrust violations** and include price fixing, division of markets, group boycotts, and tying arrangements), courts apply a **rule of reason analysis** to determine whether an antitrust violation exists. This analysis considers the geographic markets affected and the product/service market involved, the nature of the industry, the motivation for the allegedly illegal activity, and the impact of the activity on the industry.

Enforcement and Applicability to Healthcare Organizations

The Sherman Act offers both civil and criminal penalty options, while the Clayton Act offers only civil remedies. The FTC Act, on the other hand, is enforced only by the FTC and offers no private right of action at all. In any event, certain types of common activities within healthcare organizations can give rise to possible antitrust concerns:

- Health planning, which can raise restraint of trade issues

- Shared services, which can raise possible issues of price fixing or group boycott

- Utilization review, which can involve possible group boycott

- Medical staff privileging/credentialing, which can involve possible group boycott (and is discussed in greater detail below)

- Third-party payer contracts or managed care organizations, which can involve possible price fixing, group boycott, and monopolization

- Mergers and consolidations, which can involve possible monopolization of a market (Showalter 2012, 407)

In 1996 the Department of Justice and the FTC provided additional guidance for healthcare organizations by publishing "Statements of Antitrust Enforcement Policy in Health Care." The paper recognized the benefits of economy of scale in hospital mergers and set in force nine "safety zones" of activity that will ordinarily not be challenged by these federal agencies. These safety zones are outlined in figure 6.2. It is important for healthcare executives to understand the kinds of activities that can raise the specter of antitrust so that assistance can be sought in structuring these activities in ways that do not violate the law.

Figure 6.2. Healthcare antitrust safety zones

• Mergers involving small hospitals (where one has fewer than 100 beds and average census of fewer than 40 patients) • Joint ventures for expensive or high-tech equipment • Joint ventures to offer specialized services • Efforts to provide medical data • Provision of healthcare fee/price information to purchasers of health services • Surveys about prices, wages, and benefits • Joint purchasing arrangements between healthcare organizations • Exclusive and nonexclusive joint ventures with physician networks • Multiprovider networks (although these are evaluated under the rule of reason)

Source: Showalter 2012, 417.

Contract and Antitrust Issues Associated with the Medical Staff

Although the credentialing process itself is covered in chapter 16, healthcare organizations must take care to ensure that the process of credentialing and delineating privileges does not raise antitrust concerns. Antitrust-related claims sometimes grow out of a denial of staff privileges or a restriction of credentials—either denial of an individual application for privileges or credentials, or denial of an entire category or type of practitioner, such as bylaws that would deny privileges to "all chiropractors."

In this kind of litigation, the plaintiff seeks to prove anticompetitive effects from the action denying membership or privileges. The potential monetary damages associated with successful claims can be substantial. Because of this, care must be exercised not only in drafting medical staff bylaws and associated rules and regulations, but also in adhering to them at all times when considering medical staff applications and requests for privileges. Broad bylaws language that seeks to exclude an entire class of practitioners can be seen as a group boycott, which, if proven, is a per se violation of antitrust laws, as noted above. Even individual denials can raise antitrust issues when existing medical staff members seek to limit the number of certain types of potential competitors on staff (for example, the Credentials Committee chair is a neurosurgeon, and he takes action to ensure that all other neurosurgeon applications for staff membership and privileges are denied, in order to ensure his own market share).

Bylaws should clearly set forth the process for granting medical and professional staff membership and clinical privileges, and the process must require a thorough investigation of all applicable qualifications and clinical performance. Some organizations also consider the volume of certain types of cases treated by that physician or surgeon in deciding whether to grant specific privileges, sometimes because they want to secure the loyalty of that practitioner in using the hospital's facilities. This is sometimes referred to as **economic credentialing** (if that information is unrelated to clinical performance issues), and the appropriateness of using volume data is a matter of dispute. The issues of quality and volume are not completely unrelated, however. In some situations, the number of certain types of procedures performed is arguably linked to clinical performance and quality issues. Certain medical specialty societies have stated that the number of procedures performed is a relevant consideration in granting initial and renewal privileges (American Society for Gastrointestinal Endoscopy 2002).

The tension between physician loyalty and economic credentialing—and ultimately a hospital's bottom line—has been apparent in the proliferation of physician-owned hospitals, where community hospitals have resisted the referral of more profitable patients by physicians to facilities where those physicians have an ownership stake. In certain instances, physician privileges have been revoked via economic credentialing based on perceived loss of loyalty and financial conflict of interest. However, the 2010 Patient Protection and Affordable Care Act (that is, health reform) has significantly limited the ability of physicians to invest in hospitals, which may reverse the tendency for physicians to have a stake in owning a hospital.

The criteria for granting or denying specific privileges are often left to each clinical department to determine, but they must be fair, not violate the rights of any federally protected class of persons, and not be designed to favor those already on staff or restrain competition by keeping otherwise qualified practitioners off the staff. The steps should include a mechanism to request and hold a fair hearing in the event a physician wishes to challenge an adverse decision. Having some sort of internal mechanism for impartial review of the decision (by elevating those disputes to the full Medical Executive Committee and ultimately to the organization's Board of Directors) can aid in preventing antitrust-related litigation, by helping to ensure that the decision is not based on anticompetitive motivations.

Antitrust issues arise not only with independent medical staff members but also with employed physicians and other professionals. Employment agreements can be found to be anticompetitive if they are too restrictive in their terms. For example, **noncompete agreements**—in which an individual agrees not to compete directly or work for a competitor for a certain period of time after leaving his or her employment—can be subject to antitrust litigation if they are too restrictive. In *Emergicare Systems Corporation v. Bourdon*, Emergicare contracted to provide emergency physicians, including Dr. Bourdon, to Longview Regional Hospital for a period of years. In October 1991, Emergicare wrote to Bourdon to confirm that it would terminate the agreement with Longview on November 8, 1991, and accordingly, Dr. Bourdon's agreement with Emergicare would also terminate. Bourdon then contacted Longview and arranged to stay on as an emergency physician, through a new arrangement with Metroplex Emergency Physicians. Emergicare then sued Bourdon and Metroplex, alleging that Bourdon breached a covenant not to compete with Emergicare. The trial court ruled in Bourdon and Metroplex's favor, noting that the covenant sought to restrict Bourdon from working within five miles of any clinic operated by Emergicare, whether the physician ever worked in that clinic or not. The covenant also sought to restrict Bourdon from working in any emergency department where Emergicare provided services for one year following termination of Emergicare's contract. On appeal, the appellate court affirmed the trial court's decision, finding the noncompete agreement "too restrictive" and thus an unreasonable restraint of trade.

This does not mean that all noncompete agreements are invalid, but they must be narrowly drawn in order to avoid an effect that restrains trade.

Check Your Understanding 6.4

Instructions: Indicate whether the following statements are true or false (T or F).

1. Economic credentialing is the granting of medical staff privileges based on quality of care indicators.

2. Antitrust claims are valid only if they relate to an entire group of individuals who have been denied privileges at a healthcare organization.

3. A group boycott is a per se antitrust violation.

4. Courts uphold all noncompete agreements in order to protect the livelihood of organizations that have had an employee or a contractor leave for other opportunities.

5. The number of procedures performed by a provider may be linked to clinical performance and quality issues when determining medical staff privileges.

Summary

Administrators, managers, and department directors of healthcare organizations are often responsible for taking actions that have legal implications. To function under the protection of the law, healthcare organizations often define their legal status as a corporation. In so doing, they may choose to function as either a for-profit or not-for-profit entity, both of which have certain responsibilities that the organization must adhere to in order to maintain its corporate status. The benefit of a corporation is that it is a legal entity or "person" under the law. This status generally provides owners with some form of legal protection from personal liability for the debts of the corporation, although the corporation itself can both sue and be sued. To carry out the organization's business, it may enter into contracts, which are legally enforceable oral or written agreements between parties. To be legally enforceable, contracts must comply with applicable state and federal statutes and regulations, which often spell out defenses for nonperformance of the contract and remedies for breach of contract. As healthcare organizations and providers adopt EHR systems, issues related to HIT vendor contracts have surfaced regarding ways in which contracts can or cannot protect the organization or provider from problems arising from HIT applications. In addition to contracting issues, healthcare organizations may face potential antitrust or compliance implications. The Sherman Act, the Clayton Act, and the Federal Trade Commission Act are statutes that seek to protect the public from trusts and monopolies that have the power to control a market, and thereby restrict free trade and freedom of choice. Healthcare organizations must be cognizant of antitrust issues when credentialing and delineating medical staff privileges. Antitrust-related claims sometimes grow out of a denial of staff privileges or restriction of credentials. Thus, care must be exercised not only in drafting medical staff bylaws and associated rules and regulations, but also in adhering to them at all times when considering medical staff applications and requests for privileges.

References

American Society for Gastrointestinal Endoscopy. 2002. Methods of granting hospital privileges to perform gastrointestinal endoscopy. *Gastrointestinal Endoscopy* 55(7):780–783.

Fletcher, W. 1983. *Cyclopedia of the Law of Private Corporations*, section 43.10.

Gemperli, M. 2000. Rethinking the role of the learned intermediary: The effect of direct-to-consumer advertising on litigation. *Journal of AMA* 284(17):2241.

Goodman, K., E. Berner, M. Dente, B. Kaplan, R. Koppel, D. Rucker, D. Sands, and P. Wunkelstein. 2010. Challenges in ethics, safety, best practices, and oversight regarding HIT vendors, their customers, and patients: A report of an AMIA special task force. *Journal of AMIA*. http://jamia.bmj.com.

Koppel, R., and D. Kreda. 2009. Health care information technology vendors' hold harmless clause. *Journal of AMA* 301(12):1276–1278.

Leviss, J., ed. 2009. *H.I.T. or Miss: Lessons Learned from Health Information Technology Implementations.* Chicago: AHIMA.

Peregrine, M. 2009. Overview of the "community benefit" standard of federal tax exempt status. Washington, DC: American Healthcare Lawyers Association. http://publish.healthlawyers.org.

Pozgar, G. 2011. *Legal Aspects of Health Care Administration*, 11th ed. Sudbury, MA: Jones and Bartlett.

Rhodes, H., and G. Hughes. 2003. Practice brief: Letters of agreements and contracts. Chicago: AHIMA. Online extra.

Showalter, J.S. 2012. *The Law of Healthcare Administration*, 6th ed. Chicago: Health Administration Press.

Silverstein, S. 1999–2010. Contemporary issues in medical informatics: Common examples of healthcare information technology difficulties. Philadelphia: Drexel University. http://www.ischool.drexel.edu.

Silverstein, S., Y. Chen, and C. Wania. 2007. Access patterns to a website on healthcare IT failure. IST Research Day 2007 posters. Philadelphia: Drexel University College of Information Science and Technology. http://idea.library.drexel.edu.

Cases, Statutes, and Regulations Cited

Emergicare Systems Corporation v. Bourdon, 942 S.W. 2d 201 (Tex. App. 1997).

Provena Covenant Medical Center v. Department of Revenue, 2010 WL 966858, 10 (2010).

15 UCC 2-314-15: Uniform Commercial Code.

15 USC 1-7: Sherman Act. 1890.

15 USC 12-27: Clayton Act. 1914.

15 USC 41-58: Federal Trade Commission Act. 1914.

Patient Protection and Affordable Care Act (2010). Public Law 111–148.

T.C.A. 48-58-502: Authority to indemnify. 1987.

T.C.A. 48-58-601: Limitation of and immunity from actions for breach of fiduciary duty. 1986.

Chapter 7

Consent to Treatment

Jill Callahan Klaver, JD, RHIA

Learning Objectives

- Distinguish between express and implied consent

- Identify the components of informed consent

- Define and discuss the various types of advance directives

- Discuss the consent rights and limitations of competent adults and incompetent adults

- Discuss the consent rights and limitations of minors

- Describe the legal bases for challenging consent

- Discuss how consent should be documented

- Identify different types of consent forms

Key Terms

Advance directive
Consent
Do not resuscitate (DNR) order
Durable power of attorney (DPOA)
Durable power of attorney for healthcare decisions (DPOA-HCD)
Express consent
General consent

Genetic Information Nondiscrimination Act (GINA)
Good Samaritan statute
Health Insurance Portability and Accountability Act (HIPAA)
Implied consent
Informed consent
Institutional review board (IRB)
Living will

Long form
Non compos mentis
Patient Self-Determination Act (PSDA)
Power of attorney (POA)
Short form
Therapeutic privilege
Uniform Anatomical Gift Act (UAGA)
Uniform Health-Care Decisions Act (UHCDA)

Introduction

One of the most valued rights in American society is the right to control one's own body, especially when it comes to medical decision making. Individuals have the right to **consent** or refuse consent to medical treatment whether that treatment is minor or lifesaving. However, rights surrounding consent are not absolute and can be affected by factors such as age, competence, and emergency circumstances.

The law governing consent is found in both state and federal statutes as well as case law. Anyone working in healthcare must be knowledgeable about the ethical and applicable legal principles of consent. As this chapter will discuss, providing treatment without proper consent may result in liability for battery or negligence.

Types of Consent

When thinking about consent in healthcare, most people think of the patient signing a form that gives a healthcare provider permission to perform a test or procedure. However, consent is a broad process that can be in written or nonwritten form and can vary in terms of how much information is provided. In most cases, consent involves a patient's acknowledgement that he or she understands a proposed intervention, including that intervention's risks, benefits, and alternatives. In other cases, such as emergency circumstances or legal matters, consent may be provided through the operation of law rather than individual choice.

Express Consent

Express consent refers to consent that is communicated through words, whether written or spoken. An individual may show express consent through written documentation or by orally agreeing to an intervention. While both forms of express consent are valid, written consent is more desirable than oral consent from an evidentiary standpoint. The passage of time, a medical condition, or sheer forgetfulness can affect an individual's ability to recall the details of an orally expressed consent. In disputes where consent is an issue, this can lead to conflicting accounts as to the information discussed by a provider or questions raised by a patient during the oral consent process. When written consents are used, the evidence regarding the information provided is stronger. However, just because a consent is in written format does not mean that the patient's consent was informed. Express consents, whether oral or written, must provide the patient with enough information to make an informed decision regarding medical treatment. A detailed discussion of informed consent is found below.

Implied Consent

Implied consent refers to consent for medical treatment that is communicated through a person's conduct or some other means besides words. For example, most physicians do not directly ask the patient for express written or oral consent prior to conducting a basic physical examination or minor office procedure. However, the patient still communicates consent through his or her conduct: scheduling and arriving for the appointment and submitting to the exam or procedure without objection. Implied consent is most appropriate for interventions that are noninvasive and very low risk. As interventions become more invasive or risky, providers should obtain a patient's express written informed consent. For implied consent to be valid from an evidentiary standpoint, the patient's conduct and surrounding circumstances must create a reasonable belief that consent was given.

Another form of implied consent occurs in emergency situations where an individual may be unconscious or otherwise lacks capacity to communicate consent. In these cases, consent is implied by the law rather than the patient's words or conduct. The law creates a presumption that incapacitated individuals would consent to medical treatment and protects providers who treat these individuals from lawsuits based on lack of consent. Implied consent is limited in nature, and consent in this kind of situation is discussed more later in this chapter. Many states also have implied consent laws related to operating motor vehicles. These laws are aimed at protecting the public and typically state that by obtaining a license to operate a vehicle, drivers imply consent to a breath, blood, or urine test at the request of a law enforcement officer (Oregon Department of Motor Vehicles n.d.).

Informed Consent

Whether given orally or in writing, a patient's consent should be informed. In other words, an **informed consent** means the patient should have a basic understanding of what medical procedures or tests may be performed as well as the risks, benefits, and alternatives for those tests or procedures. It also implies that the individual who is being asked to give his or her informed consent is competent to give such a consent and that the consent must be voluntary. However, the amount of information provided during the consent process can vary. Sometimes information provided to the patient is tailored to a specific test or procedure and is quite detailed. In other cases, such as when it is not known what interventions may be necessary, the information provided to the patient is more generalized. For example, when patients are admitted to the hospital, they often sign a **general consent** form authorizing hospital staff to perform the underlying tests and interventions necessary for overall medical care. This general consent must be supplemented with informed consents for the more invasive tests, operations, and other interventions that care may entail.

Requirements

The type and amount of information that should be disclosed to a patient during the consent process is determined by the applicable standard of care, including the Centers for Medicare and Medicaid Services (CMS) Hospital Guidelines requirements. In other words, a provider should give the patient the same information that a reasonable provider would disclose under the same or similar circumstances. Communication between the patient and provider is paramount to obtaining informed consent. The American Medical Association suggests that physicians should disclose and discuss:

- The patient's diagnosis, if known

- The nature and purpose of a proposed treatment or procedure

- The risks and benefits of a proposed treatment or procedure

- Alternatives (regardless of their cost or the extent to which the treatment options are covered by health insurance)

- The risks and benefits of the alternative treatment or procedure

- The risks and benefits of not receiving or undergoing a treatment or procedure (AMA n.d.).

The communication process also involves answering any questions a patient may have about a proposed intervention or lack of intervention. Patients may wish to consider the questions presented in figure 7.1.

Documentation of informed consent is important to ensure a complete and accurate health record that is legally sound and evidences quality patient care. Although the informed consent process itself may span several days by being initiated before a treatment or procedure is actually scheduled, the signed consent form becomes part of the patient's health record. For quality and legal purposes, the presence of signed informed consent forms for procedures should be verified by operating room or special procedures room staff before the physician is permitted to begin the procedure. The presence of a signed consent form in a patient's health record is also important for CMS and Joint Commission surveys. The Joint Commission requires that an executed informed consent be placed in the patient's health record prior to surgery unless it is not possible to do so because of an emergency.

Figure 7.1. Questions for patients to ask regarding informed consent

- What is the condition, disease, or problem called?
- How do you recommend treating it?
- What are the risks of this type of treatment?
- What are the benefits?
- What is the complication (morbidity) rate for this treatment?
- What is the mortality (death) rate for patients in my condition using this treatment?
- What other treatments are available? Why are those not recommended?
- What will happen if I don't do anything?
- How many patients have you cared for with this problem? How many patients have you performed this surgery or this test on?
- What is your success rate in treating this problem?
- If I undergo this treatment, will it prevent me from using an alternative treatment if needed?
- Are you board certified in the specialty that treats this disease or condition?
- What can I expect if I undergo this treatment?
  —Will I be able to work and/or care for myself?
  —Will my activities be restricted?
  —How much pain or discomfort will I be in?
  —Will this treatment cause other problems?
  —What kind of side effects should I expect?
  —What should I do if I experience side effects?
  —Will you personally perform the surgery, test, or procedure?
  —Is anesthesia necessary?
  —Who will be the anesthesiologist?
- What can I expect if I don't undergo this treatment?
- What are the alternatives to this treatment?
- What are the potential risks, complications, or side effects associated with the alternative treatment?

Source: The California Patient's Guide n.d.

If a proposed medical intervention is related to a research study, then a federal law known as the Common Rule imposes specific requirements designed to protect participants in that research. Under this law, any research on human subjects must be approved by an **institutional review board** (IRB). An IRB is a committee of at least five members with varying backgrounds that determines the acceptability of proposed research in accordance with institutional policies, applicable law, and standards of professional practice and conduct (45 CFR 46.107). Among other standards, the Common Rule requires researchers to obtain informed consent from study participants. The informed consent document required by the IRB and signed by the patient is typically a separate document from the consent form for the procedure being performed. The latter consent form is to be included in the individual's health record. The basic elements of an informed consent for human subjects research include:

- A statement that the study involves research, an explanation of the purposes of the research and the expected duration of the subject's participation, a description of the procedures to be followed, and identification of any procedures which are experimental

- A description of any reasonably foreseeable risks or discomforts to the subject

- A description of any benefits to the subject or to others which may reasonably be expected from the research

- A disclosure of appropriate alternative procedures or courses of treatment, if any, that might be advantageous to the subject

- A statement describing the extent, if any, to which confidentiality of records identifying the subject will be maintained

- For research involving more than minimal risk, an explanation as to whether any compensation and an explanation as to whether any medical treatments are available if injury occurs and, if so, what they consist of, or where further information may be obtained

- An explanation of whom to contact for answers to pertinent questions about the research and research subjects' rights, and whom to contact in the event of a research-related injury to the subject

- A statement that participation is voluntary, refusal to participate will involve no penalty or loss of benefits to which the subject is otherwise entitled, and the subject may discontinue participation at any time without penalty or loss of benefits to which the subject is otherwise entitled (45 CFR 46.116)

When appropriate and required by an IRB, additional informed consent elements may be required, such as study withdrawal procedures, costs to participants, and potential conflicts of interest (45 CFR 46.116(b)).

It is important to note that consent to participate in research also involves consent to disclose medical information related to that research. In other words, study participants consent not only to the medical intervention itself, but also to the use and disclosure of their medical information for purposes of the research study. As discussed in chapter 9, the HIPAA Privacy Rule provides a framework for disclosures of medical information related to research. Medical information includes written documentation about an identifiable individual; it also includes an individual's bodily materials, such as blood and tissue samples. Unless a waiver is granted by an IRB, researchers must obtain consent prior to using human tissue specimens for research (NCI n.d.a).

IRB-approved informed consent may include restrictions on the rights of participants to access their health information during the study process. These restrictions should be noted in patients' health records.

Exceptions to Informed Consent

In most situations, healthcare providers who fail to properly obtain informed consent prior to performing a medical intervention run the risk of liability for battery or negligence. Lawsuits for battery are most often based on performing an intervention with no permission at all (such as performing a tubal ligation without consent during a Caesarean section). Negligence-based lawsuits are often based on failure to fully inform the patient of a risk, benefit, or alternative, resulting in harm to the patient (such as failing to inform a patient that nonsurgical options exist for managing a medical condition, causing the patient to undergo unnecessary surgery). Both types of lawsuits will be discussed later in the chapter. In some situations, it is not feasible for a healthcare provider to obtain informed consent prior to performing an intervention. To accommodate such situations, the law has established exceptions to the general requirement that informed consent is necessary.

Emergency Situations

As discussed earlier, the law permits a presumption of consent during emergency situations whether the patient is an adult or a minor. However, that presumption of consent is not unlimited. Healthcare providers should rely on that presumption only to address true emergencies, such as conditions posing a threat to the patient's life or the risk of permanent loss of function. Aspects of the patient's care that can await the patient's express consent should do so. For example, an emergency room physician wouldn't proceed with an elective procedure unrelated to the emergency, simply because the person accompanying the unconscious patient to the emergency room indicates that the patient would like that done too. Most states have some form of a **"Good Samaritan" statute** that protects various types of healthcare providers from liability for failing to obtain informed consent before rendering care to adults or minors at the scene of an emergency or accident. The rationale for Good Samaritan laws is that they are necessary in order to ensure that providers are not deterred from rendering aid at accident scenes for fear of being sued for battery or negligence. An example of a Good Samaritan law is provided below (Mo. Rev. Stat. 537.037; subsections 3 and 4 omitted):

> Any physician or surgeon, registered professional nurse or licensed practical nurse licensed to practice in this state . . . or licensed to practice under the equivalent laws of any other state and any person licensed as a mobile emergency medical technician . . . may:
>
> 1. In good faith render emergency care or assistance, without compensation, at the scene of an emergency or accident, and shall not be liable for any civil damages for acts or omissions other than damages occasioned by gross negligence or by willful or wanton acts or omissions by such person in rendering such emergency care;
>
> 2. In good faith render emergency care or assistance, without compensation, to any minor involved in an accident, or in competitive sports, or other emergency at the scene of an accident, without first obtaining the consent of the parent or guardian of the minor, and shall not be liable for any civil damages other than damages occasioned by gross negligence or by willful or wanton acts or omissions by such person in rendering the emergency care.

Governmental Action

Sometimes an individual's consent to a medical exam or intervention is not freely given, but is instead ordered by a court or through some other governmental action. This situation most often arises when the welfare of the public outweighs the individual's right to withhold consent.

Criminal Cases

In many states, drivers who have been pulled over must consent to blood alcohol tests when asked to do so by police officers. For example, in Oregon, if an individual refuses to consent, the government may suspend his or her driver's license for a certain period (for example, one to three years) and may use the refusal to consent as evidence against the individual in court in a driving under the influence case (Oregon Department of Motor Vehicles n.d.). This is because the government's interest in protecting the public from drivers under the influence outweighs an individual driver's right to refuse consent. This exception may also be interpreted as an implied consent, as described earlier in the chapter.

The government may also order individuals to undergo specific medical tests or interventions when certain infectious diseases may be involved (such as HIV or hepatitis B). For example, under Kansas law, if an individual has been convicted of a crime that may have involved the transmission of bodily fluids from one person to another, a court may order that individual to submit to infectious disease tests (KS Stat. Ann. 65-6009). Again, the government's interest in protecting the public from certain infectious diseases outweighs certain individuals' right to refuse consent to tests for infectious disease.

Civil Cases

In cases where the mental or physical condition of a party is at issue, courts may order a party to submit to physical or mental examinations. Courts must have "good cause" for ordering these exams and generally must specify the time, place, manner, conditions, and scope of such examinations, as well as identify the physician who will conduct the examination (for example, see MO Rev. Stat. 510.040).

Cases Involving Mental Competence

States generally have detailed laws regarding procedures for making competency determinations and committing or providing other means of treatment for mentally ill individuals. Generally, these laws provide for involuntary examinations, treatment, and detainment of individuals with mental illness who are in danger of causing harm to themselves or others (for example, see KS Stat. Ann. 59-2953, 2954). The laws also provide the framework for conducting court-ordered mental evaluations where there is a reasonable basis for the belief that an individual is **non compos mentis** (not of sound mind) and may no longer have legal competence to make their own decisions. If an individual is found to be mentally ill, then the courts may order appropriate treatment (for example, see KS Stat. Ann. 59-2966). Here, the government's interest in protecting the mentally ill individual as well as others who may be placed in danger by that mentally ill individual outweighs that individual's right to refuse medical examinations and treatment.

Courts may order psychiatric or psychological examinations of defendants in criminal cases when determining whether the defendant is competent to stand trial (for example, see KS Stat. Ann. 22-3302). Likewise, if a defendant pleads an insanity defense, he or she will be required to submit to psychiatric or psychological examinations in order to substantiate the claim of insanity (for example, see MO Rev. Stat. 522.030).

Waiver

Although legal cases have recognized the ability of a patient to waive the right to informed consent, this practice subjects a provider to legal risks that are simply better avoided altogether by securing an informed consent. Waiver of informed consent must be patient-initiated, associated only with low-risk treatments, completed only if the patient affirms that he or she would subject himself or herself to the treatment regardless of information that informed consent would provide, and carefully documented in the health record. Providers are advised to encourage patients to complete the informed consent process rather than avoiding it.

A more common type of waiver relates to individuals serving as subjects in research studies. Under the Common Rule, the informed consent requirement for human subjects research may be waived or altered if approved by an institutional review board. For approval to be granted, the IRB must find and document that (45 CFR 46.116(d)):

- The research involves no more than minimal risk to the subjects
- The waiver or alteration will not adversely affect the rights and welfare of the subjects
- The research could not practicably be carried out without the waiver or alteration
- Whenever appropriate, the subjects will be provided with additional pertinent information after participation

Regarding access to information without patient consent, an IRB may waive the informed consent requirement when a research study involves a retrospective review of charts. For example, researchers are studying whether a certain intervention has been successful for patients presenting to the emergency room, and they want to review five years of emergency department visits. Such a study may qualify for waiver of informed consent because retrospective data collection poses minimal risk to the health of subjects and locating and obtaining signatures from subjects who have visited the emergency department over the past five years may not be practicable. Again, the final decision regarding whether consent would be waived rests with the IRB.

Therapeutic Privilege

The **therapeutic privilege** is a doctrine that has historically allowed physicians to withhold information from patients in limited circumstances, stemming from the historical paternalistic nature of medicine whereby physicians had a duty to avoid things that would "discourage a patient and depress his spirits" (AMA Council on Ethical and Judicial Affairs 2006). It has been applied in extreme situations in which a provider believes that the risk of physical or psychological injury to the patient resulting from full disclosure outweighs the patient's right to be fully informed.

However, with today's emphasis on patient autonomy and individuals' right of access to their health information, the use of therapeutic privilege is discouraged in all but very extreme cases. In 2006, the AMA Council on Ethical and Judicial Affairs revised its Code of Medical Ethics to better support the patient's right of self-decision regarding healthcare thus, deemphasizing the use of the therapeutic privilege. The updated code states (AMA Council on Ethical and Judicial Affairs 2006):

> The patient's right of self-decision can be effectively exercised only if the patient possesses enough information to enable an informed choice. The patient should make his or her own determination about treatment. The physician's obligation is to present the medical facts accurately to the patient or to the individual responsible for the patient's care and to make recommendations for management in accordance with good medical practice. The physician has an ethical obligation to help the patient make choices from among the therapeutic alternatives consistent with good medical practice. Informed consent is a basic policy in both ethics and law that physicians must honor, unless the patient is unconscious or otherwise incapable of consenting and harm from failure to treat is imminent. In special circumstances, it may be appropriate to postpone disclosure of information.

> Physicians should sensitively and respectfully disclose all relevant medical information to patients. The quantity and specificity of this information should be tailored to meet the preferences and needs of individual patients. Physicians need not communicate all information at one time, but they should assess the amount of information that patients are capable of receiving at a given time and present the remainder when appropriate.

Informed Consent and GINA

The **Genetic Information Nondiscrimination Act** (GINA) is a federal law that was passed in 2008. It prohibits health insurance and employment discrimination based on genetic information and is discussed more extensively in chapter 12. Relative to genetic research, GINA generally requires that investigators include in their informed consent a description of reasonably foreseeable risks and a statement describing the degree to which the confidentiality of records identifying the subject will be maintained (HHS 2009).

GINA's antidiscrimination provisions, which include a bar on decisions based on genetic information obtained from research, apply to health insurers, group health plans, and employers with 15 or more employees. As a result, life insurers, disability insurers, long-term care insurers, and employers with fewer than 15 employees may use genetic information obtained about an individual as the result of a research study to make coverage and employment decisions (HHS 2009).

Informed Consent and HIPAA

The Privacy Rule of the **Health Insurance Portability and Accountability Act** (HIPAA), which went into effect in 2003, also addresses informed consent for research through its authorization requirements. Although a separate informed consent document for research is often preferable, HIPAA allows an organization's IRB or privacy board to permit compound authorizations that combine informed consent with an authorization for the use and disclosure of a research subject's health information. Types of authorizations permitted for research under HIPAA, including revisions per the Health Information Technology for Economic and Clinical Health Act (HITECH), are discussed more fully in chapter 9.

Advance Directives

As discussed above, communication between the physician and the patient is a key element of informed consent. However, sometimes the patient's health status may make communication impossible, such as when a patient is incapacitated by a head injury or a stroke. Through **advance directives**, the law provides a means for individuals to communicate their healthcare wishes in advance should they become incapacitated. Specifically, an advance directive is a legal document that specifies an individual's healthcare wishes in the event that he or she has a temporary or permanent loss of competence. Some advance directives appoint a specific friend, family member, or other person to make healthcare decisions on behalf of an individual should that individual lose competence. Other advance directives leave specific instructions restricting the use of ventilators, artificial nutrition and hydration, and other types of life support. Specific types of advance directives are discussed below.

Durable Powers of Attorney for Healthcare Decisions

A **power of attorney** (POA) is a legal instrument used by a principal (person) to grant legal authority to one or more agents to make certain legal and financial decisions on behalf of the principal. The principal is the individual who signs the POA and the agent is the person designated by the principal to make certain decisions or perform certain acts on the principal's behalf. The specific authority granted to the agent is listed in the POA instrument. For example, a principal may designate an agent to sign real estate contracts or transfer money on the principal's behalf. The agent's authority to act on behalf of the principal may be broad or may be limited to a specific task or transaction. Specific rules for how the POA must be drafted are defined by each state. Generally, they must be written, signed, witnessed, and executed by an adult.

Unless a POA is durable, it is only effective when the principal has capacity. Capacity indicates that an individual is mentally competent and is in control of himself or herself. If the principal becomes incapacitated, then the agent's authority is also incapacitated. So, in the above example, the agent's authority to sign real estate contracts or transfer money on the principal's behalf would be terminated upon the principal's incapacitation. This situation can be prevented by executing a **durable power of attorney** (DPOA). A DPOA is a POA that remains in effect even after the principal is incapacitated. Some DPOAs are drafted so that they only take effect when the principal becomes incapacitated. These are sometimes called springing POAs because they only "spring" into effect upon the principal's incapacitation. State law defines the specific language required to create a DPOA versus a POA, but it generally includes an express statement that the agent's authority is not terminated by the principal's incapacity.

Powers of attorney and DPOA most often deal with financial, real estate, and other legal transactions, but they generally do not cover healthcare decisions. State law creates a separate, but similar, framework for appointing agents to make healthcare decisions on behalf of principals. A **durable power of attorney for healthcare decisions** (DPOA-HCD) is a legal instrument through which a principal appoints an agent to make healthcare decisions on the principal's behalf in the event the principal become incapacitated. It is important to note that not every state calls this type of instrument a DPOA-HCD. It is sometimes referred to as a medical power of attorney or a healthcare proxy. Depending on the wording of the instrument, the agent may have power to make healthcare decisions on behalf of a principal while the principal is still competent, but often the agent's power is not effective until the principal becomes incompetent. The determination of whether a patient is incompetent is typically made by a physician or judge. Again, to be durable, the instrument must contain specific language defined by state law. For example, Kansas law requires DPOA-HCDs to contain the words, "'this power of attorney for healthcare decisions shall not be affected by subsequent disability or incapacity of the principal' or 'this power of attorney for healthcare decisions shall become effective upon the disability or incapacity of the principal,' or similar words showing the intent of the principal that the authority conferred shall be exercisable notwithstanding the principal's subsequent disability or incapacity" (KS Stat. Ann. 58-625).

In addition to the language required for durability, state law also defines other aspects of DPOA-HCDs. For example, both the principal and the agent(s) must be adults for DPOA-HCDs to be valid. A DPOA-HCD can grant the agent authority to make all healthcare decisions on behalf of the principal, or it may be limited to only certain decisions. With respect to exercising the authority granted, the agent steps into the shoes of the principal. Any decisions made by the agent are treated as though they were made by the principal. The agent not only has the power to make the healthcare decisions specified in the DPOA-HCD, but also has the power to exercise the principal's corresponding HIPAA privacy rights related to those treatment decisions.

Once executed, the principal should inform friends and family about the DPOA-HCD document and provide copies to the appointed agents as well as to any healthcare providers the principal plans on visiting. Different states tend to recognize each other's properly executed DPOA-HCDs. Therefore, providers may rely on DPOA-HCDs that were properly executed in other states. Healthcare providers should store copies of DPOA-HCDs prominently in the patient's record, and are required to do so by the laws of many states. If the provider uses an electronic health record (EHR), then the EHR must be set up to refer or link to the existence of the DPOA-HCD. Some states, such as Arizona, have created a secure advance directive registry, a website that permits individuals to store their DPOA-HCD and other advance directives online (Arizona Secretary of State 2007). Individuals then provide healthcare providers and others with passwords to access the online advance directive.

The process for revoking a DPOA-HCD varies by state law, but generally involves some form of express communication showing the principal's intent to revoke the instrument. This communication must be made to the agent as well as to healthcare providers who have been previously notified about the document's existence. In cases where spouses are appointed as agents, some DPOA-HCDs contain specific language that automatically revokes the instrument if the principal and the agent become separated or divorced. If a principal executes a second DPOA-HCD naming new agents or granting different powers, then the previous DPOA-HCD is automatically revoked. The law generally protects agents and providers who are unaware that a DPOA-HCD has been revoked and in good faith rely on the instrument to make decisions. Sample DPOA-HCDs for each state are widely available on the Internet through state government and consumer advocacy websites.

Living Wills

A **living will** is a document executed by a competent adult that expresses that individual's wishes to limit treatment measures when specific health-related diagnoses or conditions exist and the individual cannot communicate on his or her own behalf. In some states, a living will may only take effect when two or more physicians certify in writing that a patient has a terminal condition. A terminal condition generally connotes a condition where an individual is likely to die in the near future, with or without treatment. Since permanent unconsciousness or confusion caused by accidents or diseases such as Alzheimer's may not qualify as terminal, it is important to note that these conditions may be outside the scope of a living will. However, court cases have held that individuals can execute other advance directives that exceed limitations set by state terminal condition living will statutes (Missouri Bar 2006). In other states, conditions governed by living wills are broader and encompass "seriously incapacitating" illnesses or conditions, persistent unconsciousness with no reasonable expectation of recovery, or "permanent confusion." The types of treatment limited by living wills typically involve life-prolonging procedures, such as artificially supplied nutrition and hydration, cardiopulmonary resuscitation (CPR), and use of respirators.

The technical process for executing living wills varies from state to state. Common requirements are that living wills must be written, signed, and dated by the individual executing the will, executed by adults, and witnessed or acknowledged before a notary public or other witnesses not related to the individual executing the will. Not every state uses the term living will to define this type of advance directive. Sometimes the terms *healthcare directive* or *advance care plan* are used in lieu of living will. Once an individual has executed a living will, it is important that he or she communicate its existence to close friends, family, and healthcare providers. An individual should keep a copy of his or her living will in an easily accessible place, and healthcare providers must store copies of living wills in the front of a patient's paper record or make them immediately accessible in an EHR system. The process of revoking a living will varies from state to state, but generally involves some express act or statement indicating an intent to revoke. This may involve oral or written statements or physically gathering and destroying copies of the living will. In some states, healthcare providers are required to document the revocation of a living will in the patient's health records (Missouri Bar 2006).

It is common for individuals to have both a DPOA-HCD and a living will. If such an individual is incapacitated and is also diagnosed with a condition specified in the principal's living will, it can be difficult to determine whether treatment decisions should be made according to the living will or according to the agent's judgment. Some DPOA-HCDs directly address this issue by specifically stating that the agent either does or does not have the power to act in contradiction to the wishes outlined in a living will. State law may also limit an agent's ability to contradict or revoke a properly executed living will. In situations where irresolvable conflict exists, a judge may enter an order regarding treatment after being presented with evidence at a hearing.

Sample living wills and other related advance directive plans are widely available on the Internet through state government and consumer advocacy websites. Some examples include the Ohio Hospice & Palliative Care Organization Advance Directives Packet Choices Living Well at the End of Life (2004), Tennessee Department of Health's Advance Directives Resources (n.d.a) and Advance Directives for Health Care Decision Making (n.d.b) and the Kansas Bar Association's Natural Death Act Declaration (2007).

Do Not Resuscitate Orders

Generally, healthcare facility staff and paramedics will perform cardiopulmonary resuscitation (CPR) on any individual whose heart or breathing has stopped. However, individuals may wish to forego CPR for a variety of reasons, such as the belief that it will only prolong the dying process and cause unnecessary discomfort and emotional distress (State of California Emergency Medical Services Authority 2009). A **do not resuscitate (DNR) order** is a specific type of advance directive in which an individual states that healthcare providers should not perform CPR if the individual experiences cardiac arrest or cessation of breathing (NCI n.d.b).

The framework for DNR orders is addressed by state law and can vary from state to state. The individual may sign a state-approved consent form specifically tailored to requesting a DNR order. State law typically requires additional signatures from physicians and witnesses. The language required on a DNR consent form varies from state to state but generally describes CPR and indicates the individual's desire not to have CPR performed. The Joint Commission requires that all accredited acute care facilities have institutional policies regarding advance directives and DNR orders, and that they be included in the health record.

Since DNR orders are only utilized in emergency circumstances, it is important that the existence of a DNR order can be immediately communicated to healthcare providers. This is usually accomplished by issuing DNR patients an approved bracelet or some other form of identification that makes it immediately clear to healthcare providers that a valid DNR order is on file for that individual. DNR orders must be kept in the individual's health record, whether that record is paper or electronic.

Individuals have the right to revoke a DNR order at any time. The individual's revocation of the DNR order can be expressed in a variety of ways, such as writing void across the order or by removing or damaging the DNR identifier. Sometimes a DNR order can be affected by a patient's transfer from one facility to another. Some states may allow the order to transfer with the patient, while others may require a new order to be issued at the new facility. State law also addresses whether a DNR order is valid during the patient's actual transport from one facility to another. The law may also permit facilities to suspend a DNR order during surgery or when a patient's heart or breathing has stopped because of an unforeseen external event, such as choking or a car accident (Illinois Department of Public Health 2006). As part of the informed consent process, providers and patients should have detailed discussions of circumstances where DNR orders are and are not effective. Some facilities have mandated policies that require patients and physicians to reconsider the desire for a DNR order prior to certain surgeries or other medical interventions (ACS 1994).

Patient Self-Determination Act

Advance directives clearly play an important role in the informed consent process. They are the means through which individuals can ensure that their healthcare wishes are carried out even after they are incapacitated or incompetent. However, many people are not aware of their rights to execute advance directives and do not understand the differences between the various types of advance directives. In fact, studies have shown that only 10 to 25 percent of Americans have documented their end-of-life choices or appointed an agent to make their healthcare decisions (GAO 1995). Further, advance directives are not always implemented in the way individuals intend. How they are implemented depends on a variety of factors, such as whether more than one type of advance directive has been executed, the level of detail in the advance directive, and whether any family members or other individuals challenge the legal validity of the advance directive.

To raise public awareness about the use of advance directives, Congress passed the **Patient Self-Determination Act** (PSDA) as part of the Omnibus Budget Reconciliation Act of 1990. The law, which became effective in December 1991, requires healthcare institutions (that is, hospitals, nursing facilities, hospice programs, and home health agencies) that bill Medicare or Medicaid for services to provide adult patients with information about the various types of advance directives. Specifically, providers are required to:

- Provide to all adult patients, residents, and enrollees written information on their rights, under state law, to make decisions concerning medical care, including the right to execute an advance directive, as well as maintain the policies of the provider regarding implementation of advance directives

- Document in the health record whether the individual has an advance directive

- Educate the staff and the community about advance directives

- Not condition the provision of care, or otherwise discriminate, on the basis of whether an individual has an advance directive

- Ensure compliance with state law respecting advance directives (GAO 1995)

Further, the PSDA requires that the Department of Health and Human Services provide public education about advance directives and oversee provider compliance with the law's requirements.

Uniform Anatomical Gift Act

During the past several decades, medical technology has made significant improvements in the ability to harvest and successfully transplant human organs. The need for organ transplantation is great—as of January 2010 more than 105,000 individuals were on organ transplant waiting lists, according to the US government's official organ donor website, www.OrganDonor.gov. However, there is a shortage of organs available for transplantation. In 2005, 13,091 individuals died who were medically eligible to be organ donors. Of those, only 58 percent were actual organ donors. One of the key barriers to organ donation involves obtaining consent of individuals to donate their organs and enforcing such consent when individuals closely associated with the decedent object.

The legal processes for organ donation are defined by state law. However, consistency among state laws has been promoted through the adoption of the **Uniform Anatomical Gift Act** (UAGA), promulgated by the National Conference of Commissioners on Uniform State Laws (NCCUSL). The UAGA provides suggested standards for all aspects of organ donation, including who may make anatomical gifts and how intent to make anatomical gifts should be expressed. The first UAGA was created in 1968 and was adopted by all 50 states. It created an opt-in system for organ donation where individuals are not considered to be organ donors unless they have specifically indicated a desire to donate. Since then, the act has been revised several times to account for changes in medical technology and laws but has always retained the opt-in element. States have been inconsistent in the degree to which they have adopted subsequent revisions to the UAGA, resulting in confusion and barriers in the transplant process. The most recent revision to the UAGA was promulgated in 2006. The revised act is shown in figure 7.2.

The UAGA permits an anatomical gift by any person designated to make decisions about the decedent's remains, and where there is more than one person in this class of persons, so long as no objections by other class members are known. If an objection is known, the UAGA permits a majority of the members of the class of persons who are reasonably available to make the gift without having to take account of a known objection by any class member who is not reasonably available (Section 9).

Again, states are not required to adopt the revised provisions of the UAGA, and the process for obtaining informed consent for organ donation for each state must be followed. The desire to donate organs can be expressed in a number of ways, such as through registering at the Department of Motor Vehicles or leaving specific instructions in an advance directive. Where an individual has left no instructions regarding donations, state law may provide a hierarchy of persons who can consent to organ donation on behalf of the deceased. For example, Kansas law (KS Stat. Ann. 65-1734) states that when there is no notice of contrary wishes by the decedent, the following individuals (in the order of priority stated) may give all or any part of the decedent's body for donation:

- The agent for healthcare decisions established by a durable power of attorney for healthcare decisions, if such power of attorney conveys to the agent the authority to make decisions concerning organ donation

- The spouse

- The decedent's surviving adult children

- The decedent's surviving parents

- The persons in the next degree of kinship under probate law

- A guardian of the person of the decedent at the time of such person's death

- The personal representative of the decedent

Figure 7.2. Uniform Anatomical Gift Act (UAGA)

1. Honors the choice of an individual to be or not to be a donor and strengthens the language barring others from overriding a donor's decision to make an anatomical gift (Section 8)

2. Facilitates donations by expanding the list of those who may make an anatomical gift for another individual during that individual's lifetime to include health-care agents and, under certain circumstances, parents or guardians (Section 4)

3. Empowers a minor eligible under other law to apply for a driver's license to be a donor (Section 4)

4. Facilitates donations from a deceased individual who made no lifetime choice by adding to the list of persons who can make a gift of the deceased individual's body or parts the following persons: the person who was acting as the decedent's agent under a power of attorney for healthcare at the time of the decedent's death, the decedent's adult grandchildren, and an adult who exhibited special care and concern for the decedent (Section 9) and defines the meaning of "reasonably available" which is relevant to who can make an anatomical gift of a decedent's body or parts (Section 2(23))

5. Permits an anatomical gift by any member of a class where there is more than one person in the class so long as no objections by other class members are known and, if an objection is known, permits a majority of the members of the class who are reasonably available to make the gift without having to take account of a known objection by any class member who is not reasonably available (Section 9)

6. Creates numerous default rules for the interpretation of a document of gift that lacks specificity regarding either the persons to receive the gift or the purposes of the gift or both (Section 11)

7. Encourages and establishes standards for donor registries (Section 20)

8. Enables procurement organizations to gain access to documents of gifts in donor registries, health records, and the records of a state motor vehicle department (Sections 14 and 20)

9. Resolves the tension between a healthcare directive requesting the withholding or withdrawal of life support systems and anatomical gifts by permitting measures necessary to ensure the medical suitability of organs for intended transplantation or therapy to be administered (Sections 14 and 21)

10. Clarifies and expands the rules relating to cooperation and coordination between procurement organizations and coroners or medical examiners (Sections 22 and 23)

11. Recognizes anatomical gifts made under the laws of other jurisdictions (Section 19)

12. Updates the [act] to allow for electronic records and signatures (Section 25)

Source: Uniform Law Commissioners 2002.

Check Your Understanding 7.2

Instructions: Indicate whether the following statements are true or false (T or F).

1. Unless it is designated as durable, a power of attorney is only effective when the principal has capacity.

2. A durable power of attorney for healthcare decisions expresses an individual's wishes to limit treatment measures when specific health-related diagnoses or conditions exist and the individual cannot communicate on his own behalf.

3. The Patient Self-Determination Act requires hospitals that are Medicare providers to document in the health record whether an individual has an advance directive.

4. The Uniform Anatomical Gift Act permits an anatomical gift by any person designated to make decisions about a decedent's remains.

5. The technical process for executing a living will is standardized nationally.

Parties to Consent

The rights and processes surrounding informed consent operate differently depending on whether the individual is a competent adult, an incompetent adult, or a minor child. A competent adult is an individual who is mentally capable and is at or above the age of majority. The age of majority is the legal recognition that an individual is considered responsible for, and has control over, his or her actions. These actions include consenting to or refusing medical treatment, voting, entering into binding contracts, enlisting in the armed forces, marrying, buying alcohol, and other actions defined by state law. In most states the age of majority is 18 years of age (US Legal, Inc., n.d.). Exceptions include states such as Alabama and Nebraska (19 years of age) and Mississippi (21 years of age). Some states, such as Nevada, base the age of majority upon graduation from high school or a designated age, whichever occurs earlier. An incompetent adult is an individual who is no longer capable of controlling his or her actions due to illness, injury, or disability. Control over this individual is through an agent or guardian. A minor is generally defined as an individual who is under the age of majority and whose rights are usually exercised through a parent or other legal guardian. There are, however, certain circumstances that allow minors to exercise their own decision-making rights. The rights and processes surrounding informed consent are discussed in more detail below.

Competent Adults

Absent the exceptions discussed above, competent adults have a general right to consent to or refuse medical treatment. As "right to die" court decisions have ruled, a competent adult's right to refuse consent to medical treatment applies even when the treatment is lifesaving. Treatment may be refused for any reason, whether it is religious, financial, or personal. The right to refuse treatment stems from more than a century of court decisions recognizing the profound importance of bodily integrity. In 1891, the United States Supreme Court observed, "[n]o right is held more sacred, or is more carefully guarded by the common law, than the right of every individual to the possession and control of his own person, free from all restraint or interference of others, unless by clear and unquestionable authority of law" (*Union Pacific R. Co. v. Botsford*, 1891). For decades, courts have specifically applied the notion of bodily integrity in the context of medical care. In 1910, Benjamin Cardozo, who would later become a Supreme Court Justice, stated, "Every human being of adult years and sound mind has a right to determine what shall be done with his own body, and a surgeon who performs an operation without his patient's consent commits an assault, for which he is liable in damages" (*Schloendorff v. Society of New York Hospital*, 1914). When the refusal to consent is based on a religious belief, the First Amendment's freedom of religion clause provides additional authority for refusing treatment. Perhaps the most recognized example of refusing medical care based on religious beliefs occurs when Jehovah's Witnesses refuse consent to certain types of blood transfusions.

In general, the right to refuse consent to medical care has two important prerequisites: adulthood and competence. To be an adult, one must have reached the age of majority. While the standards vary from state to state, competence can generally be described as an individual's overall ability to understand, process, and communicate information adequately enough to meet essential life needs, such as food, clothing, shelter, safety, and health. Some individuals, such as those born with profound mental retardation, are never legally competent. Healthcare decisions for these individuals are generally made by parents when the individual is a minor and by court-appointed guardians after the individual reaches adulthood. Competent individuals may experience temporary or permanent loss of competence as a result of injury or illness. How healthcare decisions are made in these situations depends on whether an individual executed an advance directive such as a DPOA-HCD while he or she was still competent.

When a competent adult refuses consent to lifesaving medical treatment, two competing sets of interests arise. The first is the individual's well-established interest in privacy, due process, and self-determination. The second is the government's compelling interest in protecting and preserving human life, which has also been established through years of case law. While both interests are strong, the interests of a competent individual usually outweigh the interests of the government. *In the Matter of Robert Quackenbush* demonstrates how the two sets of interests are balanced. The case involved a 72-year-old patient who, due to his previous refusal to seek medical care for arteriosclerosis, had such advanced gangrene in his legs that one foot was literally "dangling," about to fall off. Without amputating both legs, doctors expected the patient to die within three weeks. The patient, who had refused medical care for over 40 years, was described by doctors as a "conscientious objector to medical therapy." He refused to consent to the operation because he simply wanted to return home and "live out his life." Based on the apparent irrationality of the patient's decision and the belief that infection was cognitively impairing the patient, the hospital petitioned the court to appoint a guardian who would consent to the amputation on behalf of the patient. In hearing the case, the first issue that the court addressed was whether the patient was a competent adult. The following is a summary of the evidence presented regarding competency:

- A physician who evaluated the patient on January 6th concluded that the patient was not competent to make an informed medical decision because he was disoriented as to his location, confused about who was around him, responded to questions inappropriately, and suffered visual hallucinations. The physician acknowledged that the patient's confusion could have stemmed from septicemia, which was treatable with antibiotics.

- A physician who evaluated the patient on January 11th found some fluctuations in mental lucidity, but not to such a degree that the patient was mentally incompetent. The patient and the physician thoroughly discussed his condition and the ramifications of having the operation. The physician determined that the patient had the mental capacity to make an informed choice regarding the operation. (At that point, the septicemia was better controlled, which reduced the patient's confusion.)

- The judge, who interviewed the patient on January 12, found him to be responsive and reasonably alert. The patient again expressed his wishes to forgo the surgery but left open the possibility of changing his mind if he began to experience pain (*In the Matter of Robert Quackenbush*, 1978).

Based on the evidence as a whole, the court found the patient to be mentally competent. However, the finding of competence did not end the court's inquiry—the court still needed to balance the patient's interests against the interest of the state. The hospital equated the patient's decision to refuse treatment with suicide and argued that allowing a patient to commit suicide was inconsistent with the state's compelling interest in preserving life. The court did not directly address whether the patient was committing suicide, but instead acknowledged that the ". . . State's interest weakens and the individual's right to privacy grows as the degree of bodily invasion increases and the prognosis dims, until the ultimate point when the individual's rights overcome the State's interest in preserving life." The court went on to hold that "the extensive bodily invasion involved here—the amputation of both legs above the knee and possibly the amputation of both legs entirely—is sufficient to make the State's interest in the preservation of life give way to [the patient's] right of privacy to decide his own future regardless of the absence of a dim prognosis. . . . No decision of this nature is easily made. Always present is the predominant interest in the preservation of life. But constitutional and decisional law invest [the patient] with rights that overcome that interest. [The patient], therefore, as a mentally competent individual, has the right to make his informed choice concerning the operation and I will not interfere with that choice."

In the Quackenbush case, the hospital's main argument was that the patient was committing suicide by refusing treatment and that permitting a patient to commit suicide was inconsistent with the state's interest in preserving life. When faced with this argument, courts typically distinguish between refusal of consent and suicide. The distinction is that suicide involves an act, whereas refusal of consent involves the withholding or revocation of an act. The state has a strong interest in prohibiting affirmative acts that will lead to death, such as intentionally administering a drug that will end the patient's life. However, the state's interest is not as strong when it is the patient's refusal to act (the refusal or revocation of consent) at issue. Again, the right to refuse consent is rooted in the long-standing principles of personal autonomy and self-determination.

Whenever an individual refuses consent or withdraws his or her consent, providers should clearly document that the risks, benefits, and alternatives of not administering treatment or withdrawing consent were explained to the patient. They should also obtain the individual's written acknowledgement that the risks, benefits, and alternatives of withdrawing consent were explained, and that the patient is still electing to do so.

Incompetent Adults

If an individual is no longer competent due to an illness or an injury, then that individual cannot be expected to provide informed consent for nonemergency medical treatment. An individual's incompetence may arise from a temporary problem, such as acute impairment stemming from the use of alcohol or drugs, or it may arise from a long-term or chronic condition, such as Alzheimer's disease or brain injury. Contrary to common belief, not all states have "surrogate consent" laws that automatically permit spouses or adult children and siblings to provide legal consent on behalf of an incompetent individual. Therefore, absent any advance directive, it may be necessary to appoint a guardian for the individual, especially when incompetence is likely to be long-term.

Guardianship proceedings are typically initiated by a healthcare provider or family member involved in the incompetent individual's care. At the guardianship proceeding, evidence regarding the individual's alleged incompetence is presented by qualified healthcare providers. The court will also hear testimony from a guardian ad litem, which is a lawyer appointed by the court to represent the interests of the incompetent individual during the guardianship proceedings. It may also hear evidence from other sources, such as social workers appointed to evaluate the appropriateness of a proposed guardian. After hearing the evidence, a court may appoint the spouse, adult child, or sibling as an individual's guardian or it may choose to appoint some other qualified person. Healthcare providers involved in the treatment of an individual are not usually appointed as guardians. Courts are concerned that appointing a treatment provider as a patient's guardian could give rise to a conflict of interest. For example, the treatment provider may have incentive to make consent decisions based on economic factors rather than what is in the patient's best interest. Once appointed, guardians are required to make regular reports to the court on the status of the ward (the patient).

The extent of the guardian's ability to consent to medical treatment on behalf of the incompetent individual varies from state to state (KS Stat. Ann. 59-3075). Typically, guardians have statutory authority to consent or refuse to consent to medical interventions in accordance with what is in the best interest of the ward (incompetent individual). However, states often limit a guardian's power to consent to certain interventions unless those interventions have been approved by the court. For example, nonemergency interventions involving psychosurgery, organ removal, amputation, sterilization, and experimental treatments must be approved by a court in advance.

Cases involving incompetent adults can be divided into three broad categories:

- Adults who were once competent and executed an advance directive

- Adults who were once competent but did not execute an advance directive

- Adults who never had competence

From a legal standpoint, the first category is the most straightforward. When an individual has properly executed an advance directive, then treatment decisions are generally made in accordance with that advance directive. Conflicts do not usually arise unless there is disagreement about whether the agent is acting in the principal's best interest or making decisions that are inconsistent with the principal's previously expressed wishes.

As mentioned earlier, only 10 to 25 percent of adults have preemptively expressed their wishes regarding medical treatment through advance directives. Many people simply have occasional end-of-life discussions with family and friends where they informally express their desires (that is, not to be maintained in a persistent vegetative state, or PVS). However, the absence of a formal advance directive can raise complex consent-to-treatment issues. How do healthcare providers know what treatment options an individual would consent to if he or she still had competence? Some states address this issue through surrogate consent laws that permit spouses, adult children, parents, siblings, and so on to consent on behalf of an incompetent adult. Consent decisions are made by the person who is highest in the hierarchy specified by the law. For example, if the hierarchy is spouse, adult child, adult siblings, parents, then an incapacitated individual's spouse would first provide consent on the individual's behalf. If no spouse were available, then consent decisions would be made by the individual's adult children. If there were no adult children, then any adult siblings would make consent decisions, and if no adult siblings, consent would default to parents. If the individual has no family that fit into the surrogate consent hierarchy, then a court would most likely appoint a guardian to make consent decisions on behalf of the individual. Surrogate consent laws may or may not provide a framework for addressing disagreement about consent decisions among individuals at the same hierarchal level (such as adult children or adult siblings). If conflict over treatment options exists, a hearing is held before a court. Further, surrogate consent laws often limit the kind of consent choices that can be made by surrogates in the hierarchy. For example, the law may prohibit surrogates from making consent decisions relating to mental health treatment, pregnancy care, or withdrawal of life-sustaining treatment. The Uniform Health-Care Decisions Act, a model for state-adopted surrogate consent laws, is discussed later in this chapter.

If no surrogate consent law exists or the proposed medical intervention is outside the scope of the surrogate consent law, then the treatment decision is usually made by a court-appointed guardian. Once appointed, the guardian is obligated to step into the shoes of the incapacitated individual and must attempt to make treatment decisions in accordance with what the individual would want if he or she were still competent. However, when treatment decisions by guardians involve end-of-life decisions, the courts may step in.

The first major case to deal with this kind of issue was *In re Quinlan*. The case involved a young woman who had suffered severe brain damage and entered a PVS. Her father, who was her legally appointed guardian, petitioned the court to approve the disconnection of Quinlan's respirator after her providers refused to terminate her life support. The court held that, even while incompetent, Quinlan had a constitutional right of privacy to terminate treatment. The only practical way to exercise this right was to allow her guardian and family to decide whether Quinlan would exercise her right to refuse treatment under the circumstances.

After Quinlan, courts grappled with the question of how much evidence is necessary to prove an incompetent individual's intent to consent to the withdrawal of life-sustaining treatment after he or she has become permanently incompetent. The seminal case addressing this question was *Cruzan v. Director, Missouri Department of Health*. Like Quinlan, Cruzan was a young woman who had entered a PVS. Cruzan had been in a PVS for several years when her parents, as guardians, asked that her artificial nutrition and hydration be removed. Hospital staff refused to remove the artificial nutrition and hydration because doing so would cause Cruzan's death. A state trial court authorized the withdrawal based upon the constitutional right to direct or refuse the withdrawal of life-sustaining treatment. The trial court found that a prior statement by Cruzan to her housemate that she would not wish to continue her life if sick or injured unless she could live "at least halfway normally" was sufficient evidence that Cruzan would not consent to artificial nutrition and hydration. The state supreme court reversed the decision of the trial court, finding that Cruzan's statements to her housemate were unreliable for the purpose of determining her intent.

The court went on to hold that where no advance directive exists, no person can assume an end-of-life choice on behalf of an incompetent person unless there is "clear and convincing" evidence that the person would refuse consent to life-sustaining treatment under the circumstances. Cruzan's parents appealed the decision of the state supreme court to the United States Supreme Court. The US Supreme Court affirmed the decision of the state supreme court and held that a state may require evidence of an incompetent individual's wishes as to the withdrawal of life-sustaining treatment be proved by clear and convincing evidence. After the Supreme Court decision, additional evidence of Cruzan's wishes surfaced and a new hearing was held regarding the termination of her artificial nutrition and hydration.

The trial court found that the additional evidence met the "clear and convincing" standard set by the Supreme Court and ordered the withdrawal of her artificial nutrition and hydration. No legal challenges succeeded against the order and Cruzan's artificial nutrition and hydration were ultimately removed.

The most recent and by far the most highly publicized and politically charged end-of-life case involved that of Terri Schiavo. Ms. Schiavo was a 26 year-old woman who collapsed in 1990, suffering cardiac and respiratory failure that sent her into a PVS. Eight years later, Michael Schiavo, her husband and legal guardian, sought intervention through the Florida court system (where Ms. Schiavo resided and which had jurisdiction over the case) to have her feeding tube removed. The court ordered the removal of the feeding tube in 2000, finding that testimony provided by Mr. Schiavo and other in-laws of Ms. Schiavo's constituted "clear and convincing evidence" that Ms. Schiavo would not have wished to receive life-prolonging measures given her current condition (Pinellas County Probate Court, Florida 1990). The removal was opposed by Ms. Schiavo's parents. Years of legal battles culminated in 2005 with numerous motions and petitions filed with the courts and a media frenzy that fueled the "right-to-life" versus "right-to-die" debate. Both the Florida legislature and the US Congress had passed laws that would have had the effect of precluding the removal of Ms. Schiavo's feeding tube, thus creating a seesaw effect between legislative and judicial powers and calling into question the legal authority of legislative bodies to intervene in judicial matters such as this. The legal battle came to an end on March 18, 2005, when Ms. Schiavo's feeding tube was removed per the local court's order. She died on March 31, 2005, at the age of 41 (Law Center 2005). One positive outcome of the Schiavo case was the interest it generated in the concept of advance directives and the renewed desire for individuals to memorialize their own end-of-life wishes through these documents. See table 7.1 for a comparison of the Quinlan, Cruzan, and Schiavo cases.

The clear and convincing evidence standard set forth by the Supreme Court applies to determining the wishes of a formerly competent individual. However, the standard does not apply well to circumstances where an individual has never had competence. *In Re Storar* involved a profoundly retarded 52-year-old man who had been diagnosed with bladder cancer. Part of his treatment included periodic blood transfusions, which were necessary to prolong his life. His mother, who was also his legal guardian, refused consent to the transfusions because she believed that they caused Storar too much distress. The New York Court of Appeals noted that where an individual has never been competent, "it is unrealistic to attempt to determine whether he would want to continue potentially life-prolonging treatment if he were competent" (*In Re Storar*, 1981). After hearing evidence about the transfusions, the court concluded that it should not "allow an incompetent patient to bleed to death because someone, even someone as close as a parent or sibling, feels that this is best for one with an incurable disease" (*In Re Storar*, 1981). Instead, the court applied a "best interest" standard and determined that continued transfusions were in the best interest of Storar. The transfusions did not involve excessive pain and without them, Storar's mental and physical abilities would deteriorate. Therefore, the court concluded that it was in Storar's best interest to continue the transfusions.

Uniform Health-Care Decisions Act

As the preceding discussion indicates, there has been much more attention and legislation focused on incapacitated individuals who are dying than on incapacitated individuals who are seeking recovery. As a result, the Uniform Law Commissioners of the National Conference of Commissioners on Uniform

Table 7.1. Key differences among the three end-of-life cases

Case	Quinlan	Cruzan	Schiavo
Issue	Removal of respirator	Removal of nutrition/ hydration	Removal of nutrition/ hydration
Key conflict	Conflict among family members and provider(s)	Conflict among family members and provider(s)	Conflict among family members

State Laws created in 1993 the **Uniform Health-Care Decisions Act** (UHCDA), a model law that several states have adopted. "Leaping over" state DPOA-HCD and living will legislation, it provides an additional option to the creation of these documents. Specifically, it provides that an individual who is an "adult with capacity or emancipated minor [described later in this chapter] may give an oral or written instruction to a health-care provider, which remains in force even after the individual loses capacity." Advance directives that comply with the UHCDA continue to be honored in states that have adopted the UHCDA. In the absence of an advance directive (which entails the appointment of an agent) or a court-appointed guardian, a surrogate that has been identified for the healthcare provider by the individual may make healthcare decisions on behalf of that individual. Absent the selection of a surrogate by the individual, a person related to the individual may assume that authority. Any person who acts as a surrogate must follow the individual's instructions regarding his or her healthcare or, without instructions, act in the individual's best interests. Under the model law, healthcare providers who decline to comply with a surrogate must make reasonable efforts to transfer the individual to a provider who will comply. A healthcare provider's good-faith compliance with the surrogate's instructions shields the provider from civil and criminal liability.

The Uniform Health-Care Decisions Act suggests that decision-making priority for an individual's next-of-kin be as follows, but state laws may tailor the order differently:

- Spouse
- Adult child
- Parent
- Adult sibling
- If no one is available who is so related to the individual, authority may be granted to "an adult who has exhibited special care and concern for the individual, who is familiar with the patient's personal values, and who is willing and able to make a health-care decision for the patient."
- Absent an unrelated adult who exhibits the above characteristics, a healthcare provider may seek appointment of a decision-maker by the court having jurisdiction (Uniform Law Commissioners 2002).

Minors

Although the general rule is that an individual must be a competent adult in order to consent to medical treatment, state laws allow minors to provide their own consent in certain situations. A minor is generally defined (varies by state) as an individual who is under 18 years of age and who has not been legally emancipated (declared to be an adult) by a court. By virtue of their age, minors are generally considered legally incompetent and unable to consent to their own treatment. Therefore, the consent of a parent or other legal guardian, if applicable, is sought before treatment is provided. However, special situations and exceptions related to the consent of treatment for minors are discussed below. As noted previously in this chapter, emergency situations are an exception to the consent requirement whether the patient is an adult or a minor.

Emancipated and Mature Minors

As stated above, emancipated minors are those who have been afforded legal status as an adult, generally by a situational change such as marriage. Depending on the state, statutes or judicial decisions define the parameters for emancipation. They may provide that the minor and his or her parents agree to the emancipation and the minor is self-supporting and living independently. With respect to medical treatment, parental consent should first be attempted in the absence of documentation proving emancipation. If this cannot be accomplished and a minor claims to be emancipated without supporting documentation, advice from legal counsel should be sought. It is noted that this situation applies to nonemergency situations. As described earlier in this chapter, emergencies provide an exception to the consent requirement for minors as well as adults.

Mature minors are those who meet age limits and, in some cases, other factors provided by state law that enable them to consent to their own treatment in certain situations. Many of the state laws that provide for minors to consent to their own treatment are based on public policy; that is, it is deemed more desirable for a minor to consent to his or her own treatment than to forgo that treatment because the minor does not want parents to have knowledge of a specific health condition. Such conditions, including sexually transmitted diseases and substance abuse, are detailed below.

Separated and Divorced Parents of a Minor

When parents of a minor are legally separated or divorced, issues can arise regarding the authority of either parent to consent to treatment. As with children in intact families, the consent of only one parent is generally required. However, do both parents have equal legal standing when only one of them is the custodial parent? State law should be consulted regarding the relative rights of custodial and noncustodial parents. As a matter of policy, healthcare providers may first seek consent from the custodial parent. However, care should be taken not to violate state laws that, absent a court order to the contrary, afford both parents equal legal standing regarding the medical treatment of their minor child. If a healthcare provider has reason to believe that a court has not given a parent full legal rights with respect to his or her child, documentation from the court should be required prior to honoring that parent's consent to treatment of the minor in nonemergency situations.

Treatment for Sexually Transmitted Diseases

State laws generally allow minors to seek medical interventions for the diagnosis and treatment of sexually transmitted diseases (STDs) without requiring parental consent. Therefore, providers may diagnose and treat minors for STDs without having to inform a minor's parents or guardians, and cannot be held liable for failing to obtain parental or guardian consent. The policy behind these laws is based on the presumption that many minors would not seek diagnosis and treatment of STDs if they thought their parents or guardians would find out. As a result of not seeking treatment, a minor could suffer medical complications as well as spread the STD to others. An excerpt of one such law, from Kansas (KS Stat. Ann. 65-2892), is provided below:

> Any physician, upon consultation by any person under eighteen (18) years of age as a patient, may, with the consent of such person who is hereby granted the right of giving such consent, make a diagnostic examination for venereal disease and prescribe for and treat such person for venereal disease including prophylactic treatment for exposure to venereal disease whenever such person is suspected of having a venereal disease or contact with anyone having a venereal disease. All such examinations and treatment may be performed without the consent of, or notification to, the parent, parents, guardian or any other person having custody of such person.

Treatment for Drug or Alcohol Conditions

States generally have laws permitting minors to consent on their own behalf to the diagnosis and treatment of substance abuse and related problems. The policy behind these laws is similar to that for permitting minors to consent to the diagnosis and treatment of STDs. The concern is that minors would refuse to seek medical treatment for alcohol or drug problems if they thought that their parents or guardians would be told about the treatment. By not seeking treatment, a minor is not only endangering him or herself, but also may place others in danger while under the influence. Therefore, states do not want to create barriers (such as parental consent) to minors seeking necessary diagnosis and treatment. An excerpt of a law allowing minors to consent to drug abuse or misuse or addiction is provided below (KS Stat. Ann. 65-2892a):

Any physician licensed to practice the healing arts in Kansas, upon consultation with any minor as a patient, may examine and treat such minor for drug abuse, misuse or addiction if such physician has secured the prior consent of such minor to the examination and treatment. All such examinations and treatment may be performed without the consent of any parent, guardian or other person having custody of such minor, and all minors are hereby granted the right to give consent to such examination and treatment. . . .

Treatment for Drug or Alcohol Conditions

State laws generally prohibit providers from performing abortions on minors unless certain conditions are satisfied. For example, if a minor is legally emancipated or has written consent of at least one parent or guardian, then a state may permit the abortion to be performed. Otherwise, states have varying laws that may allow a minor to petition the court for an order or permission to consent to the abortion without parental or guardian consent or knowledge. For example, in Missouri, to substitute judicial consent for parental or guardian consent for a minor's abortion, a court must determine that judicial consent is in the best interests of the minor and that the minor has been fully informed of the risks and medical consequences of an abortion (MO Rev. Stat. 188.028).

Prenatal Care

State laws may provide for a minor to receive prenatal care without her parents' consent. Such laws further the public policy purpose of promoting the health of the mother, her unborn child, and, later, her infant. It follows, then, that the consent of the parent, even if that parent is a minor, must be secured prior to treating the minor's child.

Check Your Understanding 7.3

Instructions: Indicate whether the following statements are true or false (T or F).

1. A competent adult's right to refuse consent to medical treatment applies even when the treatment is lifesaving.

2. In right-to-die cases, courts will balance an individual's right to self-determination against the interest of the state.

3. The Uniform Health-Care Decisions Act suggests that, in the absence of a surrogate, a spouse be the first person to make healthcare decisions on behalf of an individual who has lost mental capacity.

4. An emancipated minor is one who has not been afforded legal status as an adult.

5. State laws generally allow minors to seek medical treatment for sexually transmitted diseases without parental consent.

Challenges to Consents

Much of this chapter has discussed challenges to consent brought before the proposed intervention is actually performed. For example, in the *Quackenbush* case, the patient was challenging a doctor's opinion that he should consent to the amputation of his legs. The challenge was made before the amputation actually occurred. However, sometimes challenges to consent are brought after an intervention has already been performed. They are usually based on a total lack of consent or a lack of fully informed consent.

If an individual alleges that he or she never gave consent to an intervention that was actually performed, then the basis of the claim is usually battery. As discussed in chapter 5, battery consists of the intentional and nonconsensual contact with the plaintiff's person. In *Duncan v. Scottsdale Medical Imaging*, the plaintiff alleged that she informed defendants that she was allergic to certain medications and specifically stated that she only consented to the injection of morphine or Demerol. According to the plaintiff, the defendants injected her with fentanyl despite telling her that the proper medication was being used. The plaintiff further claimed that the administration of fentanyl caused severe headache, projectile vomiting, breathing difficulties, posttraumatic stress disorder, and vocal cord dysfunction. She sued the defendants for battery.

In analyzing the case, the court stated that "the battery theory should be reserved for those circumstances when a doctor performs an operation to which the patient has not consented. When the patient gives permission to perform one type of treatment and the doctor performs another, the requisite element of deliberate intent to deviate from the consent given is present" (*Duncan v. Scottsdale Medical Imaging*, 2003). The defendant argued that administering the injection did not constitute battery because the plaintiff had in fact consented to an injection, even if that injection was fentanyl. However, the court noted that the plaintiff "explicitly conditioned her consent on the use of morphine or Demerol and rejected the use of any other drug. Conduct involving the use of a sedative other than morphine or Demerol, contrary to explicit instruction and understanding, cannot be viewed as consensual." The court went on to state, "The relevant inquiry here is not whether the patient consented to an injection; the issue is whether the patient consented to receive the specific drug that was administered. Duncan could have given broad consent to the administration of any painkiller, but she gave specific instructions that she would accept only morphine or Demerol and nothing else. We hold that when a patient gives limited or conditional consent, a healthcare provider has committed a battery if the evidence shows the provider acted with willful disregard of the consent given."

Sometimes an individual consents to a procedure but later alleges that he or she was not fully informed of the risks, benefits, and alternatives associated with that procedure. Under these circumstances, a negligence claim specifically based on lack of informed consent is most appropriate. To be successful, the plaintiff must first prove that the defendant fell below the applicable standard of care. The standard of care is usually determined through expert testimony and can vary somewhat from state to state. For example, in *Hamilton v. Ashton*, the plaintiff experienced permanent facial paralysis after undergoing an ear surgery. She sued the defendant on multiple theories, including malpractice and lack of informed consent. With respect to the standard of care, the court stated, "Under the doctrine of informed consent, a doctor must disclose the facts and risks of a treatment which a reasonably prudent physician would be expected to disclose under like circumstances and which a reasonable person would want to know. This is separate and apart from the doctor's duty to 'exercise that degree of care, skill, and proficiency exercised by reasonably careful, skillful, and prudent practitioners in the same class to which he belongs, acting under the same or similar circumstances'" (*Hamilton v. Ashton*, 2006). In *Acuna v. Turkish*, the court stated, "A physician's duty of disclosure in the typical malpractice case is measured by the 'prudent patient' or 'materiality of risk' standard. The standard relates to the patient's needs, not the physician's judgment. '[A] physician must disclose to a patient all material information that a 'prudent patient' might find significant for a determination whether to undergo the proposed [medical procedure].' This standard is objective. 'The test for determining whether a particular risk must be disclosed is its materiality to the patient's decision, i.e., all risks potentially affecting the decision must be divulged.'"

Even if it is determined that the defendant fell below the applicable standard of care, the plaintiff must also prove that the defendant's failure to meet the standard actually caused the plaintiff's injury. In other words, the plaintiff must show that he or she would have made a different treatment decision if there had been full disclosure. The specific standard for establishing causation varies from state to state but usually involves the application of an objective reasonable or prudent person standard. The standard asks what a reasonable person, in the plaintiff's situation, would have done if he or she had been fully informed. For example, in *Wilson v. Merritt*, the plaintiff was a paraplegic who suffered a torn rotator cuff and a fractured shoulder during a manipulation under anesthesia procedure performed by a chiropractor. The plaintiff claimed that he would not have consented to the surgery if he had been aware that there were risks of a bone fracture or a torn rotator cuff. In applying the objective standard for causation, the court stated, "[the plaintiff] must show that a reasonable, prudent paraplegic, who had been largely paralyzed by a prior surgery and was dependent upon the use of his arms and shoulders for any mobility at all, and who, at that point, had already achieved about a 20 percent improvement in his adhesive capsulitis condition based on physical therapy alone, would have declined the procedure if informed that it could result in a torn rotator cuff and a fractured bone" (*Wilson v. Merritt*, 2006). The court went on to note, "there was sufficient evidence for a jury to conclude that, under the circumstances, a reasonable, prudent paraplegic would indeed have passed up the opportunity" (*Wilson v. Merritt*, 2006).

Documenting Consent

As a general rule, obtaining consent is a nondelegable duty. In other words, it is the responsibility of the treating provider to obtain informed consent, and it may not be delegated to some other person. When individuals enter a hospital, they are often provided with a general consent form as part of their initial paperwork. This form covers routine diagnostic procedures and medical treatment by hospital staff, as well as other activities, such as release of information for treatment purposes and disposal of human tissue and body fluids. General consent from an individual can be obtained by a staff member of the organization providing the healthcare services. However, if the patient is having a specific type of surgery (for example, open-heart surgery), the surgeon is responsible for obtaining informed consent specifically for that surgery. For both general consent and informed consent, organizational policy may provide for staff members to check for the presence of signed consent forms on patient records.

Whether consent is written or oral, it should be documented in the individual's health record. Written consent is typically provided on a separate document signed by the individual. Especially when consent is provided orally, documentation should describe the risks, benefits, and alternatives discussed by the patient and provider and reflect that patient questions were adequately answered. In certain situations, consent must be obtained in writing. For example, the Common Rule requires the written consent of research subjects, unless the consent requirement has been waived or altered by an IRB (NIH 2006). Various state laws also provide that certain medical interventions require written consent. Those interventions often pertain to the following (Foundation for Taxpayer and Consumer Rights n.d.):

- Sterilization
- Hysterectomy
- Breast cancer treatment
- Prostate cancer treatment
- Gynecological cancer treatment
- Psychosurgery
- Electroconvulsive therapy

CMS and other insurers also require written consent for specific procedures. Their requirement may include a specific form or language to be used when documenting the consent process.

Types of Consent Forms

There are three main types of consent forms: general (or blanket), short form, and long form.

General

Typically, a general consent form is used when individuals are admitted to a hospital or outpatient facility. By signing this form, an individual consents to whatever procedures, interventions, or other routine services (as compared to invasive services that require informed consent) a provider may determine to be medically necessary (Pozgar 2011). Other types of general consent forms may allow school nurses, sports coaches, and camp counselors to consent to nonmedical treatment in place of a minor's parent or guardian. These consents are limited in scope and are temporary in nature.

Short Form

In the human subjects research context, a **short form** is a written document stating that the elements of informed consent required by the Common Rule have been orally presented to and understood by the subject or the subject's legally authorized representative. When the short form is used, there must be a witness to the fact that subjects were orally provided with the requirements for informed consent. The witness must sign the short form (along with the subject) as well as a copy of an IRB-approved written summary of what was said to the subject or the subject's representative (45 CFR 46.117(b)(2)).

The same standards for a short form consent may also be applied in a nonresearch context. Providers may orally explain risks, benefits, and alternatives and have the individual sign a document acknowledging that such an explanation was provided and understood. In such cases, it is advisable for the provider to also have a witness sign the short form and acknowledge the information that was explained.

Long Form

Again in the human subjects research context, a **long form** is a consent form that includes all of the informed consent requirements included in the Common Rule (see section on informed consent requirements above). Outside of research, long consent forms should be used when a proposed medical intervention is particularly high risk, invasive, or experimental.

Check Your Understanding 7.4

Instructions: Indicate whether the following statements are true or false (T or F).

1. Battery is the usual basis of a claim for which an individual did not give consent for a procedure that was performed.

2. The basis for a lack of informed consent claim is generally negligence.

3. A treating provider should delegate the informed consent process to another person.

4. General consent allows healthcare providers to provide routine noninvasive services.

5. Both written and oral consent should be documented in an individual's health record.

Summary

An individual's right to consent or refuse consent to healthcare treatment is one of the most valued rights in American society. However, as this chapter discussed, the right is not absolute and can be affected by factors such as an individual's age and competence and the circumstances of a proposed treatment or intervention. Advance directives play a key role in consent to treatment and end-of-life decisions. Standards for advance directives and other aspects of consent are found in both state and federal statutes, regulations, and case law. Before giving consent, individuals have the right to be fully informed of a treatment's risks, benefits, and alternatives. A provider who fails to fully discuss these things with a patient may be held liable for negligence based on lack of informed consent. If an intervention is performed on a patient with no consent at all, the provider may be held liable for battery. Healthcare providers and individuals responsible for the management of health information must be familiar with the consent law applicable in their states.

References

American College of Surgeons. 1994. Statement on advance directives by patients: "Do not resuscitate" in the operating room. *Bulletin of the American College of Surgeons* 79(9):29.

American Medical Association Council on Ethical and Judicial Affairs. 2006. CEJA report 2-A-06: Withholding information from patients (therapeutic privilege). http://www.ama-assn.org.

American Medical Association. n.d. Patient physician relationship topics: Informed consent. http://www.ama-assn.org

Arizona Secretary of State. 2007. Arizona Advance Directive Registry. http://www.azsos.gov.

Department of Health and Human Services. 2009. Office for Human Research Protections. Guidance on the Genetic Information Nondiscrimination Act: Implications for Investigators and Institutional Review Boards. http://www.hhs.gov.

The Foundation for Taxpayer and Consumer Rights. n.d. The California patient's guide: Your health care rights and remedies. http://www.calpatientguide.org.

General Accountability Office. 1995. Patient Self-Determination Act: Providers offer information on advance directives but effectiveness uncertain (Letter Report GAO/HEHS-95-135). http://www.gao.gov.

Illinois Department of Public Health. 2006. Advance directives: Uniform do-not-resuscitate (DNR) advance directive. Guidance for individuals. http://www.idph.state.il.us.

Kansas Bar Association. 2007. Living Wills and Durable Powers of Attorney. http://www.ksbar.org.

Law Center. 2005. Terri Schiavo has died. http://www.cnn.com.

Missouri Bar. 2006. Living wills and other advance directives: What is a living will? http://www.mobar.org.

National Cancer Institute. n.d.a. Research on human specimens. http://www.cancerdiagnosis.nci.nih.gov.

National Cancer Institute. n.d.b. Dictionary of cancer terms. DNR order. http://www.cancer.gov.

National Institutes of Health. 2006 (Dec. 28). Office of human subjects research information sheets/forms: Sheet 6—Guidelines for writing informed consent documents. http://ohsr.od.nih.gov.

Ohio Hospice & Palliative Care Organization Advance Directives Packet Choices Living Well at the End of Life (2004), http://www.associationdatabase.com.

Oregon Department of Motor Vehicles. n.d. Suspensions and revocations. http://www.oregon.gov.

Pinellas County Probate Court, Florida. 1990. In re: The Guardianship of Theresa Marie Schiavo, Incapacitated. File No. 90-2908GD-003. http://abstractappeal.com.

Pozgar, G. 2011. *Legal Aspects of Health Care Administration*, 11th ed. Sudbury, MA: Jones and Bartlett.

State of California Emergency Medical Services Authority. 2009. Recommended guidelines for EMS personnel regarding do not resuscitate (DNR) and other patient-designated directives limiting pre-hospital care. http://emsa.ca.gov.

Tennessee Department of Health. n.d.a. Advance directives. http://health.state.tn.us.

Tennessee Department of Health. n.d.b. Advance directives for health care decision making. http://health.state.tn.us.

Uniform Law Commissioners. 2002. Uniform Health-Care Decisions Act. http://www.uniformlaws.org

Uniform Law Commissioners. 2006. Uniform Anatomical Gift Act. http://uniformlaws.org

US Legal, Inc., n.d. Age of Majority. http://minors.uslegal.com/age-of-majority/.

Cases, Statutes, and Regulations Cited

Acuna v. Turkish, 384 NJ Super. 395 (App. Div. 2006).

Cruzan v. Director, Missouri Department of Health, 497 US 261; 110 Sect. 2841 (1990).

Duncan v. Scottsdale Medical Imaging, Ltd., 70 P.3d 435; 415 AZ Adv. Rep. 43 (2003).

Hamilton v. Ashton, 846 N.E.2d 309 (IN Ct. App. 2006).

In the Matter of Robert Quackenbush, 156 NJ Super. 282; 382 A.2d 785 (1978).

In Re Quinlan, 70 NJ 10. 355 A.2d 647 (1976).

In Re Storar, 52 NY 2d 363; 420 N.E.2d 64; 52 NY 2d 382; 420 N.E.2d 73 (1981).

Schloendorff v. Society of New York Hospital, 211 NY 125; 105 N.E. 92 (1914).

Union Pacific R. Co. v. Botsford, 141 US 250; 11 Sect. 1000 (1891).

Wilson v. Merritt, 142 Cal. App. 4th 1125, 48 CA Rptr. 3d 630 (2006).

Pub. L. No. 101-508, 104 stat. 1388, codified as 42 USC 81395 cc (f): Patient Self Determination Act (1990).

45 CFR 46.107: Protection of human subjects: IRB membership. 2006.

45 CFR 46.116: Protection of human subjects: General requirements for informed consent. 2006.

45 CFR 46.117(b)(2):Documentation of informed consent. 2010.

KS Stat. Ann. 22-3302: Competency of dependent to stand trial. 1992.

KS Stat. Ann. 58-625: Powers and letters of attorney. 1989.

KS Stat. Ann. 59-2953, 2954: Care and treatment of mentally ill persons. 1998.

KS Stat. Ann. 59-2966: Order for treatment dismissal. 1998.

KS Stat. Ann. 59-3075: Guardian duties, responsibilities, power, authorities. 2002.

KS Stat. Ann. 65-1734: Order of priority of persons authorized to dispose of decedents' remains; immunity of funeral directors, funeral establishments and crematories. 2011.

KS Stat. Ann. 65-2892: Examination and treatment of persons under 18 for venereal disease, liability. 1972.

KS Stat. Ann. 65-2892a: Examination and treatment of minors for drug abuse, misuse or addiction; liability. 2009.

KS Stat. Ann. 65-6009: Persons arrested or convicted; disclosure of test results; costs of counseling and testing. 2001.

MO Rev. Stat. 188.028: Minors, abortion requirements and procedures. 2007.

MO Rev. Stat. 510.040: Court order physical and mental exams. 2007.

MO Rev. Stat. 522.030: Pleadings and proceedings. 2007.

MO Rev. Stat. 537.037: Emergency care (Good Samaritan Law). 2007.

Chapter 8

The Legal Health Record: Maintenance, Content, Documentation, and Disposition

Laurie A. Rinehart-Thompson, JD, RHIA, CHP, FAHIMA,
Rebecca B. Reynolds, EdD, MHA, RHIA, FAHIMA; and
Keith Olenik, MA, RHIA, CHP

Learning Objectives

- List the multiple purposes and content areas of the health record

- Explain the differences between the legal health record and the electronic health record

- Describe the bodies that establish documentation and maintenance standards for the health record

- Identify the documentation principles that support a legally sound health record

- Discuss the legal challenges associated with personal health records

- Describe the factors associated with the creation of health records

- Explain the various situations that lead to health record disposition

Key Terms

Abbreviations	Countersignature	Hybrid health record
Accuracy	Custodian	Initials
Addendum	Designated record set (DRS)	Joint Commission
Amendment	Destruction of records	Late entry
Authentication	Digital signature	Legal health record (LHR)
Authenticity	Disposition	Legibility
Authorship	Electronic health	Liability
Auto-authentication	record (EHR)	Master patient index (MPI)
Business record	Electronic signature	Meaningful use
Completeness	Electronic Signatures in	Medicare
Computer key	Global National Commerce	Metadata
Conditions of	Act (E-SIGN)	Personal health record (PHR)
Participation (CoP)	Handwritten signature	Physician order

Retention
Retention schedule
Revisions
Rubber signature stamps
Statutes of limitations

Timeliness
Transfer of health records
Uniform Electronic
    Transactions Act
    (UETA)

Uniform Photographic Copies
    of Business and Public
    Records as Evidence Act
    (UPA)
Version management

Introduction

Health records have existed for as long as there has been a need to deliver healthcare and communicate information about patient treatment. Patient health records are maintained by hospitals, provider offices, long-term care facilities, rehabilitation facilities, home health organizations, behavioral health organizations, and other healthcare organizations as a means to provide proof of the service and care provided. The content of health records varies according to the type of facility, but records must be maintained to meet patient care needs and to comply with standards and laws, which are often changing or evolving. While the health record has historically been paper-based, its transformation to an electronic format is "expanding the scope of patient information beyond the traditional file folder and even beyond the walls of an individual healthcare provider to include information from other providers and information provided directly by patients" (Servais 2008).

Currently, healthcare facilities maintain health records using paper or electronic formats or a combination of both (**hybrid health records**). Data captured in the health record are from source systems such as administrative, financial, and clinical information systems. The bulk of the record is usually composed of electronically stored information from numerous clinical information systems, such as laboratory, pharmacy, radiology, nursing, and other ancillary systems, along with paper documents. The data may be handwritten, may be direct voice entry captured in a word-processing system, or may come from provider wireless devices such as handheld personal computers (Amatayakul 2013).

The rapid movement from paper health records to **electronic health records** (EHRs) is aimed at promoting better patient care and reducing healthcare costs. However, health information and informatics professionals face evolving challenges in managing the confidentiality, privacy, and security of patient health records. Numerous state and federal laws, as well as accrediting and licensing standards, affect the generation and use of patient health records and the information contained within them. This in turn requires that those responsible for managing patient health records define what constitutes a legal health record and a legally sound health record in whatever format it is maintained. This chapter discusses the purposes of the health record and the concept of defining a legal health record. It also discusses the principles and guidelines related to the maintenance, content, and documentation requirements necessary to support a legally sound health record, whether that record is paper-based or electronic. The chapter concludes with a discussion of the life cycle of the health record, from creation and retention to eventual disposition.

Purposes of the Health Record

Patient health records serve several purposes, as outlined in figure 8.1. The most important purpose is to document patient treatment and continuity of care. A health record describes the reasons for a patient's encounter, background facts, observations, and treatment, or the care rendered by a provider. It serves as a communication tool that facilitates clinical decision making. Regardless of its format, the health record provides a place for the healthcare team to record information that can be used to make healthcare decisions. A team member can review the patient's status and actions taken by other team members. Thus, the health record is the healthcare team's primary reference and communication tool.

Another purpose of the health record is to provide proof of services rendered for reimbursement. Insurance companies, managed care organizations, and government programs such as **Medicare**

Figure 8.1. Purposes of the health record

- Facilitate the ongoing care and treatment of individual patients
- Support clinical decision making and communication among clinicians
- Document the services provided to patients in support of reimbursement
- Provide information for the evaluation of the quality and efficacy of the care provided
- Provide information in support of medical research and education
- Help facilitate the operational management of the facility
- Provide evidence in legal cases and information as required by local and national laws and regulations

require that specific information be documented in the health record to support the bill and to prove that the care provided was medically necessary. Documentation in the health record is also used to prove the quality and efficacy of care rendered by the healthcare provider, including information necessary for internal and external review and data required for a healthcare organization to achieve accreditation, certification, or licensure.

With the proliferation of EHRs and national emphasis on their implementation and use by physicians, a physician's ability to demonstrate **meaningful use** of the EHR will drive many physician-payment incentives. For a physician to demonstrate that he or she used data in the EHR, specific data elements must be present in the EHR system, and appropriate audit trails must exist. As this national effort continues to evolve, HIM and informatics professionals must be aware of the meaningful use definitions and ensure that the health record can support these changing documentation requirements for reimbursement.

Health records support medical research by providing information used to investigate medical conditions, treatment modalities, and prevention and control procedures, and to monitor disease trends. The health record supports the education and training of a variety of health professionals as well as healthcare consumers. Healthcare consumers may use personal health records (discussed later in this chapter) for health and wellness initiatives and to assume responsibility for their healthcare.

From an organization-wide standpoint, information from health records supports operational activities. For example, information gathered from health records may provide data on the use of services, provider patterns, and other important issues for benchmarking and strategic planning. Operationally, information in the health record also facilitates managerial decision making to improve the quality of patient care.

Finally, the health record serves as a legal document. It is the legal **business record** of the organization and serves as evidence in lawsuits or other legal actions, as discussed in chapter 4. In medical malpractice cases, the record may be used by either the plaintiff or the defendant to prove or disprove a patient's case regarding treatment rendered. It may also be used in personal injury lawsuits, workers' compensation hearings, or criminal prosecutions where the health record of a victim of a violent crime is introduced into evidence. It may provide details that witness testimony cannot.

The Legal Health Record

As just mentioned, the health record is the legal business record of an organization and serves as evidence in lawsuits or other legal actions. A business record is made and kept in the usual course of business at or near the time of the event recorded, as discussed in chapter 4. Because information that is recorded in conjunction with business practices is presumed to be trustworthy and have potential evidentiary value, it is thus generally admissible as evidence in legal proceedings. It is the record used for legal purposes and would be the record released upon a valid request. Thus, the health record serves as the **legal health record** (LHR) for an organization. The contents of an organization's LHR, however, vary depending on how the organization defines it.

Historically, the definition of the LHR focused on the paper record and its content, including radiology films and other imaging documents (AHIMA e-HIM Work Group on Defining the Legal Health Record 2005a). That definition may hold true today for organizations that function in a truly paper-based environment. However, with information technology's ability to collect, store, retrieve, and generate information electronically, the health records of most healthcare organizations are both paper and electronic, making the definition of an LHR more complex (AHIMA e-HIM Work Group on Defining the Legal Health Record 2005a). There is no one-size-fits-all definition of the LHR since laws and regulations governing the maintenance, content, and documentation requirements of a health record vary by practice setting, state and federal laws and regulations, and accrediting body standards (AHIMA e-HIM Work Group on Defining the Legal Health Record 2005a). However, the American Health Information Management Association (AHIMA) suggests that the following common principles be considered when creating a definition:

- The legal health record is generated at or for a healthcare organization as its business record and is the record that will be disclosed upon request. It does not affect the discoverability of other information held by the organization.

- Legal health records are records of care in any health-related setting used by healthcare professionals while providing patient care services or for administrative, business, or payment purposes. Some types of documentation that make up the legal health record may physically exist in separate and multiple paper-based or electronic or computer-based databases.

- The legal health record is the documentation of healthcare services provided to an individual during any aspect of healthcare delivery in any type of healthcare organization. It is consumer- or patient-centric. It contains individually identifiable data stored on any medium and collected and directly used in documenting healthcare or health status.

- Legal health records must meet accepted standards as defined by applicable federal regulations, state laws, and standards of accrediting agencies, as well as the policies of the healthcare provider.

- The **custodian** of the legal health record is usually a health information manager in collaboration with information technology personnel. Health information and informatics management professionals oversee the operational functions related to collecting, protecting, and archiving the legal health record, while information technology staff manages the technical infrastructure of the electronically stored information (AHIMA e-HIM Work Group on Defining the Legal Health Record 2005b).

If the health record is a hybrid record (partially paper and partially electronic), the healthcare organization must determine which data elements, electronic-structured documents, images, audio files, video files, and paper documents do and do not belong in the LHR. This is challenging given the unique types and amount of information that an electronic record system is capable of producing and storing. Knowledge of the source of information (paper or electronic) helps to further define each data element in the LHR and determine whether that element should be released upon request or subpoena (AHIMA e-HIM Work Group on Defining the Legal Health Record 2005b). Given the complexities of a paper- and electronic-based record environment, Servais (2008) offers eight situations to consider when defining the LHR, as summarized in figure 8.2.

Another important consideration when defining an LHR is an organization's **designated record set** (DRS). Any healthcare provider, plan, or healthcare clearinghouse that electronically transmits health information is subject to the federal Health Insurance Portability and Accountability Act (HIPAA) Privacy Rule (45 CFR 164 Subpart E). The HIPAA Privacy Rule will be discussed in much greater detail in the next chapter. However, for this chapter, it is important to understand that a DRS refers to health records and records involved in billing, insurance enrollment and coverage, and other documents "used, in whole or in part . . . to make decisions about individuals" (45 CFR 164.501). It includes records in all formats and records from other providers that are used to make decisions about an individual, including e-mail communications between a patient and a provider. The DRS encompasses more information than what is normally considered part of an LHR. Thus, a healthcare organization will need to determine which elements of the DRS will be part of its LHR and which will not.

Figure 8.2. Considerations in defining the data that constitute the LHR

1. **Sources and Secondary Data:** The same information can reside in more than one location: the source system that originally collects and receives patient information and the secondary system that receives data from the source system. For example, laboratory results may reside in both the laboratory's information system and in a clinical repository or results-reporting system. In determining which system will produce the document or data for the LHR, an organization must decide which system will be the "source of truth" or official source of data. Failure to designate a source may result in inconsistent or incomplete information being disclosed.

2. **Detail vs. Summary Data:** Findings of diagnostic studies may exist digitally in both detail and interpretive/summary form in an EHR database. Because the documents containing the findings are not identical, a decision about whether one or both will be included in the LHR must be made.

3. **Paper vs. Images:** Documents may exist both on paper and as images in a document management system. Examples include consents and "do not resuscitate" orders. The Uniform Photographic Copies of Business and Public Records as Evidence Act, which allows originals to be destroyed and reproductions to be used in their place, has been adopted by over half of the states.

4. **Data Not to Include:** Some documents or data elements, either in electronic or some other form, are not appropriate for inclusion in the content of the LHR because they do not meet the business record hearsay exception established by the Federal Rules of Evidence. For example, incident reports, insurance forms, psychotherapy notes, cancer registry data, and derived data such as accreditation reports, quality indicators, and statistical reports would not normally be included as part of an LHR.

5. **Decision Support:** Many EHR systems contain decision support documentation such as alerts, pop-up notices, and other reminders regarding orders, tests, and treatments. A healthcare organization must decide whether this documentation should be included in the LHR. Although they are not part of the healthcare documentation made in the regular course of business, actions taken in response to these reminders do affect provider treatment decisions that ultimately impact a patient's care.

6. **Sources of Communication:** Communications with patients and their family members may take place electronically through voice mails, e-mails, and Web-based portals. Whether these communications become part of the LHR depends on whether the communication provides documentation of the patient's care or justifies treatment or diagnoses. An electronic communication that establishes an appointment would not ordinarily be considered documentation of patient care and would not be considered part of the LHR and subject to disclosure. However, if the electronic communication provides documentation of patient care, treatment, or diagnosis, then it would be included in the LHR.

7. **Personal Health Records:** Patients are becoming much more involved in and educated about their own healthcare decisions. Accordingly, they are being encouraged to maintain their own personal health records (PHRs). Because information in a PHR, particularly documents compiled by patients such as immunization histories, would likely not qualify as a business record, a PHR would not be included in the LHR even though it might affect treatment decisions.

8. **Sharing of Data Between Providers:** Patient data may be transmitted electronically from one provider to another. Whether data created elsewhere becomes part of a receiving organization's LHR must be determined by the organization. If the information received is used to make decisions about the patient's care, treatment, or diagnosis, it should be included in the LHR. However, the receiving provider must document that the data were used in the health record in order for the data to be part of the LHR.

Source: Servais 2008.

Defining the LHR is important to an organization's business and legal processes. Also important is ensuring that the record is legally sound or defensible. Many principles and guidelines that support maintaining a legally sound health record, whether paper or electronic, are discussed in the remainder of this chapter.

Paper versus Electronic Health Records

For decades, the paper health record retained a relatively consistent appearance and format across many types of healthcare organizations. A provider who practiced in different types of healthcare organizations could generally pick up a paper health record and understand its organization and content.

Now many healthcare organizations function with a hybrid health record as they transition to an EHR, resulting in health records with very different appearances from one organization to another. The boundaries of the health record have expanded to include a compilation of information from a variety of media sources (paper, databases, images, text, tracings, pictures, and so forth) created both inside and outside the healthcare organization. In addition, electronic records tend to differ from paper records in six key areas, as previously discussed in chapter 4 and summarized again in figure 8.3. The differences among paper health records, hybrid health records, and EHRs add to the challenge of ensuring that an organization's health records are legally sound or defensible if called into question.

The **Uniform Photographic Copies of Business and Public Records as Evidence Act** (UPA) (28 USC 1732), of which there are both federal and state versions, states that the reproduction of any record retained in the regular course of business and kept by a process that accurately reproduces the original in any medium will be admissible as evidence. This act is important because it supports the transition from paper to electronic storage of information. It is imperative that the method used to electronically store information be reliable and able to accurately reproduce a facsimile of the original record. Healthcare organizations must consider preservation requirements of electronically stored information, including any migration of the record from one system or medium to another. Requirements of discovery and retention, as outlined in other chapters, define these expectations in greater detail.

Figure 8.3. Summary of six key areas where electronic records differ from paper records

1. Volume and duplicability (ability to replicate)—Challenges the viewer of the information to determine whether the version being viewed is valid or the most current.

2. Persistence—Electronic documents continue to exist on a computer or in a network after they have been deleted.

3. Dynamic changeable content (modifiability)—Changes, either by human intervention or by software programs, may not be visible without performing additional investigation.

4. Metadata (data about data)—Can track creation, access, revision, and printing of data.

5. Environment dependence and obsolescence (technology dependence)—Data may be inaccessible or incomprehensible outside of compatible hardware and software in which the data reside; ability to access and comprehend data is critical for the retention of electronic records.

6. Dispersion and searchability—Electronic records can be stored simultaneously in multiple locations, moved along a network both inside and outside an organization, and searched readily for specific pieces of information.

Source: The Sedona Conference 2007.

Check Your Understanding 8.1

Instructions: Indicate whether the following statements are true or false (T or F).

1. Health records using a combination of paper and electronic formats are hybrid records.

2. The most important purpose of the health record is to provide proof of services for reimbursement.

3. The health record is not permitted to serve as an organization's business record.

4. There are both federal and state versions of the Uniform Photographic Copies of Business and Public Records as Evidence Act.

5. The custodian of the LHR is responsible for collecting, protecting, and archiving the record.

Health Record Maintenance, Content, and Documentation Requirements

Standards for record maintenance, content, and documentation requirements have been established by a number of sources, including state and federal laws, accrediting bodies, and professional standard-setting organizations. State licensure requirements must be met in order for specific healthcare organizations to remain licensed. They may include specific requirements for the content, format, retention, and use of patient records. Statutes and their resulting regulations are usually under the jurisdiction of state health departments. The requirements may be specific or broad depending on the type of organization and the state. Most healthcare organizations defer to the record maintenance, content, and documentation requirements set forth by the Department of Health and Human Services (HHS), the Centers for Medicare and Medicaid Services (CMS), the **Joint Commission**, or other accreditation bodies.

Federally, CMS is responsible for developing and enforcing regulations regarding the participation of healthcare providers in Medicare and Medicaid programs, which provide healthcare services to qualified individuals. CMS sets forth health record maintenance, content, and documentation requirements in the **Conditions of Participation** (CoP) for Hospitals, as well as in the Conditions of Participation for a variety of healthcare settings, such as psychiatric hospitals and ambulatory surgical centers. The Conditions of Participation for Hospitals, for example, requires that a health record be maintained for every individual evaluated or treated as an inpatient or outpatient (42 CFR 482.24 (b)). In addition, the Conditions of Participation for Hospitals specifically requires that the content for health records "contain information to justify admission and continued hospitalization, support and diagnosis, and describe the patient's progress and response to medications and services" (42 CFR 482.24(c)).

The Joint Commission, which accredits many types of healthcare organizations, also requires that health records be maintained and that content and documentation standards be followed. The Joint Commission *Comprehensive Accreditation Manual for Hospitals* (CAMH) has standards dedicated to defining the components of a complete medical record. *CAMH* includes guidance for developing policies and procedures for the compilation, completion, authentication, retention, and release of health records. The Joint Commission's standards include specific content pertaining to health records, such as the elements to be included in the discharge summary, and content pertaining to a history and physical, operative reports, and consultations (Joint Commission 2010a, RC.01.01.01, RC02.01.01, RC02.01.03, RC.02.04.010). AHIMA also addresses maintenance, content, and documentation issues as a component of its professional practice standards.

In addition to the external standards that have been described, an organization's medical staff bylaws, rules, and regulations may also delineate requirements for the maintenance and content of health records, as well as documentation and completion standards. Medical staff bylaws and rules of individual healthcare organizations are approved by an organization's board of trustees or governing body. Bylaws usually delineate the content of health records, identify personnel permitted to document in the health record, describe time limits for record completion, and restate applicable health record requirements, such as Medicare Conditions of Participation, Joint Commission standards, and state regulations and penalties for noncompliance. State, federal, and/or Joint Commission surveyors routinely review health records, regardless of the record format or type of organization, to ensure that regulations, standards, and internal requirements as described in the bylaws are being followed (Joint Commission 2010a, MS.01.01.01).

Figure 8.4 provides a listing of standard health record content. For readers not familiar with health record content or the way the health record is compiled, see appendix 8.A (pp. 198–211). This appendix contains a detailed listing of documents typically found in a health record and information specific to various types of healthcare organizations and providers who contribute to the health record.

Documentation Principles for Health Record Entries

Just as important as complying with standards for the maintenance and content of the health record is establishing and enforcing documentation principles that not only facilitate quality patient care and

Figure 8.4. Content of the health record

Health record summary sheet (face sheet)	Ancillary reports
Administrative and demographic information	Laboratory reports
Registration data	Radiology reports
Consent to treatment	EKGs
Consent to use or disclose protected health	EEGs
information	MRIs or CT scans
Consent to special procedures	Surgical services
Advance directives	Anesthesia records
Acknowledgment of receipt of Patient's Rights	Operative report
Statement	Pathology report
Property and valuables list	Discharge summary
Birth and death certificates	Discharge plan
Clinical data	Specialized documents
Medical history	Obstetrical care
Physical examination	Neonatal care
Diagnostic and therapeutic orders	Emergency care
Special orders	Ambulatory/outpatient care
Discharge orders	Home health care
Clinical observations	Behavioral health care
Progress notes	Hospice care
Consultation reports	Rehabilitation care
Ancillary notes	Long-term care
Nursing services	
Assessment	
Care plan	
Flow sheet	
Medication administration records (MARs)	

patient safety but also provide a legally sound document. Many documentation guidelines that have historically applied to paper health records also apply to documentation in EHRs.

Language

Regardless of the medium in which a health record entry resides (that is, electronic, imaged, or paper), fundamental documentation principles apply to ensure the quality of a health record entry and reduce the risk of liability. Health record content should be specific, objective, and factual (what is known versus what is thought or presumed) and should contain complete information. Examples of generalizations and vague words that should be avoided include "patient doing well," "appears to be," "confused," "anxious," "status quo," "stable," and "as usual." If an author must speculate, the documentation must state that it is speculation. If the record documents what can be seen, heard, touched, and smelled, the entries will be specific and objective. Signs and symptoms should be described, and quotation marks should be used when quoting the patient's exact words.

A patient's response to care should be documented. Deviations from standard treatment, including the reason for the deviations, must be documented completely (AHIMA e-HIM Work Group on Maintaining the Legal EHR 2005). Situations that generate incident reports (described in chapters 4 and 14) should also be described objectively in the health record, with care taken not to assign blame or identify failures. For example, a patient fall must be recorded in the health record. However, the health record is not the appropriate place to identify the fall as being the result of "the janitor's consistent failure to put up 'wet floor' signs."

Individuals Who May Document

A governing body or board of trustees has ultimate legal responsibility for the quality of care rendered in a healthcare organization, except in organizations owned by individuals or the government. An organization's medical staff bylaws set rules for record content and who may document in the health record. Once the bylaws have been established, however, ultimate responsibility for the quality of documentation is delegated to individual providers who create and authenticate entries in the health record. The categories of personnel permitted to document in the health record will vary depending on the type of entry. Providers are permitted to create progress notes relative to their specific discipline and generally include physicians, nurses, therapists, social workers, case managers, dietitians, nurse anesthetists, pharmacists, radiology technologists, and others providing direct treatment or consultation.

Each person authorized to enter documentation into the progress notes must create his or her own note, authenticate it, provide a complete date (month, day, year) and time, and indicate authorship by signing his or her full name and title. (Authentication and authorship are discussed in greater detail later in the chapter.) Charting for a block of time (for example, 7 a.m. to 4 p.m.) is not recommended, because it does not correlate specific activities with the times they were performed by the individual who is documenting (Dougherty 2002). Documentation must be created and authenticated by the person responsible for examinations, procedures, interpretations, and other similar types of treatments. Special rules govern orders, which are discussed below.

Gaps and Omissions

A health record must reflect the chronology of the patient's care. Gaps and omissions detract from a chronology and do not contribute to quality patient care, leaving a healthcare organization susceptible to liability.

Gaps are spaces left between entries in the paper health record. Although physical gaps do not necessarily indicate that documentation has been omitted, the spaces allow subsequent entries to be made in a space previous to any entry already made. This can create confusion and hamper a patient's care. If the document is the subject of a lawsuit, such misplaced entries can create suspicion or evidence of wrongdoing. Individuals who document in paper health records must avoid leaving blank spaces between entries, to prevent information from being added out of sequence. EHR systems may not allow for gaps in the health record since all entries are timed and dated by the EHR system.

In addition to gaps in physical documentation, gaps and omissions can also occur in time. Long periods of time without documentation can also hamper patient care when necessary information is either entered late or not entered at all, particularly when such information might have already proved useful to patient care or may no longer be completely reliable due to the passage of time. Gaps and omissions in time negatively impact the timeliness of the health record, a requirement that will be discussed later in the chapter.

Orders

One of the most important pieces of documentation within the health record is the **physician order**. Physicians give orders for medical interventions such as treatments, ancillary medical services, tests and procedures, medications, and seclusion and restraint. Medication orders, which specify a particular drug, dosage, frequency, duration, and route (for example, orally or intravenously), are a source of treatment errors. Therefore, their accuracy is extremely important. Orders for the administration of medications such as narcotics and sedatives have time limits or stop orders, which automatically discontinue the medication unless the physician gives a specific order to continue.

Legibility has historically been problematic in paper records; this issue is progressively being resolved through the implementation of computerized provider order-entry (CPOE) systems that eliminate handwritten orders and reduce the risk of illegible handwriting and its associated liability. Although physicians are often the only class of healthcare professionals permitted by law to give orders, this is gradually changing as some states have granted physician assistants and nurse practitioners the ability to give orders and prescribe medications. Medical staff bylaws delineate which providers in a facility are authorized to give orders and the scope of practice for which they are authorized to give orders.

There are two types of orders, written and verbal. Verbal orders are of two types. They may be communicated in person or over the telephone to individuals authorized to receive them. The person receiving the order should sign his or her name, give his or her credential (for example, RN, PT, or LPN), and record the date and time the order was received. Because of the risks associated with miscommunication, verbal orders are strongly discouraged and are not permitted in certain health-care organizations for treatments or procedures that might put the patient at risk. When a provider is physically present, it is suggested that he or she document the order instead of dictating it to another individual. The Joint Commission has a read-back process. This mandates that, before taking action on a verbal order or verbal report of a test result, staff use a record and "read back" process to verify the information (Joint Commission 2010a, PC.02.01.03). Joint Commission standards require that the hospital identify, in writing, staff who are authorized to receive and record verbal orders (Joint Commission 2010a, RC.02.03.07).

Medical staff bylaws must specifically state the categories of personnel authorized to accept orders. Verbal orders for medication are usually required to be given to, and to be accepted only by, nursing or pharmacy personnel. Some categories of personnel that may accept verbal orders for services within their specific area of practice include physical therapists, registered nurse anesthetists, dietitians, and medical technologists.

All orders must be authenticated (verified) by the provider who gave the order or who is responsible for the patient's care. Verbal orders should be authenticated as soon as possible after they are given. Although time requirements for authentication of orders are governed by state law, accreditation standards and organizational policies are also factors for determining time frames for the authentication of verbal orders. Medicare regulations state that in the absence of state law, authentication shall occur within 48 hours. Organizations may require the ordering provider to authenticate orders within as few as 24 hours.

Some hospitals perform retrospective post-discharge reviews and analyses, in which personnel indicate orders that are lacking signatures and the responsible provider can individually authenticate them after patient discharge. However, because retrospective reviews do not affect the patient's care process, a more effective system is the review of orders while the patient is in the hospital, also known as concurrent or open-record review. Through these reviews, orders can be authenticated in a timely manner, and providers with patterns of unsigned orders can be detected. A comparison of orders with laboratory reports, other ancillary reports, and nursing documentation also ensures that orders were carried out and that the reports are included in the health record. In a paper system or a system where records are imaged after patient discharge, concurrent reviews ensure that documents are in the correct patient record. Concurrent reviews are also used for progress notes and other documents that require authentication.

Hostile Patients

When entries are made in the health record regarding a patient who is particularly hostile or irritable, general documentation principles apply, such as charting objective facts and avoiding the use of personal opinions, particularly those that are critical of the patient. These general principles are especially important because a disagreeable patient may cause a provider to use more expressive and inappropriate language. Further, a hostile patient may be more likely to file legal action in the future if the hostility is a personal attribute and not simply a manifestation of his or her medical condition.

Staff Disagreements

Professionals working in the healthcare field will not always agree on a patient's course of treatment and may need to communicate these differing professional opinions to one another. In fact, one's professional standards may require that another's decisions be questioned if it is believed that those decisions will cause harm to a patient. However, documentation of staff disagreements in the health record heightens the risk of liability for both the healthcare organization and those involved in the disagreement. Individuals documenting in the health record should avoid recording disagreements in the record so as not to raise suspicion of negligence that will result in the record becoming the centerpiece of litigation.

Organizational policy should outline the parameters for staff disagreements. General documentation principles, introduced earlier in this chapter, should be followed to ensure an objective and factual record. Besides providing a basis for liability, identifying a colleague in the record as "mistaken" or "negligent" or otherwise using inflammatory language does not further quality patient care. While the documented professional conclusions of each practitioner may be inconsistent with one another, drawing attention to those differences or the emotions associated with a disagreement is best left to conversations outside the health record itself.

Documentation of Injuries Resulting from Criminal Activity

Healthcare providers may encounter and treat individuals whom they believe to be the victims of abuse, which may constitute criminal activity. As described in chapter 13, most states require healthcare personnel to report suspected abuse of specified vulnerable classes, such as children, the elderly, and individuals with developmental disabilities. Many of these statutes also provide immunity to individuals who report their suspicions in good faith. Healthcare providers may also encounter victims of criminal activities, such as gunshot wounds and stabbings. Objective and factual documentation in the health record should accompany reports made to authorities. Documentation should include statements made by the suspected victim, the identification of injuries, a thorough description of injuries, and photographs of the injuries.

Liability for Improper Entries

As described throughout this section, inappropriate documentation may lead to **liability** for an organization and its personnel and can make the health record the focal point of legal action. Missing or incomplete information in the health record may cause a court to instruct the jury that it may infer provider negligence. Further, documentation that is present can be equally damaging if it is biased, is critical of a patient or another provider, or includes personal opinions instead of medically relevant facts. Healthcare providers must be trained to document appropriately to achieve quality patient care and minimize the risk of legal liability.

Check Your Understanding 8.2

Instructions: Indicate whether the following statements are true or false (T or F).

1. "Patient appears to be anxious" is an example of good documentation in the health record.

2. Charting for a block of time is recommended because it saves time.

3. Medical staff bylaws must state the categories of personnel authorized to accept physician orders.

4. Professional conclusions of individual practitioners should be documented in the health record so that they agree with one another.

5. A jury may be permitted to infer provider negligence based on missing or incomplete information in the health record.

Maintaining a Legally Defensible Health Record

The integrity of a health record—its accuracy and completeness—is critical to its defensibility in a court of law. The documentation or information (data) within the record must be accurate and complete (Post and Anderson 2006). Documentation guidelines are similar for both paper records and EHRs; however, there are additional issues exclusive to ensuring the integrity of electronic records, including the electronic capture, storage, and retrieval of health information. Many elements contribute to a health record's integrity and, ultimately, to patient safety: authentication, accuracy, authorship, use of abbreviations, legibility, transparent changes to the record, timeliness, completeness, and the appropriate use of the print function. All these contribute to the accuracy and legal soundness of the health record, whether paper or electronic.

Authentication

As introduced earlier in chapters 3 and 4, **authenticity** refers to the genuineness of a record, that it is what it purports to be (AHIMA e-HIM Work Group on Defining the Legal Health Record 2005b). Information is authentic if it is proved to be immune from tampering and corruption. Establishing the authenticity of documentation is critical because individuals who work with or otherwise rely on health records must be assured that the information has not been altered either intentionally or accidentally. The Federal Rules of Evidence allow reproduced business records to be admitted into evidence if there is no question about their authenticity (Federal Rules of Evidence (803(6)). As mentioned earlier, states that have adopted the Uniform Photographic Copies of Business and Public Records as Evidence Act (see figure 8.5) allow for the admissibility of a reproduced business record without the original (Kerr 2001; Hughes 2001).

Authenticity is especially important with EHRs because of the perception that electronic documentation can be manipulated and altered. Authenticity pertains not only to the information created but also to the system used to create and store the information. System reliability and perception of the system's uptime (as opposed to downtime) are important to support the information's authenticity. Controlled access to the application itself is another crucial component of ensuring authenticity. Inappropriate handling of information, from a purely technical standpoint, will result in the information being invalidated and may negate the assertion that users rely on it in the normal course of business (a component of the hearsay exception for electronic records).

Related to the concept of authenticity is **authentication** of information in the health record, which refers to the ability to verify the source of a message by identifying its author and assigning responsibility to that author for entries made within the health record (Post and Anderson 2006). Authentication can be accomplished in several ways, although state statutes and regulations should be consulted regarding the legality of each.

Figure 8.5. States that have adopted the Uniform Photographic Copies of Business and Public Records as Evidence Act

Alabama	Kentucky	New York	Vermont
Alaska	Maine	North Carolina	Virgin Islands
California	Maryland	North Dakota	Virginia
Colorado	Massachusetts	Pennsylvania	Washington
Connecticut	Michigan	Rhode Island	West Virginia
Georgia	Minnesota	South Carolina	Wisconsin
Idaho	Nebraska	South Dakota	
Iowa	New Hampshire	Tennessee	
Kansas	New Jersey	Utah	

Source: Information Requirements Clearinghouse 2005, 3–4.

The Medicare Conditions of Participation for Hospitals contains two references to authentication in medical records. Section 482.24(b) states that "the hospital must use a system of author identification and record maintenance that ensures the integrity of the authentication and protects the security of all record entries." Section 482.24(c)(1) states that "all entries must be legible and complete, and must be authenticated and dated promptly by the person (identified by name and discipline) who is responsible for ordering, providing, or evaluating the service furnished." Section (c) also requires that "the author of each entry must be identified and must authenticate his or her entry; and authentication may include signatures, written initials or computer entry." These are described later in this section. The Conditions of Participation for settings other than hospitals requires that all entries in the record be signed but does not include details about methods of authentication.

The AHIMA practice brief "Maintaining a Legally Sound Health Record—Paper and Electronic" emphasizes that "for paper records, acceptable authentication methods generally include written handwritten signature, initials, and rubber signature stamps. Acceptable authentication methods for the EHR generally include electronic or digital signatures and computer key. Acceptable methods of authenticating an imaged document may follow paper or electronic guidelines" (AHIMA e-HIM Work Group on Maintaining the Legal EHR 2005, 64B). The following section expands on the information presented in this practice brief.

Authentication of Paper Records

Handwritten signatures completed in ink are the most common method of authenticating paper health records. Medicare Conditions of Participation 482.24 (c)(1) requires, at a minimum, the authenticating individual's name and discipline (for example, physical therapy), although a healthcare organization can require additional identifying information, such as the author's title or credential.

In lieu of a full signature, **initials** may be permitted as long as they are readily identifiable as the author's through a signature legend on the same document. Initials are more practical authentication devices than full signatures on documents with limited space, such as flow sheets and medication administration records. However, they should be avoided on entries such as narrative notes or assessments and may not be used where a signature is legally required. Because authentication by initials makes it difficult to positively identify the author of an entry, particularly when other practitioners share the same initials as the author, a healthcare organization reserves the right to prohibit them (AHIMA e-HIM Work Group on Maintaining the Legal EHR 2005).

Rubber signature stamps are acceptable if allowed by state and federal law as well as by payers. Using external rules and internal considerations as a guide, healthcare organization policies should define the parameters within which the use of rubber stamp signatures is acceptable, if at all. (There isn't a reference for this statement as the individual state laws are too numerous to list.) A significant change to the acceptability of rubber stamps came about after a CMS memorandum (Transmittal #248) included the statement that stamped signatures are not acceptable on any medical record. Organizations must determine the logistics of having different standards for authentication based on the payer. Similar to the use of initials, a list of signatures should be maintained to cross-reference each signature to an individual author when rubber signature stamps are used. According to the Joint Commission, the individual identified by the signature stamp or method of electronic authentication is the only individual who uses it (Joint Commission 2010a, RC.01.02.01).

Authentication of Electronic Records

To this point, the types of authentication discussed have related to paper records or imaged (scanned) records that were authenticated when they existed in paper form. The EHR presents a separate set of issues with regard to authentication. New standards for electronic signatures have been proposed in the HL7 EHR—System Records Management and Evidentiary Support (RM-ES) Functional Profile Standard. Health Level Seven International (HL7) is a not-for-profit standards developing organization accredited by the American National Standards Institute (ANSI) that is dedicated to providing a comprehensive framework and related standards for the exchange, integration, sharing, and retrieval of electronic health information that supports clinical practice and the management, delivery, and evaluation of health services. Compliance with these standards is currently voluntary, but as they become more readily adopted, there will be expectations that functionality will be consistent among all EHR products (AHIMA e-HIM Work Group: Best Practices for Electronic Signature and Attestation 2009).

Handwritten signatures merely indicate the signer's intent, whereas signatures in the electronic environment can serve the additional purposes of identifying the signer and ensuring integrity of the document. To ensure integrity of the document, three elements must be included with the method of signature used to authenticate the document (AHIMA e-HIM Work Group on Maintaining the Legal EHR 2005, 64C):

- *Authenticity* verifies the source or origin of the information and the person who created it. The process used must guarantee that the information is valid and can be relied on for the intended purpose.

- *Integrity* is the accuracy and completeness of the information. Is the document the same after having been stored or transmitted as it was at the original time of signing? The user of the information must be confident that there has been no alteration.

- *Nonrepudiation* ensures that a document cannot later be denied by one of the parties, either the originator or the receiver.

Authentication of information produced from an EHR at the highest level of accuracy, or with information that would eliminate any question of integrity, may involve the production of metadata to validate without question the integrity. **Metadata** provides information about a certain item's content, including means of creation, purpose of the data, time and date of creation, creator or author of data, placement on a network (electronic form) where the data were created, standards used (ISO9000), and so forth (McClean 2005). An audit trail can demonstrate the actions of every individual that resulted in the creation of information within the record. Production of metadata to validate the audit trail will eliminate any questions about the reliability of this information. Verbal testament from the record custodian will most likely not be enough for attestation of the record's reliability. Organizations must evaluate their ability to produce metadata and develop appropriate policies (AHIMA e-HIM Work Group: Best Practices for Electronic Signature and Attestation 2009).

Electronic signatures (e-signatures) can be viewed as the technological corollary to the handwritten signature in the paper record. E-signatures use software to bind a signature or other distinguishable mark to a specific electronic document. They require user authentication, such as a unique code, biometric identifier, or password, that is linked to the user's name, credentials, and access rights to verify the identity of the signer in the system and create an individual signature on the record (AHIMA e-HIM Work Group on Implementing Electronic Signatures 2003a).

Because e-signatures will be applied more frequently on documents in the health record where they are produced and retained in electronic formats, they do not become part of the documents that are available in the paper record. Strong policies that ensure password security are critical to ensure data integrity. Thus, a statement ensuring that the password is controlled and used only by the responsible provider should be required to ensure that the provider understands the importance of securing his or her password and the consequences of sharing it with others. E-signatures are acceptable if allowed by state and federal law and payer requirements. EHR software that includes an e-signature feature should contain the three assurances regarding authenticity, integrity, and nonrepudiation, as described in the bulleted list above. E-signatures are frequently used to authenticate transcribed reports created by a transcriptionist from physician dictation and in CPOE systems.

A digital ink or digitized signature differs from an e-signature in that, instead of using a code or other identifier, it uses a handwritten signature on a pen pad that is converted into an electronic image. Digitized signatures are acceptable if allowed by state and federal law and payer requirements (AHIMA e-HIM Work Group on Maintaining the Legal EHR 2005).

A **digital signature** is a subset of e-signature technology. A digital signature does not produce an electronic version of a handwritten signature, but instead encrypts the document (represented by a series of numbers), identifies who performed the encryption (that is, the person who is authenticating), and validates and detects whether any subsequent changes have been made to the document (AHIMA e-HIM Work Group on Implementing Electronic Signatures 2003a). A digital signature is linked to the document in a database application where the information is stored. It "provides a digital guarantee that information has not been modified, as if it were protected by a tamper-proof seal that is broken if the content is altered" (AHIMA e-HIM Work Group on Maintaining the Legal EHR 2005, 64c).

A **computer key** (a number unique to a specific computer) or other code is an acceptable method for authenticating entries in an EHR if allowed by state and federal law and payer requirements. A legend should link each code to an individual author. Authorized users should sign a statement ensuring that they will not allow others to use the computer key and that they understand that appropriate sanctions may be taken for misuse (AHIMA e-HIM Work Group on Maintaining the Legal EHR 2005).

Electronic Signature Legislation

Laws associated with e-signatures have been passed in order to promote e-commerce. Nonuniform laws passed by Utah and California were followed by a more coordinated approach. In 1999, the National Conference of Commissioners of Uniform State Laws (NCCUSL) introduced the **Uniform Electronic Transactions Act** (UETA). Its purpose was to make electronic transactions as enforceable as paper transactions in order to remove barriers to e-commerce and increase the level of trust associated with electronic business transactions. In 2000, Congress passed the **Electronic Signatures in Global National Commerce Act** (E-SIGN), which gives e-signatures the same legality as handwritten signatures where interstate commerce is involved (15 USC 7001, et seq.). Its purpose was to facilitate e-commerce and address some of the legal barriers to electronic transactions by providing that a signature or record may not be denied legal effect solely because it was created electronically.

E-SIGN also provides guidance on how records may be stored and retained electronically. If a document is required by law to be retained, an electronic version is acceptable if the document accurately reflects the information in the record, is accessible, and can be reproduced at a later date in some format, whether by printing or electronic transmission. E-SIGN does not mandate any specific type of technology, thereby allowing other federal and state agencies to establish more specific standards governing the format of EHRs and signatures. It does not appear that an agency can require a nonelectronic format without establishing a compelling reason for doing so.

A complication with E-SIGN is inconsistency regarding the acceptability of e-signatures from state to state and even within a state (AHIMA e-HIM Work Group on Implementing Electronic Signatures 2003a). This inconsistency becomes an issue for healthcare organizations whose facilities span state lines. Without consistent regulations on e-signatures and records, organizations must strive to comply with all applicable regulations even though they may conflict with one another.

A significant legislative issue associated with e-signatures is identifying the types that meet regulatory requirements. Legislation has generally taken three different approaches: all e-signatures satisfy legal signature requirements, e-signatures satisfy legal signature requirements only when they possess certain security attributes (that is, user authentication plus a PIN), and only digital signatures satisfy legal signature requirements. With its technology-neutral requirements, the second approach is the most common. Statutes adopting this approach generally state that an e-signature will be considered legally valid if it is unique to the person using it, can be verified, is under the sole control of the person using it, and is linked to the data in such a manner that, if the data are changed, the signature is invalidated.

In 2003 AHIMA provided a state-by-state list of regulations pertaining to electronic signatures (AHIMA e-HIM Work Group on Implementing Electronic Signatures 2003b). The most recent regulations, per state, can be obtained at respective state government websites. Most websites follow the convention of http://www.statename.gov. As mentioned previously, inconsistencies exist between states in regard to E-SIGN legislation. For example, Alaska allows a stamp or computer-key signature as an acceptable substitute for a physician's signature when the physician has given a signed statement to the hospital administration that he or she is the only person who has possession of and may use the stamp or key. However, Arkansas requires at least the first initial, last name, and title. Computerized signatures may be either by code, number, or initials or by the method developed by the facility. It is important to verify the regulations of a state before adopting an e-signature process.

Authentication Issues

Several authentication issues exist regardless of whether a record is in a paper, imaged, or electronic format, or a combination of formats. It is imperative that the author of each entry in a health record be identified and that all entries in the health record be authenticated.

Countersignatures

A **countersignature** is authentication by a second provider that signifies review and evaluation of the actions and documentation, including authentication, of a first provider. The entries of individuals who are required to practice under the direct supervision of another professional should be countersigned by an individual who has authority to evaluate the entry. Once countersigned, the entry is legally adopted by the supervising professional as his or her own entry. For example, an attending physician may be required to countersign a medical student's or resident physician's entries or dictated reports. The use of countersignatures is generally dictated by state licensing or certification statutes related to the professional scope of practice. Their uses are also typically outlined in medical staff bylaws and other healthcare organization policies. The CMS Interpretive Guidelines for Hospitals (482.24(c)(1)(I)) require that medical staff rules and regulations identify the types of documents or entries that require a countersignature by a supervisor or attending medical staff member. Countersignatures in teaching hospitals are especially important to show that the attending physician responsible for the patient is actively involved in the patient's care (AHIMA e-HIM Work Group on Maintaining the Legal EHR 2005).

Multiple Authentications

Multiple staff members complete some documents, such as assessments, at different times. This can create challenges because multiple authentications are required. As with any entry, a mechanism to identify the author of each section of the document must be established. At a minimum, a signature area at the end of the document should exist for staff to sign and date. Staff completing sections of the assessment should either indicate the sections they completed at the signature line or initial the sections they completed. EHRs must allow for the capture of each person's identity within the documentation tool for the information that they entered, although situations where more than one provider must authenticate a document can be problematic for digital signature technology (AHIMA e-HIM Work Group on Maintaining the Legal EHR 2005).

At times, an individual may document in the health record for someone else. Because the individual who actually provides the care is responsible for documentation of that care, the provider must authenticate the information entered by another individual. The documentation must reflect who provided the care. Clinical information supplied by the provider to the person writing the entry should be clearly attributed to the source of the information. Electronic documentation tools must allow for documentation of who provided the care and who entered the information, delineating who performed which action. Electronic documentation should identify the person who entered the information, the date of the entry, and authentication by the actual provider of care with the corresponding date of authentication (AHIMA e-HIM Work Group on Maintaining the Legal EHR 2005).

Auto-authentication

Auto-authentication is a process by which the failure of an author to review and affirmatively either approve or disapprove an entry within a specified time period results in authentication. For example, an organization's policy may allow a physician or other provider to state in advance that dictated and transcribed reports may be considered approved and signed if the provider does not make corrections within a certain period of time. Variations of this process may exist, such as sending a list of reports to the provider and having the provider sign the list (AHIMA e-HIM Work Group on Maintaining the Legal EHR 2005).

Auto-authentication contradicts the basic premise of authentication standards, which is that the author of each entry takes specific action to verify that the entry is his or hers, takes responsibility for it, and attests that the entry is accurate. Auto-authentication that fails to require an author to review his or her reports presents a legal liability for the healthcare organization and is likely to be noncompliant with federal and state authorization requirements (AHIMA e-HIM Work Group on Guidelines for EHR Documentation Practice 2007). Further, auto-authentication does not comply with Joint Commission standards. Therefore, processes should be in place to ensure that authors review and authenticate dictated documents after they are transcribed. Joint Commission standards require that signatures entered for the purpose of authentication after transcription be dated (Joint Commission 2010a, RC.01.02.01).

Check Your Understanding 8.3

Instructions: Indicate whether the following statements are true or false (T or F).

1. Authentication refers to the ability to verify the source of an entry in a health record.

2. Author initials are prohibited as an authentication mechanism in a health record.

3. Metadata provides information about an entry's content, including date and time of creation.

4. A countersignature signifies review and evaluation of the actions and documentation of another provider.

5. Auto-authentication is favored by the Joint Commission because it is an efficient authentication tool.

Accuracy

Accuracy of information refers to the extent to which the information reflects the true, correct, and exact description of the care that was delivered with respect to both content and timing (Servais 2008). It includes identification of the patient by name and health record number on every page in the health record, whether paper or electronic (AHIMA e-HIM Work Group on Maintaining the Legal EHR 2005). The accuracy and completeness of entries in the health record are the responsibility of the author(s). Organizational policies and procedures must reflect this (Servais 2008). EHRs pose additional accuracy challenges because they may contain data from multiple databases and sources. Training providers about appropriate data entry and system use, as well as checks and balances in the system, including audits, is necessary. Some EHR systems automatically audit data with rules-based tools that compare the data being entered with data that have already been entered. Settings in the system can require that certain pieces of data be captured before moving to the next field or before exiting the system. While these requirements can be cumbersome to the user, they contribute to the accuracy and completeness of the information. Careful consideration should be given to the development of an audit plan to ensure accuracy.

Authorship

Authorship is the origination or creation of recorded information attributed to a specific individual or entity acting at a particular time. As noted earlier in the chapter, healthcare organizations have policies and bylaws that define the individuals who have the right and authority to document in the health record, regardless of record format (AHIMA e-HIM Work Group on Maintaining the Legal EHR 2005).

The ability to utilize the cut, copy, and paste functions that may exist in an EHR weakens the integrity of documentation and raises authorship questions. Although such functions were available in paper records through photocopying, gluing, cropping, or other similar mechanisms, they were not widely used because they were cumbersome to accomplish and easily observed. These barriers have been removed in the EHR, creating significant legal challenges. The risks are significant and include placing the information on the wrong encounter or wrong patient, omitting the identity of the original author of the information, using information without the original author's permission, entering information that does not reflect the current situation or that has not been validated, and accomplishing these functions without the author's knowledge or permission if safeguards are not in place. The last risk, if done intentionally, could be considered fraud if it results in documentation for services not rendered. To minimize risk, policies and procedures should define the appropriate use of the cut, copy, and paste functions: who can perform these functions and how the system tracks the original author and changes that were made (AHIMA e-HIM Work Group on Maintaining the Legal EHR 2005).

Abbreviations

Historically used in health record documentation, **abbreviations** compromise patient safety because they can have duplicate meanings and be misunderstood. The Joint Commission has established a list of abbreviations that are prohibited in all its accredited organizations. To comply with the Joint Commission's patient safety initiative, every healthcare organization should strive to limit or eliminate the use of abbreviations in health record documentation (Joint Commission 2010b). Further, the Joint Commission has a list of prohibited abbreviations, acronyms, symbols, and dose designations that its accredited facilities must include in written hospital policy (Joint Commission 2010a, IM.02.02.01). When there is more than one meaning for an approved abbreviation, only one meaning should be used, or the context in which the abbreviation is to be used should be identified. Additionally, organizations should have a list of prohibited abbreviations, acronyms, and symbols (AHIMA e-HIM Work Group on Maintaining the Legal EHR 2005; Joint Commission 2010a, IM.02.02.01). Concurrent and retrospective analyses of records should ensure that symbols and abbreviations used in documentation have been approved by the medical staff and have only one clear meaning. Because EHR systems can be designed to convert entered abbreviations into complete words, abbreviations should be eliminated as information is formatted for the EHR (AHIMA e-HIM Work Group on Maintaining the Legal EHR 2005).

Legibility

The quality of provider entries includes **legibility**, which is a focus area of accreditation and licensure bodies. The consequences of illegibility have been targeted by the Joint Commission as part of its emphasis on patient safety (Joint Commission 2010b). If an entry cannot be read, it must be assumed that it cannot be or was not used in the patient care process. Entries that cannot be read should be rewritten on the next available line, refer back to the original documentation, explain the reason for the duplicate entry, and be written legibly. The rewritten entry must be the same as the original. A long-standing problem with paper health records, illegibility has been reduced through the presence of EHRs. However, readability of images or scans can still be negatively affected by the use of color (for example, to indicate test results), low resolution, and poorly imaged documents in a document management system.

Changes to the Health Record

Documentation within the health record may need to be changed or added for many reasons. Foremost are entries that are incomplete or contain erroneous information. While changes to a record may be necessary to ensure its integrity, the manner in which the changes occur can, in fact, diminish its integrity and subject it to legal scrutiny. Because of this, policies and procedures should define the process for making changes and the time period in which they can be made, along with retention of previous versions (version management is discussed later in this chapter). Changes to entries in the health record can be used against a healthcare organization as evidence of negligence or a consciousness of guilt if they are not completed appropriately and with transparency. Original entries that are incomplete or incorrect must be changed using professional guidelines (AHIMA e-HIM Work Group on Maintaining the Legal EHR 2005; AHIMA 2009). Changes can occur in the form of revisions (also referred to as corrections or alterations), additions (late entries, amendments, or addenda), and deletions.

Revisions to the Health Record

Revisions to health record entries generally involve replacing incorrect information with correct information in a manner that ensures that the original entry is preserved and that future readers can rely on it. Corrections in paper records should be completed by drawing a line through the erroneous information so that the original information remains legible and marking it as an error. A notation of the date, time, and signature of the individual making the correction should accompany the correct information.

Errors in EHRs should be handled in a similar manner. Recommendations for standards on appropriate methods to correct information in the EHR can be found in the HL7 functional model (HL7). Information should not be deleted in paper records (for example, erasures, obliterations, or whiting out) or EHRs; however, corrections in the EHR may not be visible like they are on paper. Because of this, the ability to track changes in an EHR (such as the person making the change, the date, and the time) is critical from an evidentiary standpoint. The person making the correction should enter the correct information and reference the incorrect information. A notation or flag should be visible with the new information to indicate that there was a change, along with a link to the original incorrect information (AHIMA e-HIM Work Group on Maintaining the Legal EHR 2005).

Individuals who document in paper or electronic records must be educated about organizational policies and procedures for making appropriate document revisions, as well as sanctions for doing so inappropriately. Alterations that intentionally change the content or character of health information for less than honorable purposes, such as concealing wrongdoing, are referred to as tampering. Such alterations may constitute criminal conduct such as fraud; thus, policies and procedures should be in place to prevent such occurrences.

Additions to the Health Record

A **late entry** is documented in the health record when a pertinent entry was missed or was not written in a timely manner. Late entries should be documented as follows:

- Identify the new entry as a late entry.

- Enter the current date and time. Do not try to give the appearance that the entry was made on a previous date or time.

- Identify or refer to the date and incident for which the late entry is written.

- If the late entry is used to document an omission, validate the source of additional information as much as possible (for example, where you obtained the information to write the late entry).

- When using late entries, document as soon as possible. There is no time limit for writing a late entry; however, the more time that passes, the less reliable the entry becomes (AHIMA e-HIM Work Group on Maintaining the Legal EHR 2005).

An **amendment (addendum)** is a type of late entry in which information is added to support or clarify a previous entry. Often, more space is required, and the addition cannot be made in the same location as the original entry. The process for adding a new supporting entry or adding to an existing entry should follow the steps recommended by the AHIMA e-HIM Workgroup on Maintaining the Legal EHR (2005):

- Document the date and time of the addendum.

- Write "addendum" and state the reason for the addendum, referring back to the original or parent document or entry.

- Enter an addendum as soon as possible after the original entry.

- Link the addendum to the original entry in the EHR.

Different scenarios for making any of these changes can be found in "Amendments, Corrections, and Deletions in the Electronic Health Record: An American Health Information Management Association Toolkit" (AHIMA 2009). In addition to a change made by a provider, a patient may also request an amendment to his or her health record, as defined by the HIPAA Privacy Rule (45 CFR 164.526), which will be discussed in more detail in chapter 9.

Deletions from the Health Record

Organizational policy should define the rare occasions when documentation may be deleted from a health record. Deletion of documentation should not occur except in very specific circumstances (for example, documentation is entered in the wrong patient record and is discovered immediately after it is entered). In this case, a special procedure may allow for the removal of the incorrect information before anyone else has had a chance to view it.

In an electronic environment, appropriate deletion may be referred to as a retraction, where the information is no longer available for viewing but is available behind the scenes or through an administrative record view. For example, in an EHR the incorrect information would remain attached to the record in the background, but no indication of an error would be present. Each organization should evaluate situations where deletion (or retraction) may be appropriate and develop policies and procedures (AHIMA e-HIM Work Group on Maintaining the Legal EHR 2005).

Information may be deleted to preserve confidentiality. In adoptions, references to the birth mother's identity may be deleted from the record. A flag or other marker would indicate that the information had been deleted, and only authorized individuals would have access to the information in another location. The deleted information would not be released with the record unless permitted by state law.

Version Management

Version management refers to how an organization handles the numerous versions that may exist of a document or collection of data. If the information has been used for patient care, whether it was authenticated or not, it must be retained and managed. A decision must be made as to which version or versions of the document or information will be displayed, who will have access to the versions, and how they will be flagged in the record.

It is acceptable for a draft of a dictated and transcribed note or report to be changed before authentication unless there is a reason to believe the changes are suspect and would not reflect actual events or action or it has been relied upon for patient care. Organizational policy should define how long a document will remain as a draft. After that time period or after a document has been authenticated, any changes should follow the organization's late entry or amendment procedures. The original document must then be maintained along with the new revised document. (AHIMA e-HIM Work Group on Maintaining the Legal EHR 2005)

Check Your Understanding 8.4

Instructions: Indicate whether the following statements are true or false (T or F).

1. A Joint Commission–accredited organization may use any abbreviation in health record documentation as long as it is explained in a facility-wide key or legend.

2. Illegibility has been reduced through the presence of EHRs.

3. Incorrect information in the health record should be obliterated so that it cannot be confused with the updated, corrected information placed in the record.

4. A late entry in the health record should not be identified as such because it may lead to negligence liability.

5. Version management is how an organization handles numerous versions that may exist of a document.

Timeliness and Completeness

The final elements that contribute to the legally defensible health record are **timeliness** and **completeness** of documentation. Both are the responsibility of the author. If documentation is performed in a timely manner, the health record will ultimately be complete within the time lines established by legal and accreditation standards and by organizational policy and medical staff bylaws. Licensure and accreditation bodies mandate timeliness of entries, but timeliness is also important from an evidentiary and admissibility standpoint. Entries should be made in the health record as soon as possible after an event or observation. As described earlier, the complete date and time for each entry in a paper record must be recorded to show when the entry occurred. This will also provide the chronology of care provided to the patient. EHR users generally do not need to enter the date and time since the system will do this automatically. However, the date and time for late entries should be manually entered in an EHR to reflect when the entry should have been made. This manually entered information will exist in addition to the system's automatic time and date stamp for when the entry was made (AHIMA e-HIM Work Group on Maintaining the Legal EHR 2005).

The health record is not complete until all its parts are assembled and the appropriate documents are authenticated. Medical staff bylaws must include time limits for health record completion. Completion of a health record may be ensured by concurrent analysis (record review by HIM staff during the patient's stay in a healthcare organization to determine whether signatures or other pertinent information is missing). If documentation is missing, healthcare providers are reminded to complete and sign items in the record before the patient is discharged. Another form of record analysis is discharge analysis, which occurs after patient discharge. The patient's record is reviewed by HIM staff to ensure that the record is complete and that all information is in the correct patient record. Analysis can be greatly streamlined in EHR systems that automatically check for missing documents and signatures.

EHRs offer unique issues for determining when the record is considered complete. EHR users could potentially make changes or additions to the health record at any point in time. Organizational policy should determine the point at which no additional changes can be made to information within the health record. System functionality needs to support organizational policy to ensure and demonstrate health record integrity. Exceptions can be made for specific circumstances where a correction to information must be made or new information in the form of an addendum needs to be made for accuracy of the information (AHIMA 2009).

Printing

The AHIMA e-HIM Work Group states that printing can create a legal challenge for healthcare organizations with an EHR system if clinicians print from the EHR and then document on printouts rather than in the system. Reliance on both paper and electronic documentation will also complicate the e-discovery process. The organization must establish strict printing policies, including justification for printing paper internally, who has authority to print, how printing will be tracked in an audit trail, and the format and version of documents that may be printed. An emerging best practice for printing from an EHR for legal purposes is to create one standard print view that creates a PDF of the information. This method ensures that the output for legal purposes always produces a consistent collection of information (Rollins 2007).

Although the problem of duplicate copies is magnified in an EHR system, it is not entirely unique to the electronic environment. Photocopies of original paper documents can also create problems when providers document on them. While the original paper document is ordinarily considered the "source of truth," this is questioned when a photocopy contains additional and updated information. Whether printed from an electronic system or photocopied from a paper original, multiple copies also heighten the risk of confidentiality breaches. Thus, the creation, use, and disposal of additional copies must be monitored in settings that use EHRs, paper health records, or a combination of both (AHIMA e-HIM Work Group on Maintaining the Legal EHR 2005).

Personal Health Records

Personal health records (PHRs) offer unique challenges to the HIM and informatics professional in the management of the LHR. PHRs, also known as consumer health records or patient health records, are created, maintained, and managed by the individual or patient to whom the information pertains. The Markle Foundation's Connecting for Health collaboration defines a PHR as "an electronic application through which individuals can access, manage and share their health information, and that of others for whom they are authorized, in a private, secure and confidential environment" (Markle Foundation 2003). The discussion of PHRs in this chapter focuses on the potential legal issues created if an organization determines that PHRs should be integrated into the LHR. Inherent to that decision is the concern that, as discussed in figure 8.2, a PHR does not qualify as a business record and should not be included in the LHR even though it may affect treatment decisions. Although important to the healthcare industry, issues related to the content, media used for creation and storage, adoption, and benefits of PHRs will not be discussed here.

One challenge for the HIM and informatics professional is the inadequate structure of the current legal framework to distinguish between the health record of the provider and the PHR maintained by the patient. Current state and federal laws, including HIPAA, focus on the business and legal reasons that providers have to maintain health records. However, there is little focus on PHRs. The HIM and informatics professional must guide organizational decision making and policy analysis as to the consequences of bringing patient- or consumer-created health information into an organization's LHR (Dolan et al. 2009). The most obvious mechanism for a PHR to become integrated into an organization's LHR is via a formal request to amend the health record. The amendment request process is outlined in the HIPAA Privacy Rule provisions (chapter 9) and may be outlined in state statutes. It is imperative that HIM and informatics professionals prepare for questions from patients related to how the organization may incorporate information from their PHRs.

The lack of standards for PHRs may soon change, as several standards development initiatives have begun to focus on PHRs. They include the Certification Commission for Healthcare Information Technology (CCHIT) and Health Level 7 (HL7) System Functional Model (PHR-S FM). CCHIT was founded in 2004 and has certified EHRs since 2006. Recognized by the federal government as a certifying body, it established the first comprehensive, practical definition of what capabilities are needed in EHRs (CCHIT, n.d.). The PHR-S FM standard focuses on the consumer's right to edit information that feeds into the PHR from an EHR (HL7, n.d.). The CCHIT's PHR workgroup is using the PHR-S

FM standards to determine PHR product certification criteria. These national efforts will have a trickle-down impact on organizations that are attempting to operationalize these standards.

Another challenge created by PHRs is the existence of provider-sponsored patient portals where patients can enter health information into a system that the provider owns and controls. There are many policy decisions to be made, such as whether the PHR becomes part of the facility's LHR and who may access, amend, and disclose information from the PHR. Guidance from an HIM and informatics professional is important.

Although PHRs present a multitude of possibilities for enhancing patient care, the World Privacy Forum and consumer privacy advocates have expressed concern that PHRs threaten current privacy protections since it is unclear whether any statutory protections for PHRs exist (Gellman 2008). Provisions in the American Recovery and Reinvestment Act of 2009 (ARRA) extend protections to PHRs held by non-HIPAA-covered entities. (More information about ARRA is included in chapter 9.) Many in the healthcare industry are calling for the creation of a PHR liaison, personal health information custodian, or patient information coordinator to assist patients or consumers in managing their personal health information. This role would include consumer education regarding privacy and security issues associated with the creation of a PHR. AHIMA has developed sample job descriptions, and it is clear that HIM and informatics professionals have a vital role to play in the consumer health movement.

Health Record Identification, Retention, and Disposition

Sound policies and procedures for the identification, retention, and disposition of health records are vital to validate claims of information integrity when information is at the heart of litigation, regardless of record format. An organization must know where its information is housed, how long it should be retained, and when and whether it may be destroyed. It is important for retention policies and procedures to address the LHR, but they should also address backup tapes, voice mail, word-processing drafts, and shadow records (that is, duplicate records or copies). When an organization is ready to replace or upgrade either an EHR or a paper record system, it must consider its policies on the accessibility, retention, and destruction of information. This section discusses the legal issues associated with the creation and identification of health records, **retention** (including storage and retrieval), and **disposition** (destruction, transfer, or loss). The term "maintenance" broadly refers to the life cycle of the health record, from the time of creation through disposition.

Health Record Identification

The health record is created when a patient is first admitted to or treated in a healthcare facility organization. If the patient is admitted to a hospital or other type of care facility or is seeking treatment in an ambulatory care setting, the health record is initiated with the collection of admission or registration information. The patient is usually assigned a unique identification number or other form of identification, which is essential for future record retrieval purposes. This initial information usually becomes part of the facility's **master patient index** (MPI) or patient identifying directory. The MPI or directory is maintained in a variety of ways, using media such as index cards, microfilm rolls, or microfiche or electronic systems. The goal of an MPI or directory is to assist in maintaining a longitudinal patient health record from birth to death. The MPI or patient directory serves as a link to the patient record and facilitates patient identification that is critical to the quality and safety of patient care.

Ensuring the correct identification of patients and ensuring that one (and only one) patient is assigned a particular identifier, whether it is a number or patient name, are ongoing challenges (AHIMA MPI Task Force 2004). For example, patients may not remember previous admissions or episodes of outpatient care, or they may have been admitted under a different name or a different spelling of their name; additionally, incorrect information may have been entered that resulted in an incorrect number being assigned to the patient in subsequent encounters. It is important for the healthcare provider to identify and locate the patient's health record in a timely and efficient manner in order to support quality care and patient safety. To facilitate accurate and timely retrieval of patient health records, the concept of a universal identifier unique to each patient (similar to the concept of a Social Security number) has been debated extensively among government, public, and private groups. However, patient confidentiality concerns, especially in regard to EHRs, have stalled adoption of an identifier on a national level.

Health Record Retention

The retention of health records in any format involves mechanisms to store the records, provide for timely retrieval, and establish the lengths of times that various types of records will be retained by the healthcare organization.

Storage and Retrieval

Healthcare organizations need policies that address the storage of health records. While storage and retention are closely linked (retention and factors that affect retention periods are discussed in detail below), storage considerations for paper records include the amount of physical space available and, in the absence of policies providing for record destruction, the cost and feasibility of storing records off-site or converting them to another medium. Storage considerations for electronic records differ because a much greater volume can be stored in a smaller space. Organizations with EHRs may choose to add more storage capacity because advancements in storage technology have grown at an exceptional rate and a reasonable price, thus providing a variety of options for data retention. Additionally, the volume of data that can be put on electronic devices exceeds the capacity of early computers. Mobile devices, including smartphones and laptop computers, are viewed as a necessity by many providers. However, associated privacy and security risks such as loss, theft, and compromised confidentiality during transmission must be addressed through organizational policies (Tessier 2010). Storage decisions must also be made in conjunction with retention decisions and factors that affect those decisions.

Retrieval is quickly locating requested records and information needed for patient care or other uses. Retrieval of paper health records involves checking out records from a filing area and tracking those that are not returned within a specified period. A software system may be used to track patient records. Retrieval of EHRs includes approval of a request and placement of the record in a work queue or work list for the requestor to access. When a patient's record cannot be located, a provider cannot access prior medical information and the patient's care may be compromised due to duplicate or improper treatment.

Factors That Influence Retention Periods

Because the health record is a multifaceted document with demands placed on it by many diverse interests, policies establishing retention schedules are critical to the record management process. In addition to federal and state laws and other legal issues, such as statutes of limitations, healthcare organizations must take into account the compelling requirements of external organizations, such as the Joint Commission and the Department of Health and Human Services Office of Inspector General, and recommended retention standards published by AHIMA. Internal factors include emerging EHR technology, patient populations (for example, severity and readmission rates), institutional medical practice, research activity, educational needs, access to new technology, storage constraints or capabilities, cost, and disaster recovery plans. These external and internal factors, discussed in greater detail in this section, require the availability of a patient's health record for varying periods of time. Thus, a record retention policy that meets an organization's needs must be developed (Rinehart-Thompson 2008).

A study funded by the AHIMA Foundation on Research and Education (FORE), hereafter the AHIMA Foundation, collected record retention information in 2005 from a sample of acute care general hospitals in the United States. Table 8.1 displays results of that study relative to record retention periods for health records of adults and minors. As the study shows, approximately half the respondent facilities retain the health records of both adults and minors permanently (Rinehart-Thompson 2006).

Federal and State Laws

All applicable state and federal statutes and regulations must frequently be reviewed and compared with one another to ensure that health records are retained for the time period required. Medicare requires records to be maintained for at least five years (42 CFR 482.24(b)), including radiologist records (printouts, films, scans, and other images), home health agency records, long-term care records, laboratory records, and any other records that document information about claims for reimbursement. When state laws or licensing standards require a longer retention period, the longer requirement must be followed. Many states recommend that patient health records be retained for 10 years following patient discharge or death. Special requirements for minor patients are discussed in detail below. Some types of records, such as mammograms, may have retention periods up to 20 or 30 years.

Source data records (for example, fetal monitoring strips, EEGs, EKGs, videotapes, treadmill tests, magnetic tapes, and other images that are interpreted and/or summarized into final transcribed reports) are usually maintained in the department where they originated and must be retained for as long as they are legally required to be maintained. Fetal monitoring strips are considered part of the mother's record; however, because they relate to the newborn, they should be maintained for the same period of time that the newborn's record is maintained. State and federal agencies may also have retention requirements relative to specific types of health records. For example, the Occupational Safety and Health Administration (OSHA) requires records of employees with occupational exposure to be maintained for the duration of employment plus 30 years (Reynolds 2010).

Statutes of Limitations

Applicable **statutes of limitations**, which are the time periods in which a lawsuit may be filed, must be considered in establishing a retention schedule. There is no one statute of limitations that must be considered, as they vary by state and by the type of action being brought (for example, torts, contracts, and

Table 8.1. Retention periods for adult and minor records

Record Retention Periods	f	%
Adult Records (n = 81)		
Permanent retention	41	50.6
30–50 years	7	8.6
20–29 years	7	8.6
10–19 years	22	27.2
5–9 years	4	4.9
Less than 5 years	0	0.0
Minor Records (n = 80)		
Permanent retention	42	52.5
30 years	3	3.8
20–29 years	22	27.5
13–19 years	0	0.0
12 years or less	4	5.0
Specified number of years past age of majority	9	11.3

Source: Rinehart-Thompson 2006, table 5.

specific periods for professional malpractice lawsuits). Although it must be given primary consideration, the statute of limitations for the types of lawsuits that concern a healthcare organization ordinarily will be much shorter than the retention periods mandated by Medicare, patient care needs, and many of the organization's other operational needs.

There are exceptions:

Minors: The statute of limitations in the case of minors may exceed the time for which health records are ordinarily retained. Whereas a minor may file a lawsuit on his or her own behalf upon reaching the age of majority, the statute of limitations does not begin to run until the minor reaches the age of majority, which is often 18 years of age. If the statute of limitations for the lawsuit being brought is two years, the minor would be able to bring legal action until he or she is 20 years old. If the lawsuit related to alleged medical malpractice when the child was 2 years old, the retention period—in order to comply with the statute of limitations— would be 18 years (from the time the child was 2 years old until he or she reached 20 years of age). This can create operational burdens for a healthcare organization and must be factored into its record retention policy.

Incompetent Individuals: A state's statute of limitations may also be extended for individuals deemed legally incompetent by virtue of a mental disability. Because a person's incompetence may never be lifted (for example, an individual with a developmental disability), thus enabling a lawsuit to be filed at any time, an organization's record retention policy should specify that the records of these individuals should never be destroyed.

Accreditation Standards

The Joint Commission defers to applicable statutes, regulations, patient care purposes, and an organization's operational and legal needs for determining appropriate record retention periods. In the "Record of Care" chapter in *Comprehensive Accreditation Manual for Hospitals: The Official Handbook*, the Joint Commission states that the retention of the original or legally reproduced medical record is determined by its use and hospital policy (Joint Commission 2010a, RC.01.05.01). The Joint Commission surveys organizations to ensure that they comply with legal requirements and their own health record retention policies.

AHIMA Recommendations

Although they do not have the force and effect of law, professional practice guidelines are often valuable in making operational decisions. AHIMA has established health record retention recommendations that guide practice in many healthcare organizations. A 2005 study of individuals responsible for the management of health information in general acute care hospitals showed that nearly 50 percent of the respondents used the AHIMA recommendations, in part, to determine record retention periods (Rinehart-Thompson 2006). Figure 8.6 displays the AHIMA-recommended retention standards (Fletcher and Rhodes 2002).

Operational Needs

AHIMA recommends that healthcare organizations develop health record retention schedules that meet the organization's operational needs. The paramount need is patient care, but operational needs may also include other uses by patients, physicians, nonphysician providers, researchers, and staff or patient educators. An organization, depending on its specific needs, may have many legitimate uses that necessitate extending retention periods. In the AHIMA Foundation–funded study previously mentioned, data were also collected about factors that influence health record retention practices. Table 8.2 displays those results. Although state and federal laws had the most significant impact on retention decisions, facility operational needs such as research, cost of retention, and education played important roles as well (Rinehart-Thompson 2006).

Figure 8.6. AHIMA's recommended retention standards

Health Information	Recommended Retention Period
Diagnostic images (such as x-ray film)	5 years
Disease index	10 years
Fetal heart monitor records	10 years after the infant reaches the age of majority
Master patient/person index	Permanently
Operative index	10 years
Patient health records (adults)	10 years after the most recent encounter
Patient health records (minors)	10 years after the most recent encounter
Physician index	10 years
Register of births	Permanently
Register of deaths	Permanently
Register of surgical procedures	Permanently

Source: Fletcher and Rhodes 2002, table 1.

Table 8.2. Factors influencing record retention practices

Factor	f	%
State record retention laws	73	90.1
Medicare Conditions of Participation	49	60.5
Facility operational needs	41	50.6
Research	20	24.7
Costs of retaining records	19	23.5
Education	12	14.8
More convenient not to purge	10	12.3
Other needs or reasons	7	8.6
AHIMA recommended retention standards	40	49.4
Statute of limitations for lawsuits	38	46.9
Joint Commission or other accrediting bodies	37	45.7
Other federal laws	12	14.8
Other state laws	6	7.4

Source: Rinehart-Thompson 2006, table 7.

Record Retention Schedules

A healthcare organization must consider the previously mentioned factors when developing its health record **retention schedule**. In many cases, the schedule may not differ among record formats; however, organizations may decide to retain records for different periods of time based on the media types on which they reside. A retention schedule should specify what information should be retained, the time period for which it should be retained, and the storage medium (that is, format) on which it is to be retained (Fletcher and Rhodes 2002). Retention schedules should address the transfer of health records from one medium to another (for example, from paper to microfilm). This is discussed later in the chapter. For a list of state statutes or regulations pertaining to retention of health information and a listing of federal record retention requirements, see the AHIMA practice brief "Retention of Health Information" (Fletcher and Rhodes 2002).

EHR Retention

Many decisions pertaining to health record retention are determined by the organization's existing record formats. Retention of electronic information is a complex task. In addition to retention guidelines that govern paper records, policies and procedures should specifically outline retention of the myriad electronic media types that exist, many in portable form (for example, images, optical disks, computer disks, CDs, and DVDs). In addition to health information, data inherent to EHR systems, such as metadata, alerts, and reminders, should be addressed in a retention policy. This information will be important for certifying the integrity of the record for business and legal purposes. Organizational retention requirements should be part of the selection and management of an EHR system.

An organization must also consider permanency of records in its retention policies. Information maintained in an EHR system is subject to technology changes or obsolescence that will impact its permanency and ability to be accessed. A National Archives report on preserving electronic records stated that the average life cycle of a software system is two to five years (US General Accounting Office 1999). Procedures to protect data integrity during system conversions must be addressed and documented. A retention policy must factor in the projected life of the systems software to ensure that older information will be accessible after the original system has been upgraded or technology has changed. The National Archives report outlines three alternatives that should be considered in the development of a retention policy, although all have capacity and cost issues associated with them:

- Maintain records in a software-independent format (such as document management systems)
- Reformat and migrate records to new software systems
- Maintain necessary hardware and software to make the information accessible

Other challenges that may be encountered in maintaining electronic information and that should be considered when creating retention policies are scanned images and fetal monitoring strips. Scanned images that have been directly fed into a document management system (and are available to physicians and other providers) are not always of diagnostic quality. In these cases, retention policies should state that the ancillary departments that created the information should maintain the information for the appropriate retention period. Also, because fetal monitoring strips are often not compatible with scanning systems, specific computer software that digitally stores fetal monitoring tracings may need to be installed within the labor and delivery area so that retention requirements can be met.

Check Your Understanding 8.5

Instructions: Indicate whether the following statements are true or false (T or F).

1. A computer system's print function provides additional challenges for organizations with EHRs.
2. A patient's PHR is a business record.
3. A master patient index is a directory of patient-identifying information.
4. Statutes of limitations may not be considered when establishing a health record retention schedule.
5. When establishing a health record retention schedule, an organization must retain all records for the same period of time.

Health Record Disposition

Disposition involves the removal of records from a record storage system. Removal may occur for many reasons but is often the result of a record becoming inactive due to the cessation of patient encounters (for example, a live patient has not returned within a specified period of time or a patient has died) or achievement of the maximum retention period. Although a healthcare organization may not retain paper health records indefinitely due to reasons such as cost and storage capabilities, organizations with EHRs may also develop disposition procedures because the benefit of retaining older records may not outweigh their usefulness in treating the patient or fulfilling other organizational needs. Establishing policies that incorporate state and federal laws and other standards is part of the disposition process.

AHIMA recommends taking all of the following factors into consideration when determining the appropriate disposition of health records:

- State laws regarding record retention and disposal, as well as statutes of limitations

- State licensing standards

- Medicare and Medicaid requirements

- Federal laws governing treatment for alcohol and drug abuse (if applicable)

- Guidelines issued by professional organizations

- The needs and wishes of patients (Rhodes and Brandt 2003)

Destruction of Health Records

Not every piece of data or information needs to be kept forever. Destruction of health records should be carried out according to federal and state law and pursuant to an approved retention schedule and destruction policy. A good retention plan includes instructions and guidelines for information destruction and is included in an organization's policies and procedures manual to ensure that record destruction is part of the normal course of business and that no one particular record or group of records is singled out for destruction. Where organizations fail to apply destruction policies uniformly or where destruction is contrary to policy, a court may allow a jury to infer in a negligence suit that, if the record were available, it would have shown that the organization acted improperly in treating the patient.

Even if they are otherwise scheduled for destruction, records involved in any open investigation, audit, or litigation should not be destroyed. This ensures that spoliation of evidence does not occur. Such destruction would subject the organization to greater liability for failure to retain information. Appropriate safeguards should be implemented within electronic systems to prevent inappropriate destruction of information. (For example, a legal hold, as discussed in chapter 4, should be initiated.)

Destruction policies and procedures must ensure that paper records are destroyed so that protected health information (PHI) is not revealed and cannot be re-created. AHIMA recommends burning, shredding, pulping, or pulverizing (Hughes 2002). The HIPAA Privacy Rule mandates that agreements with shredding companies and other destruction companies include language ensuring that information will not be further disclosed (45 CFR 164.504(e)(2)). Destruction that is outsourced should be documented with a certificate of destruction once the process is complete. The certificate should include, or be accompanied by, a list of the specific documents destroyed and a description of the manner of destruction. AHIMA recommends that organizations maintain destruction documents permanently because they may be required as evidence that records were destroyed in the regular course of business. Figure 8.7 provides a list of recommendations from AHIMA regarding the **destruction of records** (Hughes 2002).

EHR destruction policies should include specific instructions about how the information will be destroyed. Deleting information from its original location or file folder does not prevent it from being

Figure 8.7.   AHIMA recommendations for destruction of records

AHIMA recommends that destruction should be documented, including:

• Date of destruction

• Method of destruction

• Description of the disposed record series of numbers or items

• Inclusive dates covered

• A statement that the records were destroyed in the normal course of business

• The signatures of the individuals supervising and witnessing the destruction

If destruction services are to be contracted, the contract should:

• Specify the method of destruction

• Specify the time that will elapse between acquisition and destruction of data

• Establish safeguards against breaches in confidentiality

• Indemnify the healthcare facility from loss due to unauthorized disclosure

• Provide proof of destruction

Source: Hughes 2002.

accessed from the hard drive or storage media. Several methods are available to permanently remove the information (Hughes 2002). Physically destroying the storage media, rendering it unusable, is the most secure means of destruction. CDs and DVDs should be destroyed with a shredder. Overwriting of hard drives utilizing Department of Defense–accepted software replaces previously stored information with a pattern of meaningless information that renders the original information unrecoverable. Hard drives may be neutralized with a magnetic field (degaussing) to erase data. Whichever methods are chosen, the organization must ensure that they are appropriate given the type of information and the storage medium (Hughes 2002). One type of electronic information that warrants special attention and must be managed is e-mail. Because healthcare organizations produce vast quantities of e-mail containing highly sensitive information, not only must e-mail information be appropriately maintained and safeguarded for confidentiality and integrity purposes, but destruction procedures must be established (Burrington-Brown and Hughes 2003). E-mail messages deleted by the user and from the server may still be in circulation.

Transfer of Health Records

The **transfer of health records** can include moving a record from one medium to another (for example, from paper to microfilm or to an optical imaging system) or to another records custodian. Because the transfer of records from one medium to another often does not include a custodial change, fewer legal implications apply. Many circumstances can lead to the transfer of health records. Although they frequently pertain to smaller businesses such as physician practices, they can also occur in larger healthcare organizations through mergers, acquisitions, and sales (Reynolds 2010). The transfer of health records may be associated with ownership changes (sale of a business to a new owner or a buyout by co-providers when another provider leaves, retires, or dies) or closure of a healthcare organization (due to retirement, cessation of practice, or death of a provider) (AMA 2005).

The HIPAA Privacy Rule, discussed in chapter 9, does not require the patient's authorization in order to carry out healthcare operations, even if an activity uses health information that identifies a patient. Because circumstances that involve the transfer of records, such as sales and transfers, are within the HIPAA definition of healthcare operations (45 CFR 164.501), healthcare organizations must refer to applicable state laws and other federal laws to determine whether requirements exist that are more stringent than HIPAA requirements before record transfer occurs.

Ownership Change

An ownership change may occur when a healthcare organization is sold. In physician or other provider practices where the providers have a shared ownership, one of the providers may retire, die, or otherwise relinquish his or her interest in a practice. In these cases, health records are considered assets and are most likely to be transferred to the successor provider(s), meaning the entity or individual(s) that purchase(s) or assume(s) responsibility for the organization.

In physician practices, patients are given the option to transfer their records to another provider of choice before their records are transferred to the successor provider. When a physician leaves a group practice, patients should be given the choice to transfer their records and move with the physician or to have the records and the responsibility for care transferred to another provider in the group. State medical associations and the American Medical Association (AMA) Code of Ethics (2, Opinion 7.03) have made it clear that patients must be given information about the practice status of a departing physician, regardless of the reason for the departure, and must be given the physician's new address and the opportunity to have their records forwarded to that physician at his or her new location in a timely manner and without interference (Reynolds 2010).

Although noncompete contracts may be in place to limit a physician's ability to treat patients within a certain geographical area upon his or her departure and relocation, such a contractual limitation does not belong to the patient. As a result, the patient must be given his or her own information. Because contracts may specify that health records are owned by the provider group, the group practice from which a provider is departing may only be obligated to provide copies of the record rather than the original. In any event, applicable state and federal laws should be consulted for the handling of records when an ownership change has occurred.

Closure

Many of the same circumstances that lead to a change in ownership (provider retirement, death, or departure from a practice) can also cause a healthcare organization to close if a successor is not identified. Although this may occur most commonly in smaller provider practices, it can also take place in larger healthcare organizations when a hospital closes as the result of financial distress or as part of corporate restructuring. Paramount in these situations are the integrity, accessibility, and continued confidentiality of patient information (Rhodes and Brandt 2003). Guidance can often be obtained from the state health department or the state agency that licenses the organization that is closing. Applicable state laws should be consulted for handling records when closure occurs, because state legal requirements may vary. They may mandate that records be transferred to another healthcare organization, permit storage in a secure warehouse, require that the state licensing agency simply be notified of the disposition that will occur (destruction or transfer of the records to a new location), or require delivery of the records directly to the licensing agency. Transfer of records to another provider is optimal; however, when this cannot be accomplished in the face of a closure, AHIMA recommends that other storage options be considered, such as archival with a reputable commercial storage firm (Rhodes and Brandt 2003). Such a firm should be considered only if it:

- Has experience in handling confidential patient information

- Guarantees the security and confidentiality of the records

- Ensures that patients and other legitimate requestors will have access to the information

If a storage firm is used, specific provisions should be negotiated and included in the written agreement. Such provisions include but are not limited to:

- Agreement to keep all information confidential, disclosing only to authorized representatives of the provider or upon written authorization from the patient/legal representative

- Prompt return of all embodiments of confidential information without retaining copies thereof upon the provider's request

- Prohibition against selling, sharing, discussing, assigning, transferring, or otherwise disclosing confidential information with any other individuals or business entities

- Prohibition against use of confidential information for any purpose other than providing mutually agreed-upon services

- Agreement to protect information against theft, loss, unauthorized destruction, or other unauthorized access

- Return or destruction of information at the end of the mutually agreed-upon retention period

- Assurance that providers, patients, and other legitimate users will have access to the information (Rhodes and Brandt 2003)

When transfer is not feasible and destruction must occur as a last resort, destruction must occur appropriately, as described earlier in this chapter.

Whether the ultimate fate of health records belonging to an organization that is closing its doors is transfer or destruction, there must be a plan to provide a patient access to his or her own information either at the new location or prior to destruction. If a record is being transferred to a new location, only copies should be given to a patient if the required record retention period has not expired. For both transfers and destruction of their health records, patients should be individually notified. If this is not possible, information about the organization's closure and the ultimate disposition of its health records should be published for distribution to the general population.

Providers that offer alcohol or drug abuse services, such as education, training, treatment, rehabilitation, or research, must dispose of records as required by federal law (AHIMA 2011). Also, record retention laws that govern the organization must be followed for transferred records. Similar to health records maintained by organizations that continue to operate, appropriate record retention schedules should be followed to allow destruction to occur as legally required for health records of organizations that have closed. An organization's malpractice insurance carrier should be apprised of the disposition status of the organization's health records (Rhodes and Brandt 2003).

For a list by state of laws and other guidelines pertaining to facility closure, see the AHIMA practice brief "Protecting Patient Information after a Facility Closure" (Rhodes and Brandt 2003).

Liability Associated with Loss or Destruction of Records

A healthcare organization is responsible for maintaining health records in its custody according to applicable laws and organizational policies. When an organization cannot produce a health record, its risk of liability increases, particularly when the record is needed for patient care or evidence in a legal action. If a healthcare organization fails to produce a health record, the burden of proof shifts to that organization to prove that the loss was unintentional and that there was no negligent treatment. As discussed earlier, however, a court may instruct that failure of a healthcare organization to produce evidence in the form of a health record creates an inference of negligence or a consciousness of guilt. Although failure to produce a health record most often conjures up images of a lost paper record, data can also be lost in electronic and document management systems, resulting in the same liability risks. Mechanisms ensuring that health information can be located will differ depending on the record format, but a carefully designed records management program is critical in all settings and will lessen the possibility of misplaced records in whatever formats they exist.

Check Your Understanding 8.6

Instructions: Indicate whether the following statements are true or false (T or F).

1. Health record disposition includes transferring records from paper to an optical imaging system.

2. When a physician closes a practice, all health records should be destroyed immediately to protect the privacy of patient information.

3. Data in a health record need to be kept forever.

4. Degaussing a hard drive involves neutralizing it with a magnetic field as a method to erase patient information.

5. When an e-mail message is deleted, it is eliminated from an organization's electronic system.

Summary

The health record is a multipurpose document that is central to any healthcare organization. The healthcare industry's revolutionary transition from paper records to EHRs prompted the need for healthcare organizations to define and identify the parameters of the LHR, the document that is released to third parties upon valid request, and to differentiate it from the EHR, the PHR, and the myriad data that an EIIR is capable of producing.

Regardless of a health record's format, there are many core documentation principles that apply to both paper and electronic environments. These principles are critical to ensure both high-quality patient care and a legally defensible health record that will be admitted as evidence in legal proceedings. Among these principles are appropriate authentication, accuracy, authorship, approved abbreviations, legibility, timeliness, completion, appropriate use of the print function, and transparent changes to the record. All these principles contribute to the integrity of the health record.

Healthcare organizations employ a variety of record formats. As technology has changed, so have the methods of maintaining health records. Every healthcare organization must consider the creation, retention, and disposition of its health records on the basis of relevant laws and organizational needs. Health record retention decisions influence the organization in many ways and must be considered with due care.

References

AHIMA. 2009. Amendments, corrections, and deletions in the electronic health record: An American Health Information Management Association toolkit. http://www.ahima.org.

AHIMA. 2011. Practice brief: Protecting patient information after a facility closure (updated). *Journal of AHIMA*: Web extra.

AHIMA e-HIM Work Group: Best Practices for Electronic Signature and Attestation. 2009. Electronic signature, attestation, and authorship. *Journal of AHIMA* 80(11):62–68.

AHIMA e-HIM Work Group on Defining the Legal Health Record. 2005a. Practice brief: Guidelines for defining the legal health record for disclosure purposes. *Journal of AHIMA* 76(8):64A–64G.

AHIMA e-HIM Work Group on Defining the Legal Health Record. 2005b. Practice brief: The legal process and electronic health records. *Journal of AHIMA* 76(9):96A–96D.

AHIMA e-HIM Work Group on Guidelines for EHR Documentation Practice. 2007. Practice brief: Guidelines for EHR documentation to prevent fraud. *Journal of AHIMA* 78(1):65–68.

AHIMA e-HIM Work Group on Implementing Electronic Signatures. 2003a. Practice brief: Implementing electronic signatures. Web extra. Chicago: AHIMA.

AHIMA e-HIM Work Group on Implementing Electronic Signatures. 2003b. Implementing electronic signatures, appendix: State-by-state review of regulations pertaining to electronic signatures. Chicago: AHIMA.

AHIMA e-HIM Work Group on Maintaining the Legal EHR. 2005. Practice brief: Maintaining a legally sound health record—paper and electronic. *Journal of AHIMA* 76(10):64A–64L.

AHIMA MPI Task Force. 2004. Practice brief: Building an enterprise master person index. *Journal of AHIMA* 75(1):56A–56D.

Amatayakul, M. 2013. *Electronic Health Records: A Practical Guide for Professionals and Organizations*, 5th ed, revised reprint. Chicago: AHIMA.

American Medical Association. 2005. Opinion E-7.03 Records of physicians upon retirement or departure from a group. http://www.ama-assn.org/.

American Medical Association Code of Ethics. n.d. http://www.ama-assn.org/.

Burrington-Brown, J., and G. Hughes. 2003. Practice brief: Provider-patient E-mail security. Web extra. Chicago: AHIMA.

Certification Commission for Health Information Technology. n.d. http://www.cchit.org/about.

Dolan, M., J. Wolter, C. Nielsen, and J. Burrington-Brown. 2009. Consumer health informatics: Is there a role for HIM professionals? *Perspectives in Health Information Management*—Summer.

Dougherty, M. 2002. Practice brief: Maintaining a legally sound health record. *Journal of AHIMA* 73(8): 64A–64G.

Fletcher, D., and H. Rhodes. 2002. Practice brief: Retention of health information. Webextra. Chicago: AHIMA.

Gellman, R. 2008. Personal health records: Why many PHRs threaten privacy. The World Privacy Forum. http://www.worldprivacyforum.org.

Health Level Seven (HL7). n.d. Personal health record system functional model. http://www.hl7.org.

Hughes, G. 2001. Facsimile transmission of health information. *Journal of AHIMA* 72(6):64E–64F.

Hughes, G. 2002. Practice brief: Destruction of patient health information. Web extra. Chicago: AHIMA.

Joint Commission. 2010a. *Comprehensive Accreditation Manual for Hospitals*. Oakbrook Terrace, IL: Joint Commission.

Joint Commission. 2010b. 2010 National Patient Safety Goals (NPSGs). http://www.jointcommission.org.

Kerr, O. 2001. Computer records and the Federal Rules of Evidence. *USA Bulletin* 49(2). http://www.justice.gov

Markle Foundation Connecting for Health. 2003. The personal health working group final report. http://www.policyarchive.org

McClean, T.R. 2005. Authenticating EHR metadata. *Journal of AHIMA* 80(2): 40–41, 50.

National Conference of Commissioners of Uniform State Laws. 1999. Uniform Electronic Transaction Act. http://www.uniformlaws.org

Post, G., and D. Anderson. 2006. *Management Information Systems*, 4th ed. Boston, MA: McGraw-Hill.

Reynolds, R., ed. 2010. *Tennessee Health Information Management Association Legal Handbook*, 11th ed. Winchester, TN: THIMA.

Rhodes, H., and M. Brandt. 2003. Practice brief: Protecting patient information after a facility closure. Web extra. Chicago: AHIMA.

Rinehart-Thompson, L. 2006. Exploring record retention practices among the nation's 'most wired' hospitals. *AHIMA 78th National Convention and Exhibit Proceedings*, 241–258. Denver, CO.

Rinehart-Thompson, L. 2008. Record retention practices among the nation's 'most wired' hospitals. *Perspectives in Health Information Management* 5(8): Summer.

Rollins, G. 2007. Printing electronic records: Managing the hassle and the risk. *Journal of AHIMA* 78(5):36–40.

The Sedona Conference. 2007. The Sedona Working Group series. Best practices: Recommendations and principles for addressing electronic document production. http://www.thesedonaconference.com.

Servais, C. 2008. *The Legal Health Record.* Chicago: AHIMA.

Tessier, C. 2010. Moving targets: Maximizing the rewards and minimizing the risks of mobile devices. *Journal of AHIMA* 81(4):38–40. http://www.ahima.org.

US General Accounting Office. 1999. National archives: Preserving electronic records in an era of rapidly changing technology: Report to the Chairman Committee on Governmental Affairs US Senate. Report no. GAO/GGD-99-94. http://www.gao.gov.

Cases, Statutes, and Regulations Cited

42 CFR 482.24(b): Form and retention of record. 2004.

42 CFR 482.24(c): Content of record. 2004.

45 CFR 164 Subpart E: Standards for privacy of identifiable health information. 2003.

45 CFR 164.501: Privacy of individually identifiable health information: Definitions. 2003.

45 CFR 164.504(e)(2): Implementation specifications: business associate contracts. 2003.

45 CFR 164.526: Amendment of protected health information. 2003.

15 USC 700l, et seq.: Electronic Signatures in Global National Commerce Act. 2000.

28 USC 1732: Uniform Photographic Copies of Business and Public Records as Evidence Act. 1977.

American Recovery and Reinvestment Act of 2009. Public Law 111-5.

Appendix 8.A

Detailed Content of the Health Record

This appendix provides an overview of the type of information contained within a health record. Health information is defined by HIPAA as any information, whether oral or recorded in any form or medium, that (1) is created or received by a healthcare provider, health plan, public health authority, employer, life insurer, school or university, or healthcare clearinghouse; and (2) relates to the past, present, or future physical or mental health or condition of an individual; the provision of healthcare to an individual; or the past, present, or future payment for the provision of healthcare to an individual (45 CFR 160.103). Specifically, the health information that makes up a health record will vary depending on the type of healthcare facility or organization providing the care and whether the patient is hospitalized or being treated as an outpatient in some capacity. The health record may be paper, electronic, or a combination of both, known as a hybrid record.

Content of the Health Record

All health records contain information that can be classified into two broad categories: administrative/demographic data and clinical data. All health record entries must be legible, complete, dated, and authenticated according to the policies of the healthcare provider.

Administrative and Demographic Information

Administrative and demographic information is generally found on the front page of the paper patient health record or located from a patient query or search menu in an electronic record system. The information entered provides facts that identify the patient and data related to payment and reimbursement and other operational needs of the healthcare facility.

Registration Data

Registration data represent one type of administrative information. Registration data are collected prior to, or at the time of, an inpatient admission treatment in an emergency department or outpatient facility or a physician or other provider office. This is the first information collected by the facility and includes payment information regarding responsibility for the bill. Administrative information also includes the various consents for treatment and information about the use of patient information, notification of patient rights, and other nonclinical information.

Demographic information, another type of administrative information, includes facts such as:

- The patient's name
- The patient's address
- The patient's telephone number
- The patient's date of birth

Information for this appendix is adopted from Reynolds, R.B., and E.D. Bowman. 2012. Paper-based and hybrid health records. Chapter 8 in *Health Information Management: Concepts, Principles, and Practice*, 4rd ed. Edited by LaTour, K.M. and S. Eichenwald-Maki. Chicago: AHIMA.

- The patient's next of kin

- Other identifying information specific to the patient

A unique identifier number, which can be called the medical record number (MRN) or the person identification number, is assigned to the health record and allows all information about the patient to be inserted into the correct paper record or to be accessed when a query about a particular patient is entered into the electronic system. This unique identifier is critical in accessing the patient's correct information within facilities and in linking information with other providers such as in health information exchange. Demographic information helps to specifically identify the patient and provides statistical information that is vital for planning, research, statistics, and other purposes within the organization.

Demographic information may be entered directly into the electronic system by admission or registration personnel. In cases where the patient is coming to the facility for elective or voluntary treatment and/or an operative procedure, he or she can provide this information prior to arrival at the facility. The patient usually provides the information directly, but in cases where the patient is a minor or is incapacitated, or in an emergency situation, another individual may provide the information. In such cases, the record must state the name and relationship of the person providing the information in case the information has to be verified or amended.

The demographic information in a totally paper-based health record environment is usually on the first page, which is called the face sheet or front sheet. The term "face sheet" is often used to refer to the computer view containing the information in facilities that have an EHR in which a printout of the computer screen becomes the face sheet of a paper or hybrid record.

Consent to Treatment

Through the consent process, the patient agrees to undergo the treatments and procedures to be performed by clinical caregivers. This general consent is often part of the admission or entry process into the healthcare facility. However, the consent does not replace the individual consent forms the patient must complete and sign for each surgical or special procedure to indicate that he or she is fully informed about the specific care to be provided. Consents signed by the patient for experimental drugs and treatment and for participation in research must be included in the health record. Refusal of treatment or procedures likewise must be included to ensure that the consequences of the decision have been explained and the patient is aware of them.

Notice of Privacy Practices and Authorization for Disclosure

The Health Insurance Portability and Accountability Act (HIPAA) Privacy Rule requires that upon admission to the facility or prior to treatment by the provider, patients must be informed about the use of protected health information (PHI). This Notice of Privacy Practices must explain and give examples of the uses of the patient's PHI for treatment, payment, and healthcare operations, as well as other disclosures for purposes established in the regulations (45 CFR 164.520). Patients must be asked to sign an acknowledgement that they received the notice. If a particular disclosure information is not covered in the Notice of Privacy Practices, the patient must sign an authorization form specific to the additional disclosure before his or her information can be disclosed.

Consent to Special Procedures

In cases where the patient is coming to the facility for a specific procedure, an informed consent spelling out the exact details of the treatment must be signed by the patient or his or her legally authorized representative. This consent must show that the patient or the person authorized to act on behalf of the patient understands exactly what the procedure, test, or operation is going to be, including any possible risks, alternative methods, and outcomes.

Advance Directives

An advance directive is a written document, such as a living will, that states the patient's preferences for care. It can also be in the form of a durable power of attorney for healthcare in which the patient names another person to make medical decisions on his or her behalf in the event he or she is incapacitated. When the patient has a written advance directive, its existence must be noted in the health record. Patients or family members may bring the document to the facility to show the patient's wishes in cases of terminal disease, traumatic injury, or cardiac arrest. The advance directive can be included as part of the health record, although its inclusion may not be required. There may be documentation by the physician of a discussion with the patient or the family about the patient's wishes, rather than a formal written document.

Patients must be informed that they have the right to have an advance directive. Further, they must be notified of the provider's policies regarding its refusal to comply with advance directives.

Acknowledgment of Receipt of Patient's Rights Statement

The Centers for Medicare and Medicaid Services (CMS) requires that patients be informed of their rights, including the right to know who is treating them, the right to confidentiality, and the right to be informed about treatment (42 CFR 482.13). The patient's rights statement also must explain the patient's right to refuse treatment, to participate in care planning, and to be safe from abuse. The patient must sign a statement that these rights have been explained, and the signed statement must be made part of the health record. States often have laws and regulations regarding the rights that must be explained to patients, such as the right to privacy in treatment, the right to refuse treatment, and the right to refuse experimental treatments and drugs.

Property and Valuables List

Although facilities encourage patients to leave jewelry and other valuables at home, patients will have personal articles such as clothing, teeth, eyeglasses, and hearing aids with them. Patients may be asked to sign a release of responsibility form to absolve the facility of responsibility for loss or damage to their personal property. This form then becomes part of the patient health record.

Clinical Data

Clinical data include information related to the patient's condition, course of treatment, and progress. The patient health record includes mainly clinical data.

Medical History

The history is a summary of the patient's illness from his or her point of view. Its purpose is to allow the patient or his or her authorized representative to give the physician as much background information about the patient's illness as possible. The physician usually tailors the physical examination to symptoms described in the patient's history and begins an assessment. Thus, the history provides a base on which the physician can develop a plan.

Documentation guidelines for histories, physical examinations, and medical decision making published by CMS affect physician reimbursement.

Components of the Medical History

The medical history has several components, including:

- Chief complaint: Told in the patient's own words (or those of the patient's representative), the chief complaint is the principal reason the patient is seeking care.

- Present illness: This component addresses what the patient feels the problem is and includes a brief description of the duration, location, and circumstances of the complaint.

- Past medical history: This consists of questions designed to gather information about past surgeries and other illnesses that might have a bearing on the patient's current illness. The physician asks about childhood and adult illnesses, operations, injuries, drug sensitivities, allergies, and other health problems.

- Social and personal history: The social history uncovers information about habits and living conditions that might have a bearing on the patient's illness, such as marital status, occupation, environment, and so on. Consumption of alcohol or tobacco products also may affect a patient's health. This section also should address the patient's psychosocial needs.

- Family medical history: The questions in this component allow the physician to learn whether other family members have conditions that might be considered genetic. Common questions concern cardiovascular diseases or conditions, renal diseases, history of cancer or diabetes, allergies, health of immediate relatives, and ages of relatives at death and causes of their deaths.

- Review of systems: This component consists of questions designed to cue the patient to reveal symptoms he or she may have forgotten, did not think were important, or neglected to mention when providing the historical information.

It is important that the person recording the history document whether the information was given by the patient or by another person in cases where the patient is unable to communicate.

Physical Examination

The physical examination is the actual comprehensive assessment of the patient by the physician. Its purpose is to obtain initial signs and symptoms so that appropriate treatment can begin. The end of the physical examination should indicate the impression based on the information obtained and the initial plan for the patient's care while in the hospital.

Components of the Physical Examination

The physical examination is conducted by observing the patient, palpating or touching the patient, tapping the thoracic and abdominal cavities, listening to breath and heart sounds, and taking the blood pressure. The patient is examined thoroughly. If the patient is admitted for a particular procedure, a more focused physical examination will take place.

Time Frame of the History and Physical Examination

The facility must have a policy that establishes a time frame for completing the history and physical. Most facilities set the timeframe as the first 24 hours following admission and require that the history and physical be completed by the provider who is admitting the patient. It is acceptable to the Joint Commission when the history and physical examination are completed within 30 days before the patient is admitted. Medicare regulations specify that the history and physical examination be completed by the physician or other qualified individual who has medical staff privileges in accordance with state law. The history and physical examination must be completed no more than 30 days before or 24 hours after admission, and the report must be in the record within 24 hours after admission. Medicare requires that if the history and physical have been completed within the 30 days prior to admission, there must be an updated entry in the medical record that documents an examination for any changes in the patient's condition, and this entry must be included in the record within the first 24 hours of admission.

The Joint Commission requires the history and physical examination to be recorded and made part of the patient health record prior to any operative procedure. When the physician chooses to dictate the history and physical, the dictated report must be transcribed and made part of the patient's health record before the procedure. When the report is dictated but not transcribed, a written preoperative note covering the history and physical is acceptable only in an emergency. The physician must write an explanation of the emergency circumstances.

The health informatics and information management professional is responsible for ensuring that the most stringent time requirements are followed so that the facility is in compliance with state and federal laws and regulations, licensure standards, Medicare Conditions of Participation, and accreditation requirements for the specific type of facility. When the patient is readmitted within 30 days after discharge for the same condition, some hospitals allow the previous history and physical examination to be updated and signed and dated by the physician. This is called an interval history and is acceptable to the Joint Commission.

Diagnostic and Therapeutic Orders

Physicians' orders drive the healthcare team. Orders may be for treatments, ancillary medical services, laboratory tests, radiological procedures, drugs, devices, related materials, restraint, or seclusion. Orders change according to the patient's needs and responses to previous treatment. In the case of drugs, the physician orders a specific drug in a particular dosage stating how often the drug is to be given, by what means (orally, intravenously, or by other method), and for how long. Certain categories of drugs, such as narcotics and sedatives, have an automatic time limit or stop order. This means that these medications must be discontinued unless the physician gives a specific order to continue administration of the medication. This prevents patients from receiving drugs for a longer period of time than is necessary.

Orders for tests and services must demonstrate the medical necessity and explain the reason for the order. The legibility of orders is important to ensure that they are clearly understood by the personnel who must carry them out. Some facilities use a computerized physician order-entry (CPOE) system. Verbal orders entered into the record or computer system by nonphysician personnel must be signed or authenticated by the provider authorized to give orders. If providers have not signed in a timely manner, the computer will not let them access the system until the orders are signed.

Clinicians Authorized to Give and Receive Orders

Orders must be written by the physician or verbally communicated to persons authorized to receive verbal orders either in person or by telephone. The person accepting the order should sign and give his or her title, such as RN, PT, or LPN, as appropriate. In some states, certified registered nurse practitioners and physician assistants are allowed to write or give verbal orders.

Medical staff policies and procedures must specifically state the categories of personnel authorized to accept orders. Verbal orders for medication are usually required to be given to and to be accepted only by nursing or pharmacy personnel. Some categories of personnel that may accept verbal or oral orders for services within the specific area of practice include physical therapists, registered nurse anesthetists, dietitians, and medical technologists.

Orders for tests and treatments must justify the condition of medical necessity, because payers may not reimburse the facility if the reason for the test or treatment is not properly documented.

The time the order is given should be recorded. Some facilities do not allow verbal orders for treatments or procedures that might put the patient at risk. Other facilities require verbal orders to be repeated by the person accepting them to verify that they are clearly understood.

Signatures on Orders

Orders must be dated and signed, or authenticated, to prove authorship by the provider or providers responsible for the patient's care who either entered or gave the orders. In the case of verbal or telephone orders, the provider should authenticate them as soon as possible after giving them. Many facilities require the ordering provider to indicate that the telephone orders are accurate, complete, and final by signing or authenticating them within 24 hours. The timing requirements for signatures on orders are governed by state law, facility policy, accreditation standards, and government regulations and may vary from facility to facility. Medicare regulations state that in the absence of state law, the time limit for authentication will be within 48 hours.

For years, personnel analyzed and reviewed each order and marked those with missing signatures so that each could be individually authenticated by the responsible provider after discharge. However, signing orders after discharge does not affect the patient's care process, so many facilities no longer routinely review orders for signatures following patient discharge. A review of orders is part of the concurrent or open-record review process while patients are in-house or in the facility; thus, orders can be signed in a timely manner, and providers with patterns of unsigned orders can be detected. A comparison of orders with laboratory and other ancillary reports and with nursing documentation is another way to ensure that all orders are carried out.

Some facilities have developed standing or standard orders for certain procedures that all physicians can use when performing the particular procedure. Other facilities require an additional order to implement the standing orders, and still others allow a registered nurse to initiate the standing orders because the medical staff has previously approved them.

Special Orders

"Do not resuscitate" (DNR) orders must contain documentation that the decision to withhold cardiopulmonary resuscitation (CPR) was discussed, when the decision was made, and who participated in the decision. This discussion is often documented in the progress notes. Generally, patients are presumed to have consented to CPR unless a DNR order is present in the record. This may be part of the advance directives in the record.

Orders for seclusion and restraint, including drugs used for restraint, must comply with facility policies and Medicare regulations, state laws, and Joint Commission requirements. These should never be standing or as-needed orders but, instead, must be ordered only when necessary to protect the patient or others from injury or harm. Specific time limits for these orders must be followed, and there must be continuous oversight of the patient under restraint or seclusion.

Discharge Orders

Discharge orders for hospital patients must be entered by a physician. When a patient leaves against medical advice, this fact should be noted in lieu of a discharge order because the patient was not actually discharged. In the case of death, some facilities require that a discharge to the morgue order be written.

Clinical Observations

Clinical observations of the patient are documented in the health record in several formats, including progress notes, consultation reports, and ancillary notes, as described below.

Medical Services

Progress notes are chronological statements about the patient's response to treatment during his or her stay in the facility. Facility procedures and policies must state exactly what categories of personnel are allowed to write or enter information into progress notes. Generally, these personnel include physicians, nurses, physical therapists, occupational therapists, respiratory therapists, social workers, case managers, dietitians, nurse anesthetists, pharmacists, radiology technologists, speech therapists, and others providing direct treatment or consultation to the patient. Each person authorized to enter documentation into the progress notes must write or enter his or her own note, authenticate and date it, and indicate authorship by signing his or her full name and title.

Each progress note reviews changes in the patient's condition, findings based on the facts of the case, test results, and response to treatment, as well as an analysis of the findings. The final part of the note contains the decisions or actions planned for future care. When writing in a paper patient record, providers must avoid leaving blank spaces between progress notes, to prevent information from being added out of sequence.

Flow charts are an effective way to illustrate the patient's progress and can be computerized to demonstrate progress or to keep track of certain data. Many physicians and other providers use hand-held personal computers to maintain ongoing flow chart information about patients, such as blood glucose levels over time.

The patient's condition determines how frequently progress notes are recorded. The frequency of the recording of progress notes is generally established by the healthcare facility or payers of care. In a hospital, the physician primarily responsible for the patient's care is often required to enter a progress note daily. Doing so shows the physician's involvement and that he or she is aware of changes in the patient's condition.

Consultations are additional opinions of specialists. The attending physician may request that the specialist see the patient and prepare a consultation report. Each consultant is responsible for writing, dictating, or entering his or her own report. The report should show evidence of the consultant's review of the record and the patient and any pertinent findings, opinions, and recommendations. Moreover, the documentation should show that the physician requesting the consultation reviewed the report.

Nursing Services

Nursing personnel have the most frequent contact with patients, and their notes provide the daily record of the patients' progress and condition and demonstrate the continuity of care. Licensed registered nurses, licensed practical nurses (sometimes called licensed vocational nurses), and nursing assistants record the facts of the physician's orders being carried out, observe the patient's response to treatment interventions, and describe the patient's condition and complaints as well as the outcome of care as reflected in the patient's status at discharge or termination of treatment.

Nursing personnel begin recording information in the health record when the patient is admitted to the facility. They coordinate the patient's care to ensure that orders are carried out. The initial nursing assessment must summarize the date, time, and method of admission; the patient's condition, symptoms, and vital signs; and other information. All nursing notes must be signed or authenticated by the individuals who provided the service or observed the patient's condition. Full names and titles are required.

Charting by exception, or focus charting, is a method of charting only abnormal or unusual findings or deviations from the prescribed plan of care. A complete assessment is performed every shift or every eight hours. When events differ from the assessment or the expected norm for a particular patient, the notes should focus on that particular event and include the data, intervention, and response. Flow sheets and care plans may be used to illustrate changes in the patient's condition. The purpose of charting by exception is to reduce repetitive recordkeeping and documentation of normal events. Bedside terminals, direct input of monitoring information, and other computerization of nursing observations and medication distribution save nurses a great deal of time because information does not have to be rewritten numerous times.

Medication administration records (MARs) or electronic MARs (eMARs) are maintained for all patients and include medications given, time, form of administration, and dosage and strength. The records are updated when the patient is given his or her medication. The health record must reflect when a medication is given in error, indicating what was done about it and the patient's response. Adverse drug reactions must be fully documented and reported to the provider and to the performance improvement or risk management program according to guidelines established by the facility.

Flow sheets are often used in addition to narrative notes for intake and output records showing how much fluid the patient consumed and how much was eliminated. In addition, blood glucose records are often flow-charted for ease of comparison. Degree of pain is another aspect of the patient's condition that is commonly flow-charted.

Nurses are responsible for maintaining records of patient transfers (to surgery, to another room, or to another level of care) as well as visits to physician or treatment offices and other locations outside the facility.

Case managers are nurses, social workers, or other personnel who are responsible for assisting the patient through the care process. The case management process improves quality of care because care is scheduled in an orderly way and fragmentation is reduced. Hospitals, managed care organizations, and other facilities use case managers to improve coordination of care, scheduling, and discharge planning. Many facilities use predetermined care paths that are specific to diagnoses or conditions; case managers ensure that patients receive care according to the care path. Care paths are also called clinical pathways, critical paths, and clinical algorithms.

Ancillary Services

Laboratory and radiology reports and reports from other ancillary services, such as EKGs (electrocardiographs) and EEGs (electroencephalographs), must be signed by the physician responsible for the interpretations. A pathologist is responsible for the work of the clinical laboratory; a radiologist is responsible for the work of the radiology department. Many states have separate retention schedules for the actual x-rays that differ from the retention timeframes for other health records. The final interpretations of the radiology or other reports become part of the health record and are kept as long as the health records are kept. Digital images may be part of a computerized picture archiving communication system (PACS).

Laboratory results in a computerized environment are available to the provider as soon as they are entered into the system. In most facilities, a laboratory summary is generated consistently throughout the patient's stay, with a final summary completed within 24 hours after discharge. These multipage summaries are printed and made part of the patient health record. Some facilities use manually completed laboratory forms divided into several sections. The original report is the one that should be included in the record. The laboratory conducts tests on blood, urine, sputum, and other body fluids. Many specialized tests are performed in the laboratory to provide information the physician can use to make a diagnosis, including analyses of specimens removed during surgery. Most facilities require the original laboratory results to be placed in the health record within 24 hours.

Healthcare facility policies and procedures must state that the practitioner approved by the medical staff to interpret diagnostic procedures, such as nuclear medicine procedures, MRIs, EEGs, and EKGs, should sign or authenticate and date his or her interpretations. The interpretations then become part of the health record. Scans and videotapes, tracings, or other actual recordings are often fed directly into the computer system. Providers may view such recordings, but the recordings do not become part of the permanent record. It is important that all tests or procedures ordered have corresponding results reported in the health record.

Orders and records of services rendered to patients from rehabilitation, physical therapy, occupational therapy, audiology, or speech pathology should be included in the record as appropriate to the patient. These reports must contain evaluations, recommendations, goals, course of treatment, and response to treatment. Nutritional care plans need to be developed in compliance with a physician order, and information on nutrition and diet should be included in the discharge plan and transfer orders.

Surgical Services

The operative section of the health record includes the anesthesia record, the intraoperative record, and the recovery record. The history and physical examination, informed consents signed by the patient or his or her authorized representative, and the postoperative progress note also are part of the documentation about the operative procedure. Every patient's chart must include a complete history and physical examination prior to surgery or an invasive procedure unless there is an emergency.

The anesthesiologist or the certified registered nurse anesthetist must write a preanesthesia evaluation or an updated evaluation prior to surgery. This evaluation must cover information on the anesthesia to be used, risk factors, allergy and drug history, potential problems, and a general assessment of the patient's condition. An intraoperative anesthesia record must be maintained of all events during surgery, including complete information on the anesthesia administration, blood pressure, pulse, respiration, and other monitors of the patient's condition. Finally, after surgery, the appropriate anesthesia personnel must enter a postoperative anesthesia follow-up report. Outpatient surgical cases also must include postanesthesia evaluations. Records of postanesthesia visits should indicate any unusual events or complications. Proposed Medicare regulations state that any individual qualified to administer anesthesia can complete the postanesthesia evaluation.

The operative report itself must be entered or dictated by the surgeon immediately after surgery and must include the names of the surgeon and assistants, technical procedures performed, findings, specimens removed, estimated blood loss, and postoperative diagnosis. The surgeon must enter a brief postoperative progress note in the record immediately after surgery, before the patient leaves the operating suite. The postoperative progress note must be completed to provide information for patient care until the typed report is made part of the patient record, usually 12 to 24 hours after surgery. Some facilities use a preprinted postoperative progress note form or template with the required elements listed to remind the surgeon of the items that must be included. The postoperative progress notes and the dictation and transcription of operative reports must be carefully monitored to ensure that they are integrated with the health record in a timely manner.

Pathology reports are required for every case in which a surgical specimen is removed or expelled during a procedure and must include a microscopic and gross evaluation of the tissue. These reports are part of the operative section of the health record and must be authenticated by the pathologist. The preoperative diagnosis and pathological diagnosis can then be compared.

Information on the patient's discharge from the postoperative or postanesthesia care unit must be documented and authenticated by the licensed independent practitioner responsible for the discharge or by the provider verifying that the patient is ready for discharge according to specific discharge criteria. The operative section also will contain data on implants, including product numbers, and additional information for follow-up.

Organ Transplantation

CMS requires hospitals to inform families of the opportunity to donate organs, tissues, or eyes. Documentation showing that the organ procurement organization has been notified regarding a patient near death must be included in the health record so that anatomical gifts can be preserved and used. In the case of living donor transplants of kidneys or other organs, an operative report must be entered for both donor and recipient following all the standards for operative records.

Conclusions at Termination of Care: Discharge Summary and Discharge Plan

The health record must summarize the patient's condition at the beginning of treatment and basic information about tests, examinations, procedures, and results occurring as a result of treatment. The conclusion at termination of care is called the discharge summary. The discharge summary, also called the clinical resume, provides details about the patient's stay in the facility and is the foundation for future treatment. It is prepared when the patient is discharged or transferred to another facility or when the patient expires. The summary states the patient's reason for admission and gives a brief history explaining why he or she needed to be hospitalized. Pertinent laboratory, radiological, consultation, and other significant findings, as well as the patient's response to treatment or procedures, are included. In addition to a description of the patient's condition at discharge, the discharge summary delineates specific instructions given to the family for future care, including information on medications, referrals to other providers, diet, activities, follow-up visits to the physician, and the patient's final diagnoses. The discharge summary must be signed and dated by the physician.

Some facilities require the final diagnoses to be recorded and the discharge summary to be dictated or entered at discharge, or they immediately consider the chart delinquent. The information in the discharge summary is extremely important for meeting the facility's coding, billing, and reimbursement needs. In some facilities, a paper discharge summary form or template with an outline of contents is used to ensure that all items are included. The form has three parts so that the part with follow-up instructions can be given to the patient or printed from the computer system.

When a patient dies in the hospital, hospitals often require the physician who pronounced death to enter a note or order that gives the time and date of death. The death note is in addition to the discharge summary required in all death cases, no matter how long the patient was in the facility. Most facilities do not require a discharge summary for normal newborns and obstetrical cases without complications, as long as there is a final progress note.

A discharge summary is not required for patients who are in the hospital for 48 hours or less. Such patients usually have a short-stay or short-service record or a final discharge progress note. This one-page form or template can be used to record the history and physical examination, the operative report, the discharge summary, and discharge instructions. When the patient is admitted to the facility, the reason for admission must be recorded. When the patient dies 48 hours or less after admission, the short-stay record is insufficient and a complete discharge summary must be prepared.

The discharge summary must be completed within 30 days after the date of discharge. When a patient is transferred, the physician should complete the discharge summary within 24 hours.

The principal diagnosis and other diagnoses should be recorded completely without symbols or abbreviations on the health record summary sheet (the face sheet) or discharge summary or on another form or template prescribed by the facility. The principal diagnosis is defined as the condition determined, after study, to be chiefly responsible for occasioning the patient's admission to the hospital.

Healthcare facilities must determine what information goes with the patient when he or she is transferred to another level of care. When the transfer is to an affiliated institution that is part of the same healthcare system, the original patient record is transferred with the patient and new orders are written at the receiving institution to initiate care. A discharge summary is generally required.

Discharge Plan

Discharge planning information regarding further treatment of the patient should be part of the acute care health record. The discharge planning process begins at admission and must include information on the patient's ability to perform self-care as well as other services needed by the patient. The case manager, the social worker, utilization review personnel, or nursing personnel may write this plan.

Records Filed with the Health Record

It is important for healthcare facilities to develop policies to determine exactly what health information that is mailed, faxed, or personally brought to the facility by the patient or patient's family becomes part of the receiving facility's designated record set. A good practice is to have the attending physician review copies and note which documents should be made permanent parts of the record. Any extraneous copies, x-rays, or other information should be returned to the patient.

Specialized Health Record Content

The content of the patient health record varies according to the type of care provided. Facilities that offer specialized services, such as behavioral health, long-term care, or physician office practice, to name a few, require documentation that is special to that area of service. Joint Commission standards and regulations often specify particular content to include in the record. The following sections describe various specialized services and their records.

Obstetrical Care

The prenatal record, which is kept in the physician's office, serves as the history and physical for an obstetrical patient. When the patient requires a Cesarean section (C-section), the record must include a full history and physical or a detailed admission progress note explaining the need for a C-section.

A labor and delivery record indicates the name of the patient, maiden name, date of delivery, sex of infant, name of physician, name of persons assisting, any complications, type of anesthesia used, name of person administering anesthesia, and names of others present at delivery. In the case of a stillborn infant, a separate patient record is not created; rather, information is recorded in the mother's delivery record. A fetal death certificate is completed on the appropriate form.

Neonatal Care

Newborns are considered separate patients with separate health records. The newborn patient record must include an admission examination and a discharge examination. Usually, special chart forms or templates for progress notes, orders, and nursing notes are included. When the patient has been in the newborn intensive care unit, a complete discharge summary is required.

Emergency Care

Emergency health records may be filed separately or incorporated into the health record when the patient is admitted to the same facility. When the records are filed separately, the emergency health record must be available when the patient is readmitted or seeks care in the future. Most of the emergency information is recorded on one form or template in a paper health record format. Additional sheets include laboratory, radiology, and other tests; consent forms; and follow-up instructions.

The content of the emergency health record should include:

- Identification data

- Time of arrival

- Means of arrival (by ambulance, private automobile, or police vehicle)

- Name of person or organization transporting patient to the emergency department

- Pertinent history, including chief complaint and onset of injury or illness

- Significant physical findings

- Laboratory, x-ray, and EKG findings

- Treatment rendered

- Conclusions at termination of treatment

- Disposition of patient, including whether sent home, transferred, or admitted

- Condition of the patient upon discharge or transfer

- Diagnosis upon discharge

- Instructions given to the patient or the family regarding further care and follow-up

- Signatures and titles of the patient's caregivers

When the patient leaves before being seen or against medical advice, this fact should be noted in the emergency health record. Consent forms for treatment must be included. In cases where there is an emergency or the patient is in critical condition or otherwise unable to sign the consent form, an explanation should be documented. A copy of the emergency record should be made available to the provider of follow-up care.

Most states require facilities to maintain an additional chronological record to register all patients visiting the emergency department with name, date, time of arrival, and record number. This registration also includes the names of patients who were dead on arrival.

Emergency patients must be made aware of their rights. Transfer and acceptance policies and procedures must be delineated to ensure that facilities comply with the Emergency Medical Treatment and Active Labor Act (EMTALA) (42 USC §1395dd) and state regulations regarding transfers. Patients cannot be transferred or refused treatment for reasons related to ability to pay or source of payment, nor can hospitals determine that space is unavailable based on ability to pay or source of payment (42 CFR 489.24). Anyone who requests or requires an examination must be provided an appropriate medical screening examination by hospital staff to determine whether a medical emergency exists. Further, the hospital must stabilize the medical emergency by ensuring an airway and ventilation, by controlling hemorrhage, and by stabilizing or splinting fractures before a patient can be transferred. The hospital must maintain screening examinations for a period of five years.

Appropriate transfer means that the receiving hospital agrees to receive the patient and provide appropriate medical treatment. Records must be provided to the receiving hospital, and the patient or responsible person must understand the medical necessity of the transfer.

Ambulatory or Outpatient Care

Ambulatory or outpatient care means that patients move from location to location. Patients arrive for treatment and leave after treatment has been administered; they do not stay overnight. Ambulatory or outpatient care may be given in a freestanding clinic, a clinic that is part of a larger hospital system, or a physician or other provider office. When patients are in a clinic affiliated with a hospital, the entire health record should be available. The Joint Commission requires ambulatory patients to have a summary list by the third visit that includes known diagnoses, conditions, procedures, drug allergies, and medications. It also requires each ambulatory care record to contain a history and physical examination, operative reports, diagnostic and therapeutic procedures, consultations, follow-up notes, observations of patients, and discharge notes at the conclusion or termination of treatment. Contents vary depending on the treatment received.

Ambulatory facilities that only perform surgery are called ambulatory surgery centers (ASCs). Patients having surgery at any type of ambulatory facility must have a history and physical examination prior to surgery, consents, an operative note, a postoperative progress note, and the same anesthesia information as an operative patient in the hospital. In addition, the record must document instructions for postoperative care and postoperative follow-up. Clinics often call patients after surgery, and these calls should be documented in the record. The Accreditation Association for Ambulatory Health Care requires that the history and physical examination, laboratory reports, radiology reports, operative reports, and consultations be signed or authenticated in a timely manner. Laboratory and other results must be included in the patient record as soon as possible.

Traditionally, physician office records have been less comprehensive than hospital medical records. Physicians must develop standardized formats and comprehensive documentation practices.

The focus of ambulatory care is to see or treat patients quickly and then move them efficiently out of the facility. Because of the brief nature of ambulatory care, rapid access to information is vital.

Behavioral Healthcare

Behavioral health records, also known as mental health records or psychiatric records, must include diagnostic and assessment information. Medicare requires that the records contain a provisional or admitting diagnosis and the reason for admission as well as the names of the persons involved in making the admission decision. In addition, a goal-oriented treatment plan must be in place.

Medicare further requires that social service records assess family and home information and community resources available to the patient. Special requirements for a psychiatric evaluation include history, mental status, information on the present illness, and intellectual and memory function. Progress notes must be recorded at least weekly for the first two months and at least once monthly thereafter. Finally, a discharge summary should be entered in the record. Special attention must be paid to orders for restraint and seclusion as noted in the discussion on orders.

Home Health Services

According to the National Association for Home Care (NAHC), the term "home care" covers many types of services "delivered at home to recovering, disabled, chronically or terminally ill persons in need of medical, nursing, social, or therapeutic treatment and/or assistance with the essential activities of daily living" (NAHC 2005). Physicians order home care services that may include visits from many types of healthcare providers, including physicians and nurses. Patient health records must contain a legible record of each visit, describing what was done to or for the patient during the visit.

The providers working with patients must develop and document periodic plans of care. Specific forms developed by CMS are used in home care to document and update the plan of care. Verbal orders must be signed before the home health agency submits a bill for payment.

Hospice Care Services

The National Hospice and Palliative Care Organization (NHPCO) defines hospice care as a "team-oriented approach to expert medical care, pain management, and emotional and spiritual support expressly tailored to the patient's needs and wishes" (2005). Because hospice care is delivered to patients with all types of terminal illnesses, the family is involved in the care and support is given by the hospice organization. Hospice services are provided in numerous types of settings, including homes, hospitals, and long-term care facilities (NHPCO 2005). Special documentation for the election of hospice care is required for CMS to reimburse for services.

Rehabilitation Services

Rehabilitation covers a wide range of services provided to build or rebuild the patient's abilities to perform the usual activities of daily life. Among these services are physical therapy, occupational therapy, and speech therapy.

Physical therapists work in numerous types of facilities, ranging from acute care to long-term care and patient homes, setting goals for patients and helping them reach their goals by building muscle strength and respiratory and circulatory efficiency. Their patients include those who have been disabled for a number of reasons, including birth defect, trauma, and illness. Treatments include exercise, manipulation, heat therapy, light therapy, the use of electricity, and therapeutic massage. In addition to setting treatment goals, physical therapists have to document patient progress.

Occupational therapists are part of the rehabilitation team and work with patients to restore their ability to perform the usual functions of daily life, such as eating, dressing, preparing food, working, and handling other activities specific to the patient. Speech therapists and other specialized therapists are important members of the rehabilitation team and work together to achieve a variety of patient goals.

Long-Term Care

Long-term care describes the care provided for extended periods of time to patients recovering from illness or injury. Long-term care facilities offer a combination of services, ranging from independent living to assisted living to skilled nursing care. Rehabilitation services are often part of the long-term care plan. The long-term care record must document a comprehensive assessment that includes items in the Minimum Data Set (MDS) to meet Medicare requirements stated in 42 CFR 483.20.

In addition, long-term care facilities must meet state requirements. Individualized patient care plans must be developed and included in the health record. These plans must cover the potential for rehabilitation, the ability to perform activities of daily living, medications prescribed, and other aspects of care.

As with acute care facilities, the frequency of notes depends on the patient's condition. The focus in long-term care is on the achievement of goals. The health information management functions are similar to those in other types of facilities, but a great deal of concurrent review is required. Paper records of patients who have been in the facility for an extended period of time must be divided, with the most current information maintained on the nursing unit and the rest filed elsewhere to save space at the nursing station.

Chapter 9

The HIPAA Privacy Rule

Laurie A. Rinehart-Thompson, JD, RHIA, CHP, FAHIMA

Learning Objectives

- Describe the purpose and goals of the HIPAA Privacy Rule

- Explain the source of law from which the HIPAA Privacy Rule is derived

- Identify to whom and what the HIPAA Privacy Rule applies

- Describe the various types of organizations governed by the HIPAA Privacy Rule

- Explain the parameters for the appropriate redisclosure of patient information

- Discuss examples of each of the individual rights granted by the HIPAA Privacy Rule

- Explain the restrictions that the HIPAA Privacy Rule places on the use of protected health information for marketing and fundraising purposes and apply them to factual situations

- Explain the HIPAA Privacy Rule's parameters on the use of protected health information for research

- Examine conflicts and determine prevailing law between the HIPAA Privacy Rule and state law

- Summarize the administrative requirements and penalties for noncompliance imposed by the HIPAA Privacy Rule

Key Terms

Access
Access report
Accounting of disclosures
Administrative simplification
Affiliated covered entities
Amendment request
American Recovery and
    Reinvestment Act (ARRA)
Authorization
Belmont Report
Breach

Breach notification
Business associate (BA)
Business associate agreement
    (BAA)
Center for Democracy and
    Technology
Clinical Laboratory
    Improvement Act (CLIA)
Compound authorization
Conditioned authorization
Conditions of Participation

Confidential communications
Consent
Covered entities (CE)
Deidentified information
Designated record set (DRS)
Disclosure
Enforcement Rule
Facility directory
Freedom of Information Act
    of 1967 (FOIA)
Fundraising

Health Information Technology for Economic and Clinical Health (HITECH) Act

Health Insurance Portability and Accountability Act of 1996 (HIPAA)

Health Privacy Project

Hybrid entity

Individual

Institutional review board (IRB)

Limited data set

Mitigation

National Research Act of 1974Notice of Privacy Practices (NPP)

Organized healthcare arrangement (OHCA)

Personal representative

Preemption

Privacy Act of 1974

Privacy board

Privacy officer

Privacy Rule

Protected health information (PHI)

Psychotherapy notes

Redisclosure

Request

Request restrictions

Retaliation and waiver

Safe Harbor method

Stand-alone authorization

Treatment, payment, and operations (TPO)

Unconditioned authorization

Use

Workforce

Introduction

April 14, 2003, marked the effective date of a law heralded by some as the most dramatic change in healthcare since the implementation of Medicare and Medicaid. The healthcare industry ushered in the portion of the Health Insurance Portability and Accountability Act (HIPAA) known as the HIPAA Privacy Rule. In the years since it went into effect, healthcare organizations and providers have continued to uphold the spirit of the law and operate within its confines. Although its requirements are immense, experts debate whether the law has increased patient privacy rights as they relate to health information or whether it has merely cloaked questionable access by others in a complex law filled with a maze of requirements. Nonetheless, the privacy of patient information has been, and continues to be, a central value in healthcare. Although the HIPAA Privacy Rule has imposed many requirements, it does not change the advocacy role that healthcare professionals have always held with respect to protecting patient information. This chapter will introduce the reader to this highly publicized law by analyzing the backdrop of patient information privacy and the need for additional privacy protections. Next, it will discuss the law's applicability, relevant terms, requirements, and—most important—the purpose for which the law was primarily created: the privacy of an individual's health information. Additionally, this chapter will discuss changes to the original HIPAA provisions that are present in the Health Information Technology for Economic and Clinical Health (HITECH) Act of the 2009 American Recovery and Reinvestment Act (ARRA) (Pub.L. 111-5).

Because the HIPAA Privacy Rule is so extensive, this chapter has been divided into three sections to organize the material: "Overview of HIPAA and Other Patient Privacy Laws; HIPAA Terminology" (Section 1); "Core Privacy Rule Documents and the Minimum Necessary Requirement" (Section 2); and "Individual Rights; Other Key Requirements; Penalties for Noncompliance" (Section 3).

Section 1: Overview of HIPAA and Other Patient Privacy Laws; HIPAA Terminology

Purpose and Goals of the HIPAA Privacy Rule

The HIPAA **Privacy Rule** is a key federal law governing the privacy and confidentiality of patient information. Although the term *patient privacy* is often used when referring to the HIPAA Privacy Rule, the concept is broader in scope because it involves patient care and the need for privacy as it relates to one's person. The effects of the HIPAA Privacy Rule, conversely, are to provide privacy protections to one's health information. The law's first goal is to provide an individual with greater rights with respect to his or her health information; the second goal is to provide greater privacy protections for one's health information, which serves to limit access by others. While navigating the Privacy Rule's key terms, concepts, and many exceptions, remember that the rule was written to accomplish these two goals.

Source of Law

The **Health Insurance Portability and Accountability Act of 1996** (HIPAA) was enacted by Congress on August 21, 1996, and became federal statutory law. As described below under "Scope and Anatomy of the Law," HIPAA is expansive and covers a broad array of issues. From the statutory requirements of the privacy portion of HIPAA, the US Department of Health and Human Services (HHS) created an administrative law that became effective April 14, 2003. The final administrative rule promulgated by HHS resulted in numerous iterations that were influenced by feedback from stakeholders. The federal government published the Standards for Privacy of Individually Identifiable Health Information, more commonly referred to as the HIPAA Privacy Rule (and also referred to as the final rule) in the Federal Register on December 28, 2000 (HHS 2000). With amendments, the final modified Privacy Rule was published August 14, 2002 (HHS 2002; Hughes 2003). Although available from many sources, including the HHS website, the regulations are officially available in the Code of Federal Regulations (45 CFR 160 and 164; HHS 2002). The American Recovery and Reinvestment Act, passed by Congress in 2009, contained changes to the HIPAA Privacy Rule as delineated in the HITECH Act. These acts are described in greater detail later in this chapter.

Scope and Anatomy of the Law

HIPAA immediately connotes privacy because that aspect of the law has been so highly publicized. However, privacy is only one portion of the entire law, albeit an extremely important aspect to the management of health information. HIPAA consists of five broad sections (titles), most of which do not specifically address the protection of patient information. Although much attention has rightfully been given to both the privacy and security aspects of HIPAA, the broader scope of the act is apparent from its name. An acknowledgment of all portions of the law is necessary to appreciate the entire breadth of this legislation. In fact, HIPAA amends three pieces of federal legislation already in existence: the Internal Revenue Code of 1986 (26 USC), the Employee Retirement Income Security Act of 1986 (ERISA) (29 USC 2001 et seq.), and the Public Health Service Act (42 USC 6A).

As shown in figure 9.1, HIPAA contains five titles and addresses more than the privacy of patient information. Title I protects individuals and their dependents from losing their health insurance when

Figure 9.1. HIPAA components

Title I	Health Care Access, Portability, and Renewability	Title III	Tax-Related Health Provision
		Title IV	Group Health Plan Requirements
Title II	Preventing Health Care Fraud & Abuse Medical Liability Reform Administrative Simplification: 1) Privacy 2) Security 3) Transactions and Code Sets 4) Unique National Provider Identifiers 5) Enforcement	Title V	Revenue Offsets

leaving or changing jobs by providing insurance continuity (portability). It also prohibits discrimination based on a person's status or that of his or her dependents in the enrollment in health insurance plans and the amount of premiums charged. Titles III, IV, and V contain tax-related provisions relevant to the Internal Revenue Code and requirements for group health plans. In particular, Title III provides certain deductions for medical insurance, and Title IV specifies group health plan coverage for individuals with pre-existing conditions and income tax requirements for specific groups (45 CFR 165.512(e), Pub. L. 104-191).

Title II is the most relevant title to the management of health information, containing provisions relating to the prevention of healthcare fraud and abuse and medical liability (medical malpractice) reform, as well as administrative simplification. The Privacy Rule resides in the administrative simplification provision of Title II along with the HIPAA security regulations (which relate to safeguards—often technical in nature—that protect the privacy of patient information and are covered in chapter 10 of this text), transactions and code set standardization requirements, unique national provider identifiers, and the enforcement rule. Because the complexity of HIPAA is well known, the term *administrative simplification* seems a misnomer. However, this term refers to HIPAA's attempt to streamline and standardize the healthcare industry's nonuniform and seemingly inefficient business practices, such as billing. A significant part of this simplification process is the creation of standards for the electronic transmission of data. This was the original intent of HIPAA. The privacy and security rules were created thereafter.

American Recovery and Reinvestment Act of 2009

On February 17, 2009, President Obama signed the **American Recovery and Reinvestment Act (ARRA)** into law. This multifaceted statute, which included significant funding for health information technology and as well as other stimulus funding, also provided for significant changes to the HIPAA Privacy Rule. These changes are located in the **Health Information Technology for Economic and Clinical Health (HITECH) Act**, a statute within ARRA. In general, the compliance date for HITECH provisions affecting HIPAA was set at February 17, 2010, one year from the date the law was signed. However, varying timelines for federal rule drafting have resulted in multiple compliance deadlines. Two interim final rules relating to breach notification and enforcement (an update to a pre-HITECH 2006 final enforcement rule) were published in 2009. On July 14, 2010, and May 31, 2011, HHS issued proposed rules with suggested modifications to the HITECH Act. The January 2013 final rule, "Modifications to the HIPAA Privacy, Security, Enforcement, and Breach Notification Rules," finalized the two interim final rules and provisions in the July 2010 proposed rule (AHIMA 2013). The May 2011 proposed rule is still pending. Major revisions, which are addressed in each relevant section in this chapter, include changes to requirements relating to business associates and their subcontractors; protected health information of deceased individuals; Notice of Privacy Practices; the sale of information; provisions affecting the minimum necessary requirement; individual rights (namely, access, accounting of disclosures, and the right to request restrictions); student immunization records; research authorizations; breach notification; provisions affecting personal health record vendors; marketing and fundraising; and increased enforcement and penalties for noncompliance.

ARRA also codified (recognized per statute) the Office of the National Coordinator for Health Information Technology (ONC), which was previously established by an executive order. It now has an expanded role in supporting the implementation of health information technology (HHS 2009a). Practical implications are the creation of an HIT Policy Committee to address technologies to promote electronic health record (EHR) privacy and security, and the establishment of an HIT Standards Committee consisting of members with expertise in healthcare privacy and security. Provisions also include the appointment of a chief privacy officer of the ONC to advise on electronic health information privacy, security, and data stewardship (AHIMA 2009a).

History and Comparison with Existing Laws

Legal protection of the privacy of patient information has historically resided within individual state laws, consequently creating a complex patchwork effect. Some states broadly addressed patient confidentiality, while others protected only specific types of health information, such as HIV/AIDS and behavioral health. Still other states were virtually devoid of patient confidentiality protections. Defined by inconsistency, state laws provided varying degrees of protection. With increasing demand for access to patient information and movement toward electronic billing transactions and an EHR, it was logical that public concern about threats to health information privacy would gain momentum and result in federal legislation directed specifically toward the privacy of patient information.

Several bills designed to create a national law protecting the privacy of patient information were unsuccessfully introduced during the 1990s. Many years ensued before federal legislation was eventually passed by Congress in the form of HIPAA. Further, limited federal laws (discussed below) existed to protect only certain types of health information (for example, drug and alcohol abuse records) or information held only by certain entities (for example, agencies of the federal government). The result of limited and inconsistent federal and state laws was that many types of health information—especially those not deemed to be of a highly sensitive nature—were left unprotected by any statute. Often, the only recourse that individuals had if their confidentiality was breached was through the court system, which is often an expensive, time-consuming, and emotionally exhausting experience with no guaranteed outcome. For example, if an individual lived in a state with statutes that protected only information related to behavioral health and HIV, the only recourse for the wrongful disclosure of that individual's highly personal plastic surgery records from a nonfederal healthcare provider was through the state court system. Under the HIPAA Privacy Rule, however, all types of health information—regardless of their nature—are treated equally. Further, HIPAA violations result in sanctions outside the judicial system. Overall, the Privacy Rule is designed to increase privacy and confidentiality of patient information and to provide a less cumbersome recourse.

Because of the broad impact of the HIPAA Privacy Rule, the privacy of patient information is a priority as individuals and organizations affected by it (that is, covered entities and their business associates, which are described later in this chapter) strive to comply with its requirements. It has also created a number of challenges for the healthcare industry and to health information management (HIM) departments in particular.

The HIPAA Privacy Rule (hereafter referred to as "the Privacy Rule") transformed the landscape of patient information by expanding the breadth of privacy protection and protecting the confidentiality of a widely defined scope of medical and personal information. The following discussion of federal laws in effect prior to the implementation of the Privacy Rule demonstrates their limited application and authority.

Freedom of Information Act of 1967

The underlying purpose of the federal **Freedom of Information Act of 1967** (5 USC 552), commonly referred to as FOIA, is not the privacy of information but, rather, the right of disclosure to and access by the public regarding federal agency records. The rationale for such openness is government accountability to its citizens and, ultimately, its taxpayers. Although the notion of the public's right to inspect the documents, and therefore the work, of its government is compelling, the sensitive and private nature of certain documents rises above the public's right to know. Built into this legislation are exceptions that govern documents such as medical records (if reasons for disclosure do not outweigh the exception), in order to preserve the privacy of the individuals about whom they are written. Application of this law to the healthcare system is relatively narrow because most healthcare organizations are not federal, although one significant exception is the Department of Veterans Affairs through its operation of federal inpatient and outpatient healthcare facilities (Department of Justice 2004).

Privacy Act of 1974

In 1974, a federal law was passed to protect privacy. In part, the **Privacy Act of 1974** (5 USC 552a) "requires federal agencies holding personally identifiable records to safeguard that information and provide individuals with certain privacy rights" (Roth 2004a), such as the right to access and request amendment to their records (Hughes 2003). Although the purpose of the legislation is nondisclosure, as opposed to FOIA's underlying premise of disclosure, this act is also narrow because it only applies to information collected by the federal government (for example, Veterans Affairs facilities); further, it is not tailored to the protection of health information. As a result, its impact on the protection of patient information is extremely limited.

Federal Drug and Alcohol Laws

The Drug Abuse Prevention, Treatment, and Rehabilitation Act of 1972 (42 USC 4541–4594; 42 CFR 2.1–2.67; orig. 21 USC 1101–1800) and the Comprehensive Alcohol Abuse and Alcoholism Prevention, Treatment, and Rehabilitation Act of 1970 are federal statutes that provide specific and highly particularized safeguards for the protection of information relating to the diagnosis, treatment, or referral for treatment of conditions relating to drug abuse or other substance abuse. While these pieces of legislation are more global than the Privacy Act of 1974 (because they apply to all federally assisted alcohol and drug abuse treatment programs—not just federal providers), they nonetheless apply to only a niche population of patients rather than to the protection of patient information generally. These laws will be discussed more extensively in chapter 12.

Medicare Conditions of Participation

The requirements that govern providers receiving Medicare and Medicaid reimbursement include specific safeguards to protect patient information and to allow patients some measure of control over their health information (Roth 2004b). As with the laws discussed above, however, the **Conditions of Participation** regulate only providers and, narrower still, only those receiving funds from the Medicare and Medicaid programs. While this includes a vast number of providers, the Conditions of Participation nonetheless are inapplicable to nonproviders holding confidential patient information and do not apply to patients insured by other payers or those not covered by insurance at all.

State Laws

As noted earlier, laws protecting the privacy of patient information and governing access, use, and disclosure largely resided with individual states and varied considerably, creating a patchwork of laws. While many states passed laws to protect highly sensitive health records such as behavioral health and HIV/AIDS, not all states possessed laws that protected health information generally. With the passage of the Privacy Rule, a minimum amount of protection (that is, a floor) was achieved uniformly across all the states through the establishment of a consistent set of requirements that affected providers, healthcare clearinghouses, and health plans.

Professional Ethical Standards and Codes of Conduct

Ethical standards and codes of conduct governing a variety of healthcare professionals, including health information management (HIM) and informatics professionals, have provided long-standing guidance regarding privacy protection of patient information. In particular, the American Health Information Management Association (AHIMA) *Code of Ethics* states that HIM professionals "preserve, protect, and secure personal health information in any form or medium and hold in the highest regards health information and other information of a confidential nature…" Although the AHIMA *Code of Ethics* does not have the force of law, it nonetheless provides ethical principles that guide the profession and bind individuals who are members of AHIMA and who hold an AHIMA credential (AHIMA 2011).

Check Your Understanding 9.1

Instructions: Indicate whether the following statements are true or false (T or F).

1. The Privacy Rule resides in the administrative simplification provision of Title II of HIPAA.

2. The HITECH Act of ARRA of 2009 made significant changes to the HIPAA Privacy Rule.

3. FOIA was enacted to address the privacy of health information.

4. Drug and alcohol abuse treatment records have received protection under federal law.

5. The Conditions of Participation regulate only providers who receive funds from the Medicare and Medicaid programs.

Applicability

The scope of the HIPAA Privacy Rule is best grasped by identifying the individuals and organizations that are subject to it (who) and the types of information that it protects (what).

The first element, *who*, consists of covered entities and their business associates. The second element, *what*, is protected health information.

Covered Entities and Workforce

The Privacy Rule defines **covered entities** (CEs) as one or more of the following:

- A healthcare provider who transmits any health information pertaining to certain transactions (financial or administrative in nature) in electronic form

- A health plan, which is an individual or group plan that provides or pays the costs of medical care

- A healthcare clearinghouse, an entity that processes billing transactions between a healthcare provider and a health plan (45 CFR 160.103(3))

Each of these categories is broad. Healthcare providers—as providers of medical or health services, or any other person or organization who furnishes, bills, or is paid for healthcare—range from individual practitioners (such as physicians, dentists, and chiropractors) to healthcare organizations (such as pharmacies, hospitals, and long-term care facilities). Additionally, CEs are responsible for their **workforce**, consisting of employees, volunteers, student interns, and trainees (45 CFR 160.103). Not limited to those who receive wages, a workforce encompasses those who work under the direct control of the CE. With this in mind, a CE would be wise to consider as workforce members even those employees of outsourced vendors who routinely work on-site in the CE's facility.

Transactions, referred to in the above paragraph, that are affected by the Privacy Rule are those that relate to:

- Health claims and encounter information

- Health plan enrollment and disenrollment (termination)

- Eligibility for a health plan

- Healthcare payment and remittance advice

- Health plan premium payments

- Health claim status

- Referral certification and authorization

- Coordination of benefits

- First report of injury

- Health claims attachments

- Other transactions as prescribed by the Secretary of HHS (45 CFR 160.103)

Business Associates

A **business associate** (BA) is a person or organization other than a member of a CE's workforce that performs functions or activities on behalf of or affecting a CE that involve the use or disclosure of individually identifiable health information (45 CFR 160.103(1)), which will be discussed later in this chapter. Per HITECH, the BA definition specifically includes patient safety organizations (PSOs), which receive and analyze patient safety issues; health information exchanges (HIEs) and health information organizations (HIOs), which share health information among providers electronically; e-prescribing gateways, which facilitate the prescribing process between physicians and pharmacies; other persons who facilitate data transmissions; and personal health record (PHR) vendors that, by contract, enable CEs to offer PHRs to their patients as part of the CE's EHR (HHS 2010a, 40872). Per HITECH, a BA's subcontractors are BAs under HIPAA if they require access to an individual's protected health information, regardless of whether a business associate agreement has actually been signed (HHS 2010a, 40873).

Once a CE identifies a person or organization as a BA, the CE is obligated to initiate a **business associate agreement** (BAA) to legally protect information handled outside the CE. It is through this written and signed contract that CEs may lawfully disclose protected health information (PHI) to BAs, such as consultants, billing companies, accounting firms, or others that may perform services for the provider. In the BAA, the BA agrees to abide by the provider's requirements to protect the information's security and confidentiality. In other words, the BA must agree not to use or disclose the PHI in ways the provider would not permit and must agree to protect patient information from unauthorized access or disclosure. Under HITECH, a BA's workforce, as with CEs, includes paid and unpaid individuals working under the BA's direct control (HHS 2010a, 40874).

At a minimum, the agreement between a CE and a BA should contain the requirements specified in figure 9.2, reflecting the updated BA requirements instituted by HITECH.

Under HIPAA as originally written, BAs were bound by the law by virtue of their association (via contract) with one or more CEs. HITECH has changed this by directly requiring organizations or individuals meeting the definition of BA to comply with certain provisions of HIPAA, including breach notification and restrictions on the sale of health information, and subjecting them to the same civil and criminal penalties that CEs face for violating the law (AHIMA 2009a). Also applicable to BAs are the administrative, physical, and technical safeguards of the HIPAA security regulations, along with the policies, procedures, and documentation requirements also imposed by the HIPAA security regulations (discussed in chapter 10) (AHIMA 2009a). Additional requirements, as explained throughout the chapter, will be addressed as being applicable to BAs. BAs are now much more vulnerable if they violate HIPAA.

Figure 9.2. BA contract specifics

The requirements placed on business associates under HIPAA and ensuing HITECH legislation have heightened the importance of business associate agreements. Covered entities cannot disclose PHI to business associates unless the two have entered into a written contract that meets HIPAA and HITECH requirements. Under HITECH, privacy, security, and breach notification requirements apply to business associates.

Such a contract would include provisions that:

- Prohibit the business associate from using or disclosing the PHI for any purpose other than that stated in the contract, and pursuant to the Privacy Rule and minimum necessary standard

- Prohibit the business associate from using or disclosing the PHI in a manner that would violate the requirements of the HIPAA Privacy Rule

- Require the business associate to maintain safeguards, as necessary, to ensure that the PHI is not used or disclosed except as provided by the contract

- Require the business associate to report to the covered entity any use or disclosure of the PHI that is not provided for in the contract

- Clarify that the business associate is responsible to report breaches of unsecured PHI

- Clarify that the business associate must adhere to policy and procedure, and documentation requirements imposed by the HIPAA Security Rule

- Establish how the covered entity would provide access to PHI to the individual whom the information is about when the business associate has made any material alterations to the information

- Require the business associate to make available its internal practices, books, and records relating to the use and disclosure of PHI received from the covered entity to the Department of Health and Human Services or its agents

- Establish how the entity would provide access to PHI to the individual whom the information is about in circumstances where the business associate holds the information and the covered entity does not

- Require the business associate to incorporate any amendments or corrections to the PHI when notified by the covered entity that the information is inaccurate or incomplete

- At termination of the contract, require the business associate to return or destroy all PHI received from the covered entity that it still maintains and prohibit the associate from retaining it

- State that individuals who are the subject of disclosed PHI are intended third-party beneficiaries of the contract

- Authorize the covered entity to terminate the contract when it determines that the business associate has repeatedly violated a term required in the contract

- State the business associate is subject to the HIPAA Security Rule, including implementation of administrative, technical and procedural safeguards, and procedural and documentation requirements

- State that the business associate will receive satisfactory assurances from its subcontractors that the subcontractors will appropriately safeguard protected health information

- State that subcontractors of the business associate are responsible for complying with HIPAA, and are directly liable for HIPAA violations, as is the business associate, even if the business associate has not entered into a contractual agreement with the subcontractor

- Clarify that the business associate is responsible to take action, possibly including termination, against a subcontractor if it violates HIPAA or provisions of the BAA

- Clarify that the business associate is subject to civil monetary penalties for violation of the Privacy Rule or the Security Rule

Source: Adapted from Cassidy 2000; updated 2010 per ARRA/HITECH requirements (NPRM 40872–40874).

CEs have historically been required to respond to BA noncompliance, but BAs are now also required (per HITECH) to respond to CE noncompliance by requiring corrective action or severing the relationship with the CE.

Per HITECH, entities meeting the definition of *business associate*, even if they have not entered into a BAA, will be obligated as BAs by definition (HHS 2010a, 40874).

Protected Health Information (PHI)

The Privacy Rule safeguards a category of information called **protected health information** (PHI). To be PHI, it first must be deemed individually identifiable by meeting the first part of a three-part test:

1. It must either identify the person or provide a reasonable basis to believe the person could be identified from the information given (including demographic information).

   It must then meet the second and third parts of a three-part test to be PHI:

2. It must relate to one's past, present, or future physical or mental health condition; the provision of healthcare; or payment for the provision of healthcare.

3. It must be held or transmitted by a CE or its BA in any form or medium, including electronic, paper, and oral forms. (45 CFR 160.103; Amatayakul 2001a).

Figure 9.3 outlines the test for determining whether the information meets the definition of PHI.

Under HITECH, individually identifiable health information of persons deceased for more than 50 years is no longer protected by the Privacy Rule (HHS 2010a, 40874).

Deidentified Information

Key to defining PHI is the first part of the above test, which requires information to either identify an individual or provide a reasonable basis to believe the person could be identified from the information given. This definition does not include deidentified information, which fails the first part of the test and therefore does not receive Privacy Rule protection.

Deidentified information is information from which personal characteristics have been removed and that, as a result, neither identifies nor provides a reasonable basis to believe it could identify an individual. Deidentified information cannot later be constituted or combined to reidentify an individual. Deidentified information is commonly used in research, in decision support, or for similar purposes.

Because of the power of current information technologies in assisting with the collection and analysis of data, it is possible to identify individuals by combining specific data. Therefore, the Privacy Rule requires the CE to do one of the following things to ensure deidentification of information:

- The CE can remove certain elements to ensure that the patient's information is truly deidentified. This is the **Safe Harbor method**. These 18 elements are listed in figure 9.4 (45 CFR 164.514(b)).

- The CE can have an expert apply generally accepted statistical and scientific principles and methods to minimize the risk that the information might be used to identify an individual.

What if the CE needs to reidentify information that has been stripped of individual identifiers? In other words, how might the entity match information back to the person it identifies? The Privacy Rule allows an entity to assign a code to deidentified information to allow for reidentification. However, in doing so, the entity must ensure that the code assigned is not derived from or related to the information about the patient and cannot be translated to his or her identity. It also has to ensure that the code is not used for any other purpose and does not disclose in any way the mechanism for reidentification.

Figure 9.3. Test for determining whether information is PHI

Individually identifiable health information in any form or medium (paper, imaged, electronic, oral) that:

1. Identifies the person or provides a reasonable basis to believe the person could be identified from the information given

AND

2. Relates to one's health condition (physical or mental health; past, present, or future), provision of healthcare, or payment for provision of healthcare

AND

3. Is held or transmitted by a covered entity or (via a business associate agreement) its business associate

Figure 9.4. Data elements to be removed for deidentification of information

The following 18 identifiers pertain not only to the in dividual but also to relatives, employers, and the individual's household members, and they must be removed:

1. Names

2. Geographic subdivisions smaller than a state, including street address, city, county, precinct, and zip code if that geographic unit contains fewer than 20,000 people. The initial three digits of such zip code may be changed to 000, or zip codes with the same three initial digits may be combined to form a unit of more than 20,000 people.

3. All elements of dates, except the year, directly related to an individual, including birth, admission, discharge, and death dates. In addition, all ages over 89 and all elements of dates (including the year) that would identify such age cannot be used. However, individuals over 89 can be aggregated into a single category of 90 or over.

4. Telephone numbers

5. Fax numbers

6. E-mail addresses

7. Social Security numbers

8. Medical record numbers

9. Health plan beneficiary numbers

10. Account numbers

11. Certificate/license numbers

12. Vehicle identifiers and serial numbers, including license plate numbers

13. Device identifiers and serial numbers

14. Web universal resource locators (URLs)

15. Internet protocol (IP) address numbers

16. Biometric identifiers, including fingerprints and voice prints

17. Full-face photographic images and any comparable images

18. Any other unique identification number, characteristic, or code, except for permissible reidentification

Source: 45 CFR 164.514(b) (2) (i).

Check Your Understanding 9.2

Instructions: Indicate whether the following statements are true or false (T or F).

1. A CE need only consider its employees when evaluating HIPAA compliance within the organization.

2. The HITECH Act has strengthened BA Privacy Rule compliance requirements.

3. In part, information must be individually identifiable to meet the definition of PHI.

4. Deidentified information receives Privacy Rule protections.

5. A BA is anyone who might have access to a CE's PHI.

Additional Privacy Rule Elements

In addition to understanding who and what the HIPAA Privacy Rule applies to, it is also important to understand additional terms of art that further explain the rule's applicability.

Individuals

The Privacy Rule refers to *individuals* as opposed to *patients* or *clients*. As defined by the Privacy Rule, an individual is the person who is the subject of the PHI (45 CFR 160.103).

Personal Representatives

The Privacy Rule also addresses **personal representatives** (45 CFR 164.502(g)) by clarifying that persons with legal authority to act on behalf of another adult, an emancipated minor, an unemancipated minor, or a deceased individual shall be treated as a personal representative under the Privacy Rule. Under the Privacy Rule, a personal representative must be treated the same as the individual regarding the use and disclosure of the individual's PHI. Although parents are generally the personal representatives of their minor children, with legal authority to exercise all the individual rights in the Privacy Rule (including access to the minor's record), parents, guardians, or others acting *in loco parentis* of a minor are not treated as personal representatives if the minor has consented to his or her own treatment. Personal representative rights may be denied if one is suspected of abusing or neglecting the individual and granting rights could endanger the individual.

Designated Record Set

The Privacy Rule (45 CFR 164.524 and 45 CFR 164.526) allows individuals to inspect, obtain a copy of, and amend information in their designated record set, including information that exists in paper, imaged, and electronic form.

A **designated record set** (DRS) is defined (45 CFR 164.501) as a group of records maintained by or for a CE that is:

- The medical records and billing records about individuals maintained by or for a covered healthcare provider

- The enrollment, payment, claims adjudication, and case or medical management record systems maintained by or for a health plan

- Used in whole or in part by or for the CE to make decisions about individuals

The preamble of the Privacy Rule states that a CE is to provide access to PHI in accordance with the rule regardless of whether the CE created the information. Further, shadow records—maintained apart from the official, or central, medical record—should be considered part of the DRS if they are retained (which they most likely are) for purposes of making decisions about an individual (HHS 2000; Amatayakul 2001b).

Because of their relationship with CEs, BAs will often hold records that meet the DRS definition. According to the preamble of the December 28, 2000, final rule, records held by a BA that meet the definition of DRS are part of the CE's DRS. According to the Privacy Rule preamble, when CEs incorporate PHI in a variety of data systems (for example, quality control and peer review analyses), not all of which will be used to make decisions about individuals, such systems are not considered part of the DRS (HHS 2000; Hughes 2003). Some state statutes additionally protect these records from discovery.

The Privacy Rule limits certain patient rights to the DRS only. This relieves organizations from retrieving information from a variety of sources (for example, telephone message pads, surgery schedules, appointment logs, and databases) where an individual's health information resides but is not used to make care or payment decisions about that person (Hughes 2003).

Figure 9.5 provides a comparison between the DRS and the legal health record, which was discussed in the previous chapter.

Disclosure, Use, and Request

With the twin goals of giving individuals greater control over their PHI and restricting access by others, the Privacy Rule affects three types of situations in which PHI is handled: disclosure, use, and request. **Disclosure** of PHI is the act of making information known, or the release or dissemination of confidential information about an identifiable person by a CE or a BA to another entity or person. While disclosure is often emphasized, the Privacy Rule is equally concerned with the appropriate degree of **use**, which is the sharing, employment, application, utilization, examination, or analysis of individually identifiable health information within an entity that maintains such information. CEs must also comply with the Privacy Rule when they request PHI. A **request** for PHI is made by a CE or its BA. Of the three, the Privacy Rule emphasizes disclosure and use.

Treatment, Payment, and Operations

Treatment, payment, and operations (45 CFR 164.501), collectively and hereafter referred to as TPO, are functions of a CE that are necessary for the CE to successfully conduct business. It is not the intent of the Privacy Rule to impose onerous rules that hinder a CE's functions. Thus, some of the Privacy Rule's requirements are relaxed or removed where PHI is needed for purposes of TPO.

Treatment usually means providing, coordinating, or managing healthcare or healthcare-related services by one or more healthcare providers (for example, the usual provision of care to patients admitted to the hospital or during an office appointment with a physician). Treatment in the Privacy Rule definition also covers healthcare provider consultations relating to a patient or the referral of a patient for healthcare from one provider to another.

Payment includes a broad set of activities. For example, it can refer to activities by a health plan to obtain premiums or to activities by a healthcare provider or health plan to obtain reimbursement for care or services provided. Billing, claims management, claims collection, review of the medical necessity of care, and utilization review are all included under payment.

The Privacy Rule provides a broad list of activities that fall under the umbrella of healthcare operations: quality assessment and improvement, case management, review of healthcare professionals' qualifications, insurance contracting, legal and auditing functions, and general business management functions such as providing customer service and conducting due diligence. It is important to distinguish activities that are operations from those that are not and to include examples of operations in the Notice of Privacy Practices, discussed later in this chapter.

Figure 9.5. Comparison of the designated record set and legal health record

Designated Record Set versus the Legal Health Record		
This side-by-side comparison of the designated record set and the legal health record demonstrates the differences between the two sets of information, as well as their purposes.		
	Designated Record Set	**Legal Health Record**
Definition	A group of records maintained by or for a covered entity that is the medical and billing records about individuals; enrollment, payment, claims adjudication, and case or medical management record systems maintained by or for a health plan; information used in whole or in part by or for the HIPAA covered entity to make decisions about individuals.	The business record generated at or for a healthcare organization. It is the record that would be released upon receipt of a request. The legal health record is the officially declared record of healthcare services provided to an individual delivered by a provider.
Purpose	Used to clarify the access and amendment standards in the HIPAA Privacy Rule, which provide that individuals generally have the right to inspect and obtain a copy of protected health information in the designated record set.	The official business record of healthcare services delivered by the entity for regulatory and disclosure purposes.
Content	Defined in organizational policy and required by the HIPAA Privacy Rule. The content of the designated record set includes medical and billing records of covered providers; enrollment, payment, claims, and case information of a health plan; and information used in whole or in part by or for the covered entity to make decisions about individuals.	Defined in organizational policy and can include individually identifiable data in any medium collected and directly used in documenting healthcare services or health status. It excludes administrative, derived, and aggregate data.
Uses	Supports individual HIPAA right of access and amendment.	Provides a record of health status as well as documentation of care for reimbursement, quality management, research, and public health purposes; facilitates business decision making and education of healthcare practitioners as well as the legal needs of the healthcare organization.

Source: Dougherty and Washington 2008.

Health Information in Personnel and Educational Records

Although a person or organization may be subject to the Privacy Rule, not all information that the person or organization holds or comes into contact with is protected by the Privacy Rule. For example, the Privacy Rule specifically excludes employment records held by the CE in its capacity as employer (45 CFR 160.103). Under this exclusion, employee physical examination reports contained within personnel files are specifically exempted from the rule. Educational records covered by the Federal Educational Records Privacy Act (FERPA), 20 USC 1232(g), are also excluded from the Privacy Rule's definition of PHI.

Organization Types

Covered entity is a term of art under the Privacy Rule and generally encompasses the neatly defined categories of healthcare providers, health plans, and healthcare clearinghouses. However, these categories are neither mutually exclusive nor all-inclusive. For example, an organization may function as a CE in one aspect of its business but not in another. Further, an organization may function as more than one type of CE. Specific examples are explored below.

A **hybrid entity** (45 CFR 164.103) performs both covered and noncovered functions under the Privacy Rule (HHS 2003). For example, a university that educates students and maintains student educational records is not covered by the Privacy Rule; however, the same university, in its operation of a medical center, is covered by the Privacy Rule as a healthcare provider.

The term *affiliated covered entity (CE)* (45 CFR 164.105) refers to legally separate CEs affiliated by common ownership or control. For purposes of the Privacy Rule, these legally separate entities may refer to themselves as a single CE. Such references must be in writing (HHS 2003).

An **organized healthcare arrangement** (45 CFR 164.103) is characterized by two or more CEs who share PHI to manage and benefit their common enterprise and are recognized by the public as a single entity (HHS 2003).

CEs may perform multiple covered functions (45 CFR 164.504(g)). They must operate each covered function separately and must not disclose PHI to a function not involved with the individual, remaining compliant with the Privacy Rule relative to each function they perform (HHS 2003). For example, a medical facility may also be a self-insured health plan. If an employee of the medical facility is a patient but not an enrollee of the health plan, that individual's PHI may only be used by the medical facility in its capacity as a healthcare provider and may not be shared with the health plan.

Check Your Understanding 9.3

Instructions: Indicate whether the following statements are true or false (T or F).

1. Under the Privacy Rule, a personal representative must be treated the same as the individual regarding the use and disclosure of the individual's PHI.

2. By definition, a DRS includes billing records.

3. A hospital employee's pre-employment physical examination is in his personnel file in Human Resources; this report is PHI.

4. A university with a medical center is a hybrid entity under the Privacy Rule.

5. Some of the Privacy Rule's requirements are relaxed or removed where PHI is needed for purposes of TPO.

Section 2: Core Privacy Rule Documents and the Minimum Necessary Requirement

Key Privacy Rule Documents

The Privacy Rule contains parameters for three key documents that serve to inform patients and give them a measure of control over their PHI. Two of these documents, the Notice of Privacy Practices and the authorization, are required, but the consent document is optional. Table 9.1 outlines differences among these three key documents.

Notice of Privacy Practices

It is important that patients have some control over—or at least knowledge of—the disclosures and uses of their health information. Ensuring that patients have knowledge about their PHI is a key purpose of the Notice of Privacy Practices.

Table 9.1. Notice of privacy practices, consent, and authorization requirements

	Notice of Privacy Practices	Consent	Authorization
Required?	Required by HIPAA	Optional	Required by HIPAA
Requirements re: TPO	Must explain TPO uses and disclosures, along with other types of uses and disclosures	Obtains patient permission to use or disclose PHI for TPO purposes only	Is used to obtain for a number of types of uses and disclosures, although is not required for TPO uses and disclosures
PHI that this document addresses	Provides prospective and general information about how PHI might be used or disclosed in the future (and includes information that may not have been created yet)	Provides prospective and general information about how PHI might be used or disclosed in the future for TPO purposes (and includes information that may not have been created yet)	Obtains patient permission to use or disclose specific information that generally has already been created and for which there is a specific need
Required for treatment?	May not refuse to treat an individual because he or she declines to sign this form	May condition treatment on individual signing this form	May not refuse to treat an individual because he or she declines to sign this form
Time limit on document validity	No time limit on validity of the document	No time limit on validity of the document	Time limit on validity of document (specified by an expiration date or event)

The Privacy Rule introduced the standard that individuals should be informed of how CEs use or disclose PHI. In general, section 164.520 of the Privacy Rule requires that, except for certain variations or exceptions for health plans and correctional facilities, an individual has the right to a notice explaining how PHI will be used and disclosed. This required document is called a **Notice of Privacy Practices** (NPP) or Notice of Health Information Practices. Further, this notice explains an individual's rights and the CE's legal duties with respect to PHI. The notice must be provided to an individual at his or her first contact with the CE (for example, first visit to a physician's office, first admission to a hospital, or first encounter at a clinic).

Hughes (2001a) outlines the requirements for the content of the notice as specified in 45 CFR 164.520. (See figure 9.6, which has been updated to reflect HITECH.) A sample NPP is located at the end of this chapter (appendix 9.A). Other models may be found on various websites, including:

- The AHIMA website (http://www.ahima.org)

- The American Hospital Association website (http://www.aha.org)

- The American Medical Association website (http://www.ama-assn.org)

Providers can also check the websites of their specific specialty group for information and sample notices.

Healthcare providers with a direct treatment relationship with an individual must provide the notice no later than the date of the first personal service encounter. Where services are provided by telephone, prompt mailing of the notice is required. Where services are provided electronically, automatic and simultaneous delivery of the notice is required. This requirement reminds CEs that the Privacy Rule recognizes more than just face-to-face visits as service encounters. Indeed, encounters such as telephone consultations and electronic prescribing may also necessitate a notice. Notices must be available at the site where the individual is treated and must be posted in a prominent place where the patient can reasonably be expected to read it. If a CE has a website with information about services or benefits, the notice must be prominently posted to it. In emergency situations, a CE must provide notice to the individual as soon as possible after the emergency has ended. In addition, notices must be provided to those individuals who request a copy. Finally, good-faith attempts must be made to obtain a written acknowledgment from the patient stating that the notice was received. Failure to obtain the acknowledgment, whether it is due to patient refusal or noncompliance or failure by the covered healthcare provider, must be documented (HHS 2003).

Consent to Use or Disclose PHI

Under the Privacy Rule, healthcare providers are not required to obtain the patient's **consent** to use or disclose personally identifiable information for TPO (45 CFR 164.506(b)). However, some providers may choose to obtain consent as a matter of policy. In such cases (except for the special circumstances discussed below), consent would be obtained at the time that healthcare services are provided. Because the consent for use and disclosure has no expiration date, in most cases it is indefinite unless specifically revoked by the individual. Further, consent cannot be used where an authorization would otherwise be required under the Privacy Rule.

Certain specifications should be followed with regard to content and language in the consent for use and disclosure of information. The consent should:

- Be expressed in plain language so that the individual can understand its content

- Inform the individual that the PHI may be used and disclosed to carry out TPO

- Refer the individual to the CE's NPP for a more complete description of the uses and disclosures and state that the individual has the right to review the notice before signing the consent

- State that the terms of the notice may change and describe how the individual may obtain a revised notice if the CE has reserved the right to change its privacy practices

- State that the individual has the right to request that the CE restrict how PHI is used or disclosed to carry out TPO (Note: The CE is not required to agree to the requested restrictions.)

- State that the restrictions are binding on the CE when it agrees to the requested restrictions

- State that the individual has the right to revoke the consent in writing, except to the extent that the CE has already taken action based on the consent. As mentioned above, an individual may revoke consent at any time. However, the revocation must be in writing, and the CE must document and retain any signed consent as well as any revocation.

- Be signed and dated by the individual

Several situations exist in which obtaining consent may be difficult or impossible. One would be an emergency treatment situation where there are substantial barriers to communicating with the individual. Another example would be when the healthcare provider is required by law to treat the individual but is unable to obtain consent. In such circumstances, the provider should document its attempt to obtain consent and the reason it was unable to do so. In emergency treatment situations, the provider should obtain consent as soon as reasonably possible after the delivery of treatment. A sample consent form is located at the end of this chapter (appendix 9.B).

Authorization

The Privacy Rule is specific about disclosures that require a patient's **authorization** and those that do not (45 CFR 164.502, 45 CFR 164.508, 45 CFR 164.510, 45 CFR 164.512). The following general rule provides a starting point to the Privacy Rule's intricate authorization requirements and exceptions:

Figure 9.6. Requirements for the content of the NPP

- A header that reads: "This notice describes how medical information about you may be used and disclosed and how you can get access to this information. Please review it carefully."
- A description (including at least one example) of the types of uses and disclosures the covered entity is permitted to make for treatment, payment, and healthcare operations
- A description of each of the other purposes for which the covered entity is permitted or required to use or disclose PHI without the individual's written authorization
- A statement describing uses and disclosures that require an authorization, providing that other uses and disclosures will be made only with the individual's written authorization, and that the individual may revoke such authorization
- A statement that most uses or disclosures of psychotherapy notes for marketing purposes require an authorization
- When applicable, separate statements indicating that the covered entity may contact the individual to provide appointment reminders or information about treatment alternatives or other health-related benefits and services that may be of interest to the individual; that the covered entity may raise funds; and that the group health plan or health insurance issuer or HMO may disclose protected health information to the sponsor of the plan (per the NPRM, it is suggested that the above statements be modified to align with the following two provisions)
- A statement that most treatment communications, where the covered entity receives financial remuneration in exchange, require the individual's advance notification and the opportunity to opt out
- A statement that (if intended) the covered entity may contact the individual to raise funds for the entity and the opportunity to opt out.
- A statement of the individual's rights with respect to PHI and a brief description of how the individual may exercise these rights, including:

  —The right to request restrictions on certain uses and disclosures as provided by 45 CFR 164.522(a), including a statement that the covered entity is not required to agree to a requested restriction unless the disclosure would be made to a health plan for payment or operations purposes (and not for treatment) and the individual has paid for the healthcare service or item completely out of pocket

  —The right to receive confidential communications of PHI as detailed in 45 CFR 164.522(b), as applicable

  —The right to inspect and copy PHI as detailed in 45 CFR 164.524

  —The right to amend PHI as detailed in 45 CFR 164.526

  —The right to receive an accounting of disclosures as detailed in 45 CFR 164.528

  —The right to obtain a paper copy of the notice upon request as detailed in 45 CFR 164.520
- A statement that the covered entity is required by law to maintain the privacy of PHI and to provide individuals with a notice of its legal duties and privacy practices with respect to PHI
- A statement that the covered entity is obligated to abide by breach notification requirements, including notification to affected individuals, the media (where applicable), and the Secretary of HHS (inclusion of a required statement in the Notice of Privacy Practices is pending per NPRM)
- A statement that the covered entity is required to abide by the terms of the notice currently in effect
- A statement that the covered entity reserves the right to change the terms of its notice and to make the new notice provisions effective for all PHI that it maintains
- A statement describing how the covered entity will provide individuals with a revised notice
- A statement that individuals may complain to the covered entity and the secretary of the Department of Health and Human Services when they believe their privacy rights have been violated, a brief description of how to file a complaint with the covered entity, and a statement that there will be no retaliation for filing a complaint
- The name or title and telephone number of a person or office to contact for further information
- An effective date, which may not be earlier than the date on which the notice is published.

Source: 45 CFR 164.520; Hughes 2001a. Updated 2010 per ARRA/HITECH requirements (NPRM 40897–40898).

General rule: Patient authorization is required for the use or disclosure of PHI unless it meets an exception where authorization is not required.

Stated another way, except for the purposes and circumstances specifically mentioned in the Privacy Rule that do not require an authorization for use or disclosure (which are outlined later in this chapter and listed in figure 9.7), all other uses and disclosures require an individual's authorization. Because PHI may be requested for medical, legal, personal, and myriad other purposes, CEs must be familiar with the Privacy Rule so that each type of disclosure and use can be sorted out to determine whether an authorization is required, how much information can be used or disclosed (to be discussed in the "Minimum Necessary Requirement" section later in this chapter), and how to handle each type of situation appropriately. CEs must consider not only the authorization requirements of the HIPAA Privacy Rule but also the authorization requirements that govern use and disclosure in the CE's particular state (see chapter 12).

Required Elements

The Privacy Rule provides specific requirements for patient authorization forms, including elements an authorization for release of information (disclosure) must contain. While these required core elements do not differ significantly from the elements historically recommended by AHIMA as professional best

Figure 9.7. Authorization requirements for use and disclosure of PHI

I. Patient Authorization Required:

All situations except those listed in Part II

II. Patient Authorization Not Required:

A. When use or disclosure is *required*, even without patient authorization

- When the individual or the individual's personal representative requests access or accounting of disclosures (with exceptions)
- Dept. of HHS investigation, review, or enforcement action

B. When use or disclosure is *permitted*, even without patient authorization

- Patient has opportunity to informally agree or object
  —facility directory
  —notification of relatives and friends
- Patient does not have opportunity to agree or object
  —Public interest and benefit (12 types)
    1. As required by law
    2. For public health activities
    3. To disclose PHI regarding victims of abuse, neglect, or domestic violence
    4. For health oversight activities
    5. For judicial and administrative proceedings
    6. For law enforcement purposes (six specific situations)
    7. Regarding decedents
    8. For cadaveric organ, eye, or tissue donation
    9. For research, with limitations
    10. To prevent or lessen serious threat to health or safety
    11. For essential government functions
    12. For workers' compensation
  —TPO
  —To the individual/patient
  —Incidental disclosures
  —Limited data set

---

practice, they now have the force and effect of federal law. Under the Privacy Rule, a valid authorization must be written in plain language and contain at least the elements listed in figure 9.8. A sample authorization form is located at the end of this chapter (appendix 9.C).

An authorization is considered invalid (defective) when any one of the following occurs (45 CFR 164.508(b)(2–4)):

- The expiration date has passed or the expiration event is known by the CE to have occurred.

- The authorization has not been filled out completely with respect to a required element or lacks a required element.

- The authorization is known by the CE to have been revoked.

- The authorization violates the compound authorization requirements, if applicable. (A compound authorization combines an individual's authorization for the disclosure of health information with informed consent for the performance of medical treatment.)

- Any material information in the authorization is known by the CE to be false.

- Completion of an authorization is required for an individual to be eligible for treatment, payment, or enrollment in a health plan, or to be eligible for benefits on an authorization (with certain exceptions to this rule delineated in 45 CFR 164.508(b)(4)).

Because of their unique nature, HIPAA specifically addresses psychotherapy notes. **Psychotherapy notes** are behavioral health notes recorded by a mental health professional who documents or analyzes contents and impressions of conversations that are part of private counseling sessions. Psychotherapy notes are not part of the health record and do not contain information such as diagnoses, prescriptions, treatment modalities, or test results (45 CFR 164.501). Authorizations are always required for the use or disclosure of psychotherapy notes except to carry out TPO or to fulfill one of the following purposes (45 CFR 164.508(a)(2)):

- Use by the originator of the psychotherapy notes for treatment

- Use or disclosure by the CE in training programs for students, trainees, or practitioners in mental health

- Use or disclosure by the CE to defend a legal action or other proceeding brought by the individual

- Use or disclosure that is required or permitted with respect to the oversight of the originator of the psychotherapy notes

When Authorization Is Required

One of the Privacy Rule's goals is to provide greater privacy protections for one's health information by limiting access by others. This includes both use and disclosure. As figure 9.7 shows, PHI may not be used or disclosed by a CE unless:

1. The individual who is the subject of the information authorizes the use or disclosure in writing; or

2. The Privacy Rule *requires or permits* such use or disclosure without the individual's authorization.

The Privacy Rule *requires* use or disclosure in only two situations:

1. When the individual or the individual's personal representative requests access to PHI or an accounting of disclosures of the PHI; and

2. When the HHS conducts an investigation, review, or enforcement action.

Figure 9.8. Privacy Rule requirements for a valid authorization

Description of Information

This description must identify the information to be used or disclosed in a specific and meaningful fashion. For example, the request should specify what is wanted, such as "the discharge summary and the operative report," rather than asking for "any and all information." Providing the time frame for the information that is to be released (for example, hospitalization from 6/1/08 to 6/5/08) also provides a more specific description of the desired information.

Name of Person or Entity Authorized to Use or Disclose

The authorization must include the name or other specific identification of the person(s) or class of persons authorized to use or disclose the information. For example, the name of a hospital that is disclosing a patient's health information must be included.

Recipient of Information

The Privacy Rule requires that the authorization include the specific person(s) or class of persons (by name or other specific identification) to whom the covered entity may make the disclosure, such as an insurance company. This information should be verified by checking the patient demographic information that is collected on admission. If the insurance company information does not match, the patient should be contacted for clarification.

Purpose of Disclosure

Although the Privacy Rule requires that this element be present on authorizations, the patient is not required to provide a statement of purpose, and "at the request of the individual" is sufficient per the Privacy Rule.

Expiration

The Privacy Rule requires that an expiration date or expiration event (for example, "at the end of the research study" or "none") that relates to the individual or the purpose of the use or disclosure be included on the authorization.

Signature and Date

The patient must sign and date the authorization. It is essential that the signature be compared with one already existing in the medical record for validation purposes. A patient's personal representative may sign the authorization in lieu of the patient provided that a statement is included that describes that person's authority to act for the patient.

Although it is best practice for an authorization to be completed and dated after the date of the service (so that information is not created after the authorization was signed), the Privacy Rule does not prohibit predated authorizations as long as the authorization encompasses the category of information that is later created and the authorization has not expired or been revoked. In summation, "the covered entity may use or disclose PHI that has been identified in the authorization regardless of when the information was created" (HHS 2007).

Statement of Right to Revoke

An authorization must contain a statement of the individual's right to revoke the authorization in writing and the exceptions to the right to revoke, together with a description of how the individual may revoke it.

Statement of Redisclosure

An authorization must include a statement that information used or disclosed pursuant to the authorization may be subject to redisclosure by the recipient and, subsequently, would no longer be protected by the Privacy Rule.

Statement of Eligibility

A statement in the authorization must specify that treatment, payment, enrollment, or eligibility for benefits cannot be denied because an individual declines to sign the authorization.

Copy Provided

A copy of the signed authorization is provided to the individual when authorization for use or disclosure is sought by the covered entity.

Source: Adapted from 45 CFR 164.508(c)(1–4).

When Authorization Is Not Required

In addition to the two situations where use or disclosure is *required* without the individual's authorization (see also figure 9.7), there are many situations where the Privacy Rule *permits* a CE to use or disclose PHI without an individual's authorization (HHS 2003). These situations are listed in figure 9.7. This significant number of exceptions to the patient authorization requirement leads critics to argue that the Privacy Rule diminishes the privacy of patient information rather than improving it. However, the Privacy Rule is only *permissive* in this respect. Its exceptions may be subject to stricter state laws or organizational policies that provide greater privacy protections. In other words, CEs may be required by state law or may choose to require patient authorization even if the Privacy Rule permits use or disclosure without it.

Two examples below illustrate the HIPAA Privacy Rule's relaxation of the authorization requirement, although many CEs continue to adhere to their more stringent pre-HIPAA practices.

Example 1: A hospital (CE), under the Privacy Rule, is not required to obtain a patient's authorization before sending records from the patient's hospital stay to a physician who is following up with that patient (treatment purposes). While many hospitals, in accordance with prior policy, will continue to require an authorization in a situation such as this, the Privacy Rule has removed that requirement. Note: The minimum necessary requirement (discussed later in this chapter) does not apply when PHI is disclosed for treatment purposes, although CEs should exercise caution.

Example 2: A healthcare provider (CE), under the Privacy Rule, is not required to obtain a patient's authorization before sending records from a patient's visit to the patient's health insurance company for payment purposes. Again, many providers will continue to require an authorization in accordance with their prior policies; however, it is not required per the Privacy Rule. The minimum necessary requirement does apply to disclosures made for payment purposes.

Uses and Disclosures that Require an Opportunity for the Individual to Agree or Object

Section 45 CFR 164.510 of the Privacy Rule lists two circumstances in which PHI can be used without the individual's written authorization, but where the individual must be informed in advance and given an opportunity to agree, prohibit (object to), or restrict the use or disclosure. These are illustrated in figure 9.7. The CE may inform the individual in a verbal communication and obtain his or her verbal agreement or objection rather than obtaining a written authorization. First, a healthcare facility may maintain a **facility directory** of patients being treated. Once the individual has agreed, the Privacy Rule permits the facility to maintain in its directory the following information about an individual: name, location in the facility, condition described in general terms, and religious affiliation. This information may be disclosed to persons who ask for the individual by name, with the exception of an individual's religious affiliation, which can be disclosed only to clergy members of the individual's religion. The CE must inform the patient of the information to be included in the directory and the people to whom the information may be disclosed. The individual must be given the opportunity to restrict or prohibit some or all of the uses or disclosures.

In an emergency situation, if it is impractical or impossible to inform the patient and obtain agreement, the facility can use and disclose PHI, but it must be consistent with the prior expressed preference of the patient, or the facility must determine that it is in the patient's best interest to do so. When it becomes possible after the emergency, the healthcare facility must inform patients and give them the opportunity to object to such use and disclosure.

Second, the Privacy Rule allows a CE, exercising its professional judgment, to disclose to a family member or a close friend PHI that is directly relevant to his or her involvement with the individual's care or payment if the individual is not present. This includes allowing a person acting on behalf of the individual to pick up prescriptions and medical supplies. Likewise, a CE may disclose PHI, including the individual's location, general condition, or death, to notify or assist in the notification of a family member, personal representative, or some other person responsible for the patient's care (45 CFR 164.510(b)).

However, if the individual is present and otherwise able to make healthcare decisions, the CE may only use or disclose the PHI in the above situations if it has done one of the following:

- Obtained the individual's agreement

- Provided the individual with the opportunity to object to the disclosure and the patient has not objected

- Reasonably inferred from the circumstances that the individual does not object to the disclosure

The CE may also use or disclose PHI to a public or private entity authorized by law or by its charter to assist in disaster relief efforts.

Uses and Disclosures for Which Authorization or Opportunity to Agree or Object Is Not Required

There are 16 circumstances (see figure 9.7) in which PHI can be used or disclosed without the individual's written authorization and for which the individual does not have the opportunity to agree or object. Section 45 CFR 164.512 of the Privacy Rule, titled "Uses and disclosures for which an authorization or opportunity to agree or object is not required," lists the first 12 circumstances (public interest and benefit activities), which have been identified as activities that serve national priority purposes (see figure 9.7). There are four remaining uses and disclosures for which authorization and the opportunity to agree or object are not required (the four bulleted items at the bottom of figure 9.7); however, they are not listed in section 164.512 of the Privacy Rule. They are TPO, disclosure to the subject individual, incidental disclosures, and limited data sets (discussed later).

In addition to the 12 public interest and benefit exceptions, Figure 9.7 also lists those situations where use and disclosure are *required*, even without patient authorization.

The Privacy Rule *permits* uses and disclosures without an individual's authorization in the 12 public interest and benefit circumstances; however, if such a use or authorization would violate a state law that otherwise protects the information more (that is, it is "more stringent") than the Privacy Rule, then the information cannot be legally used or disclosed.

Oftentimes, a disclosure may meet more than one of the following 12 public interest and benefit situations, as outlined in the Privacy Rule (45 CFR 164.512):

1. **As required by law:** Disclosures are permitted when required by laws that meet the public interest requirements of disclosures relating to victims of abuse, neglect, or domestic violence; judicial and administrative proceedings; and law enforcement purposes. These three areas are detailed more fully below.

2. **Public health activities:** Use or disclosure of PHI for public health activities serves such purposes as preventing or controlling diseases, injuries, and disabilities; reporting disease, injury (such as child abuse), and vital events such as births and deaths; and public health surveillance, investigation, or interventions.

   Examples include the reporting of adverse events or product defects in order to comply with Food and Drug Administration regulations and, when authorized by law, reporting a person who may have been exposed to a communicable disease and might be at risk for contracting or spreading it. Per HITECH, disclosure of student immunization records also constitutes a public health activity.

3. **Victims of abuse, neglect, or domestic violence:** An example is the reporting of a situation to authorities, such as Adult Protective Services, who are authorized by law to receive information about abuse or neglect. (Note: Child abuse reporting is contained within public health activities above.)

Although disclosures for the purpose of reporting abuse, neglect, or domestic violence do not require an authorization, the Privacy Rule does require the CE to promptly inform the individual that such a report has been or will be made unless it believes that doing so would place the individual at risk of serious harm if the CE would be informing the personal representative, whom it reasonably believes is responsible for the abuse, neglect, or other injury.

4. **Healthcare oversight activities:** An authorized health oversight agency may receive PHI under the Privacy Rule for activities authorized by law, such as audits, civil or criminal investigations, licensure, and other inspections.

5. **Judicial and administrative proceedings:** Disclosures for judicial and administrative proceedings are permitted in response to an order of a court or an administrative tribunal, provided that the CE discloses only the PHI expressly authorized by such an order or in response to a subpoena, discovery request, or other lawful process. With regard to subpoenas and discovery requests, the party seeking the PHI must assure the CE that it has made reasonable efforts to make the request known to the individual who is the subject of the PHI. In this situation, the entity must also be assured that the time for the individual to raise objections to the court or administrative tribunal has elapsed and that no objections were filed, all objections have been resolved, or a qualified protective order has been secured.

6. **Law enforcement purposes:** Are disclosures of PHI to law enforcement officers allowable? The Privacy Rule specifies six instances in which disclosures to law enforcement do not require patient authorization or the opportunity to agree or object:

   a. Pursuant to legal process or otherwise required by law. Examples of legal process include a court order, court-ordered warrant, subpoena, or summons issued by a judicial officer. Relative to the "as required by law" situation, for example, a law may exist that requires the reporting of certain types of wounds or other physical injuries to law enforcement.

   b. In response to a law enforcement official's request for the purpose of identifying or locating a suspect, fugitive, material witness, or missing person. In such cases, only the following information may be disclosed:

      — Name and address
      — Date and place of birth
      — Social Security number
      — ABO blood type and Rh factor
      — Type of injury
      — Date and time of treatment
      — Date and time of death, if applicable
      — Description of distinguishing physical characteristics, including height, weight, gender, race, hair and eye color, and presence or absence of facial scars or tattoos

   c. In response to a law enforcement official's request about an individual who is or is suspected to be a victim of a crime (when the individual agrees to the disclosure or when the CE is unable to obtain the individual's agreement because of incapacity or other emergency circumstance). The law enforcement official must represent that such information is needed to determine whether a violation of law has occurred, that immediate law enforcement activity depends on the disclosure, and that disclosure is in the best interest of the individual as determined by the CE.

   d. About a deceased individual when the CE suspects that the death may have resulted from criminal conduct.

e. To a law enforcement official when the CE believes in good faith that the information constitutes evidence of criminal conduct that occurred on the CE's premises.

f. To a law enforcement official in response to a medical emergency when the CE believes that disclosure is necessary to alert law enforcement to the commission and nature of a crime; the location or victims of such a crime; and the identity, description, and location of the perpetrator of such a crime. Further, it is permitted when the CE believes the medical emergency was the result of abuse, neglect, or domestic violence.

Again, the Privacy Rule is permissive in this respect, and state law can prohibit or restrict such use or disclosure.

7. **Decedents:** HIPAA's privacy protections survive an individual's death for 50 years; nonetheless, disclosures to a coroner or medical examiner are permitted in order to identify a deceased person, determine a cause of death, or accomplish other purposes as required by law.

In accordance with applicable law, disclosures to funeral directors are permitted as necessary to allow them to carry out their duties with respect to the decedent. This type of information may also be disclosed in reasonable anticipation of an individual's death.

8. **Cadaveric organ, eye, or tissue donation:** PHI may be disclosed to organ procurement agencies or other entities to facilitate the procurement, banking, or transplantation of cadaveric organs, eyes, or tissue.

9. **Research:** The Privacy Rule permits a CE to use or disclose PHI for research if an approved authorization waiver or alteration or other exceptions are met. Research is described more fully later in this chapter.

10. **Threat to health and safety:** Disclosures are allowed under circumstances where the CE believes the use or disclosure of information is necessary to prevent or lessen a serious and imminent threat to the health or safety of an individual or the public. In such cases, disclosure must be made to a person who can reasonably prevent or lessen the threat. Disclosures are also permissible when it is necessary for law enforcement officials to apprehend an individual who may have caused harm to the victim or when it appears that the individual has escaped from a correctional institution or lawful custody.

11. **Essential (specialized) government functions:** There are a number of instances with regard to specialized government functions where uses and disclosures are permitted without authorization or the opportunity to agree or object. Primarily, these include circumstances involving release of information regarding armed forces personnel for military and veterans activities, for purposes of national security and intelligence activities, for protective services for the president of the United States and others, and for public benefits and medical suitability determinations.

Disclosure of an inmate's PHI to correctional institutions or to a law enforcement official who has lawful custody is permitted by the Privacy Rule provided that the correctional institution states that the information is necessary to provide continuing healthcare; to secure the health and safety of the individual or other inmates, officers, employees, transportation personnel, or law enforcement on the premises; or to ensure the administration and maintenance of the institution's safety, security, and good order.

12. **Workers' compensation:** The Privacy Rule permits the disclosure of PHI relating to work-related illness or injury, or workplace-related medical surveillance to the extent such disclosure complies with workers' compensation laws.

In addition to the 12 public interest and benefit situations, specifically categorized in the Privacy Rule as "uses and disclosures for which authorization or opportunity to agree or object is not required," the following four types of uses and disclosures also do not require patient authorization or an opportunity for the patient to agree or object (see the four bulleted items at the bottom of figure 9.7); however, they have not been categorized as such in the Privacy Rule. They are:

1. TPO

2. Disclosure to the subject individual/patient

3. Incidental disclosures

4. Limited data set

The first two have been discussed at length in this chapter; the latter two will be examined here.

Incidental uses or disclosures occur as part of a permitted use or disclosure (45 CFR 164.502(a)(1)(iii)) and are a component of doing business. For example, calling out patients' names in a physician's office is an incidental disclosure because it occurs as part of the office operations. As long as the information disclosed is the minimum necessary (for example, the patient's name with no diagnostic information), this is permissible under the Privacy Rule without the patient's authorization or opportunity to agree or object.

A **limited data set** is PHI that excludes most direct identifiers of the individual and the individual's relatives, employers, and household members (45 CFR 164.514(e)(2)) but does not deidentify the information. Such PHI may be used or disclosed without the patient's authorization or the opportunity to agree or object, provided it is used or disclosed only for research, public health, or healthcare operations.

Authorization and the Sale of PHI

HITECH prohibits both CEs and BAs from selling PHI without patient authorization. In the authorization, the patient must declare whether the recipient of the PHI can exchange it further for payment. Exceptions to this prohibition include public health and research data; treatment and healthcare operations (including, for example, the sale or merger of a CE); a BA pursuant to a BAA; an individual who is receiving a copy of his or her own PHI; and for other exchanges deemed by the Secretary of HHS to be permissible (AHIMA 2009a). Under HITECH, disclosures are permitted in exchange for reasonable remuneration, without patient authorization, for other reasons including payment, accounting of disclosures, as required by law (HHS 2010a, 40890–40891).

Revocation

An individual may revoke an authorization at any time if it is done in writing. However, revocation does not apply when the CE has already acted on the authorization.

Check Your Understanding 9.4

Instructions: Indicate whether the following statements are true or false (T or F).

1. The HIPAA consent explains an individual's rights and the CE's legal duties with respect to PHI.

2. Per the HIPAA Privacy Rule, patient authorization is required for the use or disclosure of PHI unless it meets an exception whereby authorization is not required.

3. Although an individual must verbally agree to be included in a facility directory, written authorization is not required.

4. One of the 12 public interest and benefit exceptions to the authorization requirements is disclosure to organ procurement agencies.

5. Incidental disclosures do not require an individual's written authorization.

Redisclosure

Patient information is often created by a healthcare provider and assimilated into another healthcare provider's records. Examples include copies of reports sent by a physician to a hospital upon patient admission or a patient's hospital records sent to a nursing facility for the patient's follow-up care. **Redisclosure** is disclosure by a healthcare organization of information that was created by and received from another entity. Providers need to balance requests for patient information, which are necessary for continuity of care, with the appropriateness of redisclosing this information. Federal laws specifically protect substance abuse records from routine redisclosure and strictly limit other disclosures without patient authorization, but what about information that is not highly sensitive in nature? This topic was addressed extensively in the AHIMA practice brief "Redisclosure of Patient Health Information" and is discussed below (AHIMA 2009b).

The HHS Office for Civil Rights (OCR) provides guidance stating that it is permissible for "a provider who is a CE to disclose a complete medical record, including portions that were created by another provider, assuming that the disclosure is for a purpose permitted by the Privacy Rule, such as treatment" (HHS 2007). State laws that address the issue of redisclosure must also be read in conjunction with the Privacy Rule, as discussed in the preemption section below. In the interest of patient care, health records from other facilities should be made part of the DRS at the current facility if that information is needed for diagnosis or treatment, and if state law does not otherwise prohibit it. If conflicts of law do occur, legal counsel should be consulted. Further, facility policies and procedures must be developed regarding redisclosure, including mechanisms to verify the authority of individuals receiving PHI and identify situations where redisclosure is and is not appropriate. Appropriate redisclosures include those that:

- Facilitate patient care

- Are disclosed only after a patient has been encouraged to first attempt to obtain records from the originating facility

- Are disclosed to comply with legal process

- Include only information contained within the DRS

Further, when testifying as to the authenticity of redisclosed health information, it is necessary to state that the information was received from another facility via usual business practices, that the information was received in good faith, and that testimony regarding the recordkeeping practices at the facility that created the records is not possible (AHIMA 2009b).

Minimum Necessary Requirement

The Privacy Rule introduced the standard of minimum necessary, a "need to know" filter that is applied to limit access to a patient's PHI (45 CFR 164.502(b)(1)) and to limit the amount of PHI used, disclosed, and requested. Essentially, this means that healthcare providers and other CEs must limit uses, disclosures, and requests to only the amount needed to accomplish the intended purpose, with individuals having access only to information to which they are entitled and that they need to conduct business. For example, for payment purposes, only the minimum amount of information that is necessary to substantiate a claim for payment should be disclosed. HIM professionals have always followed policies and procedures to release the minimum amount of information requested for the specific purpose, but the Privacy Rule reinforces this traditional practice.

With respect to individuals working for a CE, the minimum necessary standard must be carefully applied to the use of information by the workforce. For example, policies and procedures should identify persons or classes of persons working for the CE who need to access PHI to perform their duties. In addition, categories of PHI that each person or class of persons can access and use should be identified.

For example, employees working in the dietary department would not have the same level of access to PHI as a nurse working in critical care.

There are certain circumstances where the minimum necessary requirement does not apply, such as:

- To healthcare providers for treatment

- To the individual or the individual's personal representative

- Pursuant to the individual's authorization

- To the Secretary of HHS for investigations, compliance review, or enforcement

- As required by law

- To meet other Privacy Rule compliance requirements (45 CFR 164.502(b)(2))

TPO as a whole is not exempted; rather, only treatment is exempted from the minimum necessary requirement. Use and disclosure of PHI for payment and operations purposes must still adhere to the requirement.

Because "minimum necessary" has been somewhat unclear depending on who is making the determination, HITECH has sought to provide clarification via guidance from the Secretary of HHS. Clarification is still pending. Until a final determination is made, CEs are to use the limited data set (that is, PHI with certain specified direct identifiers removed) as a guideline for using or disclosing only the minimum necessary information, while reverting back to the "amount needed to accomplish the intended purpose" definition when the limited data set definition is inadequate (AHIMA 2009a). Per the January 2013 final rule, the minimum necessary standard now also applies to BAs.

Section 3: Individual Rights; Other Key Requirements; Penalties for Noncompliance

Individual Rights

The Privacy Rule provides patients with significant rights that allow them some measure of control over their health information. Those rights include right of access, right to request amendment of PHI, right to an accounting of disclosures, right to request confidential communications, right to request restrictions of PHI, and right to complain of Privacy Rule violations. These rights are described below. A chart that details all individual rights except the right to complain of Privacy Rule violations is located at the end of this chapter (appendix 9.D).

Access

Section 164.524 of the Privacy Rule states that an individual has a right of **access** to inspect and obtain a copy of his or her own PHI that is contained in a DRS, such as a health record (45 CFR 164.524). The individual's right extends for as long as the PHI is maintained.

Access to information may be denied in some situations because it is specifically exempted from access by the Privacy Rule or it is not part of the DRS. The Privacy Rule preamble makes clear that individuals do not have a right of access to:

- Psychotherapy notes

- Information compiled in reasonable anticipation of, or for use in, a civil, criminal, or administrative action or proceeding

- PHI held by clinical laboratories if the Clinical Laboratory Improvement Amendments of 1988 (42 CFR 493) prohibit such access

- PHI held by certain research laboratories that are exempt from the **Clinical Laboratory Improvement Act** (CLIA) regulations (45 CFR 164.524; Hughes 2003). (Note: CLIA regulations aim to ensure quality laboratory testing.)

Why is it so important that individuals be able to access (with exceptions) their own PHI? Although the physical health record belongs to the organization that created it, the patient has an interest (or ownership) in the information about him or her that is contained within the record. To provide no specific right of access allows providers and others the ability to deny access. For example, Ohio Revised Code 3701.74 at one time required only hospitals to provide patients with copies of their health records, thus exempting physicians and other healthcare providers (as well as those CEs that are today subject to the Privacy Rule). As a result, physicians and other providers denied or ignored patient requests for their own information because there was no statute compelling them to respond. Fortunately, Ohio law subsequently changed in the face of the Privacy Rule's implementation, and patients are now dually given the right of access through Ohio law and the HIPAA Privacy Rule. Nonetheless, the past provides an important reminder of the need for a federal law that protects patients' rights with respect to their own health information. In the context of the EHR, HITECH requires CEs with EHRs to make PHI available electronically or, if the individual requests, to send PHI to a designated person or entity electronically (Nunn 2009). Consistent with HIPAA's pre-existing requirements regarding fees, a fee for providing the information is permitted if it does not exceed the CE's labor costs (AHIMA 2009a). It can encompass only the cost associated with providing the information, not including retrieval costs (AHIMA 2010a).

Grounds for Denial of Access

According to the Privacy Rule, a CE can at times deny individuals access to PHI without providing them an opportunity to review or appeal the denial. This is an unreviewable denial and is important, particularly in the release of information area.

Denials that are not subject to an appeals process include those for access to PHI contained in psychotherapy notes, as well as PHI held by CEs that are correctional institutions or providers who have acted under the direction of a correctional institution. In these situations, an inmate's request to obtain a copy of his or her own PHI may be denied under certain circumstances without an appeal. In some situations, PHI is created or obtained by a covered healthcare provider in the course of research that includes treatment. Sometimes an individual receiving treatment as part of a research study agrees to suspend his or her right to access PHI temporarily. This is usually for protection of the integrity of the research study. In such cases, the CE may deny access to PHI as long as the research is in progress.

There are two other circumstances in which a CE may deny an individual access to his or her own PHI without the benefit of an appeals process. One situation is where the PHI was obtained from someone other than a healthcare provider under a promise of confidentiality. If the CE decides that the access requested would be reasonably likely to reveal the source of the information, access might be denied without benefit of appeal. The other situation is where the PHI is contained in records that are subject to the Federal Privacy Act (5 USC 552a) if the denial of access under the Privacy Act would meet the requirements of that law.

In two instances, the Privacy Rule requires a CE to give an individual the right to review a denial of access. These are situations in which a licensed healthcare professional determines that access to PHI as requested by the individual or his or her personal representative would:

1. Likely endanger the life or physical safety of the individual or another person, or

2. Reasonably endanger the life or physical safety of another person mentioned in the PHI

According to the Privacy Rule, when a denial is made in such circumstances, the CE has certain responsibilities. First, it must write the denial in plain language and include a reason. Second, it must explain that the individual has the right to request a review of the denial. Third, it must describe how the individual can complain to the CE and must include the name or title and phone number of the person or office to contact. Finally, it must explain how the individual can lodge a complaint with the Secretary of the Department of HHS. Moreover, when access to PHI is denied on the grounds mentioned above, the individual has the right to have the denial reviewed by a licensed healthcare professional. This must be someone who did not participate in the original denial and who is designated by the CE to act as the reviewing official. The CE must then grant or deny access in accordance with the reviewing official's decision.

Requesting Access to One's Own PHI

The Privacy Rule specifies that the CE may require individuals to make their requests in writing, provided it has informed them of such a requirement. Timely response is an important part of the Privacy Rule. A CE must act on an individual's request for review of PHI no later than 30 days after the request is made, extending the response by no more than 30 days if within the 30-day time period it gives the reason for the delay and the date by which it will respond. The CE may extend the time for action on a request for access only once.

In responding to an individual's request for access to his or her PHI, the CE must arrange a convenient time and place of inspection with the individual or mail a copy of the PHI at the individual's request. Per HITECH, CEs with EHRs must provide individuals with electronic copies and must transmit the copy to the individual's designee upon request. The Privacy Rule allows the CE to impose a reasonable cost-based fee when the individual requests a copy of the PHI or agrees to accept summary or explanatory information. Generally, the fee may include the cost of:

- Copying, including supplies and labor

- Postage, when the individual has requested that the copy, summary, or explanation be mailed

- Preparing an explanation or summary, if agreed to by the individual

Retrieval fees charged to the patient (whether standard fees or based on actual retrieval costs) are not allowed under the Privacy Rule; this was made clear by the January 2013 final rule (AHIMA 2013). Retrieval fees are permissible for nonpatient requests. Per HITECH, the fee imposed for providing a copy of an EHR may not exceed labor costs incurred in responding to the request. However, what are considered labor costs has not yet been determined.

When requests for access to PHI are granted, the CE must provide access to the PHI in the form or format requested if it is readily producible in such form or format. If it is not, it must be produced in a readable hard-copy form or other form or format agreed to by the CE and the individual.

Following the January 2013 final rule, HITECH makes it easier for schools to receive student immunization records where state or other law requires it prior to student admission. HITECH permits CEs to disclose a child's immunization records (considered a public health activity) to a school with the oral consent of the parent or guardian. This contrasts with the previous written authorization requirement (HHS 2010a, 40895).

Request Amendment

Many states have laws or regulations that permit individuals to amend their health records. Section 164.526 of the Privacy Rule also permits individuals to request that a CE amend PHI or a record about the individual in a DRS (45 CFR 164.526). However, the CE may deny the request if it determines that the PHI or the record:

- Was not created by the CE

- Is not part of the DRS

- Is not available for inspection as noted in the regulation of access (for example, psychotherapy notes, inmate of a correctional institution)

- Is accurate or complete as it stands

The CE may require the individual to make an **amendment request** in writing and provide a reason for the amendment. This requirement must be communicated in advance to the individual, usually taking place in the CE's NPP.

The Privacy Rule requires a CE to act on an individual's amendment request no later than 60 days after its receipt by either allowing the requested amendment or denying it in writing. The entity may extend its response by 30 days if it explains the reasons for the delay in writing and gives a date by which it will complete its action. There can be no additional extensions.

What must a CE do when an amendment is granted? The Privacy Rule requires it to:

1. Identify the records in the DRS that are affected by the amendment and append the information through a link to the amendment's location. For example, if the diagnosis were incorrect, the amendment would have to appear and be linked to each record or report in the DRS.

2. Inform the individual that the amendment was accepted and have him or her identify the persons with whom the amendment needs to be shared and then obtain his or her agreement to notify those persons. The CE must make reasonable efforts to provide the amendment within a reasonable amount of time to anyone who has received the PHI.

What must the CE do when it denies a requested amendment? Within the required 60 days, the CE must write a denial in plain language that contains the following information (45 CFR 164.526(d)):

- The basis for the denial

- The individual's right to submit a written statement disagreeing with the denial

- The process by which the individual can submit his or her disagreement

- A statement explaining how, if the individual does not submit a disagreement to the denial, he or she may request that both the original amendment request and the CE's denial accompany any future disclosures of the PHI that is the subject of the amendment

- A description of how the individual may complain to the CE, including the name or title and telephone number of the contact person or office

The CE can prepare a written rebuttal to the individual's disagreement statement, but it must provide the individual with a copy of it.

All requests for amendments, denials, the individual's statement of disagreement, and the CE's rebuttal, if one was created, must be appended or linked to the record or PHI that is the subject of the amendment request. When any future disclosures of the information are made, this material or a summary of it must accompany them. However, if a request for amendment was denied and the individual did not write a statement of disagreement, the request for amendment and denial must only accompany future disclosures if the individual requests it.

Accounting of Disclosures

Maintaining some type of accounting procedure for monitoring and tracking PHI disclosures has been a common practice in departments that manage health information. However, the Privacy Rule has a specific standard with respect to such recordkeeping. Section 164.528 of the Privacy Rule, which provides for an **accounting of disclosures**, states that an individual has the right to receive an accounting of certain disclosures made by a CE.

The types of disclosures that must be included in the Privacy Rule's accounting requirement are limited, but do currently include public interest and benefit disclosures. The May 31, 2011 proposed rule, however, proposes excluding some public and interest benefit disclosures from an accounting. Disclosures for which an accounting is not required and which are therefore exempt include the following:

- Needed to carry out TPO (although this exception is only applicable to CEs without EHRs per HITECH and will be further discussed below)

- To the individuals to whom the information pertains

- Incident to an otherwise permitted or required use or disclosure

- Pursuant to an authorization

- For use in the facility's directory, to persons involved in the individual's care, or for other notification purposes

- To meet national security or intelligence requirements

- To correctional institutions or law enforcement officials

- As part of a limited data set

- Disclosures that occurred before the compliance date for the CE

The accounting requirement includes disclosures made in writing, electronically, by telephone, or orally. Disclosures not included in this list of exemptions are permitted by the Privacy Rule; however, per the May 31, 2011 proposed rule, HITECH proposes that items to be included in an accounting be specifically listed.

Originally, a significant change to the accounting of disclosures requirement under HITECH was that CEs that used or maintained an EHR would have to include TPO disclosures in their accounting of disclosures. HITECH established a timetable for compliance with this change depending on when CEs acquired an EHR. CEs with more recent EHR acquisitions are required to comply before those with older systems, presumably because of newer systems' capability to handle the increased volume and more complex requirements. However, the May 31, 2011 proposed rule excludes both TPO and uses from the accounting requirement for paper records and EHRs (HHS 2011). Instead, it proposes a separate "access report" for EHRs, allowing individuals to see who has viewed their DRS in the previous three years. TPO disclosures would therefore be displayed in the **access report** rather than in the accounting of disclosures, as earlier suggested. This proposal is pending. Prior to HITECH, requesters received an accounting of disclosures made during the previous six years. Per HITECH's changes, the time frame is shortened so that an individual can receive an accounting including disclosures made during only the previous three years (AHIMA 2009a).

CEs must recognize that not all of their activities meet the "healthcare operations" definition in order not to overlook disclosures that must be tracked. For example, mandatory public health reporting is not part of a CE's operations. (Such reporting includes requirements by states to report births [birth certificates]; communicable diseases; and incidents of abuse or suspected abuse of children, individuals who are mentally disabled, and the elderly.) As a result, these disclosures must be included in an accounting of disclosures. Also if a physician's office reports a patient's tuberculosis to a public health authority, that disclosure must be included if a patient requests an accounting. If a CE provides PHI to a third-party public health authority to review, but the third party does not actually review the PHI, the mere right of access must be included in an accounting of disclosures. As a corollary, erroneous disclosures (such as a facsimile transmitted to the wrong recipient) are also subject to the accounting of disclosures requirement, regardless of whether the recipient read the information. (These may also constitute breaches, discussed later in this chapter.) Disclosure pursuant to a court order without a patient's written authorization would also be subject to an accounting of disclosures. However, disclosure pursuant to a subpoena that is accompanied by a patient's written authorization would not be subject to an accounting, because the authorization exempts the disclosure from the accounting requirement.

A CE may either account for the disclosures of its BAs or provide for the BA to make its own accounting. Under HITECH, BAs must respond to accounting requests made directly to them (AHIMA 2009a).

In some situations, the individual's right to an accounting of PHI disclosure may be suspended at the written request of a health oversight agency or law enforcement official. In these situations, the written request from the appropriate agency or law enforcement official must indicate that such an accounting would impede its activities. The oversight agency or the law enforcement official must also indicate how long such a suspension is required.

The Privacy Rule requires that certain items be included in an accounting, although HITECH proposes to relax the specificity to some extent. The date of disclosure, the name and address (when known) of the entity or person who received the information, and a brief statement of the purpose of the disclosure or a copy of the individual's request for an accounting are required. Certain time limits also apply. A CE must act on a request no later than 60 days after its receipt with one 30-day extension, as long as it notifies the individual in writing of the reasons for the delay and when the accounting will be made available. Per the May 31, 2011 proposed rule, HITECH proposes to limit the response period to 30 days, with one 30-day extension.

The first accounting within any 12-month period must be provided without charge. For any other request within a 12-month period, the CE may charge a reasonable cost-based fee. However, the entity must inform individuals of the fee in advance and give them the opportunity to withdraw or modify the request. The Privacy Rule requires documentation to be maintained on all accounting requests, including the information in the accounting, the written accounting that was provided to the individual, and the titles of persons or offices responsible for receiving and processing requests for an accounting. Policies and procedures must be developed to ensure that PHI disclosed from all areas of an organization, especially those areas outside an HIM department, can be tracked and compiled when an accounting request is received.

Confidential Communications

Healthcare providers and health plans must give individuals the right of **confidential communications**, or the opportunity to request that communications of PHI be routed to an alternative location or by an alternative method (45 CFR 164.522(b)). Healthcare providers must honor such a request without requiring a reason if the request is reasonable. Health plans must honor such a request if it is reasonable and if the requesting individual states that disclosure could pose a safety risk. However, healthcare providers and health plans may refuse to accommodate requests if the individual does not provide information as to how payment will be handled or if the individual does not provide an alternative address or method by which he or she can be contacted.

An example of a request for confidential communications would be a woman who requests that billing information from her psychiatrist, from whom she is seeking treatment because of domestic violence, be sent to her work address instead of to her home.

Request Restrictions

Under the Privacy Rule, a CE must permit an individual to **request restrictions**, meaning that an individual may request the CE to restrict the uses and disclosures of PHI for carrying out TPO (45 CFR 164.522(a)). Historically, the CE has not been required to agree to these requests and may not be allowed to honor them (for example, where disclosures are required by law). When the CE does agree to a restriction, it must abide by it. The restriction can be terminated by either the individual or the CE. When the CE initiates termination of the agreement, it must inform the individual that it is doing so.

However, the termination is only effective with respect to the PHI created or received after the individual has been informed (45 CFR 164.522(a)).

Although, as noted above, HIPAA originally gave CEs discretion not to agree to restriction requests, HITECH requires they be complied with (unless otherwise required by law) if the disclosure would be made to a health plan for payment or operations (and not for treatment) and the PHI pertains solely to an item or service that has been paid for in full by other than the health plan (AHIMA 2009a). The logistics of carrying out this requirement, however, will be complex.

Submit Complaints

A CE must provide a process for an individual to complain about the entity's policies and procedures, noncompliance with them, or noncompliance with the Privacy Rule. The CE's NPP must contain contact information at the CE level and inform individuals of the ability to submit complaints to the OCR. For individuals who choose not to complain to the CE or who submit complaints at both levels, the OCR maintains regional offices that field complaints from individuals in that region. The CE must document all complaints it receives, along with the disposition of each complaint. As of March 31, 2011, more than 59,000 complaints alleging Privacy Rule violations had been filed nationally with the OCR. In 2009, the most frequent violations were impermissible uses and disclosures, followed by safeguard violations and violations relating to access and the minimum necessary requirement. The types of complaints were consistent with those of previous years (Heubusch 2010).

Check Your Understanding 9.5

Instructions: Indicate whether the following statements are true or false (T or F).

1. Under no circumstances should health records from other facilities be made part of an organization's DRS.

2. The minimum necessary principle applies to disclosures made for TPO purposes.

3. An individual has the right of access to his or her psychotherapy notes.

4. Per HITECH, an accounting of disclosures includes TPO disclosures made by covered entities with EHRs.

5. Complaints about alleged Privacy Rule violations must be submitted to the covered entity.

Breach Notification

HITECH added **breach notification** requirements for entities with custody of patient information. These requirements are significant because, unlike any imposed in the past, they place organizations on the radar of regulatory agencies and in the media spotlight when PHI is handled inappropriately. Further, they extend consequences to entities not previously bound by HIPAA.

HIPAA CEs and BAs, which may include PHR vendors, are subject to HHS-issued breach notification regulations. Non-CEs and non-BAs (including non-BA PHR vendors, third-party service providers of PHR vendors, and other non-HIPAA CEs or BAs affiliated with PHR vendors) are subject to companion breach notification regulations issued by the Federal Trade Commission (FTC). Under both sets of regulations, entities must identify breaches and make appropriate notifications. In particular, entities subject to FTC regulations must notify the FTC and the individual(s) affected by the breach. Third-party PHR service providers shall notify the PHR vendor or entity of the breach.

Other notification requirements, such as the content and nature of breach notices, parallel requirements established by HHS (AHIMA 2009a). HITECH defines a **breach** as an "unauthorized acquisition, access, use or disclosure of PHI which compromises the security or privacy of such information." It does not include disclosures to unauthorized persons if they would not reasonably be able to retain the disclosed information (American Recovery and Reinvestment Act of 2009, Title XIII, Subtitle D Sections 13400, 13402).

Further, it does not include situations where a workforce member or individual, acting under the CE's or BA's authority, unintentionally acquires, accesses, or uses the information as long as it was in good faith, within the scope of authority, and not further disclosed or used in an impermissible manner. Finally, it does not include inadvertent disclosure by an individual at a CE or BA to another authorized person at a CE, BA, or organized healthcare arrangement of which the CE is a part, and the information is not further disclosed or used in an impermissible manner (Dennis 2010). Breach notification applies only to unsecured PHI, defined as that which technology has not made unusable, unreadable, or indecipherable to unauthorized persons. The January 2013 final rule states that "an impermissible use or disclosure of PHI is presumed to be a breach unless the covered entity or business associate demonstrates that there is a low probability that the PHI has been compromised" (AHIMA 2013). Breaches are deemed to have been discovered when the breach is first known or when it reasonably should have been known. Individuals whose information has been breached must be notified without unreasonable delay, and within 60 days, by first-class mail and by a faster method (such as telephone) if there is the potential for "imminent misuse." Where more than nine individuals are affected and written notice is unsuccessful, web postings or the media are recommended. A significant threshold is 500 affected people. At that point, media outlets must be used and the Secretary of HHS must be notified immediately. For all breaches, CEs must report to HHS using an online breach reporting system (HHS 2009b).

Individuals whose PHI has been breached must be provided with the following information:

- A description of what occurred (including date of breach and date that breach was discovered)

- The types of unsecured PHI that were involved (such as name, social security number, date of birth, home address, and account number)

- Steps that the individual may take to protect himself or herself

- What the entity is doing to investigate, mitigate, and prevent future occurrences

- Contact information for the individual to ask questions and receive updates (AHIMA 2009a)

Marketing

The Privacy Rule defines marketing as communication about a product or service that encourages the recipient to purchase or use that product or service (45 CFR 164.501). Generally, the Privacy Rule requires that an individual's authorization be obtained prior to using his or her PHI for marketing. However, marketing has posed some difficulty since the Privacy Rule's inception, because CEs at times have classified a marketing activity as a healthcare operation, thus eliminating the need (in the CE's mind) to obtain an individual's authorization. HITECH clarifies that communications are considered to be marketing *unless* they:

- Describe a health-related product or service (or payment for the product or service) provided by or included in the benefit plan of the CE making the communication, including communications about participants in the health provider's or health plan's network

- Describe replacements or enhancements to a health plan

- Describe available health-related products or services that are of value, although not part of a benefit plan

- Are for treatment of the individual

- Are for case management or care coordination for the individual, or to direct or recommend alternative treatments, therapies, healthcare providers, or settings of care (45 CFR 164.501)

Therefore, although the communications just listed look like marketing, by definition they have been exempted. Rather, they are considered healthcare treatment or operations and no authorization is required.

Common communications that meet the definition of marketing, on the other hand, but do not require authorization are those that:

- Occur face-to-face between the CE and the individual; or

- Concern a promotional gift of nominal value provided by the CE (45 CFR 164.508(a)(3))

A CE must obtain patient authorization to send communications about *non-health-related* products or services, or to give or sell the individual's PHI to third parties for marketing. However, concerns exist regarding the ability of CEs to sell individuals' PHI so that third parties can market their *health-related* products or services. Under HITECH, the ability of CEs to categorize health-related communications as healthcare operations (which exempts them from marketing requirements) is limited. If a CE is to make a communication in exchange for financial remuneration, prior authorization (clearly stating that the CE is being paid for the communication) is required before the CE (or BA) makes the communication. Exceptions include communications describing currently prescribed drugs and, per HITECH, refill reminders as long as the amount of remuneration received by the CE is reasonable.

Per HITECH, subsidized communications—even if they look like healthcare operations—require individual authorization. A CE's NPP must specify the CE's intent to send subsidized communications and the individual's ability to opt out. The communication itself must disclose the remuneration and reiterate the ability to opt out (HHS 2010a, 40884–40887).

Fundraising

For **fundraising** activities that benefit the CE, 45 CFR 164.514(f) permits the CE to use or disclose to a BA or an institutionally related foundation, without authorization, demographic information and dates of healthcare provided to an individual. The CE must inform individuals in its NPP that PHI may be used for this purpose. The CE must include instructions either before the first solicitation or as part of the fundraising materials about how to opt out of receiving materials in the future. Reasonable efforts must be made to ensure the individual's wishes are honored. If a fundraising activity targets individuals based on diagnosis (for example, patients with kidney disease are targeted to raise funds for a new kidney dialysis center), prior authorization is required. Per HITECH, fundraising communications that use or disclose PHI are healthcare operations and must clearly and conspicuously provide the recipient the opportunity to opt out of communications. This opt-out is considered a revocation of authorization (AHIMA 2009a). Under HITECH, an opt-out may be applied to the current campaign only or to all future fundraising campaigns (HHS 2010a, 40896–40897).

Research

The potential to misuse human subjects in research activities and, hence, the need to protect those subjects are historical issues. The harmful use of concentration camp prisoners by Nazi physicians for experimentation without the consent of those individuals resulted in the Nuremberg Code. Although the code did not become law in the United States, it remains a powerful statement on the ethical use of human subjects. In the United States, the US Public Health Service used male African-American sharecroppers (again without their consent) for a harmful study in which treatment was often denied, in what is known as the Tuskegee Syphilis Study (1932–1972). This ultimately led to the **National Research Act of 1974** (Pub. L. 93-348), which required the Department of Health, Education, and Welfare (now the HHS) to codify its policy for the protection of human subjects into federal regulations and created a commission that generated the **Belmont Report**, a "statement of basic ethical principles that should assist in resolving the ethical problems that surround the conduct of research with human subjects" (NIH 1979). These studies and others demonstrate the international historical misuse of human subjects, against which protections are vital.

Today, research on human subjects is governed by the Federal Policy for the Protection of Human Subjects (the Common Rule), which emanated from the joint promulgation of regulations from several federal agencies and, specifically, from HHS regulations 45 CFR Part 46 (1981), based on the Belmont Report. In 1991, the portion of the HHS regulations that focused on the protection of human subjects (45 CFR 46(a)) was adopted by a number of federal departments and agencies involved in human subject research either as research bodies themselves or as agencies that fund research conducted by others. The Food and Drug Administration imposes additional requirements at 21 CFR Parts 50 and 56. Requirements of the Common Rule include (45 CFR 46.101–46.112):

- Compliance assurances by organizations conducting research

- Requirements for informed consent

- Special protections for vulnerable populations, such as prisoners, pregnant women, children, mentally disabled persons, and economically or educationally disadvantaged persons

Additionally, an institutional review board (IRB) must approve federally funded human subjects research, despite the presence of informed consent, with such approval including assurances as to the preservation of the subjects' privacy and confidentiality (Roth 2004b; Burrington-Brown and Wagg 2003). The HIPAA Privacy Rule provides additional protections where research places human subjects—and their private information—at risk.

Inherent in the humane and dignified treatment of fellow human beings is the protection of individuals' privacy during the conduct of research, regardless of whether the researchers are interacting with the subjects or merely using private information about them, if that information is identifiable. Thus, the Privacy Rule's general requirement is that authorization must be obtained for uses and disclosures of PHI created for research that includes treatment of the individual. Public information, de-identified data, or data that is recorded by the investigation so that the subject cannot be directly identified or identified through links are not subject to the Common Rule (Burrington-Brown and Wagg 2003).

The Privacy Rule expands the Common Rule's requirements by regulating both privately and federally funded research and, subsequently, requiring the creation and use of privacy boards where an IRB does not already exist (Amatayakul 2003). (Note: A **privacy board** is a group formed by a CE to review research studies where authorization waivers are requested and to ensure the HIPAA privacy rights of research subjects.) In addition to the privacy board requirement, the primary research requirement under the Privacy Rule includes:

1. When an authorization for use and disclosure of PHI is required from an individual; and

2. In what form the authorization may occur

The Privacy Rule (CFR 164.508(b)(4)) has generally prohibited CEs from conditioning treatment, payment, and health plan enrollment or benefit eligibility on an authorization (that is, **conditioned authorizations**) unless it was for purposes such as treatment-related research and health plan enrollment. This was to discourage coercing individuals to sign authorizations in order to receive services. Consequently, **compound authorizations** (which combine informed consent with an authorization) have been limited, and **stand-alone authorizations**, which include the core elements of a valid authorization (45 CFR 164.508), have been preferred. This has caused problems for researchers who collect and store biospecimens and related PHI, because tissue-banking authorizations are **unconditioned authorizations**. Per HITECH, a CE is permitted to combine conditioned and unconditioned authorizations for research, including specimen collection and associated PHI, as long as the form clearly distinguishes between the two and provides individuals with the ability to opt in to unconditioned research activities (HHS 2010a, 40892–40893).

During a blinded study, or where there is minimal risk to the individual's privacy (for example, research is limited to a medical record review), 45 CFR 164.512 also provides the option of a waived (that is, without an individual's authorization) or altered authorization (that is, if the IRB or privacy board has approved a waiver of an individual's right to access his or her own records). The Privacy Rule further permits waiver of authorization where the researcher provides assurance that:

- The use or disclosure of PHI is solely preparatory to the research itself, and it will not be removed from the CE;

- The use or disclosure is solely for research on decedents' PHI; or

- Only a limited data set will be used for research, public health, or healthcare operations, and a limited data set use agreement is in place.

Under a limited data set, 16 of the 18 identifiers listed in figure 9.4 must be removed. The only data elements permitted are items 3 (dates) and 18 (unique code for reidentification) (CFR 164.514(e); Amatayakul 2003; Burrington-Brown and Wagg 2003).

State laws that conflict with the research authorization parameters of the Privacy Rule and provide an individual with greater privacy protection must be taken into consideration, particularly regarding PHI used or disclosed preparatory to research and on decedents (Amatayakul 2003). The issue of preemption will be discussed in the following section. Where deidentified information or a limited data set is used for research, no accounting of disclosures is required.

Table 9.2 provides a detailed analysis of the responsibilities of both the IRB and the researcher under the Privacy Rule requirements.

Check Your Understanding 9.6

Instructions: Indicate whether the following statements are true or false (T or F).

1. The threshold for required media notification in the event of a privacy breach is 300 affected individuals.

2. All activities that meet the HIPAA definition of marketing must receive prior written authorization from the individual.

3. The breach notification requirement is new per HITECH.

4. Fundraising activities that target individuals based on diagnosis require prior authorization.

5. A conditioned authorization may be allowed by HITECH in certain situations.

Table 9.2.   Actions required by HIPAA for use of PHI in research

Type of Information	IRB	Researcher	Research Subject (patient or decedent)
PHI preparatory to research	None*	Representation that use is solely and necessary for research and will not be removed from covered entity	None
Deidentified health information	None*	Removal of safe-harbor data or statistical assurance of deidentification	None
Limited data set	None*	Removal of direct identifiers and data use agreement	None
Individually identifiable health information on decedents	None*	Representation that use is solely and necessary for research on decedents and documentation of death upon request of covered entity	None
PHI of human subjects (whether research is interventional or record review)	Waive authorization requirement if determined that risk to privacy is minimal	Representation that: 1. Privacy risk is minimal based on: • plan to protect identifiers • plan to destroy identifiers unless there is a health or research reason to retain • written assurance that PHI will not be reused or redisclosed 2. Research requires use of specifically described PHI 3. Justify the waiver 4. Obtain IRB approval under normal or expedited review procedures	None
	Approve alteration of authorization (e.g., to restrict patient's access during study) if determined that risk to privacy is minimal	Same as above	Sign altered authorization form
	Approve research protocol ensuring that there is an authorization for use either combined with consent for and disclosure of PHI research or separate		Sign authorization combined with consent for research or sign standard authorization for use and disclosure of PHI for research as described in authorization

*The IRB may impose requirements, but HIPAA does not.

Source: Amatayakul 2003.

Preemption

The legal doctrine of **preemption** applies to the Privacy Rule (45 CFR 160.203). Although CEs are legally obligated to comply with both state and federal privacy laws, sometimes it is impossible to follow both. To address this conflict, preemption requires a CE to comply with federal law when federal and state laws conflict (that is, federal law preempts contrary state law). A state law is contrary when (45 CFR 160.202; Hughes 2002):

1. It would be impossible for a CE to follow both the federal and state laws or;

2. Following the state law would hinder the purpose of HIPAA

However, the federal Privacy Rule provides only a floor, or minimum, of privacy requirements. As a result, it does not preempt or supersede stricter (more stringent) state statutes. Stricter or more stringent refers to state statutes that either:

1. Provide individuals with greater privacy protections; or

2. Give individuals greater rights with respect to their PHI.

In addition to the "more stringent" exception to preemption, state law will also prevail if it fulfills one or more of the following purposes (45 CFR 160.203):

A. Is determined by the Secretary of Health and Human Services as necessary to

1. Prevent healthcare fraud and abuse

2. Ensure appropriate regulation of insurance and health plans to the extent authorized by law

3. Complete state reporting on healthcare delivery or costs

4. Serve a compelling need related to public health, safety, or welfare, and the intrusion into privacy is warranted when balanced against the need

B. Regulates the manufacture, registration, distribution, or dispensing of any controlled substance as identified by state law, or

C. Provides for the reporting of disease or injury, child abuse, birth, or death, or for the conduct of public health surveillance, investigation, or intervention; or

D. Requires a health plan to report or provide access to information for management or financial audits, program monitoring and evaluation, or licensure or certification of facilities or individuals

It is important to review state legal requirements and determine which law prevails. Because state laws vary in the level of protection they afford to patient information, a preemption analysis (which compares federal and state law to determine which one prevails) in one state may yield a different outcome than one performed in another state.

Administrative Requirements

The HIPAA Privacy Rule imposes administrative requirements that govern actual implementation of the Rule. Among other mandates, the administrative requirements include policy and procedure development, designated personnel, training, and document retention. These are outlined below.

The Privacy Rule provides several important standards regarding administrative requirements, including:

- Standards for policies and procedures and changes to policies and procedures

- Designation of a privacy officer and a contact person for receiving complaints

- Requirements for privacy training

- Mitigation of wrongful use and disclosure

- Requirements for establishing data safeguards

- Prohibition against retaliation and waiver

- Requirements for documentation retention

Individuals who manage health information are likely to find that their responsibilities include essential elements of the Privacy Rule.

Policies and Procedures

A CE must implement policies and procedures to ensure compliance with all standards, implementation specifications, and other requirements of the Privacy Rule. This includes conducting an ongoing review of privacy policies and procedures and ensuring that all policy changes are consistent with changes in the privacy and security regulations. Any regulatory changes that materially affect the CE's NPP, including those introduced by HITECH, must be updated in the NPP. Too, a revision must be indicated in the organization's policies and procedures. Individuals with expertise in the management of health information are ideally qualified for developing and overseeing such policies and procedures because of their background in privacy and security issues.

Privacy Officer and Contact Person

The Privacy Rule requires CEs to designate an individual—a **privacy officer**—to be responsible for developing and implementing privacy policies and procedures. This position is ideally suited to the background, knowledge, and skills of individuals with expertise in the management of health information.

In addition to a privacy officer, the CE must designate a person as the responsible party for receiving complaints. This individual must be able to provide further information about matters covered by the entity's NPP.

Workforce Training and Management

Every member of the CE's workforce must be trained in PHI policies and procedures. New members must be trained within a reasonable period of time after joining the workforce. In addition, whenever material changes are made to policies or procedures regarding privacy, the workforce must receive additional training. A CE should be comprehensive in its workforce training, including even less apparent workforce members who do not work directly with PHI but may come into contact with it (for example, janitorial staff and outsourced vendors' employees who work routinely on the CE's premises). Under HITECH, there are heightened consequences for BAs that violate the Privacy Rule. CEs should ensure that its BAs train their workforce members, although CEs are not responsible for providing that training themselves (AHIMA 2010b).

CEs must maintain documentation showing that privacy training has occurred. BAs should also ensure that training is documented. Although not required, a signed statement of training by each workforce member would be helpful in documenting compliance.

The CE and, now, individual members of its workforce (per HITECH) are subject to the Privacy Rule and the penalties that accompany violations. It is important for the CE to take as many precautions as possible. Because the age-old health information mantra "If you didn't document it, you didn't do it" extends beyond health records, it is important for CEs to document all steps that have been taken to ensure—to the extent possible—compliance by its workforce. In addition to documentation supporting the fact that workforce members have attended training sessions, these same individuals should also complete nondisclosure agreements stating their commitment to protecting the privacy of patient information and compliance with the Privacy Rule and further affirming their understanding and the voluntary nature of this commitment.

Mitigation

The Privacy Rule (45 CFR 164.530(f)) requires CEs to mitigate, as much as possible, harmful effects that result from the wrongful use and disclosure of PHI. Because **mitigation**, in essence, requires the lessening of the effects of a wrongful use or disclosure, it is contingent upon the CE to determine possible courses of action. Although HITECH has forced one type of mitigation—breach notification—other types of mitigation may assuage the individual, including:

- Apology

- Disciplinary action against the responsible employee or employees (although such results will not be able to be shared with the wronged individual)

- Repair of the process that resulted in the breach

- Payment of a bill or financial loss that resulted from the infraction

- Gestures of goodwill and good public relations (such as awarding gift certificates)

Mitigation may result from discovery of a breach by the CE or BA, or from a complaint that an individual has filed with the organization, the OCR, or both. Determining what constitutes a breach (which must be reported to both HHS and the individual), as well as determining the level of mitigation necessary, are steps an organization must take. Appropriate development of policies and procedures, followed by complete and detailed documentation when a situation arises, is critical to a successful mitigation process (Burrington-Brown 2003).

Data Safeguards

CEs are required to have in place appropriate administrative, technical, and physical safeguards to protect the privacy of PHI from either intentional or unintentional uses or disclosures that violate the rule. These safeguards must limit incidental uses and disclosures (45 CFR 164.530(c)). They may include the shredding of paper documents containing PHI (HHS 2003), and limiting access to areas containing PHI through the use of devices such as keycards, passwords, or locks.

Retaliation and Waiver

To ensure the integrity of an individual's right to complain about alleged Privacy Rule violations, CEs are expressly prohibited from **retaliation and waiver.** First, CEs may not retaliate against anyone who exercises his or her rights under the Privacy Rule, assists in an investigation by the HHS or other appropriate investigative authority, or opposes an act or practice that the person believes is a violation of the Privacy Rule (45 CFR 164.530(g)). Further, individuals cannot be required to waive the rights they hold under the Privacy Rule in order to obtain treatment, payment, or enrollment/benefits eligibility (HHS 2003).

Documentation and Record Retention

The Privacy Rule uses six years as the period for which Privacy Rule–related documents must be retained. The six-year time frame refers to the latter of the following: the date the document was created or the last effective date of the document (45 CFR 164.530(j); HHS 2003). Such documents include policies and procedures, the NPP, complaint dispositions, and other actions, activities, and designations that must be documented per Privacy Rule requirements.

Enforcement and Penalties for Noncompliance

A number of notable changes to enforcement and penalty provisions for HIPAA violations have been brought about by the passage of HITECH. Overall, there is a notable movement away from a collaborative approach focusing on corrective action to a more punitive stance.

The OCR enforces the Privacy Rule. Complaints are filed with the appropriate OCR regional office that covers either the individual's residence or the location where the alleged violation occurred. Although compliance with the Privacy Rule has historically been monitored through a complaint-driven process (and enforcement efforts have subsequently been criticized as lacking teeth), HITECH requires the HHS to conduct audits of CEs and BAs—not unlike those used by state licensure organizations. HHS contracted with KPMG, an audit, tax, and advisory firm, to conduct pilot audits in 2012. The pilot program is being assessed, with audits to resume thereafter. BAs are slated to be included in future audits. Because complaints will also continue to initiate investigations, however, CEs and BAs should minimize situations that lead to disgruntled patients (AHIMA 2009a). Elements of Privacy Rule compliance that are visible to patients and visitors include prominent display of the NPP, training employees (and members of the medical staff) to display respect for patient information privacy to the greatest degree, and visible demonstrations of the organization's privacy awareness (Weintraub 2003).

HITECH grants state attorneys general the ability to bring civil actions in federal district court in behalf of residents believed to have been negatively affected by a HIPAA violation. Further, whereas legal responsibility for HIPAA violations was limited to CEs, employees or other individuals can now be individually prosecuted. Civil and criminal penalties may also now apply to BAs. Further, a method for compensating individuals harmed under HIPAA and HITECH provisions is to be recommended to the Secretary of HHS.

The Final HIPAA **Enforcement Rule** created standardized procedures and substantive requirements for investigating complaints and imposing civil monetary penalties (CMPs) for HIPAA violations (HHS 2010b). The requirements included "determining and counting violations, calculating and establishing liability for CMPs, and consideration of aggravating and mitigating circumstances." The HIPAA Enforcement Rule created a uniform compliance and enforcement mechanism that addresses all the administrative simplification regulations, including privacy, security, and transactions and code sets (Wilkinson 2006).

An HHS website provides information about the department's compliance and enforcement efforts, including HHS enforcement activities, frequency of complaint types, and corrective actions resulting from consumer complaints (HHS 2010b, 2013). Additionally, the director of the HHS OCR has authority to issue subpoenas as part of the investigation of alleged HIPAA Privacy Rule violations. Per the HHS website, as of March 31, 2013, 72,570 (91%) of 79,920 complaints had been resolved, with 7,350 (9%) remaining open. Of the 28,452 complaints investigated, corrective action was achieved in 19,306 cases (68%) and no violations were found in 9,146 cases (32%) (HHS 2013). Figure 9.9 provides a flow chart from OCR that outlines the Privacy and Security Rule Complaint Process.

HITECH has increased civil monetary penalties based on levels, or tiers, of intent and neglect (Dennis 2010). The nature and extent of both the violation and the harm are used to determine the amount assessed within each range. Currently, penalties for violations range as follows, with a cap of $1,500,000 for identical violations within each violation category (HHS 2009a):

- $100–$50,000 per violation for unknowing violations

- $1,000–$50,000 per violation if due to reasonable cause and not willful neglect

- $10,000–$50,000 per violation if due to willful neglect and corrected within 30 days of discovery

- $50,000 or more per violation if due to willful neglect and not corrected as required

Figure 9.9.   HIPAA Privacy and Security Rule Complaint Process

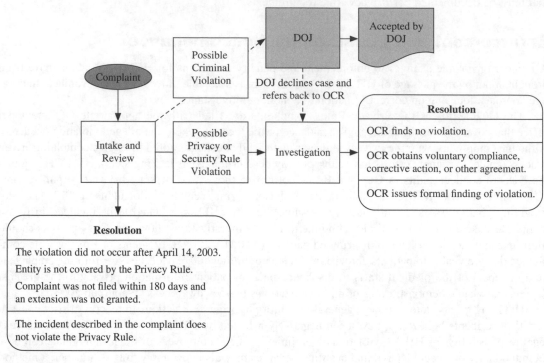

Source: HHS 2011.

The OCR may choose to pursue corrective action without assessing penalties for unknowing violations, but penalties are mandatory in all other categories. These provisions differ greatly from pre-HITECH penalties that prohibited CMPs due to reasonable cause if correction occurred within 30 days of when the CE knew or should have known of the violation (AHIMA 2009a). Penalty monies collected will support further enforcement efforts (Dennis 2010).

Privacy Advocates

As the privacy of patient information becomes more transparent to the public, privacy advocates have sprung up to support patient privacy efforts and to strengthen public awareness. Two are mentioned here. Other organizations also exist that more broadly address the issue of privacy (for example, protection of financial information).

American Health Information Management Association (AHIMA)

AHIMA is proactive both internally and externally, educating its members on privacy issues and shaping public policy and federal law to further one of the profession's central values: protecting the privacy of patient information. AHIMA serves as an instrumental privacy advocate through the functions and entities listed in figure 9.10.

Center for Democracy and Technology

Founded in 1997, the **Health Privacy Project**, a nonprofit organization that strives to raise public awareness regarding the importance of ensuring health privacy, is now part of the **Center for Democracy & Technology** (Center for Democracy & Technology n.d.). In addition to providing resources and educational materials, the organization also spotlights breaches that compromise the privacy of patient information.

Figure 9.10. AHIMA's privacy advocate functions and entities

- Policy and government relations staff
- Collaborative relationship with key privacy stakeholders, including the federal government
- Involvement with eHealth Initiative and Regional Health Information Organizations (RHIOs), addressing privacy and security concerns associated with e-HIM
- Research addressing the effectiveness of and compliance with the Privacy Rule
- Health Information Privacy and Security Week
- Advocacy Assistant on the AHIMA Web site
- Privacy workshops and seminars
- Credentials in privacy and security (Certified in Healthcare Privacy and Security [CHPS] credential and Certified in Healthcare Privacy [CHP] credential maintenance)
- Position statements regarding privacy and confidentiality of patient information
- Privacy and Security Practice Council
- Involvement in Health Information Security and Privacy Collaboration (HISPC) subcontract, with funding by Agency for Healthcare Research and Quality (AHRQ) to support 34 state projects identifying barriers that inhibit the secure flow of PHI

Check Your Understanding 9.7

Instructions: Indicate whether the following statements are true or false (T or F).

1. The Privacy Rule provides a floor, or minimum, of privacy requirements.

2. Breach notification is one type of mitigation under the Privacy Rule.

3. In order to simplify processes, individuals may be required to waive their rights under the Privacy Rule to obtain treatment or benefits eligibility.

4. Under HITECH, state attorneys general may bring civil actions in federal district court in behalf of residents believed to have been negatively affected by a HIPAA violation.

5. Enforcement of the Privacy Rule will continue to operate exclusively on a complaint-based system.

Summary

The HIM professional is and always has been an advocate and champion of health information privacy. The HIPAA Privacy Rule has not changed the values of those responsible for managing health information; rather, it has standardized a comprehensive set of requirements that incorporate those values and act to ensure the privacy of patient information and grant patient information rights. In effect since 2003, the HIPAA Privacy Rule has generated unprecedented national awareness regarding the importance of health information privacy. It is not without problems or controversy, however, including its exceptions that lessen the privacy afforded to patient information and a perceived lack of power in its enforcement. The HITECH Act of ARRA has sought to address some of those criticisms. Although it has always been the responsibility of those who manage health information to guard the values and ethics of the profession, interpreting the legal requirements as specified by the HIPAA Privacy Rule and HITECH in the context of state requirements is not an easy task. This will continue to challenge professionals responsible for managing health information for years to come.

References

AHIMA. 2009a. Analysis of health care confidentiality, privacy, and security provisions of the American Recovery and Reinvestment Act of 2009, Public Law 111-5. Chicago: AHIMA.

AHIMA. 2009b. Practice brief: Redisclosure of patient health information. *Journal of AHIMA* 80(2):51–54.

AHIMA. 2010a. Outline of the Modifications to the HIPAA Privacy, Security and Enforcement Rules under the Health Information Technology for Economic and Clinical Health Act (Title XIII of the American Recovery and Reinvestment Act of 2009). Chicago: AHIMA.

AHIMA. 2010b. HIPAA Privacy and Security training (Updated). Chicago: AHIMA.

AHIMA. 2011. *Code of Ethics*. http://www.ahima.org.

AHIMA. 2013. Analysis of Modifications to the HIPAA Privacy, Security, Enforcement, and Breach Notification Rules Under the Health Information Technology for Economic and Clinical Health Act and the Genetic Information Nondiscrimination Act; Other Modifications to the HIPAA Rules. http://www.ahima.org.

Amatayakul, M. 2001a. HIPAA on the job: Managing individual rights requirements under HIPAA privacy. *Journal of AHIMA* 72(6):16A–16D.

Amatayakul, M. 2001b. HIPAA on the job: Five steps to reading the HIPAA rules. *Journal of AHIMA* 72(8): 16A–16C.

Amatayakul, M. 2003. HIPAA on the job: Another layer of regulations: Research under HIPAA. *Journal of AHIMA* 74(1):16A–16D.

Burrington-Brown, J. 2003. Practice brief: Handling complaints and mitigation. *Journal of AHIMA* 74(10):64A–64C.

Burrington-Brown, J., and D. Wagg. 2003. Practice brief: Regulations governing research. *Journal of AHIMA* 74(3):56A–56D.

Cassidy, B. 2000. HIPAA on the job: Update on business partner/associate agreements. *Journal of AHIMA* 71(10):16A–16D.

Center for Democracy & Technology. n.d. http://www.cdt.org.

Dennis, J. 2010. *Privacy: The Impact of ARRA, HITECH, and Other Policy Initiatives*. Chicago: AHIMA.

Department of Health and Human Services. 2000. Standards for privacy of individually identifiable health information. 45 CFR Parts 160 and 164. *Federal Register* 65(250):82461–82510.

Department of Health and Human Services. 2002. Standards for privacy of individually identifiable health information; Final rule. 45 CFR Parts 160 and 164. *Federal Register* 67(157):53181–53273.

Department of Health and Human Services. 2003. Office for Civil Rights Privacy Brief: Summary of the HIPAA Privacy Rule.

Department of Health and Human Services. 2007. Office for Civil Rights. HIPAA medical privacy: National standards to protect the privacy of personal health information. http://www.hhs.gov/ocr/hipaa/.

Department of Health and Human Services. 2009a. HIPAA Administrative Simplification Enforcement. 45 CFR Parts 160. *Federal Register* 74(209):56123–56131.

Department of Health and Human Services. 2009b. Notice to the Secretary of HHS of Breach of Unsecured Protected Health Information. http://www.hhs.gov/ocr/.

Department of Health and Human Services. 2010a. Modifications to the HIPAA Privacy, Security, and Enforcement Rules under the Health Information Technology for Economic and Clinical Health Act; Proposed Rule. 45 CFR Parts 160 and 164. *Federal Register* 75(134):40868–40924.

Department of Health and Human Services. 2010b. Office for Civil Rights. HIPAA Enforcement Rule. http://www.hhs.gov/ocr/.

Department of Health and Human Services. 2011. HIPAA Privacy Rule Accounting of Disclosures Under the Health Information Technology for Economic and Clinical Health Act. 45 CFR Part 164. *Federal Register* 75 (134): 40868-40924.

Department of Health and Human Services. 2013. Office for Civil Rights. Health information privacy: numbers at a glance. http://www.hhs.gov/ocr/.

Heubusch, K. 2010. Turning 7, HIPAA tops 51,000 privacy complaints. *Journal of AHIMA:* Online extra.

Department of Justice. 2004. Freedom of Information Act Guide. http://www.usdoj.gov/.

Dougherty, M., and L. Washington. 2008. Defining and disclosing the designated record set and the legal health record. *Journal of AHIMA* 79(4):65–68.

Hughes, G. 2001a. Practice brief: Notice of information practices. *Journal of AHIMA* 72(5):64I–64M.

Hughes, G. 2001b. Practice brief: Consent for the use or disclosure of individually identifiable health information. *Journal of AHIMA* 72(5):64E–64G.

Hughes, G. 2002. Practice brief: Preemption of the HIPAA Privacy Rule. *Journal of AHIMA* 73(2):56A–56C.

Hughes, G. 2003. Practice brief: Defining the designated record set. *Journal of AHIMA* 74(1):64A–64D.

National Institutes of Health, Office of Human Subjects Research. 1979. The Belmont report: Ethical principles and guidelines for the protection of human subjects of research.

Nunn, S. 2009. Integrating ARRA: Leveraging current compliance efforts to meet the new privacy provisions. *Journal of AHIMA* 80(10):50–51.

Roth, J. 2004a. Getting "hip" to other privacy laws, part 1. *Journal of AHIMA* 75(2):50–52.

Roth, J. 2004b. Getting "hip" to other privacy laws, part 2. *Journal of AHIMA* 75(3):48–50.

Weintraub, A. 2003. Catching up with HIPAA: Managing non-compliance. *Journal of AHIMA* 74(5):67–68.

Wilkinson, W. 2006. The Office for Civil Rights and Healthcare Privacy. Remarks for the Twelfth National HIPAA Summit. Washington, DC. http://hhs.gov/ocr/.

Cases, Statutes, and Regulations Cited

21 CFR Parts 50 and 56: Prisoners, Reporting and recordkeeping requirements, Research, Safety. 1991.

42 CFR 493: Clinical Laboratory Improvement Amendments (CLIA). 1988.

45 CFR 46(a): Basic HHS Policy for Protection of Human Research Subjects. 2005.

45 CFR 46.101–46.112: Protection of Human Subjects. 2005.

45 CFR 160.103: General administrative requirements: General Provisions: Definitions. 2006.

45 CFR 160.202: General administrative requirements: Preemption of state law: Definitions. 2006.

45 CFR 160.203: General administrative requirements: Preemption of state law: General rule and exceptions. 2006.

45 CFR 164.103: Security and privacy: General provisions: Definitions. 2006.

45 CFR 164.105: Security and privacy: General provisions: Organizational requirements. 2006.

45 CFR 164.501: Privacy of individually identifiable health information: Definitions 2006.

45 CFR 164.502: Uses and disclosures of protected health information (general rules) 2006.

45 CFR 164.504: Uses and disclosures: Organizational requirements. 2006.

45 CFR 164.506: Uses and disclosures to carry out treatment, payment, and healthcare operations 2006.

45 CFR 164.508: Uses and disclosures for which authorization is required. 2006.

45 CFR 164.510: Uses and disclosures requiring an opportunity for the individual to agree or to object. 2006.

45 CFR 164.512: Uses and disclosures for which an authorization or opportunity to agree or object is not required. 2006.

45 CFR 164.514: Other requirements relating to uses and disclosures of protected health information. 2006.

45 CFR 164.520: Notice of privacy practices for protected health information. 2006.

45 CFR 164.522: Rights to request privacy protection for protected health information. 2006.

45 CFR 164.524: Access of individuals to protected health information. 2006.

45 CFR 164.526: Amendment of protected health information. 2006.

45 CFR 164.528: Accounting of disclosures of protected health information. 2006.

45 CFR 164.530: Administrative requirements. 2006.

45 CFR 165.512(e): HIPAA. 1996.

5 USC 552: Freedom of information act of 1967.

5 USC 552a (App. 3 sec. (6)(a)(4)): The privacy act of 1974.

20 USC 1232(g): Federal educational records privacy act (FERPA). 1974.

26 USC: Internal Revenue Code. 1986.

29 USC 1001 et seq.: Employee Retirement Income Security Act of 1986 (ERISA).

42 USC 6A: Public Health Service Act. 1944.

42 USC 4541–4594; 42 CFR 2.1–2.67: Drug abuse prevention, treatment, and rehabilitation act of 1972 (orig. 21 USC 1101–1800).

42 USC 4582 to 290dd-3: Comprehensive alcohol abuse and alcoholism prevention, treatment, and rehabilitation act of 1970.

American Recovery and Reinvestment Act of 2009, Title XIII—Health Information Technology, Subtitle D Sections 13400, 13402.

OH Rev. Code 3701.74: Patient or representative may request access to medical record. 2003.

Cases, Statutes, and Regulations Resources

Health Insurance Portability and Accountability Act of 1996. Public Law 104-191. Available online from http://www.cms.gov.

Appendix 9.A

Sample Notice of Privacy Practices

THIS NOTICE DESCRIBES HOW INFORMATION ABOUT YOU MAY BE USED AND DISCLOSED AND HOW YOU CAN GET ACCESS TO THIS INFORMATION. PLEASE REVIEW IT CAREFULLY.

Understanding Your Health Record/Information

Each time you visit a hospital, physician, or other healthcare provider, a record of your visit is made. Typically, this record contains your symptoms, examination and test results, diagnoses, treatment, and a plan for future care or treatment. This information, often referred to as your health or medical record, serves as a:

- basis for planning your care and treatment
- means of communication among the many health professionals who contribute to your care
- legal document describing the care you received
- means by which you or a third-party payer can verify that services billed were actually provided
- a tool in educating health professionals
- a source of data for medical research
- a source of information for public health officials charged with improving the health of the nation
- a source of data for facility planning and marketing
- a tool with which we can assess and continually work to improve the care we render and the outcomes we achieve

Understanding what is in your record and how your health information is used helps you to:

- ensure its accuracy
- better understand who, what, when, where, and why others may access your health information
- make more informed decisions when authorizing disclosure to others

Your Health Information Rights

Although your health record is the physical property of the healthcare practitioner or facility that compiled it, the information belongs to you. You have the right to:

- request a restriction on certain uses and disclosures of your information as provided by 45 CFR 164.522
- obtain a paper copy of the notice of information practices upon request
- inspect and obtain a copy of your health record as provided for in 45 CFR 164.524
- amend your health record as provided in 45 CFR 164.528
- obtain an accounting of disclosures of your health information as provided in 45 CFR 164.528
- request communications of your health information by alternative means or at alternative locations
- revoke your authorization to use or disclose health information except to the extent that action has already been taken

Our Responsibilities

This organization is required to:

- maintain the privacy of your health information
- provide you with a notice as to our legal duties and privacy practices with respect to information we collect and maintain about you

Source: Hughes, G. 2001 (May). Practice brief: Notice of information practices. *Journal of AHIMA* 72(5):64I–64M.

- abide by the terms of this notice
- notify you if we are unable to agree to a requested restriction
- accommodate reasonable requests you may have to communicate health information by alternative means or at alternative locations.

We reserve the right to change our practices and to make the new provisions effective for all protected health information we maintain. Should our information practices change, we will mail a revised notice to the address you've supplied us.

We will not use or disclose your health information without your authorization, except as described in this notice.

For More Information or to Report a Problem

If have questions and would like additional information, you may contact the director of health information management at [phone number].

If you believe your privacy rights have been violated, you can file a complaint with the director of health information management or with the secretary of Health and Human Services. There will be no retaliation for filing a complaint.

Examples of Disclosures for Treatment, Payment, and Health Operations

We will use your health information for treatment.

For example: Information obtained by a nurse, physician, or other member of your healthcare team will be recorded in your record and used to determine the course of treatment that should work best for you. Your physician will document in your record his or her expectations of the members of your healthcare team. Members of your healthcare team will then record the actions they took and their observations. In that way, the physician will know how you are responding to treatment.

We will also provide your physician or a subsequent healthcare provider with copies of various reports that should assist him or her in treating you once you're discharged from this hospital.

We will use your health information for payment.

For example: A bill may be sent to you or a third-party payer. The information on or accompanying the bill may include information that identifies you, as well as your diagnosis, procedures, and supplies used.

We will use your health information for regular health operations.

For example: Members of the medical staff, the risk or quality improvement manager, or members of the quality improvement team may use information in your health record to assess the care and outcomes in your case and others like it. This information will then be used in an effort to continually improve the quality and effectiveness of the healthcare and service we provide.

Business associates: There are some services provided in our organization through contacts with business associates. Examples include physician services in the emergency department and radiology, certain laboratory tests, and a copy service we use when making copies of your health record. When these services are contracted, we may disclose your health information to our business associate so that they can perform the job we've asked them to do and bill you or your third-party payer for services rendered. To protect your health information, however, we require the business associate to appropriately safeguard your information.

Directory: Unless you notify us that you object, we will use your name, location in the facility, general condition, and religious affiliation for directory purposes. This information may be provided to members of the clergy and, except for religious affiliation, to other people who ask for you by name.

Notification: We may use or disclose information to notify or assist in notifying a family member, personal representative, or another person responsible for your care, your location, and general condition.

Communication with family: Health professionals, using their best judgment, may disclose to a family member, other relative, close personal friend or any other person you identify, health information relevant to that person's involvement in your care or payment related to your care.

Research: We may disclose information to researchers when their research has been approved by an institutional review board that has reviewed the research proposal and established protocols to ensure the privacy of your health information.

Funeral directors: We may disclose health information to funeral directors consistent with applicable law to carry out their duties.

Organ procurement organizations: Consistent with applicable law, we may disclose health information to organ procurement organizations or other entities engaged in the procurement, banking, or transplantation of organs for the purpose of tissue donation and transplant.

Marketing: We may contact you to provide appointment reminders or information about treatment alternatives or other health-related benefits and services that may be of interest to you.

Fund raising: We may contact you as part of a fund-raising effort.

Food and Drug Administration (FDA): We may disclose to the FDA health information relative to adverse events with respect to food, supplements, product and product defects, or post marketing surveillance information to enable product recalls, repairs, or replacement.

Workers compensation: We may disclose health information to the extent authorized by and to the extent necessary to comply with laws relating to workers compensation or other similar programs established by law.

Public health: As required by law, we may disclose your health information to public health or legal authorities charged with preventing or controlling disease, injury, or disability.

Correctional institution: Should you be an inmate of a correctional institution, we may disclose to the institution or agents thereof health information necessary for your health and the health and safety of other individuals.

Law enforcement: We may disclose health information for law enforcement purposes as required by law or in response to a valid subpoena.

Federal law makes provision for your health information to be released to an appropriate health oversight agency, public health authority or attorney, provided that a work force member or business associate believes in good faith that we have engaged in unlawful conduct or have otherwise violated professional or clinical standards and are potentially endangering one or more patients, workers or the public.

Effective Date: [DATE]

Note: The above form is not meant to encompass all the various ways in which any particular facility may use health information. It is intended to get readers started insofar as developing their own notice. As with any form of this nature, the document should be reviewed and approved by legal counsel prior to implementation.

Appendix 9.B

Sample Consent for the Use and Disclosure of Health Information

I understand that as part of my healthcare, this organization originates and maintains health records describing my health history, symptoms, examination and test results, diagnoses, treatment, and any plans for future care or treatment. I understand that this information serves as:

- a basis for planning my care and treatment

- a means of communication among the many health professionals who contribute to my care

- a source of information for applying my diagnosis and surgical information to my bill

- a means by which a third-party payer can verify that services billed were actually provided

- and a tool for routine healthcare operations such as assessing quality and reviewing the competence of healthcare professionals

I understand and have been provided with a Notice of Information Practices that provides a more complete description of information uses and disclosures. I understand that I have the right to review the notice prior to signing this consent. I understand that the organization reserves the right to change their notice and practices and prior to implementation will mail a copy of any revised notice to the address I've provided. I understand that I have the right to object to the use of my health information for directory purposes. I understand that I have the right to request restrictions as to how my health information may be used or disclosed to carry out treatment, payment, or healthcare operations and that the organization is not required to agree to the restrictions requested. I understand that I may revoke this consent in writing, except to the extent that the organization has already take action in reliance thereon.

❏ I request the following restrictions to the use or disclosure of my health information.

_____

_____   _____
Signature of Patient or Legal Representative   Witness

_____   _____
Date   Notice Effective Date or Version

❏ Accepted   ❏ Denied

_____   _____
Signature   Title   Date

Source: Hughes, G. 2001 (May). Practice brief: Consent for the use or disclosure of individually identifiable health information. *Journal of AHIMA* 72(5):64E–64G.

Appendix 9.C

Sample Authorization to Use or Disclose Health Information

Patient Name: _____

Health Record Number: _____

Date of Birth: _____

1. I authorize the use or disclosure of the above named individual's health information as described below.

2. The following individual(s) or organization(s) are authorized to make the disclosure:

3. The type of information to be used or disclosed is as follows (check the appropriate boxes and include other information where indicated):

   ❑ problem list

   ❑ medication list

   ❑ list of allergies

   ❑ immunization records

   ❑ most recent history

   ❑ most recent discharge summary

   ❑ lab results (please describe the dates or types of lab tests you would like disclosed):

   _____

   ❑ x-ray and imaging reports (please describe the dates or types of x-rays or images you would like disclosed): _____

   ❑ consultation reports from (please supply doctors' names): _____

   ❑ entire record

   ❑ other (please describe): _____

4. I understand that the information in my health record may include information relating to sexually transmitted disease, acquired immunodeficiency syndrome (AIDS), or human immunodeficiency virus (HIV). It may also include information about behavioral or mental health services, and treatment for alcohol and drug abuse.

5. The information identified above may be used by or disclosed to the following individuals or organization(s):

   Name: _____

   Address: _____

   Name: _____

   Address: _____

Source: Hughes, G. 2002 (October). Practice brief: Required content for authorizations to disclose. *Journal of AHIMA*.

6. This information for which I am authorizing disclosure will be used for the following purpose:

❑ my personal records

❑ sharing with other healthcare providers as needed

❑ other (please describe): _____

7. I understand that I have a right to revoke this authorization at any time. I understand that if I revoke this authorization, I must do so in writing and present my written revocation to the health information management department. I understand that the revocation will not apply to information that has already been released in response to this authorization. I understand that the revocation will not apply to my insurance company when the law provides my insurer with the right to contest a claim under my policy.

8. This authorization will expire (insert date or event): _____

If I fail to specify an expiration date or event, this authorization will expire six months from the date on which it was signed.

9. I understand that once the above information is disclosed, it may be redisclosed by the recipient and the information may not be protected by federal privacy laws or regulations.

10. I understand authorizing the use or disclosure of the information identified above is voluntary. I need not sign this form to ensure healthcare treatment.

_____   _____
Signature of Patient or Legal Representative   Date

If signed by legal representative, relationship to patient _____

_____   _____
Signature of Witness   Date

Distribution: Original to provider; copy to patient; copy to accompany use or disclosure

Note: The types of documents listed on the authorization form may need to be modified depending on the particular health care setting. Authorizations for marketing need to disclose whether remuneration was received by the covered entity. This form was developed by AHIMA for discussion purposes only. It should not be used without review by your organization's legal counsel to ensure compliance with other federal and state laws and regulations.

Appendix 9.D

Individual Rights under the HIPAA Privacy Rule

Source: Adapted from Amatayakul 2001a and AHIMA 2009a.

Patient Rights at a Glance

Right	Request	Acceptance	Termination	Timeliness	Fee	Denial	Review
Right to request restriction of uses and disclosures	Provider must permit request, but does not have to be in writing.	Provider generally not required to agree, but if accepted, must not violate restriction except for emergency care. However, requests must be complied with (unless otherwise required by law) if disclosure would be to a health plan for payment or operations purposes and has been paid for the service or item completely out of pocket.	Provider may terminate if individual agrees or requests in writing, or oral agreement is documented. Termination only applies to information created or received after the individual has been informed. Restrictions cannot be terminated relative to disclosures to a health plan if the item or service has been paid for In full other than by the health plan out of pocket.	There is no provision for addressing timeliness.	There is no provision for a fee.	There are no requirements associated with denying restriction.	Not applicable
Right to receive confidential communications	Provider may require written request for receiving communications by alternative means or locations.	Provider must accommodate reasonable requests and may condition how payment will be handled but may not require explanation.	There is no provision for termination.	There is no provision for addressing timeliness.	There is no provision for a fee.	Not applicable	Not applicable
Right of access to information	Provider must permit request for copying and inspection and may, upon notice, require requests in writing. Provider may supply a summary or explanation of information, instead, if individual agrees in advance. Covered entities with EHRs must make information available electronically or must send it electronically upon the individual's request.	Provider may deny access without opportunity for review if information is: psychotherapy notes, compiled for legal proceeding, subject to CLIA, about inmate and could cause harm, subject of research to which denial of access has been agreed, subject to Privacy Act, or obtained from someone else in confidence. Provider may deny access with opportunity to review if licensed professional determines access may endanger life or safety, there is reference to another person and access could cause harm, or request made by personal representative who may cause harm. The covered entity must provide the individual with access to PHI in the form and format requested, if readily producible as such; if not readily available, must be provided in readable hard copy or other form and format agreed upon by the covered entity and the individual. The individual may direct the covered entity to transmit an electronic copy of their information in the DRS to an other entity or person. Covered entities must ensure reasonable safeguards are in place to protect the ePHI in transit.	Individuals have right of access for as long as information is maintained in designated record set.	Provider must act upon a request within 30 days. If information is not maintained on site, provider may extend by no more than 30 days if individual is notified of reasons for delay and given date for access.	Provider may impose reasonable, cost-based fee for copying, postage, and preparing an explanation or summary.	If access is denied, provider must provide timely written explanation in plain language, containing basis for denial, review rights if applicable, description of how to file a complaint, and source of information not maintained by provider if known. Provider must also give individual access to any part of information not covered under grounds for denial.	An individual may request a review of a denial by a different healthcare professional.

Patient Rights at a Glance

Right	Request	Acceptance	Termination	Timeliness	Fee	Denial	Review
Right to amend information	Provider must permit requests to amend a designated record set and may, upon notice, require request in writing and a reason.	If amendment is accepted, provider must append or link to record set and obtain and document identification and agreement to have provider notify relevant persons with which amendment needs to be shared. Provider may deny amendment if information was not created by the provider unless individual provides reasonable basis that originator is no longer available to act on request, is not part of designated record set, would not be available for access, or is accurate and complete.	Amendment applies for as long as information is maintained in designated record set.	Provider must act upon a request within 60 days of receipt. If unable to act on request within 60 days, provider may extend time by no more than 30 days provided individual is notified of reasons for delay and given date to amend.	There is no provision for a fee.	If amendment is denied, provider must provide timely written explanation in plain language, containing basis for denial, right to submit written statement of disagreement, right to request provider include request and denial with any future disclosures of information that is subject of amendment, and description of how to file a complaint.	Provider must accept written statement of disagreement (of limited length). Provider may prepare written rebuttal and must copy individual. Provider must append or link request, denial, disagreement; and rebuttal to record and include such or accurate summary with any subsequent disclosure. If no written disagreement, provider must include request and denial, or summary, in subsequent disclosures only if individual has requested such action.
Right to accounting of disclosures (subject to revision if "access report" is made final)	Provider must provide individual with written accounting including date of disclosure, name and address of recipient, description of information disclosed, purpose of disclosure or copy of individual's written authorization or other request for disclosure.	Provider must provide accounting and retain documentation of written accounting of disclosures of PHI made in three years prior to date of request, except for disclosures (1) to carry out treatment, payment, and healthcare operations (this exception will not apply to covered entities with EHRs); (2) to the individuals themselves; (3) incident to a use or disclosure otherwise permitted or required; (4) pursuant to an authorization; (5) for the facility's directory or to persons involved in the individual's care or other notification purposes; (6) for national security or intelligence purposes; (7) to correctional institutions or law enforcement as permitted; (8) as part of a limited data set; or (9) that occurred prior to the compliance date for the covered entity. As proposed in May 2011 (HHS 2011), uses and TPO disclosures would be excluded from an accounting. Instead, an access report would be available from covered entities with EHRs. This report would allow individuals to see a record of every person who viewed the individual's DRS during the previous three years. This is pending.	Not applicable.	Provider must act upon request within 60 days of receipt. If unable to provide accounting, provider may extend time by no more than 30 days provided individual is notified of reasons for delay. (A 30-day response period, with one 30-day extension, is proposed per HITECH.)	First accounting in any 12-month period must be provided without charge. A reasonable, cost-based fee may be charged for subsequent accountings in 12-month period if individual is notified in advance.	Provider must temporarily suspend right to receive an accounting of disclosures to health oversight agency or law enforcement official if agency or official provides written statement that accounting would impede their activities.	There is no provision for review of temporary suspension.

Source: Adapted from Amatayakul 2001a and AHIMA 2009a.

Chapter 10

The HIPAA Security Rule

Rebecca B. Reynolds, EdD, MHA, RHIA, FAHIMA; Melanie S. Brodnik, PhD, RHIA, FAHIMA; and Keith Olenik, MA, RHIA, CHP

Learning Objectives

- Describe the purposes of the HIPAA Security Rule
- Explain the sources of law from which the HIPAA Security Rule is derived
- Discuss the differences between the HIPAA Security Rule and the Privacy Rule
- Identify entities covered by the HIPAA Security Rule and discuss how HITECH affects business associates
- Discuss business processes to ensure security compliance
- Summarize the key components of the Security Rule
- Explain the safeguards of the HIPAA Security Rule

Key Terms

Administrative safeguards
American Recovery and
    Reinvestment Act of 2009
    (ARRA)
Automatic log-off
Business associate (BA)
Compliance
Confidentiality
Covered entities (CE)

Electronic protected health
    information (ePHI)
Encryption
Health Insurance Portability
    and Accountability Act
    (HIPAA) of 1996
Health Information Technology
    for Economic and Clinical
    Health (HITECH)

Integrity
Person or entity authentication
Physical safeguards
Security
Security officer or chief
    security officer
Technical safeguards

Introduction

The **Health Insurance Portability and Accountability Act** (HIPAA), signed into law April 21, 1996, requires the use of standards for electronic transactions containing healthcare data and information as a way to improve the efficiency and effectiveness of the healthcare system. Title II of the law was designed to protect not only the privacy of healthcare data and information but also the security of the data and information. **Security** refers to protecting information from loss, unauthorized access, or misuse, along with protecting its confidentiality. This chapter introduces the HIPAA Security Rule, which closely aligns with the Privacy Rule. Although the rules complement each other, the Privacy Rule governs the privacy of protected health information (PHI) regardless of the medium in which the information resides, whereas the Security Rule governs PHI that is transmitted by or maintained in some form of electronic media (that is, **electronic protected health information**, or **ePHI**). The chapter begins with a discussion of the purposes of the rule, its source of law, scope, and to whom the law applies. The chapter suggests a process for complying with the rule and outlines the five key components of the rule. Where appropriate, the chapter also discusses changes to the Security Rule as a result of the **Health Information Technology for Economic and Clinical Health** (HITECH) provisions of the **American Recovery and Reinvestment Act of 2009** (ARRA). It concludes with a discussion of the role of a security officer, how the rule is enforced, and the penalties for noncompliance with the rule.

Purposes of the HIPAA Security Rule

The security standards in HIPAA were developed for two primary purposes: to implement appropriate security safeguards to protect electronic healthcare information that may be at risk, and to protect an individual's health information while permitting appropriate access and use of that information. The standards ultimately promote the use of electronic health information in the industry, which is an important goal of HIPAA (HHS 2007a). The HIPAA Security Rule requires covered entities (CEs) to ensure the integrity and confidentiality of information, to protect against any reasonably anticipated threats or risks to the security and integrity of information, and to protect against unauthorized uses or disclosures of information. As a reminder, CEs are the individuals and organizations that must comply with HIPAA, as discussed below under *Applicability*. The Security Rule defines **integrity** as data or information that has not been altered or destroyed in an unauthorized manner and **confidentiality** as 'data or information that is not made available or disclosed to unauthorized persons or processes (45 CFR 164.304). Ultimately, the Security Rule seeks to ensure that CEs implement basic safeguards to protect ePHI from unauthorized access, alteration, deletion, and transmission, while at the same time ensuring data or information is accessible and usable on demand by authorized individuals.

Source of Law

As discussed in chapter 9, HIPAA (of which security is only one piece) was enacted by Congress in 1996 and became federal statutory law. The Department of Health and Human Services (HHS) published the final Security Rule in the *Federal Register*, Health Insurance Reform, Security Standards, Final Rule (45 CFR Parts 160, 162, 164(a), and 164(c)) on February 20, 2003 (HHS 2003). The rule established security standards to protect ePHI. CEs were expected to be in **compliance** with the rule by April 20, 2005, and small health plans by April 20, 2006. Changes to the HIPAA Privacy and Security Rules were passed in February 2009 as part of the HITECH Act of the ARRA Act of 2009 (ARRA 2009). The HITECH Act was designed to promote widespread adoption of electronic health records (EHRs) and electronic health information exchanges (HIEs) to improve patient care and reduce healthcare costs. To achieve these goals, HITECH identified requirements to strengthen the privacy and security protections under HIPAA to ensure patients and healthcare providers that their electronic health information is kept private and secure. In July 2010 and May 2011, HHS published proposed rules to implement some of the HITECH provisions and modify other HIPAA requirements (HHS 2010a). The 2010 proposed rule went into effect with publication of the January 2013 final rule titled "Modifications to the HIPAA Privacy, Security, Enforcement, and Breach Notification Rules Under the Health Information Technology for Economic and Clinical Health Act and the Genetic Information Nondiscrimination Act; Other Modifications to the HIPAA Rules." The 2011 proposed rule is still pending (AHIMA 2013).

Until 2009, the Centers for Medicare and Medicaid Services (CMS) was responsible for oversight and enforcement of the Security Rule, while the Office of Civil Rights (OCR) within HHS oversaw and enforced the Privacy Rule. In the latter half of 2009, authority for oversight and enforcement of the HIPAA Privacy and Security Rules was consolidated under the OCR (HHS 2009a). CMS continues to have authority for enforcement of administrative simplification regulations other than privacy and security (preventing healthcare fraud and abuse, and medical liability reform).

Scope and Anatomy of the Security Rule

HIPAA consists of five titles. The Security Rule is one of five administrative simplification provisions in the law (privacy, security, transaction code sets, unique national provider identifiers, and enforcement). The scope of the Security Rule is to protect individually identifiable health information that is transmitted by or maintained in any form of electronic media. The Security Rule defines electronic media to mean electronic storage media including memory devices in computer hard drives and any removable or transportable digital memory medium, such as magnetic-type storage or disk, optical disk, or digital memory card; or transmission media used to exchange information already in electronic storage media, such as the intranet, extranet, leased lines, dial-up lines, private networks, and physical, removable, transportable electronic storage media (45 CFR 160.103).

Congress published the first set of security standards for public comment in 1998. At that time, many of the public comments concluded that the rules were too prescriptive and not flexible enough. As a result, the final rule includes standards defined in general terms, focusing on what *should* be done rather than *how* it should be done. Efforts were made to make the rule technology-neutral and flexible so that CEs could choose the security measures that best meet their technological capabilities and operational needs to comply with the standards. The flexibility and scalability of the standards make it possible for any CE, regardless of size, to comply with the Rule.

The Security Rule itself comprises five general rules and a number of standards that encompass (a) general requirements; (b) flexibility of approach; (c) standards related to administrative, physical, and technical safeguards; organizational requirements; policies, procedures, and documentation requirements; (d) implementation specifications; and (e) maintenance of security measures (see figure 10.1), all of which will be discussed later in the chapter.

History and Comparison with Existing Laws

Until HIPAA was enacted, there were no generally accepted security standards for protecting health information. There were, however, a number of state and federal initiatives that addressed privacy, as discussed in chapter 9. With increased reliance on the use of information technology to electronically capture, store, retrieve, transmit, and exchange health information, Congress recognized the need for national security standards, resulting in the HIPAA Security Rule. The Privacy and Security Rules work in tandem to protect health information. The Privacy Rule set standards for how PHI should be controlled by establishing uses and disclosures that are authorized or required and what rights patients have in regard to their health information.

The Security Rule was written to protect ePHI and to provide guidance for how electronic health information can be accessed appropriately. There are two primary distinctions between the HIPAA Security Rule and the HIPAA Privacy Rule:

- **Electronic vs. paper vs. oral:** The Privacy Rule applies to all forms of PHI, whether electronic, written, or oral. In contrast, the narrower Security Rule covers only PHI that is in electronic form. It does not cover paper or verbal PHI.

Figure 10.1. HIPAA Title II Administrative Simplification—Security Rule

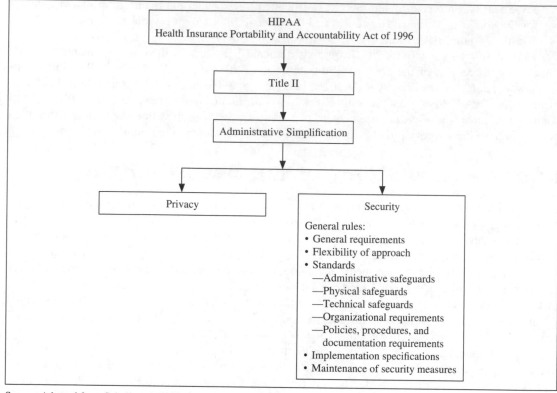

Source: Adapted from Scholl et al. 2008.

- **"Safeguard" requirement in Privacy Rule:** The Privacy Rule contains provisions that require CEs to adopt administrative, physical, and technical safeguards for PHI. While Security Rule compliance was required in 2005 at the earliest, actions taken by CEs to implement the Privacy Rule may have addressed some security requirements. However, the Security Rule provides far more comprehensive and detailed security requirements (HHS 2007a, 4).

For example, to address the growing concern for the use of devices and tools that enable access to or use of ePHI outside the CE's physical purview, HHS issued a HIPAA Security Guidance report on remote access (HHS 2006a). The report lists risks of offsite use or access and possible risk management strategies for identified risks. It also contains potential security strategies for conducting business activities through (1) portable media/devices (such as USB flash drives) that store ePHI and (2) offsite access or transport of ePHI via laptops, personal digital assistants (PDAs), home computers, and other personal equipment. The report also encourages rigor in policy and procedure development for offsite use or access to ePHI (HHS 2006a).

Applicability

The Security Rule applies to individuals or organizations identified as CEs and, with the recent enactment of the HITECH provisions, **business associates** (BAs) and the subcontractors of BAs. The Security Rule applies to the following **covered entities** (CEs):

- Covered healthcare providers—Any provider of medical or other healthcare services or supplies that transmits any health information in electronic form in connection with a transaction for which HHS has adopted a standard

- Health plans—Any individual or group plan that provides or pays the cost of healthcare (for example, a health insurance issuer or Medicare and Medicaid programs)

- Healthcare clearinghouses—Public or private entities that process another entity's healthcare transactions from a standard format to a nonstandard format or vice versa

Prior to enactment of the HITECH provisions, BAs were not held to the same standards as CEs in regard to protection of health information. BAs became BAs by contract only, not by virtue of the types of functions they carried out. Further, they were only obligated to follow the requirements set forth in their BA agreement or contract with a CE. HITECH moved to correct this weakness and now has made BAs subject to compliance with the Security Rule provisions mandating administrative, physical, and technical safeguards, in addition to adherence to the terms of their BA agreements. They must also adhere to Privacy Rule requirements, which were discussed in chapter 9. BAs that violate the provisions are subject to civil and criminal penalties (Dennis 2010).

The definition of a BA has been revised to include subcontractors of BAs, who must also follow the Security Rule or be held liable for violations. BAs must execute BA agreements with their subcontractors as well (HHS 2010a). In addition, the definition of a BA has been expanded to include entities that manage the exchange of PHI through networks, including patient locator services, e-prescribing gateways, others that provide data transmission services of PHI to a CE and require routine access to such information, or vendors that contract with CEs to offer personal health records to patients as part of the CEs' EHRs (HHS 2010a). Thus, the Security Rule now applies to a broader range of individuals and organizations (CEs, BAs, and BA subcontractors) in an effort to further protect the privacy and confidentiality of ePHI.

Ensuring Security Compliance

Security is not a one-time project but an ongoing process that requires constant analysis as the business practices of the CE and BA change, technologies advance, and new systems are implemented. To assist CEs, and now BAs, in implementing the Security Rule, the following process is recommended (HHS 2007a):

1. Assess current security, risks, and gaps
2. Develop an implementation plan
3. Implement solutions
4. Document decisions
5. Reassess periodically

CEs and BAs must decide which security measures to implement, using a risk analysis to determine circumstances that leave them open to unauthorized access and disclosure of ePHI. An ongoing security analysis will assess what security measures are already in place and what measures are still necessary. Compliance with the Privacy and Security Rules should be included in the organization's compliance assurance program. More information about corporate compliance programs is included in chapter 15.

A CE or BA should also conduct a financial analysis to determine the cost of compliance since implementing the Security Rule may be a challenge for a CE and especially for a BA who is new to the rule. Appendix 10.A provides useful information related to the planning and evaluation of a security program (AHIMA 2010). Figure 10.2 provides a summary of the main components that comprise the checklist. In addition, in 2003 the Centers for Medicare and Medicaid Services (CMS) published a series of educational documents called the HIPAA Information Series to assist with the implementation

Figure 10.2. Key components of an information security checklist

• Access control and management	• Mobile and portable device security
• Audit and accountability	• Personnel security procedures
• Awareness and training	• Physical and environmental protection
• Business associates and other nonemployees	• Policies, procedures, and plans
• Computer workstation	• Remote access
• Contingency and disaster recovery planning	• Risk analysis and management
• Incident reporting and response	• Transmission security
• Media protection and controls	

Source: AHIMA 2010.

of HIPAA requirements (CMS 2003). Additional educational papers specifically tailored to the Security Rule and implementation requirements were published by CMS in 2007 but now reside on the HHS ORC website (HHS n.d.).

Check Your Understanding 10.1

Instructions: Indicate whether the following statements are true or false (T or F).

1. The Security Rule requires CEs to ensure the integrity and legality of patient information.

2. The goal of the Security Rule is to ensure that patient information is protected from unauthorized access, alteration, deletion, and transmission.

3. CMS is the enforcement agency for the Security Rule.

4. CEs can decide to comply with only the Privacy Rule and don't have to comply with the Security Rule.

5. Only healthcare providers are required to comply with the Security Rule.

Key Components of the Security Rule

In this section of the chapter, key components of the Security Rule are presented, including modifications to the rule as a result of the HITECH Act. The HIPAA Security Rule consists of five general rules (164.306) that encompass (a) general requirements, (b) flexibility of approach, (c) standards, (d) implementation specifications, and (e) maintenance of security measures. Each of the general rules will be discussed.

Section (a), General Requirements, consists of four actions that a CE and a BA must take:

1. Ensure the confidentiality, integrity, and availability of all ePHI created, received, maintained, or transmitted by the CE and BA

2. Protect the security or integrity of ePHI from any reasonably anticipated threats or hazards

3. Protect against any reasonably anticipated uses or disclosures of ePHI not permitted or required under the Privacy Rule

4. Ensure compliance with the Security Rule by its workforce

Section (b), Flexibility of Approach, allows a CE and a BA to implement the standards and their implementation specifications reasonably and appropriately. The section lists four factors to be taken into account when deciding on the most appropriate security measures:

1. The CE's or BA's size, complexity, and capabilities

2. The security capabilities of the CE's or BA's hardware and software

3. The costs of security measures

4. The probability and criticality of potential risks to ePHI

Section (c), Standards, requires CEs or BAs to comply with the standards as found in 45 CFR 164.308–316 and BAs to comply with all standards except 164.314, Organizational Requirements. The standards are divided into five categories:

1. Administrative Safeguards (164.308)

2. Physical Safeguards (164.310)

3. Technical Safeguards (164.312)

4. Organizational Requirements (164.314)

5. Policies, Procedures, and Documentation (164.316)

The specific standards are discussed later in this chapter. The safeguards outline contains an overlap in the sections. For example, contingency plans are covered under both administrative and physical safeguards, and access controls are addressed in several standards and specifications.

Section (d), Implementation Specifications, contains detailed instructions for implementing a particular standard. Specifications are either required or addressable. Some standards include all the necessary information for implementation and are required to be implemented as published in the Security Rule. A required specification must be present for the CE or BA to be in compliance. Other standards are considered "addressable implementation specifications" to provide the CE or BA flexibility. The CE or BA is in compliance with an addressable specification if it

1. Implements the addressable specification as written, or

2. Implements an alternative, or

3. Documents that the risk for which the addressable implementation specification was provided either does not exist in the organization or exists with a negligible probability of occurrence.

The Security Rule requires CEs and BAs to evaluate their risks and vulnerabilities and implement policies and procedures to address them. Based on the CE's or BA's risk assessment, the CE or BA must address how it plans to comply with the standards. A CE or BA may decide not to implement an addressable standard. Some literature suggests that appropriate security protections vary based on the impact of the security measure on the individual's job and the type of healthcare organization (for example, single-entity versus multiple-hospital system) (Stevenson and Valenta 2009). The HIPAA Security paper "Guidance on Risk Analysis Requirements under HIPAA Security Rule" outlines the scope of a risk analysis and is a reference for CEs and BAs to determine their level of risk (HHS 2010b). Another resource is the HIPAA Security Series "Basics of Risk Analysis and Risk Management" (HHS 2007b).

Section (e), Maintenance, requires a continuing review of the reasonableness and appropriateness of a CE's or BA's security measures. It requires a CE or BA to review and modify security measures if necessary and to update documentation of such measures.

Security Rule Safeguards and Requirements

The HIPAA Security Rule's third general rule, Standards, is divided into five categories. Three standards are identified as safeguards (administrative, physical, and technical); the remaining two deal with organizational requirements; and policies, procedures, and documentation. An overview of the standards is found below. Implementation specifications that are required are marked with **R**, and those that are addressable are marked with **A**. HHS OCR offers a group of educational papers to assist CEs and now BAs with implementing the Security Rule, along with the HIPAA Security Guidance reports (referenced earlier) for risk analysis and remote use of and access to ePHI (HHS n.d.).

Administrative Safeguards (614.308)

There are nine **administrative safeguard** standards (see table 10.1) (HHS 2007c):

1. *Security management process (164.308 (a)(1))* requires the implementation of policies and procedures to prevent, detect, contain, and correct security violations. There are four implementation specifications in this section:

   — Risk analysis **R**—must conduct an accurate and thorough assessment of potential risks and vulnerabilities to the confidentiality, integrity, and availability of ePHI

   — Risk management **R**—must implement security measures that reduce risks and vulnerabilities to a reasonable and appropriate level to comply with the security standards

   — Sanction policy **R**—must apply appropriate sanctions against workforce members who fail to comply with their security policies and procedures

   — Information system activity review **R**—must implement procedures to regularly review records of information system activity, such as audit logs, access reports, and security incident tracking reports

2. *Assigned security responsibility (164.308 (a)(2))* requires the identification of the security official responsible for overseeing development of the organization's security policies and procedures. There are no implementation specifications with this standard. **R**

3. *Workforce security (164.308)(a)(3))* requires the implementation of policies and procedures to ensure that all members of its workforce have appropriate access to ePHI and to prevent those workforce members who do not have access from obtaining access. There are three implementation specifications in this standard:

   — Authorization and/or supervision **A**—must have procedures for ensuring that the workforce working with ePHI has adequate authorization and/or supervision

   — Workforce clearance procedures **A**—there must be a procedure to determine what access is appropriate for the workforce

   — Termination procedures **A**—there must be a procedure for terminating access to ePHI when a workforce member is no longer employed or responsibilities change

4. *Information access management (164.308)(a)(4)* requires the implementation of policies and procedures for authorizing access to ePHI. There are three implementation specifications within this standard:

   — Isolating healthcare clearinghouse functions **R**—may or may not apply to all healthcare organizations but may apply to a CE or BA that is a provider and also submits claims for other providers

   — Access authorization **A**—must have policies and procedures for granting access to ePHI through a workstation, transaction, program, or other process

Table 10.1. Administrative safeguards

Standard	Section	Implementation Specifications R = Required, A = Addressable	
1. Security Management Process	164.308(a)(1)	Risk Analysis	R
		Risk Management	R
		Sanction Policy	R
		Information System Activity Review	R
2. Assigned Security Responsibility	164.308(a)(2)		R
3. Workforce Security	164.308(a)(3)	Authorization and/or Supervision	A
		Workforce Clearance Procedures	A
		Termination Procedures	A
4. Information Access Management	164.308(a)(4)	Isolating Healthcare Clearinghouse Functions	R
		Access Authorization	A
		Access Establishment and Modification	A
5. Security Awareness Training	164.308(a)(5)	Security Reminders	A
		Protection from Malicious Software	A
		Log-In Monitoring	A
		Password Management	A
6. Security Incident Reporting	164.308(a)(6)	Response and Reporting	R
7. Contingency Plan	164.308(a)(7)	Data Backup Plan	R
		Disaster Recovery Plan	R
		Emergency Mode Operation Plan	R
		Testing and Revision Procedures	A
		Applications and Data Criticality Analysis	A
8. Evaluation	164.308(a)(8)		R
9. Business Associate Contracts & Other Arrangements	164.308(b)(1)	Written Contract or Other Arrangement	R

Source: HHS 2007b.

— Access establishment and modification **A**—must have policies and procedures (based on the access authorization) to establish, document, review, and modify a user's right to access a workstation, transaction, program, or process

5. *Security awareness training (164.308)(a)(5)* requires the implementation of awareness and training programs for all members of its workforce:

— Security reminders **A**—should conduct periodic security updates

— Protection from malicious software **A**—should have procedures for guarding against, detecting, and reporting malicious software

— Log-in monitoring **A**—should have procedures for monitoring log-in attempts and reporting discrepancies

— Password management **A**—should have procedures for creating, changing, and safeguarding passwords

6. *Security incident reporting (164.308)(a)(6)* requires the implementation of policies and procedures to address security incidents:

— Response and reporting **R**—identify and respond to suspect or known security incidents; mitigate, to extent practicable, harmful effects of security incidents that are known to the CE or BA; and document security incidents and their outcomes

7. *Contingency plan (164.308)(a)(7)* includes five implementation specifications:

— Data backup plan **R**—must have procedures to create and maintain an exact retrievable copy of ePHI

— Disaster recovery plan **R**—must include procedures to restore any lost data

— Emergency mode operation plan **R**—must have procedures that provide for the continuation of critical business processes needed to protect ePHI while operating in emergency mode

— Testing and revision procedures **A**—should have a procedure to test and modify all contingency plans periodically

— Applications and data criticality analysis **A**—should assess the relative criticality of specific applications and data in support of contingency plans

8. *Evaluation (164.308)(a)(8)* requires the periodic performance of technical and nontechnical evaluations in response to environmental or operational changes affecting the security of ePHI. **R**

9. *Business associate contracts and other arrangements (164.308)(b)*

— CE may permit a BA to create, receive, maintain, or transmit ePHI on the CE's behalf only if the CE obtains satisfactory assurances in accordance with 164.314(a) that the BA will appropriately safeguard the information. A CE is not required to obtain such assurances from a BA that is a subcontractor.

— BA may permit a BA that is a subcontractor to create, receive, maintain, or transmit ePHI on the BA's behalf only if the BA obtains satisfactory assurances that the subcontractor will appropriately safeguard the information.

— Written contract or other arrangement R—must document satisfactory assurances through a written contract or other arrangement with the business associate that meets the applicable requirements of the contract

Physical Safeguards (614.310)

There are four **physical safeguard** standards (see table 10.2) (HHS 2007d):

1. *Facility access controls (164.310)(a)(1)* requires the implementation of policies and procedures to limit physical access to its electronic information systems and the facilities in which they are housed to authorized users. There are four implementation specifications within this standard:

— Contingency operations **A**—should have procedures to allow facility access to support the restoration of lost data under the disaster recovery plan and emergency mode operations plan

— Facility security plan **A**—must have policies and procedures to safeguard the facility and equipment from unauthorized access, tampering, and theft

Table 10.2. Physical safeguards

Standard	Section	Implementation Specifications R = Required, A = Addressable	
1. Facility Access Controls	164.310(a)(1)	Contingency Operations	A
		Facility Security Plan	A
		Access Control and Validation Procedures	A
		Maintenance Records	A
2. Workstation Use	164.310(b)		R
3. Workstation Security	164.310(c)		R
4. Device and Media Controls	164.310(d)(1)	Disposal	R
		Media Reuse	R
		Accountability	A
		Data Backup and Storage	A

Source: HHS 2007c.

— Access control and validation procedures **A**—should have procedures to control and validate access to facilities based on users' roles or functions

— Maintenance records **A**—should have policies and procedures to document repairs and modifications to the physical components of a facility as they relate to security

2. *Workstation use (164.310)(b)* requires the implementation of policies and procedures that specify the proper functions to be performed, the manner in which those functions are to be performed, and the physical attributes of the surroundings of a specific workstation or class of workstation that can be used to access ePHI. **R**

3. *Workstation security (164.310)(c)* requires the implementation of physical safeguards for all workstations that are used to access ePHI and to restrict access to authorized users. **R**

4. *Device and media controls (164.310)(d)(1)* requires the implementation of policies and procedures for the removal of hardware and electronic media that contain ePHI into and out of a facility, as well as movement within a facility. There are four implementation specifications with this standard:

— Disposal **R**—must have policies and procedures for the final disposition of ePHI and/or hardware or electronic media on which it is stored

— Media reuse **R**—must have procedures for removal of ePHI from electronic media before the media can be reused

— Accountability **A**—must maintain a record of movements of hardware and electronic media and any person responsible for it

— Data backup and storage **A**—must create a retrievable, exact copy of ePHI, when needed, before movement of equipment

Technical Safeguards (164.312)

There are five **technical safeguard** standards (see table 10.3) (HHS 2007e):

1. *Access control (164.312)(a)(1)* requires the implementation of technical policies and procedures for electronic information systems that maintain ePHI to allow access only to those

Table 10.3. Technical safeguards

Standard	Section	Implementation Specifications R = Required, A = Addressable	
1. Access Control	164.312(a)(1)	Unique User Identification	R
		Emergency Access Procedure	R
		Automatic Log-off	A
		Encryption and Decryption	A
2. Audit Controls	164.312(b)		R
3. Integrity	164.312(c)(1)	Mechanism to Authenticate Electronic Protected Health Information	A
4. Person or Entity Authentication	164.312(d)		R
5. Transmission Security	164.312(e)(1)	Integrity Controls	A
		Encryption	A

Source: HHS 2007c.

persons or software programs that have been granted access rights as specified in the administrative safeguards. There are four implementation specifications with this standard:

— Unique user identification **R**—must assign a unique name or number for identifying and tracking user identity

— Emergency access procedure **R**—must establish procedures for obtaining necessary ePHI in an emergency

— Automatic log-off **A**—must implement electronic processes that terminate an electronic session after a predetermined time of inactivity

— **Encryption** and decryption **A**—should implement a mechanism to encrypt and decrypt ePHI as needed

2. *Audit controls (164.312)(b)* requires the implementation of hardware, software, and/or procedures that record and examine activity in the information systems that contain ePHI. **R**

3. *Integrity (164.312)(c)(1)* requires the implementation of policies and procedures to protect ePHI from improper alteration or destruction and a corroborating electronic mechanism. **A**

4. *Person or entity authentication (164.312)(d)* requires the implementation of procedures to verify that a person or entity seeking access to ePHI is the person or entity they claim to be. **R**

5. *Transmission security (164.312)(e)(1)* requires the implementation of technical measures to guard against unauthorized access to ePHI that is transmitted across a network. There are two implementation specifications with this standard:

— Integrity controls **A**—must implement security measures to ensure that electronically transmitted ePHI is not improperly modified without detection

— Encryption **A**—should encrypt ePHI whenever it is deemed appropriate

Organizational Requirements (164.314)

Organizational requirements include two standards (see table 10.4) (HHS 2007f):

Table 10.4. Organizational requirements

Standard	Section	Implementation Specifications R = Required, A = Addressable	
1. Business Associate Contracts or Other Arrangements	164.314(a)(1)	Business Associate	R
		Other Arrangements	R
2. Group Health Plans	164.314(b)(1)	Implementation Specifications	R

Source: HHS 2007e.

1. *Business associate contracts or other arrangements (164.314)(a)(1)* as required by 164.308(b) (4) must meet the requirements of (a)(2)(i-iii) as applicable. There are three implementation specifications:

   — Business associate contracts **R**—contract must provide that BA complies with applicable requirements of subpart and ensure that subcontractors that create, receive, maintain, or transmit ePHI on behalf of BA agree to comply with the applicable requirements by entering into a contract or arrangement that complies with this section; must report to CE any security incident of which it becomes aware, including breaches of unsecured PHI

   — Other arrangements **R**—CE is in compliance if it has another arrangement in place that meets requirements of 164.504(e)(3)

   — Business associate contracts with subcontractors **R**—requirements as previously required between a CE and a BA apply to the contract or arrangement between a BA and a subcontractor in the same manner

2. *Group health plans (164.314)(b)* requires the plan sponsor to reasonably and appropriately safeguard the confidentiality, integrity, and availability of ePHI. There is one implementation specification:

   — Plan document **R**—plan documents of group health plan must require sponsor to implement administrative, physical, and technical safeguards that protect the confidentiality, integrity, and availability of ePHI that it creates, receives, maintains, or transmits on behalf of the group plan; separation of ePHI is supported by security measures; ensure that any agent to whom it provides information agrees to implement security measures to protect information and report to the health plan any security incident of which it is aware

Policies, Procedures, and Documentation (164.316)

There are two standards for policies, procedures, and documentation (see table 10.5) (HHS 2007f):

1. *Policies and procedures (164.316)(a)* requires the establishment and implementation of policies and procedures to comply with the standards, implementation specifications, and other requirements. A CE or BA may change its policies and procedures at any time, provided that those changes are documented and implemented.

2. *Documentation (164.316)(b)* requires the maintenance of the policies and procedures implemented to comply with the Security Rule in written form. There are three implementation specifications:

   — Time limit **R**—must retain the documentation for six years from the date of its creation or the date when it was last in effect, whichever is later

   — Availability **R**—must make the documentation available to those persons responsible for implementing the policies and procedures

   — Updates **R**—must review the documentation periodically and update it as needed

Table 10.5. Policies, procedures, and documentation requirements

Standard	Section	Implementation Specifications R = Required, A = Addressable	
1. Policies and Procedures	164.316(a)	Not Applicable	
2. Documentation	164.316(b)(1)	Time Limit	R
		Availability	R
		Updates	R

Source: HHS 2007e.

Security Officer Designation

The administrative safeguards of the Security Rule (164.308)(a)(2) contain an implementation specification that requires a single individual to be responsible for overseeing the information security program. This parallels the Privacy Rule, which requires an individual in the organization to be designated responsible for overseeing privacy policies and procedures. Generally, this person is identified as a **security officer or chief security officer**. The chief security officer may report to the chief information officer (CIO) or another administrator in the healthcare organization. The role of security officer may be 100 percent of an individual's job responsibilities or only a fraction, depending on the size of the organization and the scope of its use of health information technology and information systems. Regardless of the actual reporting structure, the chief security officer must be given authority to effectively manage the security program, apply sanctions, and influence employees. Security officers must periodically evaluate their organization's electronic information systems and networks for proper technical controls and processes. It is important to remember the physical security safeguards and ensure they are considered as frequently as network security, because one server room door left unlocked can cause more loss of ePHI than an external intrusion.

Enforcement and Penalties for Noncompliance

On February 16, 2006, the HHS published a final rule for imposing civil monetary penalties on CEs that violate any of the HIPAA administrative simplification requirements (HHS 2006b). The 2006 HIPAA Enforcement Rule created a uniform compliance and enforcement mechanism that addresses all the administrative simplification regulations, including privacy, security, and transactions and code sets (Wilkinson 2006). As previously mentioned, oversight and enforcement of the Security Rule was the responsibility of CMS, but as of July 27, 2009, the responsibility transitioned to the OCR (HHS 2010c). Notable changes to enforcement and penalty provisions for HIPAA have occurred due to the passage of the HITECH Act, as discussed in chapter 9. These revisions are essentially the same for both the Privacy and Security Rules.

To reiterate, the HITECH Act established four categories of violations that reflect increasing levels of culpability, with corresponding tiers of penalty amounts. The nature and extent of both the violation and the harm are used to determine the amount assessed within each range. The OCR may choose to pursue corrective action without assessing penalties for unknowing violations, but penalties are mandatory in all other categories. Penalty monies collected will support further enforcement efforts (Dennis 2010).

As with the Privacy Rule, the enforcement of penalties for noncompliance begins with a complaint from a patient, some other consumer, or an employee, or by a CE or BA compliance review results. Individuals may file a formal complaint with the OCR if they believe a CE or BA has violated the Security Rule. If OCR accepts the complaint, it will investigate. If it determines that the CE or BA is not in compliance, it will work with the entity to obtain voluntary compliance, corrective action, or resolution agreement. If the entity does not act to resolve the issue, OCR may impose civil monetary penalties.

If OCR believes that the actions of the entity are a violation of the criminal provision of HIPAA (42 USC 1320d-6), OCR may refer the complaint to the Department of Justice. See figure 9.9, p. 255, for the OCR flow chart of the Privacy and Security Rule Complaint Process. HITECH has also authorized random audits, which serve to detect noncompliance. These were discussed in chapter 9.

An HHS website provides information about the department's compliance and enforcement efforts, including HHS enforcement activities, frequency of complaint types, and corrective actions resulting from consumer complaints (HHS 2010b, 2010c). Additionally, the director of HHS OCR has the authority to issue subpoenas as part of the investigation of alleged HIPAA violations.

Currently, penalties for violations range as follows and can increase significantly for each violation, with a cap of $1.5 million for identical violations within each violation category in a calendar year (HHS 2009b):

- $100–$50,000 per violation for unknowing violations

- $1,000–$50,000 per violation if due to reasonable cause and not willful neglect

- $10,000–$50,000 per violation if due to willful neglect and corrected within 30 days of discovery

- $50,000 or more per violation if due to willful neglect and not corrected as required

---

Check Your Understanding 10.2

Instructions: Indicate whether the following statements are true or false (T or F).

1. The Security Rule contains provisions that CEs can ignore.

2. The Security Rule is completely technical and requires computer programmers to address.

3. The Security Rule contains both required and addressable standards.

4. The Security Rule contains encryption specifications that all CEs must comply with.

5. The Conditions of Participation restrict payment to providers that are not compliant with the Security Rule.

Summary

The HIPAA Security Rule, which governs the security of ePHI, has been in effect since April 2005. As a result, most CEs and their employees are familiar with its requirements and continue to work toward organizational compliance. However, the ARRA's HITECH provisions have expanded the Security Rule to require organizations and individuals previously untouched by the rule to come into compliance. Overall, the purpose of the Security Rule is to minimize risk and protect ePHI. Its standards focus on what *should* be done to ensure health information security rather than *how* it should be done. The rule attempts to establish an information security floor through a set of technology, policy, and business process requirements related to administrative, physical, and technical safeguards; organizational requirements; and policies, procedures, and documentation. The next chapter discusses security mechanisms that can be employed to ensure compliance. These include data security mechanisms as well as system security mechanisms. It is important that health information management and informatics professionals realize that successfully securing information is less about technology and more about business policies and practices and changes in individual behaviors.

References

AHIMA. 2013. Analysis of Modifications to the HIPAA Privacy, Security, Enforcement, and Breach Notification Rules Under the Health Information Technology for Economic and Clinical Health Act and the Genetic Information Nondiscrimination Act; Other Modifications to the HIPAA Rules. http://www.ahima.org.

AHIMA. 2010 (updated). Information security—An overview. Chicago: AHIMA. Web extra.

Centers for Medicare and Medicaid Services. 2003. HIPAA Information Series for Providers. http://www.cms.gov/.

Dennis, J. 2010. *Privacy: The Impact of ARRA, HITECH, and Other Policy Initiatives*. Chicago: AHIMA.

Department of Health and Human Services. 2003. Health insurance reform: Security standards. Final rule. 45 CFR 160, 162, and 164. *Federal Register* 68(34):8333–8381.

Department of Health and Human Services. 2006a (December). HIPAA security guidance. Remote access. http://www.hhs.gov/ocr/.

Department of Health and Human Services. 2006b. HIPAA administrative simplification: Enforcement; Final rule. 45 CFR 160 and 164. *Federal Register* 71(32):8390–8433.

Department of Health and Human Services. 2007a. HIPAA security series: Security 101 for covered entities. Volume 2, paper 1. http://www.hhs.gov/ocr/.

Department of Health and Human Services. 2007b. HIPAA security series: Basics of risk analysis and risk management 2(6). http://www.hhs.gov/ocr/.

Department of Health and Human Services. 2007c. HIPAA security series: 2—Security standards: Administrative safeguards 2(2). http://www.hhs.gov/ocr/.

Department of Health and Human Services. 2007d. HIPAA security series: 3—Security standards: Physical safeguards 2(3). http://www.hhs.gov/ocr/.

Department of Health and Human Services. 2007e. HIPAA security series: 4—Security standards: Technical safeguards 2(4). http://www.hhs.gov/ocr/.

Department of Health and Human Services. 2007f. HIPAA security series: Organizational, policies and procedures and documentation requirements 2(5). http://www.hhs.gov/ocr/.

Department of Health and Human Services. 2009a. News release: HHS delegates authority for the HIPAA Security Rule to Office for Civil Rights. http://www.hhs.gov/.

Department of Health and Human Services. 2009b. HIPAA administrative simplification enforcement. 45 CFR Parts 160. *Federal Register* 74(209):56123–56131.

Department of Health and Human Services. 2010a. Modifications to the HIPAA privacy, security, and enforcement rules under the Health Information Technology for Economic and Clinical Health Act; Proposed rule. 45 CFR Parts 160 and 164. *Federal Register* 75(134):40868–40924.

Department of Health and Human Services. 2010b. Office for Civil Rights. Guidance on risk analysis requirements under the HIPAA Security Rule. http://www.hhs.gov/ocr/.

Department of Health and Human Services. 2010c. Office for Civil Rights. HIPAA enforcement rule. http://www.hhs.gov/ocr/.

Department of Health and Human Services. n.d. Office for Civil Rights. Security rule guidance material. http://www.hhs.gov/ocr/.

Scholl, M., K. Stine, J. Hash, P. Bowen, A. Johnson, C. Smith, and D. Steinbery. 2008. An introductory resource guide for implementing the HIPAA Security Rule. National Institute of Standards and Technology, Department of Commerce. Gaithersburg, MD. http://www.hhs.gov/ocr/.

Stevenson, G., and A. Valenta. 2009. Securing ePHI: Can clinicians and IT ever agree? *Journal of Healthcare Information Management* 23(4): 46–53.

Wilkinson, W. 2006. The Office for Civil Rights and Healthcare Privacy. Remarks for the Twelfth National HIPAA Summit. Washington, DC. http://hhs.gov/ocr/.

Cases, Statutes, and Regulations Cited

45 CFR 160: Definitions. 2006.

45 CFR 160.103: Definitions 2006.

45 CFR 162: Administrative requirements. 2006.

45 CFR 164: Security and privacy. 2006.

45 CFR 164.304: Definitions. 2006.

45 CFR 164.306: General rules. 2006.

45 CFR 164.308: Administrative safeguards. 2006.

45 CFR 164.308(a)(1): Security management functions. 2006.

45 CFR 164.308(a)(2): Assigned security responsibility. 2006.

45 CFR 164.308(a)(3): Workforce security. 2006.

45 CFR 164.308(a)(4): Information access management. 2006.

45 CFR 164.308(a)(5): Security awareness and training. 2006.

45 CFR 164.308(a)(6): Security incident reporting. 2006.

45 CFR 164.308(a)(7): Contingency plan. 2006.

45 CFR 164.308(a)(8): Evaluation. 2006.

45 CFR 164.308(b)(1): Business associate contracts and other arrangements.2006.

45 CFR 164.310: Physical safeguards. 2006.

45 CFR 164.310(a)(1): Facility access controls. 2006.

45 CFR 164.310(b): Workstation use. 2006.

45 CFR 164.310(c): Workstation security. 2006.

45 CFR 164.310(d)(1): Device and media controls. 2006.

45 CFR 164.312: Technical safeguards. 2006.

45 CFR 164.312(a)(1): Access control. 2006.

45 CFR 164.312(b): Audit controls. 2006.

45 CFR 164.312(c)(1): Integrity. 2006.

45 CFR 164.312(d): Person or entity authentication. 2006.

45 CFR 164.312(e)(1): Transmission security. 2006.

45 CFR 164.314: Organizational requirements. 2006.

45 CFR 164.314(a): Business associate contracts or other arrangements. 2006.

45 CFR 164.314(b): Group health plans. 2006.

45 CFR 164.316: Policies, procedures, and documentation. 2006.

45 CFR 164.316(a): Policies and procedures. 2006.

45 CFR 164.316(b): Documentation. 2006.

42 USC 1320d-6: Wrongful disclosure of individually identifiable health information.

American Recovery and Reinvestment Act of 2009, Title XIII—Health Information Technology, Subtitle D. Public Law 111-5.

Appendix 10.A

Information Security: A Checklist for Healthcare Professionals

The following list, although not exhaustive, outlines basic tenets of an information security program. Healthcare professionals may use this as a tool for evaluating their organization's information security program.

Access Control and Management

- Access control processes such as request, authorization, establishment, periodic review, and modification are addressed in policies and procedures.

- Access privileges are assigned based on a worker's role within the organization to ensure access is restricted to only the information needed to do the job.

- Access privileges based on roles are well documented and approved by management.

- Clinical applications have internal controls to limit the amount of patient information that the average user can print or download. Social Security numbers of patients are masked or not displayed to any worker who does not have a business need to see them.

- Password management rules (length, complexity, expiration, etc.) are consistent for applications and systems that process and store PHI. Exceptions to password rules are documented and approved by management.

- An individual's identity is verified before his or her password is reset. Wherever possible, avoid using or migrate away from using any part of an individual's Social Security number as an identifier for validating a user's identity to reset his or her password.

- Workers are logged off or locked out of a clinical application automatically after a predetermined period of inactivity, such as 10 minutes. This function triggers an event (audit) log entry that can be reviewed and reported.

- Access is removed or deactivated promptly when a user is terminated, resigns, or ends his or her affiliation with the organization and/or is disabled automatically after a predefined period of inactivity, such as 60 days. Ongoing monitoring of the termination process is used to verify that this process is being accomplished.

- Based on a report provided by the system administrator, managers periodically (at least annually) validate that worker access privileges are appropriate.

- Work with physician office managers on periodically reviewing user access privileges and roles to determine if access is appropriate; disable user accounts that have been inactive for long periods of time (e.g., 30 or more days). Management should review accounts that have been inactive for extended periods of time to determine if termination processes are not working effectively.

- Real patient identifiers are not used in test and training environments. If any test reports or temporary files use real patient identifiers, the files are deleted as soon as the testing or training is completed.

- IT personnel, including service (help) desk personnel, understand their responsibility for maintaining the confidentiality of patient information and cannot take control of a computer screen remotely without an individual's knowledge or permission.

- Appropriate mechanisms are in place to protect highly sensitive patient and employee health information, which may include information relating to HIV test results, lifestyle, substance abuse, psychological profiles, cosmetic surgery, or behavioral health records.

- Outside vendors and third parties can access only the information needed to perform their required service, and, wherever feasible, access to PHI or other confidential information is limited to read only.

Audit and Accountability

- Audit logs contain sufficient detail to verify which patient records were viewed or updated and by whom.

- The responsibility for reviewing audit logs has been assigned formally.

- Periodically, random audits of user activities are conducted to maintain a culture of accountability.

- Periodically, audits of particular activities are conducted to identify breaches of confidentiality; examples include, but not be limited to, VIPs, employees who are patients, audits of new employees, employees viewing records outside their area of responsibility (emergency room accesses), and when suspected activity occurs or a complaint has been filed.

- Ongoing audit log reviews are conducted for potential security breaches (such as failed log-in attempts) at the network, server, and application levels.

- Audit logs are secured and protected from unauthorized modifications so that only individuals with a job-related need can view the logs.

- Warning banners and/or other awareness methods are used to notify and remind workers that their activities are being audited and monitored.

Awareness and Training

- There are organizational records or documents demonstrating that information security awareness is being conducted. Annual refresher training is required. Issues involving individuals who have not completed their annual security awareness training are brought to management.

- Security awareness is linked to user provisioning. Employees, temporary workers, contractors, and some vendors complete initial security awareness training before gaining access to PHI.

- Annually, management reviews and provides feedback for both the initial and the refresher security awareness training to ensure the content is current and addresses newly discovered threats or risks.

- All workers (employees and nonemployees such as students, volunteers, contractors, etc.) sign a confidentiality agreement.

- The organization's medical staff bylaws or rules outline physician responsibilities for protecting the confidentiality of health information.

- Staff members of physician offices with remote access are trained adequately on use of the clinical system and their responsibilities for protecting confidential information.

- Employees should be aware of the HITECH Act and HIPAA penalties and fines that could be levied on healthcare workers if they violate organizational policies and breach PHI with willful intent.

Business Associates and Other Nonemployees

- Business associate agreements have been updated as a result of the HITECH Act to include the new HIPAA security rule requirements, the new definition of breach, and the details for breach notification, including:

  — How to report
  — When to report
  — Who to report to

- Satisfactory assurances of compliance are obtained from business associates and any of their agents or subcontractors (chain of trust agreement).

Computer Workstation

- Policies and procedures are in place that outline workers' responsibilities for securing workstations, laptops, and other portable devices.

- Security practices include workers consistently logging off before leaving their work area. Screen savers are activated after a predetermined period of inactivity to prevent incidental disclosure of PHI.

- An accurate inventory is maintained for computer equipment (laptops, desktops, tapes, flash drives, etc.) and biomedical devices that store PHI. General security safeguards and controls also are implemented for biomedical devices storing PHI to maintain security consistency.

Contingency and Disaster Recovery Planning

- Information systems are backed up periodically, and the back-up data is maintained off-site in a secure location. The frequency of the back-up procedure is determined by the organization's needs.

- Information needed to treat patients is available at the bedside in the event of a loss of data-processing capabilities.

- Departments have their own documented contingency plan in place in the event of planned or unplanned downtimes of critical applications and systems.

- A formal business impact analysis is conducted to identify critical applications and data. The business impact analysis identifies the recovery point objective and recovery time objective for each of the critical applications and systems.

- The disaster recovery plan meets the recovery point objective and recovery time objective for the organization.

- There is documented evidence of a recent exercise or a test of the disaster recovery plan.

Incident Reporting and Response

- Employees are instructed how to detect and report known or suspected information incidents and privacy breaches.

- The organization has an incident response team, and its core members have received training, especially on collecting and handling evidence during an investigation.

- A tabletop exercise is conducted periodically to test incident response capability.

- The organization follows breach reporting requirements as specified under the HITECH Act and has an objective process in place for analyzing the potential risk of harm in the event of an incident.

Media Protection and Controls

- PHI stored on media, including back-up media, is encrypted in accordance with the National Institute of Standards and Technology's Special Publication 800-111, "Guide to Storage Encryption Technologies for End User Devices."

   Note: Although encryption is addressable and not required, it is highly recommended to avoid breach notifications and lower enforcement penalties by exercising reasonable diligence for protecting PHI.

- Voice technology that is produced digitally from or stored on an information system is included in policies, safeguards, and controls used to protect electronic media.

- Policies and procedures addressing patient requests to obtain copies of their medical information in an electronic format include appropriate media controls to reduce risks.

- When printed reports containing confidential information are no longer needed, they are disposed of in a manner that protects their confidentiality (shredding, pulping, or burning).

- Hard disk drives are sanitized, meaning all confidential information is erased permanently from the drive, before being disposed of or reused. Documentation of destruction is maintained.

Mobile and Portable Device Security

- An accurate inventory of laptops, tablets, and other portable devices that store PHI is maintained.

- Steps have been taken to secure laptops, tablets, and mobile devices, such as smartphones and flash drives, including the following security controls:

   — Power-on password protection or biometric authentication to prevent unauthorized access in the event the device is lost or stolen
   — Automatic lockout set to enable after a predefined period of inactivity, such as 10 minutes
   — Encryption to protect data at rest
   — Automatic synchronization of stored data
   — Memory wipe to erase all data automatically either after a predetermined number of unsuccessful log-on attempts or when a remote wipe command is issued

Personnel Security Procedures

- Photo identification badges are used to distinguish employees and workforce members from contractors, sales representatives, and visitors.

- Procedures are documented for performing background investigations of workforce members, including some nonemployees working in key positions, before allowing access to PHI. The types of background checks performed are appropriate to a worker's level of access to PHI and other confidential information.

- Additional background checks may be conducted for individuals in trusted positions, such as a system administrator or network engineer.

- A reinvestigation process is conducted for positions identified as high risk.

Physical and Environmental Protection

- A facility security plan (also known as an environment of care plan) outlines the physical security procedures and controls for office buildings and addresses:

  — Access to restricted areas, such as the data center, network operations, and other areas where large volumes of PHI are stored in electronic or paper format

  — Equipment control into and out of the organization

  — Sign-in sheets for visitors to restricted access areas such as data centers

  — When and where visitors must be escorted

  — Maintenance records of changes or work performed on physical access controls (e.g., work on door locks, changing of combination door locks, etc.) that are related to security, which could be addressed by using copies of facility work orders

- Privacy and security walkthrough inspections are conducted and documented to ensure that PHI and electronic PHI are secured properly when not in use, to evaluate physical security controls, and to identify any issues or weaknesses in the implementation of the information security program.

Policies, Procedures, and Plans

- Information security policies are reviewed periodically by management to ensure that the policies are in line with accreditation standards and state and federal laws and that they are updated as needed.

- Tools may be used to manage and distribute policies and procedures centrally and to verify that workers have reviewed the policies that pertain to them.

- Periodic evaluations are conducted, either internally or by engaging a third party, to assess the effectiveness of policies and procedures and their compliance with the HIPAA security rule.

Remote Access

- Appropriate measures are in place to protect systems from unauthorized remote access.

- An automatic disconnect of a log-in session is enabled after a specific period of inactivity.

- Two-factor authentication may be used for remote connectivity, especially for anyone with system administrator privileges.

Risk Analysis and Management

- A well-defined risk assessment process is documented. The process is followed to identify threats and vulnerabilities and to present the results in a formal risk analysis report.

- Periodic risk analysis is conducted and covers systems and applications that store, process, or transmit PHI. Risk analysis is an ongoing process to evaluate which security controls are appropriate and should be accomplished whenever there is a significant change in the computing environment. The US Department of Health and Human Services released "Guidance on Risk Analysis Requirements under the HIPAA Security Rule" in the summer of 2010, which states, "The frequency of performance will vary among covered entities. Some covered entities may perform these processes annually or as needed (e.g., bi-annual or every 3 years) depending on circumstances of their environment."[1]

- Risk analysis reports (the findings and recommended corrective actions as a result of conducting a risk analysis) are reviewed and signed by management.

- The latest network vulnerability scanning and penetration test results are available for review. The risks associated with the discovered vulnerabilities are managed appropriately.

Transmission Security

- PHI and other confidential information being transmitted outside of the organization (via the Internet) are encrypted using a method that meets Federal Information Processing Standards 140-2.

    Note: Although encryption is addressable and not required, it is highly recommended to avoid breach notifications and lower enforcement penalties by exercising reasonable diligence for protecting PHI.

- Outbound e-mail is scanned, and e-mails detected as containing sensitive and confidential information are encrypted automatically to protect them from unauthorized access, alteration, and disclosure.

- Wireless networks use Wi-Fi Protected Access (WPA2) encryption to secure transmissions from mobile devices such as laptops mounted on carts in clinical areas to the applications and systems within the internal network.

    Note: As encryption technology continues to advance, WPA2 may be replaced in the future with stronger encryption standards when those are developed.

---

1. Department of Health and Human Services. "Guidance on Risk Analysis Requirements under the HI-PAA Security Rule." July 14, 2010. Available online at www.hhs.gov.

Chapter 11

Security Threats and Controls

Keith Olenik, MA, RHIA, CHP; Melanie S. Brodnik, PhD, RHIA, FAHIMA; Rebecca B. Reynolds, EdD, MHA, RHIA, FAHIMA; and Laurie Rinehart-Thompson, JD, RHIA, CHP, FAHIMA

Learning Objectives

- Identify potential internal and external security threats, distinguishing human threats from natural and environmental threats

- List mechanisms to prevent and detect identity theft

- Identify types of medical identity theft and mechanisms to prevent, detect, and mitigate such theft

- Distinguish access controls from systems controls and provide examples of each

- Discuss entity authentication methods, including termination of access and remote-access controls

- Detail methods of transmitting electronic protected health information and explain security risks associated with each

- Recognize the importance of contingency planning or disaster recovery planning in securing health information

Key Terms

Audit trail
Authentication
Automatic log-off
Biometric identification
  systems
Computer viruses
Context-based access control
  (CBAC)
Contingency planning
Creditor
Cryptography
Data encryption
Disaster recovery planning
Encryption
Entity authentication

External security threat
Fair and Accurate Credit
  Transactions Act (FACTA)
Firewall
Identity theft
Information system
Internal security threat
Medical identity theft
Password
Pretty good privacy (PGP)
Red flags
Red Flags Rule
Required standards
Role-based access control
  (RBAC)

Security incident
Social media
Telephone callback
  procedures
Termination of access
Tokens
Trojan horse
Unique identifier
User-based access control
  (UBAC)
Wired equivalent privacy
  (WEP)
Worm

Introduction

To protect the privacy and security of patient information, a healthcare organization must address the circumstances that threaten the information and implement ways to secure the information from wrongful access. The Health Insurance Portability and Accountability Act (HIPAA) Security Rule requires that selected security safeguards be implemented to protect electronic protected health information (ePHI). The rule identifies administrative, physical, technical, organizational, and procedural standards that must be followed. Although the rule is written to be "technology neutral," common controls can be employed to meet the **required standards**. This chapter discusses not only the threats to the security of ePHI with a focus on identity theft, including medical identity theft, but also the more common mechanisms used to protect ePHI in terms of access and systems controls. Suggestions for preventing identity theft and medical identity theft are offered, along with issues to consider when transmitting ePHI via fax, e-mail, Internet, or other wireless devices. The importance of establishing policies and procedures for a complete security program are discussed. The chapter closes with a discussion of contingency or disaster recovery planning. Privacy and security of ePHI are intertwined, thus making it difficult to protect the privacy of ePHI without some form of security in place.

Internal and External Security Threats

In general, threats to the privacy and security of health information fall into two broad categories: human threats and natural or environmental threats. Both types can be either **internal security threats** or **external security threats**. Internal human threats are caused by individuals within the organization, such as employees, whereas external human threats are caused by individuals outside the organization. Internal natural or environmental threats include fire or water damage that originates within the organization, whereas external natural or environmental threats include flooding, lightning, and tornadoes. This section of the chapter provides an overview of human threats and natural or environmental threats. It then goes into greater detail to discuss the human threats of identity theft and medical identity theft.

Human Threats

A survey of HIPAA Security Rule compliance found that the majority of respondents (70 percent) considered humans to be the greatest threat to ePHI (Davis et al. 2006). Human threats can be unintentional or intentional. Unintentional threats include employee errors that may result from lack of training in proper system use. When users share passwords or download information from a nonsecure Internet site, for example, they create the potential for a breach in security. Intentional threats include attacks from outside the network or internal malicious actions by workforce members. Computer viruses are among the most common and virulent forms of intentional computer tampering. They pose a serious threat to electronic patient data and healthcare applications. Intentional threats also include theft, intentional alteration of data, and intentional destruction of data. The culprit of an intentional act could be a disgruntled employee, a computer hacker, or a prankster. In a Florida case, the daughter of a hospital employee accessed confidential information through an unattended computer workstation in the facility's emergency room. She wrote down names and addresses of recent patients and then called to tell them that they had tested positive for HIV when, in fact, they had not (*Washington Post* 1995).

Internal security breaches are far more common than external breaches. However, with increased use of information technology, breaches are occurring as a result of external hackers. Some of the more common forms of internal breaches to security across all industries are the installation or use of unauthorized software, use of the organization's computing resources for illegal or illicit communications or activities (porn surfing, e-mail harassment, and such), and the use of the organization's computing resources for personal profit. In November 2010, Ponemon Institute published the results of an in-depth study on actual data loss and data theft experienced by 65 healthcare organizations (Ponemon 2010). The results indicated that (1) data breaches were costing study participants approximately $2 million over a two-year period, and (2) organizations did not have adequate resources to prevent and detect data breaches, nor was protecting patient data a priority (Ponemon 2010). Figure 11.1 provides additional

Figure 11.1.   Security breach examples

An Oklahoma State Department of Health (OSDH) laptop computer and other items were stolen from a personal vehicle while an agency employee was in Yukon, Oklahoma, on April 6, 2011. A database related to the Oklahoma Birth Defects Registry was on the laptop computer. The Oklahoma Birth Defects Registry (OBDR) provides statewide surveillance of birth defects to reduce the prevalence of birth defects through prevention education, monitoring trends, and analyzing data. The laptop was used to record data from hospital medical records. The data includes information on nearly 35,000 children with birth defects. In addition, 50 paper files containing abstracted medical information were also taken in the theft. The OSDH is notifying nearly **133,000** individuals that their names and some personal information may have been contained on the laptop computer. (Oklahoma State Department of Health. 2011. http://www.ok.gov)

The New York City Health and Hospitals Corporation (HHC) on February 9, 2011, began to notify **1.7 million** patients, staff, contractors, vendors, and others who were treated by and/or provided services during the past 20 years for or at Jacobi Medical Center, North Central Bronx Hospital, or their offsite clinics, which comprise the North Bronx Healthcare Network. The notification is about a recent reported theft of electronic record files that contained their personal information, protected health information (PHI), or personally identifiable employee medical information (PIEMI). Personal information can include Social Security numbers, names, addresses, and other information that may be used to identify individuals. PHI can include personal information and patients' medical histories. PIEMI can include personal information and employees' health information. (New York City Health and Hospitals Corporation, Data Theft Notification. 2011. http://www.nyc.gov)

Computer security breaches at two University of North Carolina Greensboro (UNCG) clinics allowed unauthorized access to information about more than **2,500** individuals. The university has mailed letters to the last known addresses of those whose personal information was exposed and posted notices on the clinics' websites. The two computers infected with malware via the Internet were in the university's Speech and Hearing Center and Psychology Clinic, which provide services to the public. (SPAMFighter, 2009. http://www.spamfighter.com/News-11832-UNCG-Suffers-a-Computer-Virus-Infection.htm).

A laptop computer with health and personal information on **21,000** patients was stolen from an office at Thomas Jefferson University Hospital in Philadelphia in June 2010. The patients whose unencrypted records were on the password-protected laptop were notified last Friday of the theft in a letter from hospital president Thomas J. Lewis, who offered identity-theft monitoring and protection. Lewis said the hospital would do all it could to protect the patients whose information, including Social Security numbers, had been exposed and take steps to prevent similar incidents in the future. (*Philadelphia Inquirer.* 2010. http://articles.philly.com/2010-07-29/news/24970387_1_social-security-numbers-laptop-patient-records)

The US Department of Health and Human Services (HHS) maintains a list of all breaches of unsecured protected health information affecting 500 or more individuals, which must be reported to HHS. This searchable list is available at http://www.hhs.gov/ocr/privacy/hipaa/administrative/breachnotificationrule/breachtool.html.

examples of security breaches as related to human theft. The Health Information Technology for Economic and Clinical Health (HITECH) Act enhances the HIPAA Privacy and Security Rules as related to data breaches caused by individuals. HITECH specifically addresses requirements and penalties related to breaches, as discussed in chapter 9.

Natural and Environmental Threats

Natural and environmental threats such as hurricanes, tornados, floods, fire, power surges, lightning, and water damage can be significant factors in the loss of PHI, whether in electronic or paper format. Healthcare providers must have a process in place for protecting and recovering their information, not only to adhere to HIPAA and HITECH requirements but also to comply with Joint Commission standards.

Public health officials have learned many lessons from perhaps the worst public health disaster in US history in regard to protecting PHI. As a result of Hurricane Katrina, which struck New Orleans and the surrounding states in 2005, over a million people were displaced. Patient records, especially paper records, of many healthcare providers were lost, destroyed, or rendered inaccessible. Some providers that used electronic health records (EHRs), however, were able to recover patient records. Certain parts of the HIPAA Privacy Rule had to be suspended at the time to allow healthcare providers to treat displaced persons without fear of breaking the law. The disaster also brought attention to the importance of disaster recovery and contingency planning, which is now part of the HIPAA Security regulation. A more detailed discussion of contingency planning and disaster recovery planning appears below.

Identity Theft

Identity theft is a fast-growing crime made possible for the most part by the ease with which information can be stolen in electronic environments. Because patient demographic, financial, and healthcare information is collected, transmitted, and maintained in the course of operations of a healthcare provider, that provider has an obligation to protect such information. Employees or disgruntled former employees may be the source of patient identity theft. For example, in 2004, Richard Gibson, an employee of the Seattle Cancer Center Alliance, was convicted of using a patient's name, Social Security number, and date of birth to obtain four credit cards, which he used to purchase $9,100 worth of personal items. Gibson was convicted under the HIPAA Privacy Rule, sentenced to 16 months in prison (plus three years of supervised release), and ordered to pay more than $9,000 in restitution (Health Data Management 2004).

In October 1998, Congress passed the Identity Theft and Assumption Deterrence Act (18 USC 1028) (Identity Theft Act), making it a federal crime to commit an act of identity theft. The act defines identity theft as when someone "knowingly transfers or uses, without lawful authority, a means of identification of another person with the intent to commit, or aid or abet, any unlawful activity that constitutes a violation of federal law, or that constitutes a felony under any applicable state or local law" (18 USC 1028). The Federal Trade Commission (FTC) has oversight responsibility for identity theft regulations and requires financial institutions and creditors to develop and implement written identity theft prevention programs. It is the clearinghouse for complaints related to identity theft. If a person is found guilty of identity theft the maximum penalty is 15 years in prison and up to $250,000 in fines. Unfortunately, identity theft has not been confined to just the wrongful use of someone's identity for financial gain. In recent years there has been an increase in medical identity theft.

Medical Identity Theft

Like identity theft, **medical identity theft** is a crime. It is a type of identity theft and a type of financial fraud that involves the inappropriate or unauthorized misrepresentation of one's identity. It is "when someone uses an individual's identifying information, such as their healthcare insurance information or Social Security number, without the individual's knowledge or permission, to obtain medical services or goods, or to obtain money by falsifying claims for medical services and falsifying medical records to support those claims" (Dixon 2006, 16). Its victims include patients, providers, and insurers.

The World Privacy Forum has identified two primary types of medical identity theft (Dixon 2006). The first type is the use of a person's name and, at times, other identifiers (for example, Social Security number), without the knowledge or consent of the victim, to obtain medical services or goods. In a subset of this first type, a person's name or other identifier may be used with that individual's consent but without the individual's full understanding of the ramifications (for example, allowing an uninsured family member to use one's insurance card so that medical services will be covered). The second type is the use of a person's identity to obtain money by falsifying claims for medical services.

Medical identity theft does not include situations where patient information is altered but the patient's identity is not abused. Likewise, if a patient's financial information is used to purchase goods or services that are not medical in nature, this is not medical identity theft, because the consequences are financial in nature only.

Medical identity theft is either internal or external. Internal medical identity theft is committed by organization insiders, such as clinical or administrative staff with access to patient information. Sophisticated crime rings may infiltrate an organization to commit internal medical identity theft, posing or functioning as staff while stealing patient-identifying information until they are either caught or exit the organization undetected. There is concern that the EHR may assist perpetrators by granting them broad access to patient information. Therefore, adequate preemployment and ongoing background checks are important.

External medical identity theft is committed by individuals outside an organization. Although the extent to which uninsured Americans are committing external medical identity theft out of a sense of need (that is, to obtain covered medical services) may be increasing, the World Privacy Forum suggests that internal crimes occur more frequently than external ones (Dixon 2006).

Implications of Medical Identity Theft

Medical identity theft is distinguished from other types of identity theft because it creates negative consequences to both the victim's financial status and medical information. A victim may face financial consequences such as debt collection, monetary losses, damaged credit, and insurance denials (if lifetime caps are reached). A victim could also receive improper medical treatment if incorrect medical information (that of the perpetrator) is inserted in the victim's health record. For example, if the medical identity theft victim is given a blood transfusion based on the different, and incompatible, blood type of a perpetrator whose medical information was wrongfully entered into the victim's health record, the result could be life-threatening.

Although many states have data breach notification laws, very few address medical information, and while financial industry regulations protect consumers against lost or stolen credit cards, no corollary exists for medical identity theft victims. HIPAA presently does not address medical identity theft. Further, the right to request an accounting of disclosures does not detect the insertion of a perpetrator's medical information into a victim's health record. Under the HITECH Act as originally written, healthcare entities with EHRs would be required to provide an accounting of payment disclosures (upon patient request), which could detect disclosures to payers for services the victim did not receive (AHIMA 2013). A subsequent rule issued in 2011, however, proposes to exclude uses and TPO from an accounting for both paper and electronic records. Instead, individuals (upon request) would be able receive an access report from covered entities with EHRs, allowing an individual to see a record of every person who viewed the individual's designated record set during the previous three years. TPO disclosures would therefore be displayed in the access report rather than in an accounting of disclosures (HHS 2011). The proposed rule regarding accounting of disclosures and access reports has not been finalized. However, for detection to occur via either an accounting of disclosures or an access report, a victim must take the initiative to request an accounting or access report and study the disclosures and other access that occurred. In the absence of a suspicion of illicit activity involving the victim's medical account, such a request may not occur.

Of greater significance is the HITECH breach notification requirement, which requires patients to be notified if their protected health information (PHI) has been breached. This has the potential to inform victims of medical identity theft. Also, HITECH states personal health record vendors and third-party service providers that serve as business associates are subject to the breach notification requirement (AHIMA 2013).

Fair and Accurate Credit Transactions Act and the Red Flag Rule

As previously mentioned, the FTC has oversight responsibility for identity theft issues. In 2007, Identity Theft Red Flags and Address Discrepancies Rules were enacted as part of the federal **Fair and Accurate Credit Transactions Act** (FACTA) of 2003. FACTA requires financial institutions and creditors to develop and implement written identity theft programs that identify, detect, and respond to red flags that may signal the presence of identity theft. A **red flag** is defined as a "pattern, practice, or specific activity that could indicate identity theft" (Gellman and Dixon 2009, 4). Although this law does not specifically address medical identity theft, it is significant because many healthcare organizations meet the definition of **creditor,** which is anyone who regularly, and in the ordinary course of business, meets one of the following criteria:

- Obtains or uses consumer reports in connection with a credit transaction;

- Furnishes information to consumer reporting agencies in connection with a credit transaction; or

- Advances funds to, or on behalf of, someone (except for funds for expenses that are incidental to a service provided by the creditor to that person)

The compliance date for the **Red Flags Rule** was December 31, 2010. The law consists of five categories of red flags (16 CFR Part 681), which include the following:

- Alerts, notifications, or warnings from a consumer reporting agency

- Suspicious documents

- Suspicious personally identifying information such as a suspicious address

- Unusual use of, or suspicious activity relating to, a covered account

- Notices from customers, victims of identity theft, law enforcement authorities, or other businesses about possible identity theft in connection with an account

The red flags should be used as triggers to alert an organization that an identity theft problem may exist. To assist healthcare providers that are creditors and may also be victims of medical identity theft, the World Privacy Forum recommends that providers incorporate red flags specifically related to patients and insurers into their policies and procedures for preventing, detecting, and mitigating theft. See figure 11.2 for examples of red flags for healthcare providers.

Prevention, Detection, and Mitigation of Medical Identity Theft

Healthcare organizations can be victimized by both identity theft and, more specifically, medical identity theft. As a result, they need to take appropriate steps to prevent and detect both crimes, whether committed by their employees, business partners, or others. Many of the challenges and the remedies applicable to identity theft also apply to medical identity theft. References to identity theft, below, can be extended to medical identity theft as well.

Davis and others (2005) posited that preventing identity theft poses many challenges, including the following:

- Ensuring that preventive safeguards are in place to protect the privacy and security of patient information

- Balancing patient privacy protections with disclosure of identity theft events to victims, law enforcement officials, and federal agencies

- Identifying resources to assist healthcare organizations, providers, and patients who are victims of identity theft

To help prevent identity theft, healthcare providers should consider the following measures as outlined by Davis and others (2005):

1. Ensure appropriate background checks of employees and business associates who may have access to business and patient PHI.

2. Minimize the use of Social Security numbers for identification; whenever possible, redact or replace some of the digits in the number; avoid displaying the entire number on any document, screen, or data collection field.

3. Store patient information in a secure manner, ensuring that physical safeguards such as restricted access and locks are in place. Consider securing a release of liability from patients who refuse to use facility-provided lockboxes or other storage for personal items.

4. Implement and comply with organizational policies for the appropriate disposal, destruction, and reuse of any media used to collect and store patient information.

5. Implement and comply with organizational policies and procedures that provide safeguards to ensure the security and privacy of patient information collected, maintained, and transmitted electronically. At a minimum:

   — Limit access to electronic patient information to a need-to-know basis and establish minimum necessary access controls.

   — Require unique user identification and password controls.

   — Implement encryption practices for transmitting patient information.

   — Install appropriate hardware and software protective mechanisms such as firewalls and protected networks.

   — Perform routine audits to determine appropriate access to information, including access to patient information by newly hired staff.

6. Train staff on organizational policies and practices developed to provide protection and appropriate use and disclosure of patient information, as well as appropriate responses to identity theft events.

Figure 11.2.   Examples of red flags for healthcare providers

• A complaint or question from a patient based on the patient's receipt of:
  —A bill for another individual
  —A bill for a product or service that the patient denies receiving
  —A bill from a healthcare provider that the patient never patronized
  or
  —A notice of insurance benefits (or Explanation of Benefits) for health services never received
• Records showing medical treatment that is inconsistent with a physical examination or with a medical history as reported by the patient
• A complaint or question from a patient about the receipt of a collection notice from a bill collector
• A patient or insurance company report stating that coverage for legitimate hospital stays is denied because insurance benefits have been depleted or a lifetime cap has been reached
• A complaint or question from a patient about information added to a credit report by a healthcare provider or insurer
• A dispute of a bill by a patient who claims to be the victim of any type of identity theft
• A patient who has an insurance number but never produces an insurance card or other physical documentation of insurance
• A notice or inquiry from an insurance fraud investigator for a private insurance company or a law enforcement agency

Source: Gellman and Dixon 2009, 5–6.

7. Develop a proactive identity theft response plan or policy that clearly outlines the response process and identifies the organization's obligations to report or disclose to law enforcement or government agencies information related to such crimes.

— Identify federal and state laws applicable to identity theft, reporting, and disclosing.

— Complete a preemption analysis addressing HIPAA's permitted disclosures to law enforcement (164.512(2)) versus state law, determining when there is a need for a court order, subpoena, or patient authorization.

To further comply with administrative safeguards, if an incident of identity theft or unintentional release of identifying information occurs, the healthcare provider should initiate a process of notification that an incident has occurred. Breach notification requirements (discussed in chapter 9) must also be followed if applicable. At a minimum, Davis and others (2005) suggest that the following steps be taken:

1. Initiate an internal investigation to review the facts for both investigation and communication.

2. Determine internal operational steps based on results of the investigation, including the following:

   a. Identification and sequestering of pertinent medical records, files, and other documents

   b. Suspension of billing processes until the matter has been resolved

   c. Processing of appropriate amendments or corrections once the matter has been resolved

3. Notify local law enforcement authorities and other agencies based on federal and state law requirements. Authorization from the patient may be needed unless the notification is being done in response to a court order or in accordance with state law.

4. Notify the individual, unless it was the individual who brought this to your attention. Consider the following factors when deciding if notification is warranted:

   a. Nature of the compromise

   b. Type of information taken

   c. Likelihood of misuse

   d. Potential damage arising from misuse

5. Determine a communication response in collaboration with law enforcement and legal counsel to determine the need for a media release or response to an identity theft event.

In addition to mandated red flags, healthcare providers must take steps to prevent, detect, and mitigate both external and internal medical identity theft. Employee awareness and training, and implementation of organization-wide policies and procedures are important.

Certain types of external medical identity theft can be detected when a perpetrator presents for service or seeks to obtain benefits such as medical equipment. Providers may require a driver's license to verify a patient's identity, and registration personnel may take photographs of patients to include in their health records for future reference. More sophisticated options include biometric identifiers such as a fingerprint, a handprint, or retinal scans. Patient signatures from previous encounters may also be compared with the signature of the patient presenting for the current episode of care. All these measures, however, are dependent on valid baseline information. If the information the provider relies on is the perpetrator's signature, photograph, or biometric identifier, all future encounters will be based on fraudulent information, decreasing the chances of detecting the fraud. This may also wrongfully identify the true patient as the perpetrator when and if he or she goes to that provider for treatment (Rinehart-Thompson and Harman 2009).

Measures that verify patient identity are ineffective for internal medical identity theft. The AHIMA e-HIM Work Group on Medical Identity Theft has identified best practices to minimize internal medical identity theft (AHIMA e-HIM Work Group on Medical Identity Theft 2008). These include background checks for employees and business associates; minimizing the temporary hiring of individuals who are not licensed, credentialed, or bound by professional codes of ethics; minimizing Social Security numbers as patient identifiers; and avoiding Social Security numbers on any data collection field.

Other ways to protect electronic patient data include stringent application of security access and systems controls, which are discussed in more detail below. The AHIMA Work Group (AHIMA e-HIM Work Group on Medical Identity Theft 2008) further recommends that three areas of the HIPAA Security Rule—administrative, technical, and physical safeguards—be included in a risk analysis to identify system vulnerabilities that could subject an organization to medical identity theft. Other areas it recommends in a risk analysis include the following:

- Limiting access to the minimum necessary

- Requiring user identification and passwords

- Implementing encryption devices for transmitted data

- Installing protective hardware and software devices, including firewalls

- Eliminating open network jacks in unsecured areas

- Routinely auditing access to patient information through audit trails

When medical identity theft occurs, a response plan is necessary. An organization's compliance office is crucial in maintaining an ongoing review and revision of plans that address breach notification requirements and mitigation efforts, including the separation of intermingled health information of a victim and a perpetrator. Such plans are necessary to minimize damage. As medical identity theft continues to challenge the healthcare industry and is centered in the management of health information, effective prevention, detection, and mitigation protocols are essential (Rinehart-Thompson and Harman 2009).

Check Your Understanding 11.1

Instructions: Indicate whether the following statements are true or false (T or F).

1. Internal security breaches are far more common than external breaches.

2. The Identity Theft and Assumption Deterrence Act of 1998 makes it a federal crime to commit an act of identity theft.

3. Medical identity theft includes the use of a patient's financial information to purchase goods or services even if they are not medical in nature.

4. Healthcare organizations are excluded from the definition of "creditor" under FACTA.

5. Red flags are used to help a healthcare provider detect medical identity theft.

Security Access and Systems Controls

To adequately protect ePHI and avoid **security incidents** that breach or threaten an electronic system, an organization must employ both access controls and systems controls. This section explains the difference between the two and provides examples of each.

Access Controls

Access controls are designed to prevent unauthorized individuals from retrieving, using, or altering information. "Preventive controls try to stop harmful events from occurring, while detective controls identify if a harmful event has occurred and corrective controls are used after a harmful event to restore the system" (AHIMA 2012, 49). To prevent unauthorized access, only individuals with a "need to know" should have access to ePHI. With the ease with which ePHI can be shared through EHRs and network exchanges, healthcare entities must establish processes that identify access rights to ePHI. Often, users of ePHI are assigned network access rights that give them the ability to use basic programs such as e-mail and other business applications. Separate application access rights must be granted based on the user's role and needed functions before they are able to access the more specific components of the systems.

As healthcare entities define what constitutes their legal health record (LHR), the time factor in electronic information systems should be considered. Best practices include systems' coordination of time and date stamps to accurately capture when an event occurred, including access, and audits to detect suspicious activity. This also becomes a compliance issue. As data sharing increases, it is important to have accurate time stamps and log files to support efficient network operations and the latest **encryption** and authentication standards (Klimasewski 2007).

Access Rights

Access to ePHI can be controlled through the use of one of the following:

- User-based access

- Role-based access

- Context-based access

Before we discuss each of these options, a brief explanation of access rights is necessary. Traditional user-based and role-based access rights have two parameters—*who* and *how*. *Who* is a list of users with rights to access electronic information. This list, called an access control list, can be organized by individual users or by groups of users. Groups are generally defined by role or job function. All coders within the health information management (HIM) department would be granted the same access rights, all RNs within a particular job classification would be granted the same access, and so on.

How specifies the ways that a user can access a resource. Examples include read, write, edit, execute, append, and print. Only so-called owners and administrators would be granted full rights so that they can modify, delete, or create new components. Clearly, owner and administrative privileges for health **information systems** should be carefully monitored.

User-based access control (UBAC) is defined as "a security mechanism used to grant users of a system access based upon the identity of the user" (Health and Human Services n.d.). With **role-based access control** (RBAC), access decisions are based on the roles individual users have as part of an organization. "With RBAC, rather than attempting to map an organization's security policy to a relatively low-level set of technical controls (typically, access control lists), each user is assigned to one or more predefined roles, each of which has been assigned the various privileges needed to perform the role" (HHS n.d.). One of the benefits of RBAC over user-based access is that, as new applications are added, privileges are more easily assigned. Discretionary assignment of access by an administrator is limited with RBAC. Users must be assigned to a specific role in order to be assigned access to a specific application (Kissel 2011).

Context-based access control (CBAC) is the most stringent of the three options. A CBAC scheme begins with the protection afforded by either a user-based or role-based access control design and takes it one step further. Context-based access control takes into account the person attempting to access the data, the type of data being accessed, and the *context* of the transaction in which the access attempt is made. In other words, context-based access has three parameters to consider—who, how, and in what context the data are being accessed. The following example illustrates the differences in the three types of access control.

Mary Smith is the director of the HIM department. Under a UBAC scheme, Mary would be allowed read-only access to her hospital's laboratory information system because of her personal identity—that is, because she is Mary Smith and uses the proper log-in and password(s) to get into the system. With an RBAC scheme, Mary would be allowed read-only access to her hospital's lab system because she is part of the HIM department and all department employees have been granted read-only privileges to this system. If the hospital were to adopt a CBAC scheme, Mary might be allowed access to the lab system only from her own workstation or another workstation in the HIM department. If she attempted to log in from the emergency room or another administrative office, she might be denied access. The CBAC could also be based on time of day. Since Mary is a daytime employee, she might be denied access if she attempted to log in at night.

Most access control schemes used by healthcare organizations are a mixture of the three types—UBAC, RBAC, and CBAC.

Entity Authentication

Access control mechanisms are effective in controlling what and how users access an electronic health information system, but only if there is a system for ensuring the identity of the individual attempting to gain access. **Entity authentication** is defined as "the corroboration that an entity is the one claimed" (HHS n.d.). This means the computer reads a predetermined set of criteria to determine if the user is who he or she claims to be.

To authenticate the legitimate user of ePHI, the user must be assigned a **unique identifier**. This identifier is a combination of characters and numbers assigned and maintained by the security system. It is used to track individual user activity. This identifier is commonly called the user ID or log-on ID. It is the "public" or known portion of most user log-on procedures. For example, many organizations assign a log-on identifier that is the same as the user's e-mail address, or a combination of the user's last and first names. It is generally fairly easy to identify a user by the log-on. John Doe's log-on identifier might be *doej*, for example.

Because of the public nature of the log-on ID or user ID, there is a need to authenticate the identity of the user. The three **authentication** methods are listed below (Walsh 2011).

- Something you know, such as a password or a personal identification number (PIN)

- Something you have, such as an ATM card, a secure token, a telephone number (for callbacks), or a swipe/smart card

- Something you are, such as a biometric identifier (for example, a fingerprint, a voice scan, or an iris or retinal scan)

Combining a user name with one of the authentication methods is single-factor authentication. A combination of any two of the preceding mechanisms constitutes a two-factor system and is recommended by Walsh. Single-factor authentication that is based on what the user knows (for example, user name and password) is the least secure form of protecting information from unauthorized access.

Security methods can be used alone or in combination with other systems. Security experts often encourage layered security systems that use more than one security mechanism, even if the solutions are individually fallible.

User IDs and Passwords

The most commonly used method for controlling access to an electronic information system is through a combination of a user ID and a password or PIN. A **password** is a sequence of characters used to verify that a computer user requesting access to a system is actually that particular user. Typically, a password is made up of between 4 and 16 characters. User IDs and passwords are maintained either as part of the access control list of the network or local operating system or in a special database that is searched before the user is allowed to access the system requested. While the user ID is not secret, the password or PIN is. Although passwords are generally stored in an encrypted form, software programs exist (called password crackers) that can identify an unknown or forgotten password for legitimate purposes. Unfortunately, unauthorized persons seeking to gain access to computer systems can also use these applications. For this reason, and due to individual behaviors described below, password and PIN systems are the least secure form of entity authentication.

One common problem with passwords is that they are often simple to remember and are selected for that very reason. As a result, however, they are also simple enough for someone else to guess. To combat this, some systems automatically generate passwords that are difficult to guess or force users to select passwords that are not too easy or already in use. Unfortunately, because they are then more difficult to remember, users are more likely to write the password down or publicly display it by taping it to a workstation. A preferable strategy is to teach users to create a pass phrase that consists of eight or more words, and then use the initial letters of the words to create a password. Use uppercase for some words, such as nouns, and use lowercase letters for the rest. Substitute numbers for words where possible. Passwords created in this way are easy to remember but difficult to crack. For example, a pass phrase might be, "My mother likes to eat strawberry birthday cake," and the password developed from this might be "MMltesbc." Then add a number to the end (for example, a year), and the password becomes "MMltesbc07." The pass phrase needs to be something the user will remember.

It is essential that healthcare organizations implement clear policies on creative selection, as well as appropriate use and maintenance of passwords; employee education; and meaningful sanctions for policy violations (including prohibiting the sharing of passwords). Tips for the effective selection of passwords are included in figure 11.3.

Tokens

Tokens are devices, such as key cards, that are inserted into doors or computers. A special type of token is the RSA SecurID. This device features a number generator that runs in sync with an identical generator in a host server. The device generates a pseudorandom number every 60 seconds that, in addition to a secret PIN, can be used to authenticate the holder. With token authentication systems, identification is based on the user's possession of the token, combined with a user name and password (RSA Security 2007). The disadvantage of tokens is that they can be lost, misplaced, or stolen. When tokens are used in combination with a password or PIN, it is essential that the password or PIN not be written on the token or in a location near where the token is stored. Tokens generate a password to access the system once the user name and PIN are entered into the system. A secure token is one type of dual-factor (two-factor) authentication because the user must possess the token (something the user has) along with the user name and password (something the user knows).

Figure 11.3.   Guidelines for choosing passwords

DO

- Pick a combination of letters and at least one number.
- Create a password with at least eight characters, mixing upper- and lowercase letters if your computer system is case sensitive, and symbols, if allowed by your system.
- Choose a word or text string that you can easily remember.
- Change your password often if not automatically prompted by your computer network.

DON'T

- Create a password that someone could easily guess if they know who you are—for example, your Social Security number, birthday, maiden name, pets' names, children's names, or model of your car.
- Choose a word that can be found in the dictionary. Cracker programs can rapidly try every word in the dictionary.
- Pick a word that is currently newsworthy.
- Create a password that is similar to your previous password.
- Share your password with others or write it down in a visible location, such as on a sticky note on your desk.

Source: Adapted from Wager, Lee, and Glaser 2009.

Telephone Callback Procedures

Telephone callback procedures are another form of entity authentication and are used primarily when employees have access to health information systems from home. When a modem dials into the system, a special callback application asks for the telephone number from which the call has been placed. If this number is not an authorized number, the callback application will not allow access.

Biometric Identification Systems

Because of the inherent weaknesses in password systems, other identification systems have been developed. **Biometric identification systems** analyze biological data about the user, such as a voiceprint, fingerprint, handprint, retinal scan, face print, or full-body scan, and are likely to play an increasing role in ePHI security.

Biometric devices consist of a reader or scanning device, software that converts the scanned information into digital form, and a database that stores the biometric data for comparison. IBM, Microsoft, Novell, and other computer companies are currently working on a standard for biometric devices called BioAPI. This standard will allow different manufacturers' software products to interact with one another.

Automatic Log-off

Automatic log-off is a security procedure that causes a computer session to end after a predetermined period of inactivity, such as 10 minutes. Multiple software products are available to allow network administrators to set automatic log-off parameters. Like other password-protected screen savers, log-off systems automatically activate after a period of inactivity. However, unlike password-protected screen savers, automatic log-off mechanisms require users to enter their network passwords to access the system. Generally, there is an installed device driver that prevents rebooting to deactivate the log-off system. Other security measures that may be included with automatic log-off products prevent users from changing the screen saver or being able to set local password options in case the user is not connected to the network. Failed log-in attempts may be recorded and reported as well as statistics on user log-ins, elapsed time, and user IDs. Generally, automatic log-off from an application session closes access to data and offers protection to the database and protection against unauthorized access. This should be differentiated from automatic timeout of the workstation, which could leave the database open and its session still running (for example, a password-protected screen saver).

Termination of Access

Healthcare organizations should safeguard themselves with policies and procedures for terminating the current level of access when an employee changes roles or terminates employment with the organization. Personnel within each organizational unit should be responsible for notifying the appropriate departments to carry out **termination of access** as it currently exists when an employee is terminated or when job responsibilities change. Failure to terminate access rights creates the potential for unauthorized access to PHI. An employee who continues with the organization but in a different capacity should be prevented from having access rights no longer needed. This can be accomplished by terminating the current level of access immediately and requesting that the user's new manager establish appropriate access for the user based on the new job responsibilities.

Audit Trails

An **audit trail** is a record that shows who has accessed a computer system, when it was accessed, and what operations were performed. Audit trails are generated by specialized software that has multiple uses in securing information systems. These uses can be categorized as follows (Gopalakrishna 2000):

- Individual accountability—When an employee or another individual's actions are tracked with an audit trail, the person becomes accountable for his or her actions, which can be a strong deterrent to violating acceptable policies and procedures.

- Reconstructing electronic events—Audit trails can also be used to reconstruct how and when a computer or application was used. This can be quite useful when there is a suspected security breach, whether it is internal or external.

- Problem monitoring—Some types of auditing software allow problems such as disk failures, overutilization of system resources, or network outages to be detected as they occur.

- Intrusion detection—When there are attempts to gain unauthorized access to a system, an audit system can detect and record it.

The length of time that audit trails are retained is a legal factor that should be considered as part of an EHR functionality. Previous chapters that discussed the LHR and evidence established the importance of producing information that will justify one's actions or validate the integrity of the record. Audit trail information should be considered an ancillary portion of the LHR and retained according to record retention requirements. Many new requirements in the HITECH Act place greater importance on the ability to document actions for legal proceedings based on information contained in audit trails (Nunn 2009).

Employee Nondisclosure Agreements

Under HIPAA's administrative safeguards, a healthcare entity must ensure that its workforce members have appropriate access to ePHI while not having access to ePHI when it is not appropriate or necessary. Many organizations require employees to sign nondisclosure agreements. These are particularly important if employees work in remote locations or telecommute. Appendix 11.A contains an example of an employee nondisclosure agreement that could be used for employees who have access to confidential patient information.

Security Awareness and Training

HIPAA administrative safeguards require that a covered entity (CE) implement a security awareness and training program for all its workforce members. As with other security standards, the awareness and training requirement is nonspecific, allowing the CE to design a training program to meet its particular needs. Raising awareness and subsequently changing individual behaviors about security issues is one of the single most effective tools a CE has to ensure compliance with the HIPAA Security Rule and prevent data breaches. Because the human factor can be either the strongest or the weakest part of an information security program, efforts must be made to engage the workforce to be in compliance with security policies and procedures (Beaver 2003). With increased implementation of EHRs, the human factor must also be supported by systems that preserve the confidentiality of information.

Because the HITECH Act extended many of the HIPAA privacy and security requirements, organizations should consider expanding their existing training programs to cover more individuals. They must also address the breach notification requirements that were outlined in the previous chapter. Training programs should continually be evaluated for effectiveness and must incorporate the most recent HIPAA/HITECH requirements. AHIMA (2010a) suggests combining HIPAA privacy and security training because of topic overlaps.

As a complement to workforce awareness and training, consumer education will assist in compliance with established programs. Consumers who are knowledgeable about a healthcare organization's preventive measures will be more receptive to the organization's efforts than if they just hear about actions taken after a security breach. Through collaboration, all parties can benefit from training (Parmigiani 2009).

Remote Access Control

Organizations that allow personnel to work from home or access ePHI while at home or traveling have additional security issues and must set clear guidance regarding appropriate use of organization computer resources, including hardware, software, and web access. Kelly (2004) offers the following recommendations for keeping the remote working environment (for example, employees working from their homes) secure:

- Facilitate remote working with the support of human resources and information technology departments.

- Create a security policy and educate remote workers.

- Issue corporate equipment for work purposes only.

- Deploy virtual private networks with two-factor authentication.

- Utilize thin-client applications that do not store any information locally.

- Install tools that monitor the status of all computers.

- Check virus updates regularly.

- Require the use of personal firewalls.

- Insist on shredders for any information that is printed.

- Balance security with ease of access to eliminate subversive behaviors.

The AHIMA practice brief "Establishing a Telecommuting or Home-Based Employee Program" (Dougherty and Scichilone 2002) outlines many aspects of managing remote workers. One section outlines what should be incorporated into an organization's security policies for remote workers. The major categories include the following:

- Policy and guidelines

- Identification and authorization

- Access control

- Auditing

- Integrity

- Physical security

- Security administration

- Architecture and topology

- Education/awareness/enforcement

Each of these categories must be evaluated by the organization, and existing requirements must be considered.

Remote work may involve individuals who are traveling. This requires additional security for devices that are taken off-site (for example, laptops, personal digital assistants [PDAs], mobile phones, and other types of mobile devices) and the information they contain. Physical security of the device is the first step to ensure that information is not inappropriately released or accessed. Several tips to keep laptops more secure include avoiding the use of a computer bag, always carrying the laptop, using a physical security device such as a cable, and never leaving the laptop visible in any location (for example, a car or hotel room). Desktop firewall, antivirus, and intrusion software are other tools that can be implemented to protect not only the laptop from external threats such as viruses but also the organization's network once the laptop is reconnected. Files maintained on the laptop should be encrypted to protect them from unauthorized access or alteration.

Selection of strong passwords, as discussed previously, with a combination of more than seven alphanumeric characters should be required. Passwords should never be stored on the device or written down. All these recommendations should be considered when developing the organizational policy and education plan for remote and mobile workers. The best protection against loss of data or laptop theft is user compliance with organizational policies and procedures (Narasimman 2005).

Check Your Understanding 11.2

Instructions: Indicate whether the following statements are true or false (T or F).

1. CBAC is less stringent than RBAC.

2. Biometric identifiers signify something that the user knows.

3. An audit trail is a record that shows when a particular user accessed a computer system.

4. Employee nondisclosure agreements are particularly important for employees who work in remote locations or telecommute.

5. Employee training programs are not necessary to protect the security of PHI.

Systems Controls

In addition to access control mechanisms, several common administrative, physical, and technical systems controls can be used to further ensure protection of ePHI. These controls relate to systems hardware or software and functions such as transmission of ePHI via fax or e-mail. This section of the chapter addresses some of these controls.

Workstation Use and Security

Workstations include both hardware and software that allow access to ePHI. Workstations should be placed in areas that are secure or monitored at all times and should be positioned so that visitors or others cannot read screens in public areas (for example, a reception area). A screen device can be placed over the workstation monitor to prevent anyone other than the person directly in front of it from reading it. Clear policies should be developed for workstation use. They should delineate, among other things, the appropriate functions to perform on the workstation and rules for sharing workstations.

Data Encryption

Data encryption ensures that data transferred from one location on a network to another are secure from eavesdropping data interception. This becomes particularly important when sensitive data, such as health information, are transmitted over public networks such as the Internet or across wireless networks. Secure data are data that cannot be intercepted, copied, modified, or deleted while in transit or at rest in a file system (for example, on a disk or tape).

Cryptography is the study of encryption and decryption techniques. It is a complicated science that has vast numbers of techniques associated with it. Only the basic concepts and a few current authentication technologies will be discussed in this chapter. Two common forms of encryption used in healthcare today are "pretty good privacy" and "wired equivalent privacy." The first form, **pretty**

good privacy, is used to encrypt e-mail messages and refers to encryption that uses a serial combination of hashing, data compression, symmetric-key cryptography, and public-key cryptography. **Wired equivalent privacy** is used to protect information on wireless networks. These forms of encryption are used to authenticate the sender and the receiver of messages over networks, particularly data transmission involving the Internet. To be effective, the encryption scheme should provide three things: authentication (both the sender and the recipient are known to each other), data security (data are safe from interception), and data nonrepudiation (data that were sent have arrived unchanged).

Some of the basic encryption terminology includes *plaintext, encryption algorithm, ciphertext*, and *key*. Plaintext is data before any encryption has taken place. In other words, the original data or message is recorded in the computer system as plaintext. An encryption algorithm is the computer program that converts the plaintext into an enciphered form. The ciphertext is the data after the encryption algorithm has been applied. The key in an encryption and decryption procedure is unique data that are needed to both create the ciphertext and decrypt the ciphertext back to the original message. The length of the key is commonly used to measure the strength of the key.

The earliest encryption systems used a single, private key. In other words, the same key (code) was needed to generate the ciphertext and to decrypt it. A problem with these systems was that they required both the sender and the receiver to have the key; in addition, the key also had to be protected from interception or tampering.

Public key cryptography addresses the basic problem with single, private key systems. A public key system has two keys, a private key and a public key. In the two-key system, data encrypted with the public key can be decrypted only by a private key, and data encrypted by the private key can be decrypted only by the public key. With public key cryptography, the encrypted data become very difficult to break. Single-key encryption is much more efficient than public-private key encryption, and thus is better suited to encrypting large text documents and files. Therefore, modern public key cryptography systems create a single-use key called a session key to encrypt the message and then send the session key and message together after encrypting again with the public key algorithm.

Public key cryptography today is used as a component of public key infrastructure (PKI), an entire system designed to make the use of public key cryptography practical. PKI is actually a combination of encryption techniques, software, and services.

A CE can adopt an in-house PKI model or contract with an application service provider (ASP) to host and manage its PKI. One potential use of PKI in healthcare is sending secure e-mail. To send a secure e-mail within the PKI environment, the sender needs to retrieve the recipient's public key from a directory within his or her organization. After obtaining the public key, the sender encrypts the e-mail message (by selecting the "encrypt" button, for example) and then sends it with the recipient's public key. When the recipient receives the e-mail, the recipient's private key will automatically decrypt the message.

There are other potential uses for PKI technology in healthcare, such as ensuring secure access to web-based health records or other health information systems. One example, recently reported in *Health Management Technology*, is Marconi Medical Systems, a picture archiving communications system (PACS). Marconi is integrating PKI into its web-based products to allow remote access through a standard web browser. Another example of a health-related organization using PKI is an online prescription service. PKI is expensive, and many of the systems are proprietary and will not interact with other systems. However, with HIPAA and HITECH standards demand a higher level of security for online healthcare transactions, the use of PKI technology in healthcare is likely to increase.

Firewall Protection

A **firewall** is either a hardware or software device that examines traffic entering and leaving a network. It prevents some traffic from entering or leaving based on established rules. The term *firewall* can be used to describe the software that protects computing resources or to describe the combination of the software, hardware, and policies that protect the resources. The most common place to find a firewall is between the healthcare organization's internal network (trusted network) and the Internet (untrusted network). A firewall limits users on the Internet from accessing certain portions of the healthcare network and also limits internal users from accessing various portions of the Internet. As important as firewalls are to the overall security of health information systems, they cannot protect a system from all types of attacks. Many viruses, for example, can hide within documents that will not be stopped by a firewall.

Routers are computers that link two different networks and are responsible for routing or sending the network traffic to the correct destination. Although not as robust as firewalls, routers may be programmed to filter certain types of network traffic. Intrusion detection systems (IDS) serve as the alarm system for the network and warn of possible inappropriate attempts to access the network by examining and analyzing network traffic. Intrusion prevention systems (IPS), which identify malicious network traffic like an IDS and then apply rules to block its passage across the network like a firewall, are now available. Both an IDS and an IPS require significant human intervention to monitor the alarms and rules and check for false positives. As with all computer tools, they require people to monitor them and make sense of the messages they produce.

Virus Checking

Computer viruses come in many varieties. The common types are classified as the following:

- File infectors, which attach to program files so that when a program is loaded the virus is also loaded

- System or boot-record infectors, which infect system areas of diskettes or hard disks

- Macro viruses, which infect Microsoft Word applications, inserting unwanted words or phrases

A **worm** is a special type of computer virus that stores and then replicates itself. Worms usually transfer from computer to computer via e-mail. A **Trojan horse** is a destructive piece of programming code that hides in another piece of programming code that looks harmless, such as a macro or an e-mail message.

Because virus attacks are very common and can cause extensive damage and loss of productivity, virus checking is an important component of a health information security program. Fortunately, there are antivirus software packages on the market that are effective as long as the virus catalog is updated frequently. Publication of defects has led to the phenomenon of "zero-day exploits." This means that a defect may be exploited to produce a virus, worm, or Trojan horse attack the same day it is published; thus, antivirus companies may not be able to stop it before it circles the globe on the Internet and does considerable harm.

Most software packages can be set to automatically obtain updated virus definitions and scan the user's computer system periodically to detect and clean any viruses found. It is important for users to also keep their workstation patch updates current, as this will enhance the security features of the operating system. Many of these operating system patches fix known and exploitable vulnerabilities in the software.

Transmission of ePHI

The ability of a healthcare provider to access all relevant healthcare information on a patient is important to the overall quality of care rendered to that patient. Electronic communications used to transmit ePHI, such as facsimiles, the Internet, electronic mail, and wireless communication devices that enable functions such as text messaging, are the business records of an organization and are therefore subject to the same storage, retention, retrieval, privacy, and security provisions as any other patient-identifiable health information (Burrington-Brown and Hughes 2003). Some commonly approved methods of transmitting ePHI, emerging technological trends such as social media, and controls necessary to ensure the privacy and security of ePHI are discussed below.

Facsimile or Faxing ePHI

A facsimile (fax) machine is a common tool used for sending either paper or electronic information over telephone lines. Fax equipment and software can enhance the quality of care by expediting the transmission of information from one provider to another, but they also increase the risk of information being misdirected or intercepted by someone other than the intended recipient. Some state laws address the topic of faxing healthcare information as related to a specific part of state code, such as faxing information pertaining to a given disease to a state health department. Many states have adopted rules based on the federal Uniform Rules of Evidence (URE) that allow business records created in the normal course of business to be considered trustworthy and admissible as evidence. The URE allows that a duplicate record such as a fax is admissible to the same extent as an original unless:

1. A genuine question is raised as to the authenticity or continuing effectiveness of the original, or

2. In the circumstances it would be unfair to admit the duplicate in lieu of the original. (Uniform Rules of Evidence)

Some states have also adopted the Uniform Photographic Copies of Business and Public Records as Evidence Act or the Uniform Business Records as Evidence Act, both of which address the admissibility of record reproductions, making it appropriate to accept faxes in lieu of original health records (Davis et al. 2005).

The faxing of patient information is not specifically mentioned in regulations; however, the Centers for Medicare and Medicaid Services (CMS) addressed the faxing of physician orders to healthcare facilities in Letter No. 90-25 from the Bureau of Policy Development. The letter states that faxed copies of physician orders are permissible and do not need to be countersigned but should be retained as a permanent part of the patient's record. A healthcare provider should take precautions to ensure that the faxed copy of the order is legible (Davis et al. 2006). The HIPAA Privacy and Security Rules do not specifically address fax use, but the Department of Health and Human Services (HHS) does address it in a limited manner in its response to questions related to faxes. The guidance offered by HHS suggests that providers can use a fax to disclose PHI to another provider as long as safeguards are in place, such as placing the fax machine in a secure place, confirming the correct fax number between providers, and periodically auditing fax numbers in use. The guidance also indicates that a valid signed authorization for disclosure of PHI may be a copy received by fax (Davis et al. 2006).

Fax machines are commonplace, and PHI will continue to be faxed between provider(s) and patient. See figure 11.4 for recommendations for controlling the fax process (Davis et al. 2006). While a fax can be an extremely convenient and efficient means of transmitting PHI, there are concerns, because fax machines are not a very secure means of communication. Thus for maximum protection, whenever possible, faxing of PHI should be limited to emergency situations. It is best not to transmit highly sensitive information unless it is encrypted or transmitted only within the organization through a virtual private network.

Internet

The Internet is used in a variety of healthcare functions, such as refilling prescriptions, scheduling appointments, communicating with physicians, researching medical conditions, and performing telemedicine activities—all of which put ePHI at risk for unauthorized disclosure. Concern for Internet security depends on how the healthcare provider or patient is using the Internet and how the user is connected to it. Security risks commonly associated with Internet access are unauthorized access to the organization's information systems and networks, unauthorized disclosure of confidential patient information or the organization's proprietary information and PHI, and the introduction of computer viruses or other contaminants (Miller 1996). To address these Internet security risks, a number of security measures can be taken.

Figure 11.4. Fax privacy recommendations

1. Establish fax policies and procedures based on federal and state laws and regulations and consultation with legal counsel.

2. Include in your organization's notice of information practices uses and disclosures of individually identifiable health information made via fax machine or software where appropriate (see the AHIMA practice brief "Notice of Privacy Practices").

3. Obtain a written authorization for any use or disclosure of individually identifiable health information made via fax machine or software when not otherwise authorized by the individual's consent to treatment, payment, and healthcare operations or federal or state law or regulation.

4. Take reasonable steps to ensure the fax transmission is sent to the appropriate destination. Pre-program and periodically audit and test destination numbers whenever possible to eliminate errors in transmission from misdialing and outdated fax numbers. Periodically remind those who are frequent recipients of individually identifiable health information to notify you if their fax number is to change (for example, include a reminder in medical staff newsletters, include it as part of the credentialing process, or remind transcriptionists who often automatically fax reports to physician offices). Train staff to double-check the recipient's fax number before pressing the send key.

5. Provide education and training to workforce members on the organization's fax policies and procedures. Take reasonable operational safeguards to alert staff of faxing procedures. For example, brightly colored stickers may be affixed to fax machines, reminding staff of key fax policy issues (e.g., does the information really need to be faxed, is there a cover sheet, verify recipient's fax number, who to call if an incoming fax has been received in error).

6. Require that all fax communications be sent with a cover sheet that contains the sender's and recipient's names and contact information, confidentiality disclaimer statement, and instructions on what to do if the document is received in error, such as stated below.

   Sample Confidentiality Notice

   The documents accompanying this fax transmission contain health information that is legally privileged. This information is intended only for the use of the individual or entity named above. The authorized recipient of this information is prohibited from disclosing this information to any other party unless required to do so by law or regulation and is required to destroy the information after its stated need has been fulfilled.

   If you are not the intended recipient, you are hereby notified that any disclosure, copying, distribution, or action taken in reliance on the contents of these documents is strictly prohibited. If you have received this information in error, please notify the sender and the privacy officer immediately and arrange for the return or destruction of these documents.

7. If a facsimile transmission fails to reach the recipient, check the internal logging system of the facsimile machine to obtain the number to which the transmission was sent. If the sender becomes aware that a fax was misdirected, contact the receiver and ask that the material be returned or destroyed. Investigate misdirected faxes as a risk management occurrence or security incident; include the accidental disclosure of patient health information in the accounting of disclosures log. Mitigate the accidental disclosure and determine the need to contact the patient, organization's legal counsel, and risk management carrier.

8. Place fax machines in secure areas.

9. Establish guidelines to address retention of information transmitted via facsimile and whether it should become part of the patient's health record (e.g., is the document part of a designated record set or a business record?).

10. Take precautions to preserve the quality of faxed documents. Fax copies may fade and may need to be photocopied. Extra precautions are necessary when thermal paper is used to ensure legible copies are retained as long as the medical record is retained.

Source: Davis et al. 2006.

The first step is determining how the Internet is being used. Internet usage usually falls into one of three categories: as an information resource or library, as a communication vehicle (sending e-mails, discussion groups), or as an extension of the organization's network (that is, applications such as a transcription system hosted by a vendor that are totally web based). The second step is determining the speed of the organization's Internet connection. High-speed connections pose the greatest risk of allowing outside connections. Miller (1996) suggests that the information systems department assume responsibility for establishing and maintaining the organization's link to the Internet and limiting the use of the Internet to patient care or business functions. The organization's connection should be protected by a firewall that is monitored on an ongoing basis.

Access to the organization's systems and network should be stringently controlled, which would include preventing remote log-ins or other access functions unless authorized by the department. Guidelines concerning file transfer protocols should be defined, because file transfers from outside the organization run the risk of infecting the system or violating copyright laws.

The organization's security program should also address the use of electronic mail, which has become a major source of provider-patient communication. A more detailed discussion of e-mail is found in the next section. The risks associated with using the Internet for transmitting ePHI are likely outweighed by the benefits. Healthcare providers must understand the issues and ensure that all systems and networks that store and process patient information with links to the Internet are adequately protected, and that security policies and procedures are in place.

Electronic Mail

E-mail has become a primary means of communication for business and personal purposes. It is increasingly requested in response to litigation and is discoverable under e-Discovery rules. The American Medical Informatics Association (AMIA) defined provider-patient e-mail communication as "computer-based communication between clinicians and patients within a contractual relationship in which the health care provider has an explicit measure of responsibility for patient care" (Kane and Sands 1998, 104). Its use in provider-patient communication has become more popular. In 2008, a survey of Florida physicians indicated that 20.4 percent of physicians had used e-mail to communicate with patients (Menachemi et al. 2011). Advantages of using e-mail communication include the following:

- Efficient way to respond to multiple nonurgent messages

- Messages can be retrieved remotely and from any location

- Eliminates the telephone-tag problem

- Messages can be saved and stored in a way that telephone and face-to-face communications cannot

- Test results and treatment recommendations can be sent

- Clarification of treatment or medication instructions can be provided

- Referrals to other information resource locations can be sent (Burrington-Brown and Hughes 2003)

However, communicating highly sensitive information through e-mail, whether patient- or business-related, poses the following privacy and security risks:

- E-mail may be intercepted, which compromises patient privacy or proprietary rights of an organization. Message content can be altered or forwarded to unintended recipients.

- The true identity of the person sending the e-mail may be difficult to establish or confirm with any degree of certainty.

- Use of group e-mail messages can compromise the confidentiality of individuals when all recipients are able to see the list of names or e-mail addresses for the entire group.

- Answering e-mail from an unsecured location may compromise the privacy of the information, especially if information is stored on the unsecured device.

- Opening e-mail attachments could infect the computer or network with viruses and cause serious damage. (Burrington-Brown and Hughes 2003)

Staff training regarding the risks of using e-mail, especially to communicate PHI, must be mandatory. Staff should be trained on how to use and manage e-mail and be given specific templates for e-mail content and business functions that are routinely handled through e-mail, such as scheduling appointments, communicating lab results, and providing additional treatment information. E-mail related to patient care should be incorporated into the patient medical record.

In addition, common recipients of e-mail should sign user confidentiality agreements that prohibit forwarding e-mail to multiple users and guard against such breaches as printing out multiple unauthorized copies, leaving messages onscreen for unauthorized viewing, storing messages in an unsecured file, altering the original message, and so on. Patients should also be educated regarding their responsibility for handling their information in a secure manner. They should understand the risk of using e-mail for communication and should be encouraged to maintain copies for their own personal health record (AHIMA 2003). Guidelines specific to provider-patient e-mail communications are offered by the American Medical Association (AMA) and displayed in figure 11.5.

Figure 11.5. Summary of AMA physician-patient communication guidelines recommended for e-mail

---

- Establish turnaround time for messages. Exercise caution when using e-mail for urgent matters.
- Inform patient about privacy issues.
- Patients should know who besides addressee processes messages during addressee's usual business hours and during addressee's vacation or illness.
- Whenever possible and appropriate, physicians should retain electronic and/or paper copies of e-mails communications with patients.
- Establish types of transactions (prescription refill, appointment scheduling, etc.) and sensitivity of subject matter (HIV, mental health, etc.) permitted over e-mail.
- Instruct patients to put the category of transaction in the subject line of the message for filtering: prescription, appointment, medical advice, billing question.
- Request that patients put their name and patient identification number in the body of the message.
- Configure automatic reply to acknowledge receipt of messages.
- Send a new message to inform patient of completion of request.
- Request that patients use autoreply feature to acknowledge reading clinicians' message.
- Develop archival and retrieval mechanisms.
- Maintain a mailing list of patients, but do not send group mailings where recipients are visible to each other. Use blind copy feature in software.
- Avoid anger, sarcasm, harsh criticism, and libelous references to third parties in messages.
- Append a standard block of text to the end of e-mail messages to patients, which contains the physician's full name, contact information, and reminders about security and the importance of alternative forms of communication for emergencies.
- Explain to patients that their messages should be concise.
- When e-mail messages become too lengthy or the correspondence is prolonged, notify patients to come in to discuss or call them.
- Remind patients when they do not adhere to the guidelines.
- For patients who repeatedly do not adhere to the guidelines, it is acceptable to terminate the e-mail relationship.

Source: AMA 2002.

From a technical standpoint, several safeguards can be used to protect e-mail communication, such as anti-spam and antivirus software, filtering of outbound e-mail, encryption software, and archive solution and retention management programs (AHIMA 2003). Anti-spam and antivirus software can be provided by an outsourced provider or installed internally on an organization's servers and desktops. Filters can be applied to detect proprietary, business, or confidential patient information that also needs to be protected with encryption. In addition to identifying e-mails that require encryption, filters can also trigger an alert if there is an inappropriate or unauthorized transmission of information. Filtering of outbound e-mail is effective only if the organization enforces the use of the tools and prevents employees from using personal e-mail, which could also contain protected or private information and bypass the network filters.

Having a process for archiving e-mail messages is important since such messages are now subject to e-Discovery rules. In fact, in a 2005 study conducted by the Enterprise Strategy Group, 77 percent of organizations involved in electronic data discovery were asked to produce e-mail messages (Babineau 2007). Options for archiving e-mail are numerous. Damoulakis (2006) offers some sample questions that should be asked to determine the best archiving solution for the organization:

- Frequency: When and how often must data be archived?

- Retention: How long will the data be kept?

- Retrievability: How often and in what ways will archived data be accessed or searched?

- Taxonomy: What is the methodology by which archived data will be identified and indexed?

- Ingestion: Do pre-existing or historical data need to be entered into the archive?

- Security: What are the physical (site) and logical (encryption) security requirements?

- Authentication: What levels of access controls are required?

- Immutability: Is there a requirement to prove that the data are unchanged?

- Render options: Is it acceptable for the data to be transformed for rendering purposes?

- Future options: Do the data need to be retained in a common format (for example, PDF, XML) to ensure future readability?

- Refresh criteria: What considerations need to be given to expiration of media life?

- Purge: When are archived data no longer required, and how will they be destroyed?

Along with an archive solution, the organization should also develop an e-mail retention policy and schedule based on the content of the e-mail. A sample retention schedule could contain three retention periods: immediate destruction, limited retention, and archival retention. All applicable laws and regulations should be researched prior to determining which types of messages can be placed in what category. Information related to patient care should be incorporated into the patient's record and retained according to the organization's health record retention guidelines. Business-related e-mails should be kept according to applicable record retention requirements found in state or federal laws and regulatory guidelines. Implementation of the retention schedule removes the employee from having to make decisions about the importance of e-mail messages and whether the message should be deleted or kept (see chapter 8, pp. 191–192).

In addition to the HIPAA Security Rule, other federal laws and some state laws also provide protection for electronic communications. The Electronic Communications Privacy Act of 1986 (ECPA) (18 USC 2510) was enacted by the US Congress to extend government restrictions on wiretaps from telephones to include electronic transmissions of electronic data by computer. According to the regulation, electronic communications "means any transfer of signs, signals, writing, images, sounds, data, or intelligence of any nature transmitted in whole or in part by a wire, radio, electromagnetic, photo electronic or photo optical system that effects interstate of foreign commerce" (18 USC 2510). ECPA amended Title III of the Omnibus Crime Control and Safe Streets Acts of 1968 (42 USC 3711), otherwise known as the "wiretap statute," with the intent of preventing unauthorized government access to private electronic communications. However, subsequent changes related to some provisions of the USA Patriot Act weakened this act.

Questions exist as to whether electronic communications are protected in temporary storage during transmission, which would apply to every electronic communication. Protection does exist for government surveillance conducted without a court order; from third parties with no legitimate access to the messages; and from the carriers of the messages, such as Internet service providers.

Wireless Communication Devices

Wireless networking allows a cell phone, a portable handheld device (for example, a PDA), a computer, a laptop, or a notebook computer equipped with a network card to access the network from any location within the range of the wireless transmitter.

Organizations that allow the use of wireless communication devices that include PHI should incorporate strict guidelines as to the types of devices that may be used and installed. PDAs, smartphones, pocket PCs, tablets, and cell phones are just a few of the mobile devices healthcare providers use to create, store, and access PHI. These devices are making the practice of medicine more efficient by improving the availability of clinical information from just about any location. At a minimum, data on the devices should be encrypted and the device locked, with password access required. Users of this technology must assume an added level of responsibility to protect the device along with the information.

Some additional protection is afforded wireless communication through the Federal Communications Commission regulations (47 CFR Part 15.37(f)) that prohibit the manufacture or import of devices that can pick up frequencies used by cellular phones. Several federal laws (18 USC 1029, 2511, 2701) specifically outline sanctions for intentional interception of cordless and cellular communication. These sanctions can range from fines to imprisonment, depending on the circumstances. The Communications Assistance for Law Enforcement Act of 1994 (CALEA) requires telecommunications carriers to ensure that their equipment will comply with authorized electronic surveillance by law enforcement.

Telehealth/Telemedicine

Telemedicine is defined by the American Telemedicine Association as "the use of medical information exchanged from one site to another via electronic communications to improve patients' health status (American Telemedicine Association n.d.). Closely associated with telemedicine is the broader term '**telehealth**,' which is the digital use of technologies to deliver medical care, health education, and public health services, by connecting multiple users in separate locations (i.e., videoconferencing, transmission of still images, patient portals, remote monitoring of vital signs) (Center for Connected Health Policy 2013).

A number of legal issues surround telehealth/telemedicine, privacy being first and foremost, since patient information can be transmitted anywhere in the world in a matter of seconds. Telemedicine consults routinely contain PHI about the patient that is transmitted over the Internet, by e-mail, or possibly by fax, depending on the system's capability. Requirements regarding expectations for privacy and security should be incorporated into policies and procedures for telehealth/telemedicine services. Most important, appropriate technical safeguards must be put in place before any information is transmitted or received. The Internet can act as a conduit for sending information, but appropriate forms of encryption must be utilized to protect the information.

Social Media

Social media is a collection of online technologies and practices that people use to share opinions, insights, experiences, and perspectives. Tools that take the form of text, video, images, and audio expedite conversations and allow all users to participate in creating and developing content. Healthcare organizations have begun to officially adopt some of these tools as a means of marketing and communicating with consumers or patients.

Privacy and security risks are inherent with social media tools, which were not created with health-care in mind. Organizations must evaluate the risks associated with the use of new communication tools and respond appropriately. At a minimum, organizations must develop clear policies on the appropriate use of any social media tool. Employees should be told that discussion of patient or other work-related information is strictly prohibited. The risk for inadvertent disclosures is just as great as intentional disclosures if employees do not understand the risk of posting information that does not include specific names. Organizations must perform periodic risk analysis to ensure that information has not been posted to a social medial site. Results from the assessments should drive continued education and employee awareness. Because an organization alone cannot monitor every social media site, employees should be responsible for reporting inappropriate postings of information they discover.

Contingency Planning or Disaster Recovery Planning

Contingency planning or **disaster recovery planning** is an important component of protecting ePHI mandated by the HIPAA Security Rule. Healthcare providers need plans in the event of a power failure, disaster, or other emergency that limits or eliminates access to facilities and ePHI. They should also implement a business continuity plan that will "preserve business in the wake of a disaster or disruption in service" (AHIMA 2012, 49). A continuity plan ensures that critical business functions can withstand a variety of emergencies, whereas a contingency or disaster plan includes technical, procedural, and organizational implementation components that should be followed during and after a loss (Nutten and Mansueti 2004; AHIMA 2012). A well-designed contingency or disaster plan can "protect health information from damage, minimize disruption, ensure stability, and provide for orderly recovery" (AHIMA 2010b). The plan should outline the essential components that encompass ePHI as well as other types of health information. Several key components to a contingency or disaster plan are required by the HIPAA Security Rule (45 CFR 164.308(a)(7)) and are designed to protect ePHI:

- Data backup
- Data recovery
- Emergency mode of operations

Data Backup

Information technology departments should have ongoing data backup mechanisms for all patient information. A variety of technical methods, including backup servers or storage media such as backup tapes, can be employed for data backup. Backup plans for an impending natural disaster, such as a hurricane or flood, may involve a massive data "dump" onto tapes or other media and loading it onto trucks and removing it from the vicinity.

Data Recovery

Generally, if data backup procedures are followed, the need for extensive data recovery should be minimal. However, in the event that electronic data are damaged in a disaster, a healthcare provider might seek the services of a company that specializes in electronic data recovery. Healthcare providers or organizations may opt to contract with such a company to perform the data recovery. Specific points that should be outlined in any contract with a data recovery company include the following (AHIMA 2010c):

- Specify the method of recovery.

- Do not use or further disclose the information other than as permitted or required by the contract.

- Use appropriate safeguards to prevent use or disclosure of the information other than as provided for by the contract.

- Report to the contracting organization any inappropriate use or disclosure of the information of which it becomes aware.

- Ensure that any subcontractors or agents with access to the information agree to the same restrictions and conditions.

- Indemnify the healthcare facility from loss due to unauthorized disclosure.

- Return or destroy all health information received from the contracting organization and retain no copies upon termination of the contract.

- Specify the time that will elapse between acquisition and return of information and equipment.

- Authorize the contracting entity to terminate the contract if the business partner violates any material term of the contract.

If electronic records cannot be restored, it may be necessary to reconstitute a record to the extent possible. This may involve the following (AHIMA 2010b):

- Uploading documents from any undamaged databases, such as admission, transcription, laboratory, and radiology databases or data backup services

- Re-transcribing documents from the dictation system

- Obtaining copies from recipients of previously distributed copies, such as physicians' offices, other healthcare facilities, or the business office

Emergency Mode of Operations

Another important aspect of contingency or disaster planning is to outline a set of emergency operations. These may include plans for recording clinical information in the event of a power outage. For example, how will this information be protected? If a natural disaster prevents employees from reporting to work, how will the patient information be secured? Who is responsible for ensuring the security of data and systems during an emergency? Do all employees know how to report system outages, including power, telephone, network, and others? In developing a contingency plan for securing ePHI in the event of an emergency, the healthcare organization should (AHIMA 2010b):

- List the various types of disasters that might impair the operation of the facility. For example, healthcare facilities along the coast will certainly list hurricanes; facilities in the northeast would potentially list ice storms.

- List the department (agency or organization) core processes. These processes will vary. For a large hospital health information department, core processes might include master patient index (MPI), transcription, and chart tracking.

A specific contingency plan should be developed for each identified disaster and core process. Also, consideration should be given for temporary versus long-term effects of disasters and the ability to access the facility and perform departmental functions with and without electricity.

Figure 11.6 is a sample disaster plan development checklist. Figure 11.7 is a sample contingency plan.

Figure 11.6.   Sample disaster plan development checklist

Major Function	Extended Power Outage	Fire	Flood	Hurricane	Explosion
1. MPI					
2. Assembly					
3. Deficiency analysis					
4. Coding					
5. Abstracting					
6. Release of information					
7. Transcription of dictation					
8. Chart tracking/location/ provision					
9. Birth certificates					

For each plausible disaster and major function, develop a contingency plan. As plans are completed, place a check mark in the corresponding box.

Source: Walsh et al. 2009, 178.

Figure 11.7.   Sample contingency plan

1. Facility name:

2. Department name:

3. Plan originator:

4. Date:

5. Major function: Maintenance of an accurate MPI

6. Disaster: Extended power outage

7. Assumptions: An ice storm has resulted in an extended power outage. The majority of the staff is able to report to work.

8. Existing process detail: The MPI contains the patient's name and medical record number. When a patient is admitted, the registration staff accesses the MPI to determine whether the patient already has a medical record number or whether a new number must be generated. HIM staff also accesses the MPI when they need a medical record number to pull medical records for a current hospitalization, to accompany a bill for payment, for continuing care, for quality monitoring or legal action, and to number documents for placement in the paper record. The MPI is generated by entries made by patient registration staff into the admission/discharge tracking system. The accuracy of the numbers assigned is verified by HIM.

9. If-then scenarios: If patient registration staff does not have access to the MPI when admitting a patient, the following might result:

   —the registration system or registrars will assign new numbers, creating duplicates that may cost $20 per set to correct

   —the registrars will issue no numbers and patient health information will have to be matched to patients using account numbers, admission or discharge dates, or birth dates. Medical record numbers will have to be assigned and entered into the database at a later date

If HIM staff members do not have access to an MPI, records cannot be pulled for any reason or provided to anyone.

(continued on next page)

Figure 11.7. Sample contingency plan *(continued)*

10. Interdependencies: Registration staff, patient care areas, transcription, billing, and external customers including the patient, third-party payers, attorneys, and accreditation and standards organizations have a need for the patient medical records and therefore need a functional MPI.
11. Solutions/alternatives:

Potential Solutions/Alternatives	Limitations	Benefits
Auxiliary power will be used to access an electronic copy of the MPI on disk.	• Will not work without auxiliary power • Cumbersome • Generation of some duplicate medical record numbers likely • Human resources to correct duplicate numbers are costly	• Admitting staff are accustomed to this process • Fewer duplicates than with no backup system • Less cumbersome than a totally manual system
Staff will have to depend on a paper MPI.	Printouts will be cumbersome Printouts will probably be located in HIM Generation of duplicate or no numbers likely Manual systems to correct duplicate numbers will be costly	• Provides a mechanism to look up a patient's number and pull a chart when critical

12. Tasks to be performed for selected alternatives (before, during, and after disaster)

Activity	Responsibility
Verify availability of MPI on disk	Associate director, HIM
Implement processes where disk is updated daily	Associate director, HIM
Develop contingency plan procedures and training materials	Associate director, HIM
Train patient registration and HIM staff to use contingency plan	Associate director, HIM
Post disaster and implementation contingency plan, check accuracy of record numbers assigned during disaster and correct as needed	HIM data quality coordinator
OR	
Schedule production and delivery of paper MPI on a routine basis	Associate director, HIM
Create contingency procedures and training materials for manual system	Associate director, HIM
Train patient registration and HIM staff	Associate director, HIM
Post disaster and implementation contingency plan, check accuracy of record numbers assigned during disaster and correct as needed	HIM data quality coordinator
Implementation notification schedule	

Contact	Phone number
HIM director	
HIM associate director	
HIM coordinators	
Admitting director	

Source: Walsh et al. 2009, 180–181.

Resources to Assist with Security Threats and Controls

In addition to previously mentioned access and systems controls and suggestions for addressing internal and external threats (including medical identity theft), there are other helpful security tips and cyber-security tests available from organizations. The Computer Security Resource Center of the National Institute of Standards and Technology (NIST) provides numerous resources specifically designed to address both privacy and security issues in healthcare (NIST n.d.). The National Cyber Security Alliance (NCSA), while not directly related to compliance with the HIPAA Security Rule, provides information that is easily understood by all individuals in an organization and includes tips about using antivirus software to help keep computers secure and using strong passwords and strong authentication technology to protect personal information (NCSA n.d.). Another source of help is the SANS Institute, which is a cooperative research and education organization and a trusted international source of information security training and certification (SANS n.d.). SANS research is based on consensus from network administrators, security managers, and information security professionals on the best security fundamentals and technical aspects of security. It is important for security officers as well as others responsible for managing and protecting healthcare data and information to avail themselves of such resources as the reliance on health information technology continues to grow.

Check Your Understanding 11.3

Instructions: Indicate whether the following statements are true or false (T or F).

1. Data encryption ensures that data transferred from one location on a network to another are secure from eavesdropping or data interception.

2. An organization's firewall limits external Internet users from accessing portions of the healthcare network, but it does not limit internal users from accessing portions of the Internet.

3. Facsimile machines provide a highly secure method of communication.

4. E-mail related to patient care should be kept separate from the patient medical record.

5. Disaster recovery and contingency plans related to ePHI are nice to have but not necessary.

Summary

Internal and external security threats are very real, whether intentional or unintentional or whether produced by humans, nature, or the environment. Particularly perplexing is the growing crime of identity theft, including medical identity theft. While identity theft usually results in financial consequences, victims of medical identity theft face both financial and personal safety consequences. Federal regulations such as FACTA require organizations to implement identify-theft programs that include red flags that may signal the presence of theft. Identification of red flags specific to patients offers healthcare providers additional assistance in identifying potential medical identity thefts. A variety of security access and systems controls can be employed to protect ePHI and avoid security incidents that breach or threaten a healthcare entity's electronic information system, and to promote organizational compliance with the HIPAA Security Rule and the implications of the HITECH Act. Many of the controls discussed in the chapter address administrative, physical, technical, organizational, and procedural safeguards for protecting ePHI. Healthcare providers and organizations are challenged to implement successful information security initiatives that comply with federal and state requirements but most of all provide security for ePHI.

References

AHIMA. 2003. Practice Brief: E-mail as a provider-patient electronic communication medium and its impact on the electronic health record. Web extra. Chicago: AHIMA.

AHIMA. 2010a. HIPAA Privacy and Security training (updated). Web extra. Chicago: AHIMA.

AHIMA. 2010b. Practice brief: Disaster planning for health information (updated). Web extra. Chicago: AHIMA.

AHIMA. 2013 (January 25). Analysis of Modifications to the HIPAA Privacy, Security, Enforcement, and Breach Notification Rules under the HITECH and Genetic Information Nondiscrimination Act: Other Modifications to the HIPAA Rules. Chicago: AHIMA.

AHIMA. 2012. 10 security domains (updated). *Journal of AHIMA* 83(5):48-52.

AHIMA e-HIM Work Group on Medical Identity Theft. 2008. Mitigating medical identity theft. *Journal of AHIMA* 79(7):63–69.

American Medical Association. 2002. Guidelines for physician-patient electronic communications. http://www.ama-assn.org/resources/doc/code-medical-ethics/5026a.pdf American Telemedicine Association. n.d. Nomenclature. http://www.americantelemed.org/practice/nomenclature.

Babineau, B. 2007. Mimosa expands electronic discovery beyond e-mail. (March 14, Brief). Milford, MA: Enterprise Strategy Group. http://www.esg-global.com.Beaver, K. 2003. Information security issues that healthcare management must understand. *Journal of Healthcare Information Management* 17(1):46–49.

Burrington-Brown, J., and G. Hughes. 2003. Practice brief: Provider-patient e-mail security. Web extra. Chicago: AHIMA.

Center for Connected Health Policy. 2013. What is Telehealth. http://cchpca.telehealthpolicy.us/what-is-telehealth.

Damoulakis, J. 2006. Opinion: Twelve questions to answer before buying e-mail archiving. http://www.computerworld.com.

Davis, N., et al. 2006. Practice brief: Facsimile transmission of health information. Web extra. Chicago: AHIMA.

Davis, N., C. Lemery, and K. Roberts. 2005. Practice brief: Identity theft and fraud—the impact on HIM operations. *Journal of AHIMA* 76(4):64A–64D.

Department of Health and Human Services. 2011. HIPAA Privacy Rule Accounting of Disclosures Under the Health Information Technology for Economic and Clinical Health Act. 45 CFR Part 164. *Federal Register* 76 (104): 31426–31449.

Department of Health and Human Services. n.d. Addendum 2: HIPAA security and electronic signature standards glossary of terms. http://www.aspe.hhs.gov/admnsimp/nprm/sec15.htm.

Dixon, P. 2006. Medical identity theft: The information crime that can kill you. World Privacy Forum. http://www.worldprivacyforum.org/medicalidentitytheft.html.

Dougherty, M., and R. Scichilone. 2002. Practice brief: Establishing a telecommuting or home-based employee program. *Journal of AHIMA* 73(7):72A–72L.

Gellman, R., and P. Dixon. 2009. Red Flag and address discrepancy requirements: Suggestions for health care providers. Version 2. Cardiff by the Sea, CA: World Privacy Forum. http://www.worldprivacyforum.org/pdf/WPF_RedFlagReport_09242008fs.pdf.

Gopalakrishna, R. 2000. Audit trails. http://homes.cerias.purdue.edu/~rgk/at.html.

Health Data Management. 2004. Feds get first HIPAA conviction. http://www.healthdatamanagement.com/news/10103-1.html.

Kane, B., and D. Sands. 1998. White paper: Guidelines for the clinical use of electronic mail with patients. *Journal of the American Medical Informatics Association* 5(1):104–111.

Kelly, L. 2004. Remote workers could be your weakest link. London: Incisive Media. http://www.computing.co.uk.

Kissel, R., ed. 2011. *Glossary of Key Information Security Terms*. NIST publication IR 7298, Revision 1. National Institute of Standards and Technology (NIST) Computer Security Resource Center. http://csrc.nist.gov.

Klimasewski, T. 2007. Watching the clock, part 2. HHN Most Wired. http://www.hhnmostwired.com/hhnmostwired_app/jsp/articledisplay.jsp?dcrpath=HHNMOSTWIRED/PubsNewsArticleMostWired/data/07Winter/070307MW_Online_Klimasewski&domain=HHNMOSTWIRED.

Menachemi, N., Prickett, C., and R. Brooks. 2011. The use of physician-patient e-mail: A follow-up examination of Adoption and Best Practice Adherence 2005–2008. *Journal of Medical Internet Research* 13(1):e23.

Miller, D. 1996. Internet security: What health information managers need to know. *Journal of AHIMA* 67(8):56–58.

Narasimman, R. 2005. Laptop security. http://whitepapers.hackerjournals.com.

National Cyber Security Alliance. n.d. http://www.staysafeonline.org/.

National Institute of Standards and Technology. n.d. http://www.nist.gov/index.html.

Nunn, S. 2009. Managing audit trails. *Journal of AHIMA* 80(9):44–45.

Nutten, S., and C. Mansueti. 2004. An IT contingency plan to meet HIPAA security standards. *Journal of AHIMA* 75(2):30–37.

Parmigiani, J. 2009. Communicating security efforts: Informing consumers of data protection programs helps build trust. *Journal of AHIMA* 80(11):56–57.

Ponemon Institute. 2010. Benchmark study on patient privacy and data security. http://www2.idexpertscorp.com.

Rinehart-Thompson, L., and L. Harman. 2009. Medical identity theft: The latest information crime. Prepared with funding from 3M per contract with AHIMA.

RSA Security. 2007. Securing your future with two-factor identification. http://www.rsa.com/products/securid/sb/10695_SIDTFA_SB_0210.pdf.

SANS Institute. n.d.. http://www.sans.org.

Wager, K.A., F.W. Lee, and J.P. Glaser. 2009. *Health Care Information Systems: A Practical Approach for Health Care Management*, 2nd ed. San Francisco: Jossey-Bass.

Walsh, T., B.C. Sher, G.A. Roselle, and S.D. Gamage. 2009. *Medical Records Disaster Planning: A Health Information Manager's Survival Guide.* Chicago: AHIMA.

Walsh, T. 2011. Practice brief: Security risk analysis and management: An overview (updated). Web extra. Chicago: AHIMA.

Washington Post. 1995 (March 1). Hospital clerk's child allegedly told patients that they had AIDS.

Cases, Statutes, and Regulations Cited

16 CFR Part 681: Fair and Accurate Credit Transaction Act. 2003.

45 CFR 164.308(a)(7): Contingency plan. 2005.

47 CFR Part 15.37(f): Telecommunication radio frequency devices. 1994.

18 USC 1028: Fraud and related activities in connection with identification documents and information. 1998.

18 USC 1029: Fraud and related activity in connection with access devices. 2006.

18 USC 2510: Electronic Communication Privacy Act. 1986.

18 USC 2511: Interception and disclosure of wire, oral, or electronic communications prohibited. 2002.

18 USC 2701: Unlawful access to stored communications. 2006.

42 USC 3711: Title III Omnibus Crime Control and Safe Streets Acts of 1968.

Appendix 11.A

Confidentiality and Nondisclosure Agreement (for Employees)

As an employee/contracted employee affiliated with the [name of organization], I understand that I must maintain the confidentiality of any and all data and information to which I have access in the course of carrying out my work. Organizational information that may include, but is not limited to, financial, patient identifiable, employee identifiable, intellectual property, financially non-public, contractual, of a competitively advantageous nature, and is from any source or in any form (i.e., paper, magnetic or optical media, conversations, film, etc.), may be considered confidential. The value and sensitivity of information is protected by law and by the strict policies of [name of organization]. The intent of these laws and policies is to ensure that confidential information will remain confidential through its use as a necessity to accomplish the organization's mission. Special consideration is expected for all information related to personally identifiable health information accessed in the course of your work.

As a condition to receiving electronic access and allowed access to a [system, network, or files] and/or being granted authorization to access any form of confidential information identified above, I agree to comply with the following terms and conditions:

1. My computer sign-on code is equivalent to my LEGAL SIGNATURE and I will not disclose this code to anyone or allow anyone to access the system using my sign-on code and/or password.

2. I am responsible and accountable for all entries made and all retrievals accessed under my sign-on code, even if such action was made by me or by another due to my intentional or negligent act or omission. Any data available to me will be treated as confidential information.

3. I will not attempt to learn or use another's sign-on code.

4. I will not access any online computer system using a sign-on code other than my own.

5. I will not access or request any information for which I have no responsibility.

6. If I have reason to believe that the confidentiality of my user sign-on code/password has been compromised, I will immediately notify [responsible party] by calling the helpdesk at [helpdesk phone number].

7. I will not disclose any confidential information unless required to do so in the official capacity of my employment or contract. I also understand that I have no right or ownership interest in any confidential information.

8. While signed on, I will not leave a secured computer application unattended.

9. I will comply with all policies and procedures and other rules of [name of organization] relating to confidentiality of information and access procedures.

10. I understand that my use of the [name of employer or organization] system may be periodically monitored to ensure compliance with this agreement.

11. I agree not to use the information in any way detrimental to the organization and will keep all such information confidential.

12. I will not disclose protected health information or other information that is considered proprietary, sensitive, or confidential unless there is a need-to-know basis.

13. I will limit distribution of confidential information only to parties with a legitimate need in performance of the organization's mission.

14. I agree that disclosure of confidential information is prohibited indefinitely, even after termination of employment or business relationship, unless specifically waived in writing by an authorized party.

15. This agreement cannot be terminated or canceled, nor will it expire.

16. I will follow the organizational compliance plan for use of confidential information.

I further understand that if I violate any of the above terms, I will be subject to disciplinary action, including discharge, loss of privileges, termination of contract, legal action, or any other remedy available to [name of organization].

User's Name: _____

Department: _____

Adapted from the AHIMA Home Coding Community of Practice Community Resource Posting—Sample Confidentiality Policy.

This sample form was developed by AHIMA for discussion purposes only. It should not be used without review by your organization's legal counsel to ensure compliance with local and state laws.

Source: Dougherty, Michelle, and Rita A. Scichilone. 2002 (July/August). Practice brief: Establishing a telecommuting or home-based employee program. Journal of AHIMA 73(7):72A–72L.

Chapter 12

Access, Use, and Disclosure/ Release of Health Information

Melanie S. Brodnik, PhD, RHIA, FAHIMA, and
Marcia Sharp, MBA, RHIA

Learning Objectives

- Discuss the issues surrounding ownership of health information

- Explain the access and disclosure rights of patients

- Discuss the rights and obligations of the healthcare workforce regarding access and disclosure of health information

- Summarize the access and disclosure procedures

- Summarize the issues related to managing the release of information

Key Terms

Access
Active record
Adoption
Age of majority
Americans with Disabilities
    Act (ADA)
Autopsy
Behavioral health
Clinical Laboratory
    Improvement Amendments
    (CLIA)
Competent adult
Confidentiality of Alcohol and
    Drug Abuse Patient Records
    Regulation
Court order
Disability determination
    services
Disclosure
Durable power of attorney
    (DPOA)
Durable power of attorney for
    healthcare decisions
    (DPOA-HCD)

Duty to warn
Electronic Records Express
    (ERE)
Emancipated minor
Employee health record
Fair and Accurate Credit
    Transactions Act (FACTA)
Freedom of Information Act
    (FOIA)
Health information exchange
    (HIE)
Health information handler
    (HIH)
Health information
    organization (HIO)
Homeland Security Act
Human Genome Project
Human immunodeficiency
    virus (HIV)
Incompetent adult
Inpatient
Legal guardian
Medical emergency
Minor

National Human Genome
    Research Institute
    (NHGRI)
Next-of-kin
Noncustodial parent
Nondisclosure agreement
Occupational safety and
    health record
Open records laws
Outpatient
Ownership (of health record,
    information)
Patriot Act
Personal representative
Primary data source
Privilege statutes
Protected health information
    (PHI)
Psychotherapy notes
Public records laws
Regional health information
    organization (RHIO)
Release of information (ROI)
Secondary data

Social Security Administration (SSA)	Mental Health Services Administration (SAMHSA)	Uniform Health-Care Decisions Act (UHCDA)
Subpoena	Sunshine laws	Use
Substance Abuse and	Syndromic surveillance	

Introduction

The challenge of managing protected health information (PHI) is to ensure access, use, and disclosure of PHI are handled according to state and federal rules and regulations. The HIPAA Privacy and Security Rules along with HITECH provisions were discussed in chapters 9 and 10. This chapter focuses on special circumstances in which access, use, and disclosure or release of patient information, are appropriate with or without patient authorization. As a reminder, HIPAA defines **access** as the right of an individual to inspect and obtain a copy of his or her own health information that is contained in a designated record set, while **use** is defined as the sharing, employment, application, utilization, examination, or analysis of individually identifiable health information within an entity that maintains such information. **Disclosure** is defined as "the release, transfer, provision of, access to or divulging in any other manner of information outside the entity holding the information" (45 CFR 160.103). In general **release of information** refers to providing access to PHI to an individual or entity authorized to receive or review it (Dunn and Edelstein 2008).

The chapter opens with a discussion of ownership of health information and how previously held beliefs about ownership may change as the industry increases its reliance on health information technology. Core to the issue of a patient's right to access or disclose his or her health information is the question of whether the patient is competent to make such a decision. The chapter addresses the rights of competent and incompetent adult patients as well as the rights of individuals deemed as minors. The chapter continues with an overview of workforce members who have access rights to patient information and for what reasons. Issues surrounding highly sensitive information related to behavioral health, substance abuse, HIV/AIDS, genetic information, and adoption are discussed, including their relationship to the HIPAA Privacy Rule and its recent modifications. Similarly, a number of situations involving requests for patient information are discussed. The chapter concludes with a discussion of the practical aspects of managing the process of releasing health information.

Ownership and Control of the Health Record and Health Information

Ownership of the health record has traditionally been granted to the healthcare provider who generates the record. The record as the **primary data source** contains information about the patient documented by the professionals who provided the care or services to the patient (Bowman 2010, 330). Because the health record serves as both a medical document and a legal document that provides proof of care, it is the "business" record of the healthcare provider. State and federal laws have long upheld the right of the patient to control the information within the record (Russell and Bowen 2010). The HIPAA Privacy Rule is silent on who owns the patient's record, but it does set forth the patient's right to access, view, copy, or amend the record, as discussed in chapter 9 (45 CFR 164.524, 526).

Data from the record or "primary data source" are used for many purposes, including public health reporting, research, quality and safety measures, payment, provider certification and accreditation, marketing, and other business activities. Data may be patient-specific, identifiable data such as what might be found in a state cancer registry, or they may be de-identified aggregate data about patients that is used for statistical purposes. When data from the record are used for purposes other than what was intended, those data are referred to as **secondary data** (AMIA 2007a; AMIA 2007b).

The question of who owns the health data in the record and the secondary data gleaned from the primary data source is complicated. While some state laws grant providers ownership of health records, many state laws grant patients the rights to their health information, which may also be viewed as "ownership" rights (Waller and Alcantara 1998). These rights include the right to access, obtain copies of, and request correction of patient information as well as the right to privacy. Providers, even though they may own the physical health record, have a duty to the patient and to patients' privacy rights, which means that ownership of patient-identifiable information does not reside with any one person or entity. Waller and Alcantara point out that:

> Individual[s'] rights in their medical information will exist independent of any contracts. For this reason, providers and others cannot assume "ownership" of patient records permit them to share or sell patient-identified medical information as they see fit. It is wise to avoid contract provisions that purport to transfer ownership of patient-identified data in a manner that violates patient rights or providers' obligations with respect to the information. (1998, 29)

This is an important issue as the healthcare industry relies heavily on information technology to collect, store, retrieve, and disseminate health information and adopts electronic health record (EHR) systems. Health information is captured and stored electronically not only by providers but also by health plans, clearinghouses, payers, technology and service vendors, researchers, employers, financial service firms, and public health agencies, all of which may use the information for purposes other than direct patient care. This complicates the issue of who owns health information, regardless of whether it is primary or secondary data (Burrington-Brown et al. 2007, 63). Waller and Alcantara (1998) address the issue of electronic health information in regard to ownership of de-identified and aggregate data, multiprovider systems integration arrangements, and information systems vendors and clearinghouses. Figure 12.1 provides a summary of the salient points in their discussion.

Burrington-Brown et al. suggest that there is a need to "redefine ownership in terms of access, use, and control of health data by any entity that originates, creates, produces, or holds health information whether that information is identifiable or not" (2007, 63). The American Recovery and Reinvestment Act (ARRA) provides financial incentives to promote the use and electronic sharing of personal health information through the implementation of EHRs and **health information exchanges** (HIEs). A HIE may refer to an organization that has been formed to create an electronic framework that connects hospitals, physicians, pharmacies, and other healthcare entities for the purpose of sharing patient information to facilitate timely, efficient, and effective patient care (HHS 2009a). The term is also used to denote the process of exchanging health information among entities. Another term used to describe an organization that oversees and governs the exchange of health-related information among organizations is **health information organization** (HIO); if the organization brings together other stakeholders within a geographic area, it is termed a **regional health information organization** (RHIO) (HHS 2009a).

Unfortunately, the HITECH provisions that focus on privacy and security remain silent on the issue of who owns the information generated through HIEs, HIOs, and RHIOs. "This legal uncertainty presents a major obstacle to integrating and using information about a single patient from various clinicians and hospitals" (Hall and Schulman 2009, 1282).

However, the Department of Health and Human Services (HHS) Office of the National Coordinator for Health Information Technology (ONC) is addressing the issues of access, use, and disclosure of PHI among HIEs and organizations, including what rights patients may have to allow or deny disclosure of their PHI to these entities or for secondary data uses. In 2008, the ONC published a "National Privacy and Security Framework for Electronic Exchange of Individual Identified Health Information" for the purpose of "establishing a single, consistent approach to address the privacy and security challenges related to electronic health information exchange through a network for all persons, regardless of the legal framework that may apply to a particular organization" (HHS 2008, 2). The ONC Privacy and Security Workgroup continues to address issues including consumer rights in regard to consenting for the exchange of their information; these issues are available for review on the ONC website (HHS n.d.).

Thus, the question of ownership remains under study and open for debate (Demster 2012). In an effort to encourage transparency, the American Medical Informatics Association (AMIA) has suggested that healthcare organizations develop a full disclosure policy that informs patients that while they do not have exclusive ownership of their information, they do have the right to know what is collected

Figure 12.1. Summary of salient points related to ownership of health information in an information age

Ownership of Masked and Aggregated Data

1. When medical record information is cleansed of identifiers, the law generally places few restrictions on the use of this information and generally terminates patient rights.

2. If the identity of individuals cannot be determined from data, whether by itself or combined or cross-matched with other data or databases, the general rule is that anyone who has acquired a legitimate right in the data can own it. This rule is implied by statutory definitions of the medical information protected by confidentiality statutes.

3. Data is patient-identified if the subject of the information is disclosed by the data. Patient-identifiable data need not explicitly identify the patient; rather, if the identity of the patient can be derived or inferred from the data, with or without the assistance of computers and artificial intelligence, data is patient-identifiable.

4. The question arises whether data from records in which the identity of individuals has been masked, but which still exists in discrete individual records, may be freely sold or transferred. Masking the identity of individuals in the information age may require more than merely stripping the data . . . it is possible to associate information with the identity of an individual, even when the information has been stripped of obvious identifying data elements. Thus, masking the most obvious identifiers in individual records may not always be sufficient to make the information truly anonymous.

5. If a patient's address, zip code, or telephone number are left unmasked, cross-matching becomes much easier than if these elements are masked.

6. If there are compelling reasons to permit a vendor or other party to use masked data, it may be preferable to grant a license to use the data, subject to an obligation of the licensee not to manipulate or permit manipulation of data to determine the identity of any subject of a record included in the licensed data, rather than transferring ownership of the data outright. This preserves some control by the licenser over what the licensee does with the licensed data.

7. In instances where data has been masked or aggregated so that the identities of individuals cannot be determined from the data . . . the individual's rights in the data will generally terminate, and a person with a legitimate claim to such data can own, sell, and license it. This makes copyright protection and contractual provisions spelling out ownership and rights in anonymized and aggregated data very important.

Multiprovider Systems Integration Arrangements

1. Hospitals, physicians, other healthcare providers, and, in many cases, health plans have come together in integrated delivery systems to provide seamless care to patients across the continuum of care and to manage the health of populations. Healthcare organizations are integrating their information systems and acquiring and developing shared information systems (e.g., clinical data repositories and master patient indexes).

2. The integration of patient information and information systems raises complex questions as to the relative rights in the data of the provider originating patient data, the entity operating the shared or integrated information system, and the integrated delivery system or network entity (if there is one).

3. In fashioning contracts to support multiprovider systems integration initiatives, it is important that participants avoid the pitfalls that ill-advised contractual provisions concerning information ownership can create. It is advisable for the contract among participants in the systems integration initiative to state that, as among the parties, each party shall be deemed to own the data it originates. In some instances, it may be advisable to tag certain data, such as laboratory results, to multiple "owners" to mirror what would be included in the medical records maintained by participating providers in a paper record environment.

4. Contracts among providers participating in systems integration arrangements should also specify the procedures to be followed when one participant receives a subpoena, court order, or other demand for a compulsory disclosure of data originating with another. A provision that a party receiving a demand for compulsory disclosure of data originating elsewhere must promptly notify the party originating the data of the demand and must cooperate with the originating provider in contesting disclosure.

5. To address the problems that could arise when one provider participating in a shared clinical information system relies on data originating with another provider to provide care to a patient who suffers a therapeutic misadventure, it is also wise for a contract among participating providers to grant the entity operating the shared or integrated system a perpetual license to maintain the data in the system. The licensee also should agree to make available to any participating provider information necessary to defend or respond to any claim or suit involving allegations of malpractice or to respond to any governmental or other investigation.

(continued on next page)

Figure 12.1. Summary of salient points related to ownership of health information in an information age *(continued)*

6. Ownership provisions in contracts among providers integrating or sharing information systems should further address rights to the data in the event that one provider within the network withdraws or is otherwise terminated. At a minimum, the systems integration or network agreement should provide that, upon termination or withdrawal, a participating provider is entitled to copy the data originated by such provider and documentation of the chain of copying.

7. Contracts among participating providers should set forth clearly whether any mining of the data of another party is permitted and, if so, under what circumstances, for what purposes, and subject to what restrictions on dissemination of the results.

8. Because the data of providers sharing or integrating information systems will often have value when viewed in the aggregate, the contract among participating providers should also provide a mechanism whereby the parties can collectively exploit the value of their data and state a formula or mechanism for allocating such value among the participants. So long as such data are not patient-identifiable, participating providers are free to enter into sales or licensing arrangements to realize the value of their aggregate information.

Information Systems Vendors and Clearinghouses

1. All agreements between healthcare providers' external computer service or data organizations should address whether the outside entity will be permitted to use patient information or create comparative databases or other proprietary information products for distribution to third parties.

2. The vendor's manipulation of such data for purposes of conducting statistical analysis or for constructing comparative databases will be substantially different from the way the vendor processes data for purposes of performing its obligations under its contract with the provider or the integrated delivery system. Permitting vendors to process patient data in this manner may expose participating providers to potentially serious liability for the vendor's improper disclosure of patient-identifiable information. Such use should be permitted by contract only if the contract includes detailed vendor confidentiality obligations also applicable: to the vendor's agents, employees, and subcontractors and protecting patient-identifiable data; and to information identified as proprietary information of the provider, system, or network and to practitioner- or provider-identified data.

3. The contract should also include detailed procedures and protocols the vendor must follow in processing all such data. The vendor should be required to provide indemnification for all losses resulting from breach of these obligations, including the provider's or integrated delivery system's attorneys' fees and costs.

4. It is inadvisable to grant vendors ownership rights in data composed of masked individual patient records. If a delivery system or provider wants to permit the vendor to utilize such data in creating data products, it should consider granting the vendor a license to use the data, subject to the vendor's continuing obligations not to manipulate or permit manipulation of the data in any manner that would reveal the identity of any patient and not to disclose to any third party the licensed data (unless it has been further aggregated to make it truly anonymous).

5. If a third party (such as a clearinghouse) will perform the data masking, it is important that a contract be executed prior to any transfer of patient-identifiable data to the entity charged with performing the masking. The contract should require the entity to preserve the confidentiality of all patient-identifiable data in perpetuity and to use such data only to perform its contractual obligations. The contract should also provide for return or destruction of all patient-identifiable data in the possession of the third party in any form at the conclusion of the contract.

Source: Waller and Alcantara 1998.

about them and what secondary uses may be made of the information (AMIA 2007b). Laws and standards surrounding the question of ownership are evolving and will be tested as situations arise. In the meantime, the responsibility for adhering to laws and accrediting body standards for protecting health information from its creation to final disposition, remains with providers and others who access, use, and disclose patient information.

Access to Patient Health Information

An individual has the right to control his or her own body and the right to consent or refuse consent to medical treatment as defined by federal and state laws. Similarly, an individual has certain rights to access, use, and disclose his or her PHI as defined by federal and state laws. The HIPAA Privacy Rule defines PHI as "individually identifiable health information that is transmitted by electronic media, maintained in electronic medium, or transmitted or maintained in any other form or medium" (45 CFR 160.103). The rule is specific about the access, uses, and disclosures of PHI that require patient authorization and those that do not (45 CFR 164.508). It also allows individuals to receive an accounting of disclosures, as discussed in chapter 9 and later in this chapter. Recent investigations into state health record access laws surrounding the privacy and security of interoperable HIEs, sponsored by the Agency for Healthcare Research and Quality and the ONC, revealed (RTI 2009):

> Few states have medical privacy access provisions as extensive as those found in the HIPAA Privacy Rule. However, most states have moderately detailed laws governing access to medical records held by doctors and/or hospitals including provisions that expressly address: individuals' right of access to their health information; the maximum time doctors and/or hospitals have to respond to such a request; and the maximum copying fees doctors and/or hospitals may charge for furnishing the record. The right to amend health information is the standard least likely to be addressed by state law.

Most state statutory and regulatory provisions provide patients with the right to access their health information and also provide for protecting the confidentiality of patient information. State statutes related to patient access and confidentiality of health records can be found on the website of the National Conference of State Legislatures (NCSL), which hosts a state legislative website directory (NCSL 2010). Another source for state health record laws can be found on the FindLaw website (Thomson Reuters 2012). While there are many issues related to access, use, and disclosure rights, the following discussion focuses on common situations that require oversight by those who manage the privacy and security of patient information.

Competent Adult

A **competent adult** is an individual who is mentally and physically competent to tend to his or her own affairs and has reached the **age of majority**. The age of majority in most states is 18 years or older, as discussed in chapter 7. Just as a competent adult may consent to treatment, the adult may authorize the access or disclosure of his or her health information. A competent adult may also wish to appoint another person to be his or her **personal representative**. A personal representative is someone who is legally authorized to make healthcare decisions on an individual's behalf or to act on behalf of a deceased individual or that individual's estate. A personal representative could include, for example, a spouse or next-of-kin as defined by state law, an agent, or an individual who holds a **durable power of attorney** (DPOA) or a **durable power of attorney for healthcare decisions** (DPOA-HCD) for the patient. The personal representative has the right to request and receive information about the adult's personal affairs and physical and mental health, including legal and health records.

Some states have implemented the **Uniform Health-Care Decisions Act** (UHCDA), which allows a competent adult to communicate to a supervising healthcare provider the selection of a "surrogate" (personal representative) who may make healthcare decisions for the adult (Uniform Law Commission 2010). If a surrogate has not been named, then a person related to the adult, the **next-of-kin**, can step forward and assume responsibility. The UHCDA suggests the decision-making priority order for an individual's next-of-kin, which is basically the same for decisions related to medical treatment as well. Chapter 7 has additional information on consents and a discussion of advance directives related to DPOA and DPOA-HCD. The UHCDA priority-order list is as follows:

1. Spouse

2. Adult child

3. Parent

4. Adult sibling

5. If no one is available who is so related to the individual, authority may be granted to an adult who has exhibited special care and concern for the individual, who is familiar with the patient's personal values, and who is willing and able to make a healthcare decision for the patient.

6. Absent an unrelated adult who exhibits the above characteristics, a healthcare provider may seek appointment of a decision maker by the court having jurisdiction.

The adult patient or the personal representative of the adult patient has the right to request, receive, examine, copy, amend, and authorize disclosure of the patient's healthcare information. However, before disclosing any information, the healthcare organization must identify and verify that the requester is who he or she purports to be and that the requester has the authorization to access the information. If the requester is the competent adult patient, then the requester should be asked for identification. If the requester is a personal representative, this person should be asked to produce a copy of the appropriate legal documentation to verify their right to access and disclose the patient's information. This documentation should be a witnessed DPOA or DPOA-HCD. It is a good practice to require an additional statement explaining the requester's relationship to the patient and stating why the patient is unable to sign (Reynolds 2010).

Incompetent Adult

When an individual who is at or above the age of majority becomes incapacitated due to illness or injury, either permanently or temporarily, he or she may be designated as an **incompetent adult**. When this occurs, another person should be designated to make decisions for that individual, including decisions about the use and disclosure of the individual's PHI. That person may be a parent, sibling, agent, attorney, or surrogate. Whoever serves as the incompetent adult's personal representative should, at a minimum, hold the incompetent adult's DPOA or DPOA-HCD. In the absence of an advance directive, the court system, with support from the appropriate medical community, will declare the individual incompetent. The court will then appoint a **legal guardian** to handle the matters of the incompetent adult.

The guardian may be the spouse, adult child, or sibling of the individual, or another designated person. It is important to avoid the assumption that individuals with mental illnesses are also mentally incompetent. They must be formally deemed mentally incompetent by the court. In acting for the incompetent adult, the personal representative has the right to request, receive, examine, copy, and authorize disclosure of the incompetent adult's PHI. However, as noted above, before disclosing any information, the healthcare organization should require legal documentation of the incompetent adult's legal position and the reason the adult is unable to sign the authorization, along with documentation of the personal representative's authority to access or authorize disclosure of the incompetent adult's PHI (Reynolds 2010).

Minors

A **minor** is defined as an individual under the age of 18 who has not been legally emancipated (declared an adult) by the court. By virtue of their age, minors are generally deemed legally incompetent—unable to consent for their own medical treatment or to access, use, amend, or disclose their health information. However, special situations and exceptions that allow minors to do so are explained below. Because HIPAA defers to state law on the issue of minors, applicable state laws must be consulted regarding who has authorization to access, use, or disclose a minor's PHI.

Parental Authorization Required

Because minors are, as a general rule, legally incompetent and unable to make decisions regarding the access, use, and disclosure of their own healthcare information, this authority usually belongs to the minor's parent(s) unless an exception applies. However, several categories of parents are recognized by laws, including the following:

- Married biological parents

- Separated or divorced biological parents

- Stepparents

- Adoptive parents

- Foster parents

- Grandparents (children living with grandparents who are not legal guardians)

- Legal guardians

- Others, such as a parent in the service or overseas who has transferred guardianship to a relative or friend with whom the child is temporarily living (Reynolds 2010)

Generally, only one parent's signature is required to authorize the access, use, or disclosure of a minor's PHI. In some states, only the mother's signature, regardless of the mother's age, is required, and in other states it is the custodial parent (as determined by the court) who is responsible for authorizing the access, use, and disclosure of the minor patient's PHI.

Parental Authorization Not Required

Minor patients may authorize the access, use, or disclosure of their PHI without parental authorization in several situations, most of which are defined by state statutory or regulatory provisions. An **emancipated minor** is one who is under the age of majority and self-supporting with parents who have surrendered their rights of custody, care, and support. Emancipated minors generally may authorize the access, use, and disclosure of their own PHI. If the minor is married, previously married, or in the military, the minor controls his or her PHI. If the minor is under the age of 18 and is the parent of a child, the minor may authorize the access, use, and disclosure of his or her own PHI as well as that of his or her child. In this case the minor falls under the provisions set forth for parental authorization as discussed above.

Generally, if the patient is a minor at the time of treatment or hospitalization and reaches the age of majority during this time period, the patient may authorize the access, use, or disclosure of his or her PHI. The fact that the parents, parents' insurance, or other third-party payer is paying the bill does not matter; the patient retains control over his or her PHI (Reynolds 2010).

Many state laws allow a minor to be treated for drug or alcohol dependency, mental health, sexually transmitted diseases (STDs), or HIV/AIDS or be given contraceptives and prenatal care without prior parental or legal guardian consent or knowledge. Federal rules specific to alcohol and drug abuse further define the right of minors to authorize the access, use, or disclosure of their information and will be discussed in more detail later in the chapter. Minors may also seek judicial (court) permission for an abortion in states in which it is permissible by law. In any of these situations, the minor must authorize the access, use, or disclosure of his or her PHI. Depending on the medical condition and state law, however, healthcare providers may be legally permitted to decide whether to notify the parent(s) or legal guardian(s) concerning the condition or treatment of the minor. In doing so, the parent(s) or legal guardian(s) will have access to the minor's PHI since the information was disclosed by the healthcare provider (Reynolds 2010).

Access and Authorization Rights of Noncustodial Parents and Others

State laws generally address situations involving the rights of divorced or separated parents as well as grandparents with respect to accessing and authorizing the use or disclosure of a minor's PHI. A **noncustodial parent** is a parent who does not have legal custody of the child. Noncustodial parents are legally endowed with parental rights, which generally allow them to access the healthcare information of their minor children subject to the situations stated above regarding minors. This right, which is explicitly stated in state laws and the HIPAA Privacy Rule, may be overridden if a court determines that denial of the parental right is in the best interests of the child. In the absence of a "best interests of the child" determination by the court, state laws should be consulted regarding the specific rights granted to noncustodial parents. For example, Tennessee law requires that a copy of the child's health records be furnished to the noncustodial parent by the treating physician or the treating hospital upon a written request by the noncustodial parent (TN Code Ann. 36-6-103).

In some states, either parent may authorize the release of information; however, best practice dictates that authorization should be first sought from the custodial parent whenever possible (Reynolds 2010). If state law distinguishes between custodial and noncustodial parents' rights of access, persons working with health records of minors should review requests from noncustodial parents to determine that the disclosure complies with state law. It is often the duty of the parent who is holding the restriction against a noncustodial parent to make a healthcare provider aware of the restriction order. In the case of a grandparent, other family member, or friend, this individual should produce proof of guardianship in order to authorize the access, use, or disclosure of the minor's PHI.

Providers of pediatric services may wish to include information about the rights of minors and noncustodial parents in their Notice of Privacy Practices and on all authorizations for disclosure of information as a way of providing information to patients and custodial parents or guardians about the access rights of noncustodial parents. Obtaining information about the minor patient's custody, limitations on parental rights, or special circumstances when patients are first seen or admitted can often help providers avoid problems later (Reynolds 2010).

Minors in Foster Care or Allegedly Abused

In some states, an authorization for the access or disclosure of the PHI of a child in a foster care system may be signed by the appropriate department of human services or children's services personnel. Some states delegate this responsibility to the department's designated representative. Depending on the state, a foster parent may authorize the access, use, or disclosure of a child's PHI; however, legal documentation of the relationship is required. Healthcare organizations and providers should not release any information to persons alleged to have abused the child, if known, regardless of the relationship of the person to the child (Reynolds 2010).

Employer, Employee, and Other Members of the Workforce

The HIPAA Privacy Rule broadly defines "workforce" as employees, volunteers, trainees, and other persons, whether paid or not, who work for and are under the direct control of the covered entity (CE) (45 CFR 160.103). Access to and disclosure of patient information to various workforce members varies by the job and responsibility.

Employers

Employers that may or may not be HIPAA-covered healthcare entities may request patient information for a number of reasons, including family medical leave certification, return to work certification for work-related injuries, and information for company physicians. Patient authorization is required for such disclosures, but in some states, the patient's employer, employer's insurer, and employer's and employee's attorneys do not need patient authorization to obtain health information for workers' compensation purposes.

Employees

Employees of a HIPAA-covered entity are categorized as either directly involved or not directly involved in a patient's care. Although those involved directly in a patient's care (nurses, nurse's aides, case managers, physical therapists, respiratory therapists, and so on) do not require authorization to access the health record, job descriptions and procedures must document patient care responsibilities and justify an employee's need to access the information. Employees in hospital or healthcare organization departments, who are not involved directly in patient care, will vary in their need to access patient information. The HIPAA "minimum necessary" principle must be applied to determine what access employees legitimately have to PHI (45 CFR 164.502(b)). The HIPAA security regulations should also identify facility access controls on electronic PHI (45 CFR 164.310(a)(1)). As discussed in chapter 11, employees and others discussed in this section of the chapter should be required to sign a **nondisclosure agreement** relating to the confidentiality and privacy of patient information as a condition of employment.

Physicians

Physicians are classified in numerous ways and thus must be considered according to their classifications for access purposes: attending physicians, fellows, residents, interns, house staff members in the postdoctorate programs, researchers, physicians of record versus referring physicians, consulting physicians versus follow-up physicians, treating physicians versus non-treating physicians. Physicians who are on the medical staff or part of the organized healthcare arrangement and who are treating a patient should be given access to the patient's information for treatment and payment purposes following verification of their treatment relationship. Referral or follow-up physicians may also access a patient's information following verification of the treatment relationship with the patient. In each case, the patient's authorization is not required, but verification of the treatment relationship is required.

A physician should have access to patient information if he or she is treating a specific patient. The physician should not have access to patient information of individuals that he or she is not treating unless the physician is performing designated healthcare operations such as research, peer review, or quality improvement activity. Physician office staff and personnel to whom the physician or group has outsourced billing services may access patient information or records for payment purposes.

Students

Students in medical, nursing, allied health, and counseling educational programs who are involved in direct or indirect patient care should have access to patient health records without patient authorization. A contract or letter of agreement between the student's educational institution and healthcare provider that outlines the student's access and responsibilities to maintain patient privacy and confidentiality should be maintained by both parties.

Attorneys

Attorneys may or may not be employees of a healthcare organization. Those who are employed by a healthcare organization (for example, privacy officer, risk manager, compliance officer) are considered members of the workforce and do not require authorization prior to accessing a patient's healthcare information for such purposes as defending lawsuits, handling collections, and dealing with other legal issues. A nonemployee attorney who is retained to provide legal representation to a healthcare organization or provider does not require patient authorization prior to accessing patient information; however, a business associate agreement is required per the HIPAA Privacy Rule in order for access to occur. If a patient has hired an attorney and requests that his or her attorney receive the patient's information, then the attorney must present a signed authorization from the patient that authorizes the release of the patient's information to the attorney.

Vendors

Vendors present in a healthcare organization will often have access to patient information in the course of their work. Such vendors include consultants, those who sell equipment and supplies, those who perform release-of-information functions and transcription services, and those who provide laundry, food, or equipment repair services. If the vendor meets the definition of a business associate (that is, it is using or disclosing an individual's PHI on behalf of the healthcare organization), a business associate agreement must be signed. If a vendor is not a business associate, employees of the vendor should sign confidentiality agreements and undergo HIPAA training because of their routine contact with and exposure to patient information. Neither situation requires patient authorization.

Check Your Understanding 12.1

Instructions: Indicate whether the following statements are true or false (T or F).

1. Ownership of a health record has traditionally been granted to the patient.

2. A competent adult may wish to appoint another person to be his or her personal representative.

3. A minor who is emancipated must still have his or her parents authorize for disclosure of health information.

4. A noncustodial parent has the right to access the healthcare information of their minor child subject to other mitigating circumstances related to the minor's rights to access.

5. Attorneys have automatic access to patient information because they are officers of the court.

Highly Sensitive Health Information

There are certain types of patient information that require special handling in regard to access, requests, uses, and disclosures due to the sensitive nature of the information. Information related to such issues as behavioral healthcare, substance abuse, communicable diseases, genetic testing, and adoption birth records often requires additional protection. HIPAA affords protection to all types of health information; it does not distinguish between highly sensitive health information and other types of health information but instead defers to state laws and existing federal regulations to address specific protections.

Behavioral (Mental) Health Information

Behavioral or mental health treatment is delivered though a broad array of services provided in acute and long-term hospitals, ambulatory care clinics, publicly funded community mental health centers, and group homes. **Behavioral health** encompasses the treatment of mental disorders, mental retardation, and other developmental disabilities. Patient information generated through behavioral health treatment is highly sensitive. In addition to containing very private information related to personal thoughts and relationships, the very fact that an individual is receiving behavioral health treatment is associated with a powerful and unfortunate stigma that influences an individual's life. "Our society tends to develop limited, and often negative, perceptions about that individual's intellectual capabilities, educability, employability, social skills, ability to be a good neighbor, propensity for violence, and ability to lead a productive life" (Randolph and Rinehart-Thompson 2006, 465).

Patients with mental illness, mental retardation, and developmental disabilities are given access rights to their psychiatric and health records through the HIPAA Privacy Rule and individual state statutory and regulatory provisions (45 CFR 164.524). A caveat to this access right is if the patient's healthcare provider has restricted access by documenting such restriction in the patient's treatment plan with clear reasons as to why access should be denied. Aside from providing general access rights and restricting psychotherapy notes, HIPAA does not address behavioral health records specifically. **Psychotherapy notes** are a mental health professional's documentation or analysis of private counseling conversations that are kept separate from the remainder of a behavioral health record, which usually contains information such as diagnosis, prescriptions, treatment modalities, and test results (45 CFR 164.501). The access, use, and disclosure of behavioral health records are mainly addressed by individual state statutes. Most state statutes identify records or reports related to a mentally ill, mentally retarded, or developmentally disabled person as confidential, requiring patient or appointed designee authorization before information is disclosed unless for treatment, payment, or healthcare operation purposes. Authorizations that could reveal an individual's behavioral health diagnosis or treatment should specifically state so in a manner that is obvious to the individual legally authorized to sign the authorization form.

Because of the highly sensitive nature of behavioral health information, state statutes generally include the identity of an individual as confidential information as well as the treatment information itself. Healthcare organizations that maintain a facility directory as designated by the HIPAA Privacy Rule must take care to develop protocols that specifically describe facility directory disclosures and explain to patients that such disclosures could result in a requester knowing an individual's status as a behavioral health patient (45 CFR 164.510(a)). An organization may omit the facility directory altogether for behavioral health patients, taking care to develop protocols so that the process of withholding information does not also breach an individual's confidentiality (Randolph and Rinehart-Thompson 2006).

Provider-patient privilege statutes exist in many states. Privilege statutes may include a variety of providers such as physicians, psychologists, psychiatric or mental health nurses, certified social workers, marital therapists, licensed counselors, pastoral therapists, and others. **Privilege statutes** legally protect confidential communications between provider and patient related to diagnosis and treatment from disclosure during civil and some criminal misdemeanor litigation. The mental health professional cannot be compelled to testify or disclose information without the authorization of the patient in a judicial situation. Exceptions to such statutes usually include the following situations:

- The patient brings up the issue of the mental or emotional condition.

- The health professional performs an examination under a court order.

- A psychiatrist in an involuntary commitment procedure recommends admission and confinement of the patient to avoid harm to the patient or others. (Reynolds 2010)

However, there are situations where there is a legal "**duty to warn,**" a required disclosure of information to an intended victim when a patient threatens to harm an individually identifiable person or persons and the psychiatrist or other mental health provider believes that the patient is likely to actually harm the individual(s). The healthcare provider may warn the victim and/or begin commitment proceedings to ensure that the patient is admitted and receives inpatient mental health treatment. State reporting laws also require that law enforcement be informed of the situation. Most states require that all mental health providers testify in commitment hearings. These laws generally include the duty to warn.

The most familiar case regarding the duty to warn is *Tarasoff v. the Regents of the University of California*. A therapist was told by a patient that he wanted to kill his girlfriend, Tatiana Tarasoff. No one warned Ms. Tarasoff and the patient ultimately killed her. The court ruled that the therapist had a duty to let Tarasoff know of the threat. The case established that the duty to warn consists of three aspects: first, there is a relationship between the therapist and the client; second, the therapist has a responsibility to control the actions of the client; and third, there is an identifiable potential victim (Schlossberger and Hecker 1996). Because later rulings have somewhat limited the requirements of Tarasoff, applicable case and statutory law must be consulted to determine a state's duty to warn.

As behavioral health and substance (alcohol and drug) abuse programs (discussed in more detail below) migrate from paper to EHR systems and engage in HIEs, the HHS's **Substance Abuse and Mental Health Services Administration** (SAMHSA) is working in collaboration with the ONC to ensure programs have a complete understanding of their responsibilities regarding the access, use, and disclosure of PHI, especially in regard to HIEs. In June 2010, SAMHSA and the ONC released frequently asked questions (FAQ) on applying substance abuse confidentiality regulations to HIEs which uphold the requirements as found in 42 CFR 2.11 Part 2 discussed below (SAMHSA 2010).

Substance Abuse Records

Special privacy protection is given to patients treated for substance (alcohol and drug) abuse to encourage individuals to seek treatment. Because of the highly sensitive nature of this treatment, the identity of the patient is confidential as well as the treatment information itself. Congress enacted the **Confidentiality of Alcohol and Drug Abuse Patient Records Regulation** for the purpose of encouraging individuals to seek substance abuse treatment without fear of their health information being disclosed. The regulations define facilities covered by the law as those institutions providing a federally assisted alcohol and drug program. "Program" is defined in 42 CFR 2.11 Part 2 as:

1. An individual or entity (other than a general medical care facility) which holds itself out as providing and which actually provides alcohol or drug abuse diagnosis, treatment, or referral for treatment

2. An identified unit within a general medical facility which holds itself out as providing and which actually provides alcohol or drug abuse diagnosis, treatment, or referral for treatment

3. Referral or medical personnel or other staff in a general medical facility whose primary function is the provision of alcohol or drug abuse diagnosis, treatment, or referral for treatment and who are identified as such providers. A program may provide other services in addition to alcohol and drug abuse services, for example, mental health or psychiatric services, and nevertheless be an alcohol or drug abuse program within the meaning of these regulations.

Special access and disclosure procedures must be followed in handling health records that contain the identity, diagnosis, prognosis, and treatment of patients having a primary or secondary diagnosis of alcohol or drug abuse or, within the patient records of federally assisted programs, any mention of alcohol or drug abuse.

When the HIPAA Privacy Rule and Security Rule were enacted, they did not change the current responsibility of a federally assisted program in adhering to the alcohol and drug abuse regulations regarding confidentiality and release of information. In 2004, SAMHSA published a guidance document explaining the relationship between the two sets of regulations. The guidance document states,

Substance abuse treatment programs must comply with both rules. Generally, this will mean that they will continue to follow Part 2's general rule and not disclose information unless they can obtain consent or point to an exception to that rule that specifically permits the disclosure. Programs must then make sure that the disclosure is also permissible under the Privacy Rule. (SAMHSA 2004)

Because the information in the alcohol and drug abuse patient's health record is protected, disclosures from the records are prohibited without the patient's written authorization. Both HIPAA and substance abuse laws require that patients be notified of the healthcare provider's privacy practices. A healthcare provider can combine the requirements of both programs into a single notice (SAMHSA 2004, 12). See figure 12.2 for the elements required in a single notice.

Authorization for Disclosure (Release) of Information from Substance Abuse Facilities

The regulations under 42 CFR 2.11 Part 2 are specific regarding who can authorize disclosure of patient information.

Figure 12.2. Elements required for a notice of privacy practices

- A statement, prominently displayed, stating: "This notice describes how medical information about you may be used and disclosed and how you can get access to this information. Please review it carefully";
- A detailed description of the types of uses and disclosures that may be made without the patient's consent or authorization. For substance abuse treatment programs, these would include uses and disclosures:

  —In connection with treatment, payment or health care operations (include at least one example of each);

  —To qualified service organizations or business associates who provide services to the program's treatment, payment or health care operations;

  —In medical emergencies;

  —Authorized by court order;

  —To auditors and evaluators;

  —To researchers if the information will be protected as required by Federal regulations;

  —To report suspected child abuse or neglect; and

  —To report a crime or a threat to commit a crime on the premises or against staff

- A statement that other disclosures will be made only with the patient's written consent or authorization which can be revoked, unless the program has taken action in reliance on the consent or authorization;
- A statement that the program may contact the patient to provide appointment reminders or information about treatment alternatives or other health-related benefits and services that may be of interest to the patient;
- A statement that it is required by law to maintain the privacy of PHI and to notify patients of its legal duties and privacy practices, including any changes to its policies;
- A statement that the program must abide by the terms of the notice currently in effect; a statement that the program reserves the right to change the terms of its notice and to make the new notice provisions effective for all information it maintains; and a statement describing how it will provide patients with a revised notice of its practices;
- The name or title and telephone number of a person or office the patient can contact for further information;
- A statement of the patient's rights with respect to PHI and a brief description of how the patient may exercise those rights, including:

  —The right to request restrictions on certain uses and disclosures of PHI, including the statement that the program is not required to agree with requested restrictions;

  —The right to receive confidential communications of PHI (such as having mail and telephone calls be limited to home or office location);

  —The right to access and amend PHI;

  —The right to receive an accounting of the program's disclosures of PHI;

  —The right to complain—free from retaliation—to the program and to the Secretary of Health and Human Services (HHS) about violations of privacy rights, and information on how to file a complaint with the program; and

  —The right to obtain a paper copy of the notice upon request

- The effective date of the notice. See 45 CFR 164.520(b)

[1]The Privacy Rule also requires that the notice contain information about any more restrictive law. For example, if State law further limits disclosure of HIV-related information, that restriction should also appear in the notice.

[2]Programs often need to provide PHI to criminal justice agencies that mandate patients into treatment. Under Part 2, such disclosures may be made pursuant to a non-revocable consent that complies with 42 CFR §2.35. Under the Privacy Rule, such disclosures may be made pursuant to an authorization or pursuant to a court order. In order to comply with both rules, programs may find it helpful to ask the court in such a situation to issue an order that the program disclose necessary information to the court and other law enforcement personnel.

[3]A substance abuse treatment program engaging in these kinds of activities must be careful in contacting the patient that it does not make any patient-identifying disclosures to others. If the program does not intend to contact the patient, they do not need to include this statement.

[4]This is also voluntary. However, if this statement is not included, any changes in privacy practices described in the notice will apply only to PHI the program created or received after issuing a revised notice reflecting such changes. 45 CFR §164.520(b)(1)(v)(C).

Source: SAMHSA 2004.

Programs may not use or disclose any information about any patient unless the patient has consented in writing (on a form that meets the requirements established by the regulations) or unless another very limited exception specified in the regulations applies. Any disclosure must be limited to the information necessary to carry out the purpose of the disclosure. (SAMHSA 2004, 5)

The Part 2 authorization form must include the elements listed below in addition to a written statement that the information cannot be redisclosed:

- Name or general designation of the program or person permitted to make the disclosure

- Name or title of the individual or name of the organization to which disclosure is to be made

- Name of the patient

- Purpose of the disclosure

- How much and what kind of information is to be disclosed

- Signature of patient (and, in some states, a parent or guardian)

- Date on which authorization is signed

- Statement that the authorization is subject to revocation at any time except to the extent that the program has already acted on it

- Date, event, or condition upon which authorization will expire if not previously revoked (SAMHSA 2004, 5)

In order for the substance abuse program authorization form to also be in compliance with the Privacy Rule, the program should include additional elements required by the Privacy Rule (45 CFR 164.508). These are listed in figure 9.8 (p. 232).

The patient is generally the only person who can authorize the disclosure of information. In the case of minors, the minor patient who consented to treatment must always sign the authorization for a program to disclose information even to his or her parents or guardians (SAMHSA 2004, 7). In states that require parental permission before treating a minor, both parent and minor authorization must be obtained to disclose information (42 CFR 2.14(c)(2)). In Tennessee, for example, where a minor may be treated for drug or alcohol dependency without prior parental consent, the minor must authorize the disclosure of information (TN Code Ann. 33-8-202).

Permissible Disclosures under Federal Drug and Alcohol Regulations

Situations in which information can be disclosed without the patient's written authorization include medical emergencies and scientific research, audits, and program evaluations where the individual patient is not identified. A court may authorize disclosure to avoid death or serious bodily harm to a patient or other individual.

HIV/AIDS, STDs, and Other Communicable Disease Information

Healthcare organizations must comply with applicable state laws to protect the privacy and confidentiality of patients with **human immunodeficiency virus** (HIV) or acquired immune deficiency syndrome (AIDS), sexually transmitted diseases (STDs), and in some cases hepatitis B virus or other communicable diseases. Because of the highly sensitive nature of these health conditions, the identity of the patient is confidential as well as the treatment information itself. However, each state has laws for the control of STDs, including the reporting of certain STDs and the isolation and quarantine of infected persons. State laws require physicians, clinics, hospitals, laboratories, penal institutions, and others who find a diagnosis of HIV/AIDS or certain STDs and other infectious diagnoses to report these diagnoses to the state department of health or other appropriate agency. Required reporting of these diseases is discussed further in chapter 13. The requirement to report such diseases and viruses to state health agencies is an effort to protect third parties and curtail the spread of the disease or virus.

HIPAA regulations do not provide specific privacy protection for patients with these conditions; thus, healthcare providers must follow the HIPAA Privacy and Security Rules as for other PHI unless preempted by state law. However, many states do have laws that specifically protect the confidentiality of HIV/AIDS and STD information. In addition, traditional privacy practices of healthcare organizations have provided extra protection, as a way to encourage individuals to seek treatment (Reynolds 2010).

Confidentiality Protections for HIV/AIDS

Most state laws have special procedures for the handling of HIV/AIDS patient information in regard to subpoenas, discovery, and search warrants. Release for epidemiological studies when the patient is not identified is generally allowable. Laws for minors may vary as child abuse laws may require STD testing. Most state laws also require a specific written authorization that must include the purpose or need for information and a very specific description of the extent or nature of the information to be disclosed regarding HIV/AIDS patients (for example, AIDS test results or diagnosis and treatment with inclusive dates of treatment). Unauthorized disclosure of HIV/AIDS information on a patient can result in civil or criminal penalties depending on state law, especially if the individual who released the information is found to have done so maliciously. Thus, it is important for a healthcare provider to have policies and procedures in place to ensure that the HIV/AIDS information of a patient is handled appropriately.

The following discussion offers suggestions regarding the handling of HIV/AIDS information. Attention must be paid to the process for the authorization and eventual disclosure of HIV/AIDS information. Individuals responsible for protecting the information should be sure that the authorization contains the information as required for disclosure of PHI and that information disclosed to authorized individuals or agencies is strictly limited to that information required to fulfill the purpose stated on the authorization (AHIMA 1987; Carpenter 1999). Authorizations specifying "any and all information" or other such broadly inclusive statements should not be honored, and information that is not essential to the stated purpose of the request should not be disclosed. A process should be in place that enables the healthcare provider to retain the signed authorization with notation of the specific information released, the date of release, and the signature of the individual who released the information (AHIMA 1987; Carpenter 1999). Disclosure of information from the records of HIV/AIDS patients or those tested for the HIV virus must be carefully handled, since test results may appear in many sections of the health record.

Records of HIV/AIDS patients that are in a paper format should be maintained in a secure area with restrictive access; however, special handling or marks such as stickers on the record folder that indicate the patient's HIV/AIDS status are discouraged. However, when using an EHR, the electronic system should provide flags or warning messages related to HIV/AIDS test results or treatment as a way to protect against the release or copying of HIV/AIDS information without appropriate authorization (AHIMA e-HIM Work Group on Security of Personal Health Information 2008). It is important that screening programs provide for confidential testing and communication of test results and that specific written informed consent be obtained from the patient or authorized representative of the patient prior to voluntary testing, as specified in general consent for treatment rules and guidelines. Out of courtesy to patients, the healthcare organization may wish to establish a policy that no claim for medical benefits for patients with HIV can be submitted without first ensuring the patient is aware of the diagnosis, and that the diagnosis must be submitted in order for the benefit to be paid. A patient may request that his or her information not be submitted for medical benefits if he or she chose to pay for the testing or treatment out of pocket.

State law may impose criminal liability for knowingly infecting another with HIV and, likewise, may provide immunity from liability for informing another person of potential HIV infection. For example, Tennessee Code Annotated 68-10-115 (1993) states, "A person who has a reasonable belief that a person has knowingly exposed another to HIV may inform the potential victim without incurring any liability. A person making such disclosure is immune from liability for making disclosure of the condition to the potential victim."

Additionally, many state laws provide for mandatory HIV testing upon the request of a notification of HIV test results to certain classes of individuals who may have been exposed to blood in a high-risk situation. Categories of individuals who may make such a request include law enforcement officers, paramedics, emergency response employees, firefighters, first response workers, emergency medical technicians, and volunteers making an authorized emergency response. In Ohio, the results of such testing are confidential, but the individual who was exposed has the right to request the results, and the person who provides the results is immune from liability (OH Rev. Code 3701.24.3, 3701.243).

Two other important areas healthcare providers must address relate to whether HIV/AIDS information should be disclosed to patients who are treated by healthcare workers who are HIV-positive or become HIV-positive, and whether information should be released to individuals who have contracted the virus through a blood transfusion. In the first situation, the Centers for Disease Control and Prevention (CDC) offers guidelines that recommend that a healthcare worker inform a prospective patient of his or her HIV status before the patient undergoes any type of exposure-prone procedure such as surgery. If the healthcare worker learns of his or her HIV-positive status after caring for a patient, the decision to disclose information about the worker should be handled on a case-by-case basis (Roach et al. 2006). The issue of whether to disclose information related to a donor's HIV status has not been easily resolved. Court decisions are split as to whether information should be disclosed and under what circumstances. The decision to disclose HIV/AIDS information in regard to donors remains at the discretion of a state's judicial system (Roach et al. 2006).

Check Your Understanding 12.2

Instructions: Indicate whether the following statements are true or false (T or F).

1. HIPAA does not distinguish highly sensitive health information from other types of health information.

2. Privilege statutes legally protect confidential communications between provider and patient related to diagnosis and treatment from disclosure during civil and some criminal misdemeanor litigation.

3. The duty-to-warn obligation enables a physician to disclose information to a third party who may be the victim of harm perpetrated by a patient.

4. In order for a substance abuse program to be in compliance with the Privacy Rule, the authorization of disclosure of information should include specific elements required by the Privacy Rule.

5. The health records of HIV/AIDS patients should be clearly marked as such.

Genetic Information

Genetic information provides insight into human disease and is both powerful and subject to misuse. While the term "genetic information" once referred to diseases or conditions that an individual had been diagnosed with, it now encompasses information about an individual's potential to develop a disease or condition in the future. The responsibility associated with protecting this information and using it legally and ethically is immense.

The ability to capture genetic information is the result of the **Human Genome Project** led by the **National Human Genome Research Institute** (NHGRI) of the National Institutes of Health (NIH). The project involved the identification and mapping of all human DNA. According to Fuller and Hudson (2006, 424–425):

> The Human Genome Project has given us the technology to decipher what were once an individual's most personal and intimate "family secrets"—that is, the information contained in our DNA. The instructions encrypted in our genes affect nearly every function the human body carries out, from fighting infection to thinking. Research to understand those instructions offers the promise of better health because it gives researchers and clinicians critical information to work out therapies or other strategies to prevent or treat a disease. In addition, genetic testing can alert individuals to a heightened risk of some health problems and the need to screen for them more frequently and thoroughly and to take more preventive measures.

While the genome project and the subsequent availability of genetic testing are meant to improve healthcare for all, concern has surfaced regarding the potential power of genetic information to be used against an individual. Fears exist that genetic information could be used by insurers to deny, limit, or cancel health insurance or raise premium rates and by employers to discriminate against individuals in the workplace. Some insurers may choose not to insure people who are currently healthy but are genetically predisposed to a future disease onset. Since these people might have higher health costs, insurance companies may not want to insure them and companies might not hire or keep workers who have the risk of a disease in the future (Fuller and Hudson 2006). Other difficult questions surrounding genetic testing and counseling have been addressed by the NHGRI (2007); for example:

- Should physicians and health counselors tell patients that they might be at high risk for developing an illness because of their genetic makeup when there is no effective treatment or cure for that disease now?

- Should healthcare practitioners perform genetic testing of an unborn fetus when the results might lead the parents to abort the pregnancy?

- Does the nature of genetic information create a need to revisit issues of informed consent and other ethical questions in the use of human subjects in genetics research?

- How can the biomedical community use genetic information to improve standards of patient care?

As a result of the challenges and complexities of the above issues and questions, lawmakers, scientists, and health advocacy groups worked to pass federal legislation known as the Genetic Information Nondiscrimination Act (GINA) of 2008 (Asmonga 2008). GINA prohibits discrimination by health insurers and employers based on genetic information, which is defined as:

> . . . Information about an individual's genetic tests and the genetic tests of an individual's family members, as well as information about the manifestation of a disease or disorder in an individual's family members (i.e., family medical history). . ... Genetic information also includes an individual's request for, or receipt of, genetic services, or the participation in

clinical research that includes genetic services by the individual or a family member of the individual, and the genetic information of a fetus carried by the individual or by a pregnant woman who is a family member of the individual and the genetic information of any embryo legally held by the individual or family member using an assisted reproductive technology. (EEOC n.d.)

Final regulations for Title I of GINA were effective as of December 7, 2009. Title I focuses on genetic nondiscrimination in health insurance and states that health plans may not use genetic information to make eligibility, coverage, underwriting, or premium-setting decisions. Plans cannot ask family members to undergo genetic testing or to provide genetic information. Genetic information obtained intentionally or unintentionally cannot be used for decisions related to plan enrollment. The Medicare supplemental policy and individual health insurance markets are prohibited from imposing pre-existing condition exclusions on the basis of genetic information. Title I modified the HIPAA Privacy Rule to state that genetic information is health information and prohibits the use and disclosure of genetic information by covered health plans for underwriting purposes (AHIMA 2013a; HHS 2009b). There are two exceptions to Title I, which state:

- Health insurers may request genetic information in the case that coverage of a particular claim would only be appropriate if there is a known genetic risk.

- When working in collaboration with external research entities health insurers may request (but not require) in writing that an individual undergo a genetic test. The individual may do so voluntarily, but refusal to participate will have no negative effect on his or her premium or enrollment status. The collected genetic information may be used for research purposes only, and not for underwriting decisions. (NHGRI 2009)

Title II of GINA is the responsibility of the Equal Employment Opportunity Commission (EEOC), which issued final regulations on November 9, 2010, with an effective date of January 10, 2011 (29 CFR Part 1635). Title II "prohibits the use of genetic information in making employment decisions, restricts employers and other entities covered by Title II (employment agencies, labor organizations and joint labor-management training and apprenticeship programs—referred to as "covered entities") from requesting, requiring or purchasing genetic information, and strictly limits the disclosure of genetic information" (EEOC n.d.). GINA specifically addresses the confidentiality of genetic information by stating that:

It is also unlawful for a covered entity to disclose genetic information about applicants, employees or members. Covered entities must keep genetic information confidential and in a separate medical file. (Genetic information may be kept in the same file as other medical information in compliance with the Americans with Disabilities Act.) There are limited exceptions to this non-disclosure rule, such as exceptions that provide for the disclosure of relevant genetic information to government officials investigating compliance with Title II of GINA and for disclosures made pursuant to a court order. (EEOC n.d.)

Many states have enacted statutory or regulatory provisions that safeguard genetic information and prohibit discrimination in employment and insurance benefits based on genetic information and mandatory genetic testing for employment and insurance purposes. However, the degree of protection provided by states varies. Some state provisions are less protective than GINA, and some more protective. All entities that are subject to GINA must, at a minimum, comply with applicable GINA requirements as well as more protective state laws.

The National Conference of State Legislatures (NCSL) maintains information about current issues facing states, including those surrounding genetic privacy laws. Current state genetic privacy laws are summarized in a table on the NCSL website, which includes what protections are offered for genetic information and penalties for privacy violations. The site also outlines consent requirements for performance of genetic tests, accessing genetic information, the retention and disclosure of genetic information, and the personal property rights for genetic information and DNA samples (National Conference of State Legislatures 2008).

Adoption Information

Adoption is a legal status in which the parental rights and responsibilities of one set of parents are legally terminated and a new parental relationship is established by law (Jones 2006). Parties to an adoption are the adopted individual (adoptee), the biological (natural, birth) parents, and the adoptive parent(s). The rights of each must be considered in light of access to health information. Adoption records include public and nonpublic documents such as the original sealed birth certificate, court documents relating to the adoption process, and records of the adoption agency and/or attorneys involved in the adoption (Adoption.com 2007). Most state laws deem these records to be confidential and allow their release only with a court order. While health records may not be included in the definition of adoption records, they are nonetheless crucial because of the identifying information and health information they contain.

Adoption presents a unique challenge to those charged with protecting health information. Previously shrouded in secrecy, many adoptions are now open so that the parties involved know one another's identities. Even in closed adoptions, more emphasis is being placed on blood relatives eventually identifying one another due to health considerations, personal desire, or mere curiosity.

Release of Information to Adopted Persons

A right of access exists for an adoptee's own health records, including the birth record, with all information that identifies the biological parents redacted (removed). Until the adoptee reaches the age of majority, this right of access belongs to the adoptive parents. (When the biological parents' parental rights are terminated, their right of access to the adoptee's health record is also terminated.) Once the adoptee reaches the age of majority, the right of access belongs to the adult adoptee. Policies for the collection and maintenance of adoption information vary from state to state; however, all states have provisions in statutes that allow access to nonidentifying information by an adoptive parent or guardian of an adoptee who is still a minor and then to the adoptee once they reach the age of majority (HHS 2009c). Some state statutes provide that information regarding the adoptee's physical and mental health be given to the adoptive parents at the time of adoption.

The identity of the biological parents remains confidential unless a registry (often called a mutual consent registry) has been established either by the adoption agency or by state statute that allows adoptees and biological parents to agree to have their identities disclosed (Hughes 2000). For example, the State of Ohio maintains the Ohio Adoption Registry, which was established by the Ohio General Assembly to provide a confidential and voluntary way for adopted Ohioans and their biological families to find one another. The registry resides in the Ohio Department of Health, Office of Vital Statistics (ODH 2010). Unless mandated by court order, health records are not the usual mechanism for parties to an adoption to identify and locate one another. However, requests of this nature may occur, which requires that the healthcare provider have a process in place for preserving the privacy of both parties of concern.

As described above, genetic information has become much more detailed and powerful. Access to the health information of an adoptee's biological parents or siblings can prove critical in identifying risk factors and providing background information to assist with diagnosing and treating the adopted child. Courts in a variety of states have established different thresholds as to what meets a "good cause" requirement that would justify access to information, including health information, about one's biological parents or siblings. A court will further specify whether the identifying information must be removed if access is granted to the record. A summary of state laws related to accessing adoption records can be found at the Child Welfare Information Gateway website sponsored by HHS (HHS 2009d).

Special Access, Request, and Disclosure Situations

Requests for health information vary in terms of what is requested and who is requesting the information. Such requests may be external or internal to an organization and may or may not require patient authorization. Although the general rule for the access, use, or disclosure of patient information is to first obtain the individual's authorization as noted above, there are many exceptions that are based on legal requirements, the best interests of the patient or other parties, or both. The HIPAA Privacy Rule exceptions to the authorization requirement were outlined in chapter 9. Individuals responsible for responding to requests must be trained to deal with each request in accordance with federal and state laws and organizational policy and procedure. This section discusses a variety of situations related to the access, request, and disclosure of health information that have not been discussed elsewhere in this book.

Disclosure of Active Records of Currently Hospitalized or Ambulatory Care Patients

At times, a currently hospitalized patient (**inpatient**) or a patient currently being seen in a clinic setting (**outpatient**) or their personal representative may wish to access, inspect, obtain a copy of, or disclose PHI from the patient's record. The term **active record** is often used to denote the health records of individuals who are currently hospitalized inpatients or outpatients. The Privacy Rule grants individuals the right to access, copy, and disclose their PHI in Section 164.524,526, which also states exceptions to these rights. Individual rights to PHI with exceptions are discussed in detail in chapter 9. If an active inpatient or outpatient wishes to access, copy, or disclose his or her PHI, then the healthcare provider should follow the same policies and procedures that are in place for allowing the access, copying, and disclosure of PHI for patients not currently hospitalized or being treated as an outpatient.

If no exceptions apply, a convenient time and place must be identified where the patient can inspect his or her PHI and obtain copies if requested. If such a request is made, an authorization to release health information must be signed by the patient or his or her personal representative. Because the record is active, the patient should be advised that additional information will be added to the record as the patient continues to receive care while hospitalized or treated as an outpatient. It is suggested that a patient who wishes to access or view his or her record while an inpatient or under current treatment should be provided with the assistance of a physician or other healthcare provider to help the patient in reviewing and understanding the record. If the patient wishes to have copies of the record sent to another individual, the facility should follow its normal release of information procedure for complying with the request. The procedure usually entails recordkeeping that includes the date a request was made or received; who made the request; the date the request was honored, and if not honored, why not; what was disclosed; and to whom. Such a procedure may also encompass the process for adhering to the HIPAA accounting of disclosures requirements discussed in chapter 9 and in more detail below.

Deceased Patients

HIPAA states that an individual has the same privacy rights in death as they did in life but leaves it up to the states in terms of who qualifies as the deceased person's legal or personal representative for access, use, and disclosure purposes. HITECH modifications to HIPAA provides for additional flexibility in the disclosure of a decedent's PHI by: 1. removing the PHI status from health records 50 years following the patient's death and 2. permitting covered entities to disclose decedent records to family members and others involved in the patient's care or payment of care unless doing so would be inconsistent with any known preference of the patient (Hofman 2013). Usually the legal executor or administrator of the estate has first rights to access the deceased's PHI or records. In the absence of an executor, some states may rely on the UHCDA as a guide in identifying a next-of-kin priority such as a spouse, adult child, or significant other. Other states require that these individuals become the deceased's official personal representative through appointment by a probate court or court order (Dimick 2009). In some states an individual may authorize for disclosure of his or her PHI, which is valid for two years after the death of the individual, and in other states an authorization is not valid after the individual's death. Thus, state law should be consulted to determine how long after death an authorization remains effective.

The final rule is murky on how to determine if records should be released, It leaves the responsibility up to the covered entity to have "reasonable assurance" that the person requesting the record has a legitimate right to access it. To avoid conflict, best practices suggest that healthcare providers require requesters to show proof of their relationship to the decedent or present court-authorized documentation showing authority to access the deceased individual's PHI (Dimick 2009). Although some providers may not require proof of the surviving spouse or other next-of-kin in this situation (Herrin 2007, 60), it is still good practice to require identification of the requester and to follow the provider's procedure for releasing information.

Disclosure of Information for Autopsy

Upon death, an **autopsy** may be required to determine the patient's cause of death. The reasons for determining the cause of death are numerous; they include verifying that the death was related to a criminal act, substantiating the cause of death for payment benefits, sudden unexplained or unattended death, accidents, public health hazards, research, and family history. The Privacy Rule allows the release of PHI without authorization to a medical examiner or coroner for the purpose of identifying a deceased person, determining cause of death, and other authorized purposes (45 CFR 164.512(g)(1)). State laws define which deaths are reportable to medical examiners and coroners and under what circumstances these public officials may require that an autopsy be performed. Authorization by the family or executor of the estate to conduct an autopsy is not required in these situations. If the death of the individual is not a medical examiner or coroner's case, the surviving spouse or descendents of the deceased may authorize the autopsy. The healthcare organization should require that an authorization form be completed and retained in the health record for evidentiary purposes (Roach et al. 2006, 290–291).

Open Records, Public Records, or Freedom of Information Laws

Open records laws, sometimes called **public records laws**, **sunshine laws,** or freedom of information laws, exist at the federal level and in all 50 states and the District of Columbia. The **Freedom of Information Act** (FOIA) of 1967, amended in 1996 (5 USC 552) to include electronic information, codifies what information is subject to public disclosure, including whether the information is in paper or electronic form. The FOIA specifically provides for public disclosure upon request of many types of information in the possession of federal agencies, except those files that would constitute a clear, unwarranted invasion of personal privacy (5 USC 552(b)(6)). This exemption is used to deny any FOIA requests that include PHI, as was previously discussed in chapter 9.

All 50 states and the District of Columbia have public record laws that provide public disclosure upon request of any information from any public body in a state except as otherwise exempted by state regulations. Each state defines its exemptions or exclusions, which often include the withholding of identifiable personal and health information. For example, some exemptions to the Ohio Public Records Law (OH Rev. Code 149.011), as reported in the Reporters Committee for Freedom of the Press' *Open Government Guide* (2006), include:

> Any record, except births, deaths, and the fact of admission or discharge from a hospital, that pertains to the medical history, diagnosis, prognosis, or medical condition of a patient that is generated and maintained in the process of medical treatment is exempt (Ohio Rev. Code 149.43(A)(1)(a)). Also, records of hospital quality assurance committees and hospital boards or committees reviewing professional qualifications of present or prospective members of the hospital medical staff are exempt from mandatory disclosure (Ohio Rev. Code 2305.251, 2305.25; *State ex rel. Fostoria Daily Review Co. v. Fostoria Hosp. Ass'n*, 44 Ohio St. 3d 111, 541 N.E.2d 587 (1989)). Records containing a trauma center's description of its ability to respond to disasters, mass casualties, and bioterrorism are not public records (Ohio Rev. Code 149.43(A)(1)(x), 3701.072).

There are many other exemptions to the laws, which include issues related to adoption, abortion, law enforcement, and more. What is important is for the healthcare provider to understand that while the intent of the open records laws is to keep society informed of government activities at the federal, state, and local levels, there is a responsibility for agencies that collect and maintain personally identifiable health information to protect the privacy rights of those they serve. These federal and state agencies include government-supported hospitals such as Veterans Affairs hospitals, state-funded or state-supported university medical centers, county and local hospitals and clinics, public health agencies, public health oversight agencies, and public health departments, to name a few.

Employee Health or Occupational Safety and Health Records

An **employee health record** or **occupational safety and health record** is a record kept on an employee as part of employment that contains any and all information related to such items as medical tests, drug tests, examinations, physical abilities, immunizations, screenings required by law, biohazardous exposure, and physical limitations. The employee health record should be kept separately from the personnel record of the employee due to the nature of information contained in the health record. Employers are entitled to information about an employee's medical work fitness but not to a diagnosis or specific details except as permitted by law. Supervisors and managers may be informed about necessary work restrictions and recommended accommodations.

First aid and safety personnel may be informed, when appropriate, if a condition might require emergency treatment. There are numerous federal and state regulations that govern employee health records. For example, according to the federal **Americans with Disabilities Act** (ADA) (28 CFR Part 35, 36), information regarding medical evaluations is confidential and employers may only access information related to fitness for duties, work restrictions, and accommodations. Title II of GINA also offers protection to employees as discussed above (29 CFR Part 1635).

Employee health records may contain the results of drug tests required as part of an employer's employee drug testing programs. Programs of this nature started in the 1980s when the federal government enacted drug-free work programs for federal employees. Drug testing programs serve as a preventative and deterrent method of supporting a safe, drug-free work environment. Employee drug testing programs may be required for pre-employment, prepromotion, annual physicals, post-accident follow-up, treatment follow-up, or reasonable suspicion. Random drug testing may also occur during employment. These tests may be conducted under contract or may require employees to independently undergo drug testing. All policies that require testing must be written and communicated to employees in advance. An employer must designate a medical review officer (usually a physician) as the individual who will receive drug test results and report results to appropriate management officials. Drug test results are confidential, but positive results can be cause for termination. Both the results and the subsequent action taken are confidential (SAMHSA 2007).

In all situations, employees have the right to access the results of drug testing as well as their employee health record under applicable state laws and federal Occupational Safety and Health Administration (OSHA) regulations (29 CFR 1910.20), which ensure that an employee (or designated representative) is given access to his or her own health and exposure records within 15 days of a request. Other state regulations may be stricter and preempt the OSHA rule.

Employees should be advised in advance regarding what health records are maintained on them and notified of any release of such records. Occupational health providers who are covered entities must abide by HIPAA rules and obtain patient authorization (or make reasonable efforts to do so) before disclosing health information from an employee health record. Specific authorization may be required for the disclosure of health information relating to HIV/AIDS, substance abuse, and mental health if more strictly defined by state law. Additionally, many state laws protect the confidentiality of information obtained through employee assistance programs, which provide assessment, intervention, referral for appropriate diagnosis and treatment, and follow-up services to employees whose job performance is impaired by personal concerns such as health, family, financial, alcohol, drug, legal, emotional, or other stressors.

Antiterrorism Initiatives

The federal government enacted two laws in its effort to thwart terrorism and terrorist attacks in the United States, both of which provide access to PHI under certain circumstances. The **Patriot Act** of 2001 was enacted to deter and punish terrorist acts in the United States and around the world and to enhance law enforcement investigations. The goal of the **Homeland Security Act** of 2002 is to prevent terrorist attacks in the United States while reducing vulnerability to terrorism, minimizing its damages, and assisting in recovery from attacks in the United States. Both acts give government authorities the right to access information needed to investigate and deter terrorism (AHIMA 2010).

The Patriot Act allows the director of the Federal Bureau of Investigation or a designee to apply for a production order through the court system to produce tangible items such as documents and records. It also provides sanctions for any unauthorized disclosures of the information obtained by others not involved in the investigation. A healthcare provider who in good faith provided information requested under order would not be held liable for releasing the information (AHIMA Homeland Security Work Group 2004, 56A). In contrast, the Homeland Security Act gives the secretary of Homeland Security authority to access information that would include PHI without the authorization of the patient or personal representative (AHIMA Homeland Security Work Group 2004, 56A). This act, however, specifically states that PHI is protected from unauthorized disclosure and should be used for the purpose for which it was obtained and that the redisclosure should be restricted to only those involved in the case (AHIMA Homeland Security Work Group 2004, 56A, B).

In essence, the federal government is permitted access to any and all information it deems necessary to protect the country. The healthcare provider should provide the PHI to the requesting authority without delay if appropriate identification of the official is obtained and verified. This should include making a copy of the requester's identification and noting the office location where the information will be taken and the branch of government requesting the information (AHIMA Homeland Security Work Group 2004, 56B).

In addition to the above antiterrorism regulation, state and public health authorities engage in **syndromic surveillance**. This type of surveillance refers to the "systematic gathering and analysis of pre-diagnostic health data to rapidly detect clusters of symptoms and health complaints that might indicate an infectious-disease outbreak or other public health threat" (Drociuk et al. 2004). Federal and state mandatory reporting laws related to births, deaths, child and elder abuse, treatment related to criminal acts, cancer cases, and communicable and other types of diseases have been in existence for years and are discussed in more detail in chapter 13. These laws provide public health officials with necessary information to help detect bioterrorism threats and sudden outbreaks of diseases such as West Nile virus, severe acute respiratory syndrome (SARS), and H1N1 influenza. Public health entities rely on access, use, and disclosure of syndromic surveillance information using the Electronic Surveillance System for the Early Notification of Community Based Epidemics (ESSENCE). While certain uses of the syndromic surveillance data are nonidentifiable, the majority of systems often require medical providers to disclose identifiable health information to state or federal public health agencies (Drociuk et al. 2004).

While the HIPAA Privacy Rule allows disclosure of health information without patient authorization for public interest and benefits such as public health and safety, it does not compel disclosure. However, the majority of states have regulations that do compel disclosure, with confidentiality controls in place as well. To ensure information is protected, healthcare organizations should implement policies and procedures for disclosing patient information as a result of antiterrorism legislation and other public health syndromic surveillance activity.

Consumer Reporting Agencies

A consumer reporting agency is a company that regularly assembles or evaluates consumer information for the purpose of producing reports. The information collected may be credit information or, in the case of the Medical Information Bureau (MIB), health histories and related issues. Companies that collect credit information are called credit bureaus. Equifax, Experian, and TransUnion are three of the more prominent companies that collect and report on consumer credit (Avery et al. 2003). Insurance companies exchange confidential information with the MIB on individuals who apply for life, health, disability, long-term care, or critical illness insurance. This nationwide specialty consumer reporting agency specializes in fraud detection data, risk management, and actuarial analytics for the insurance industry. Its purpose is to alert a member company when a potential client who has applied for insurance either knowingly or unknowingly omits information from his or her insurance application (MIB 2011). To provide consumers protection against misuse of their health information, the **Fair and Accurate Credit Transactions Act** of 2003 (FACTA) was enacted.

FACTA amended the Fair Credit Reporting Act (FCRA) (15 USC 1681), related to obtaining and using medical (health) information in connection with credit eligibility determination (Privacy Rights Clearinghouse 2011). The rule prohibits a creditor from obtaining and using medical information to decide a consumer's credit eligibility. However, a creditor can obtain and use financial information related to medical debts, expenses, or income (16 CFR 604(g)(2)). A consumer (a patient) must authorize for a consumer reporting agency to share medical information with employers for employment or insurance purposes. Consumer reporting agencies may not report the name, address, or telephone number of any medical information furnisher (such as a healthcare provider) unless the information is coded so as not to identify or infer the provider of care or the individual's medical condition. This restriction does not apply to insurance companies selling only property and casualty insurance (16 CFR 605(a)(6)).

Duty to Warn

As previously discussed in the section on behavioral health information, state laws may permit or even compel psychologists and psychiatrists to use their discretion to warn intended victims of potential harm without the patient's authorization. Such exceptions to state laws that traditionally consider patient–psychologist and patient–physician communications to be privileged serve the public interest by protecting individuals and are compliant with the HIPAA Privacy Rule. Mental health professionals and other healthcare providers have a duty to exercise reasonable care by warning a patient's intended victim, and the duty to warn supersedes the duty of confidentiality.

Laboratory Test Results

The federal **Clinical Laboratory Improvement Amendments** (CLIA) of 1988 (42 CFR 493.3(a)(2)) were enacted to ensure the accuracy and reliability of all laboratory testing. CLIA permits clinical laboratories to release test results to the individuals responsible for ordering the test and the laboratory that initiated the request. In March 2010, the Centers for Medicare and Medicaid Services (CMS) clarified that laboratories can electronically exchange test data but must ensure that an EHR format configures the lab results in the correct format and that lab results are sent to the correct provider (Wiedemann 2011). HIPAA defers to CLIA in regard to access, use, and disclosure of laboratory data. CLIA provides that clinical laboratories are only to disclose test results or reports to an "authorized person," which is the person who ordered the test, unless state law states otherwise. As a result, the individual who is the subject of the information is not authorized to immediately and directly receive his or her laboratory test results unless defined by state law. Instead, access to the individual's clinical laboratory information will occur through the provider who ordered the test(s). However, efforts to allow individual access are currently under consideration at the federal level.

Payment Requests from Insurance Companies and Government Agencies

Insurance companies commonly request patient information. In accordance with the HIPAA Privacy Rule, requests for payment purposes, including utilization review and medical necessity review, do not require authorization if the information is for the payment of a specific episode of care (45 CFR 164.506). However, other information requests (for example, for life insurance determinations) require patient authorization. An insurance company acting on behalf of the healthcare organization (for example, obtaining information in a lawsuit in which the insurance company represents the defendant healthcare organization or provider) does not require an authorization. In such a case, the insurance company would function as a business associate. Medicare and Medicaid and agencies working on their behalf, such as Quality Improvement Organizations and fiscal intermediaries, do not require the patient's authorization if the information is required for payment. If the information is required for enrollment, however, patient authorization is required.

The purpose of the request must be determined in order to comply with HIPAA regulations and accounting of disclosures including additional accounting requirements as defined in the HITECH provisions. Requirements under HITECH will be discussed later in this chapter under "Accounting of Disclosures and Tracking Releases."

Medical Emergencies

In **medical emergency** situations, the obligation is to treat the patient and provide whatever information is necessary. This usually entails disclosing patient information without authorization. If such a disclosure occurs, it is prudent to document the content and nature of the disclosure (for example, telephone conversation or electronic transmission) in the health record. Although the HIPAA Privacy Rule does not require authorization for disclosures made for treatment reasons, providers may elect to enforce policies that do require authorization.

An additional consideration associated with medical emergencies is the log or "run sheet" generated by emergency medical personnel as a result of their response to calls for assistance. The run sheet may contain information such as patient-identifying information, cause for service, condition of individual attended, and where the individual was taken for medical services. This information may be used for reimbursement purposes. Because these documents may be subject to a state's public records laws, state law should be consulted in conjunction with the HIPAA Privacy Rule to ensure proper disclosure.

Public Figures or Celebrities

News media personnel (and others) may have an interest in obtaining information about a public figure or celebrity who is being treated or about individuals involved in events that have cast them in the public eye. The media is not exempt from restrictions imposed by the Privacy Rule facility directory requirement. A healthcare organization may wish to exercise even greater restraint than that mandated by the directory requirement with respect to the media in order to ensure patient confidentiality for noted public figures and celebrities. For example, it is recommended that no information be provided about the location of a patient who is the subject of media inquiry. Special care should be taken to ensure that patients who are the subjects of media inquiry give authorization for any information to be disclosed or for photographs and interviews (Ohio Hospital Association 2005).

A healthcare organization may consider implementing policies and procedures for assigning an alias to patients who are public figures or celebrities and placing their health records in a separate secure area. If information is stored electronically, a process that restricts access on a need-to-know basis should be considered. Media representatives who appear at the organization should be escorted at all times and restricted from patient care areas. The healthcare organization should appoint a designated spokesperson to address media questions, ensure that staff training occurs regarding the privacy rights of public figures and celebrities, and have staff sign nondisclosure statements (Amatayakul 2003). While individuals who have willingly placed themselves in the public eye have a reduced expectation of privacy, it is nonetheless the obligation of the healthcare provider to take additional precautions to protect the privacy of these individuals and their health information.

Social Security Administration and State Disability Determination Services

Federal and state governments offer rehabilitation and disability services to help people suffering from physical or mental disabilities that affect their ability to work or return to work in a timely manner. These services are administered through the **Social Security Administration** (SSA) and state **disability determination services**. The SSA regulations require that state disability determination services responsible for providing medical evidence must determine whether a resident of a state is or is not disabled under the Social Security disability law. When an individual files a disability application with the SSA, it is transmitted to the state agency that will make the medical decision regarding the claim. The agency sends letters to every medical provider the claimant has listed on their application. The claimant is asked to voluntarily authorize the sending of all medical, school, and other records and information related to his or her case to the SSA and the state agency authorized to process the case by signing disclosure form SSA-827. The SSA has revised the form to comply with the HIPAA Privacy Rule on authorization for use and disclosure of health information.

In 2005 alone, the SSA processed over 15 million health records for disability claimants and paid over $130 million to medical providers for records. To defray costs and expedite the review process, the SSA and state disability determination services implemented the **Electronic Records Express** (ERE) initiative, which offers providers secure electronic options for submitting records related to disability claims. When a request for records concerning a disability claim is received, the provider may choose to submit the information electronically via the SSA's secure website or fax the information to the state agency handling the disability determination services. The records sent are automatically associated with the applicant's unique disability claim folder (SSA 2010). In addition, the SSA has entered into an agreement with the MedVirginia HIE to process patient disability claims. This has enabled the SSA to reduce the amount of time spent preparing, receiving, and processing patient health records or disability claims from 83 days to 32 days (HIMSS 2009). Key to the processing of this information is the patient authorization for access and disclosure of PHI. From a practice perspective, the Healthcare Information and Management Systems Society (HIMSS) offers a document that provides direction on sending records efficiently and securely to the SSA's disability claims system (HIMSS 2007). A link to the document is provided in the references section.

Health Information Handlers: Payment Integrity Review Contractors, Health Information Exchanges

A **health information handler** (HIH) is any organization that handles information on behalf of a provider. For example, most healthcare organizations and providers use an HIH to submit their claims for reimbursement purposes (CMS n.d.a). Some examples of HIHs are release of information vendors, HIEs, and EHR vendors. Some HIHs are considered covered entities, business associates, or business associate subcontractors that have agreements with providers to access, use, and/or disclose PHI. However, HIHs that provide payment oversight for federal government programs such as the Medicare Fee-for-Service program are not required to provide authorization for disclosure of PHI since they fall under the HIPAA exception that allows access and disclosure without authorization for purposes of treatment, payment, and operations (45 CFR 164.501).

Given the massive amount of information and claims handled through the Medicare Fee-for-Service program, CMS has contracted with payment integrity review contractors such as Recovery Audit Contractors (RACs), Medicare Administrative Contractors (MACs), and Zone Program Integrity Contractors (ZPICs) to measure, prevent, identify, and correct incorrect payments and identify fraudulent claims activity (CMS n.d.b). These contractors have access to patient information that is submitted to them by healthcare organizations and providers who receive letters requesting that certain medical documentation be released to the review contractors. The healthcare organization may disclose information via paper, disk, or fax. In 2010, CMS implemented a pilot program effective March 2011 that will enable providers to respond to review contractors online as well as via paper, disk, or fax through a new mechanism called Electronic Submission of Medical Documentation (esMD) (CMS n.d.b). Phase 2 of the pilot will enable review contractors to send their requests for medical documentation electronically, thus eliminating the paper request. Entities that function as HIEs that have a contract, grant, or cooperative agreement with a federal agency may also participate in the esMD pilot by submitting medical documentation electronically through a gateway service (CMS n.d.c).

Check Your Understanding 12.4

Instructions: Indicate whether the following statements are true or false (T or F).

1. In absence of a legal executor or administrator of an estate, states may follow the UHCDA to allow access to the health records of a deceased patient.

2. The Freedom of Information Act, along with open records laws including public records or sunshine laws, requires that federal or state entities make information generated in the normal course of business, including health information, public and subject to access by whoever requests the information.

3. An employer is entitled to information about an employee's medical work fitness but not to a diagnosis or other specific health details.

4. The Patriot Act of 2001 and the Homeland Security Act of 2002 allow government agents to access PHI upon request in order to protect the country.

5. The Electronic Records Express initiative, sponsored by the Social Security Administration to process disability claims, does not require patient authorization for release of PHI.

Managing the Release of Information Process

Managing the release of information (ROI) process is essential to ensuring that a healthcare organization or provider is providing the appropriate safeguards necessary for protecting the privacy, confidentiality, and security of PHI. Complicating the process is whether the information is in paper, electronic, or hybrid form. Whether ROI is handled internally by employed staff or externally by HIHs (which are also business associates) such as copy service vendors or HIEs, it can be costly in terms of time to process requests and address problems resulting from an inadequate management process. It is important that an organization have policies and procedures in place that support the management practices for access, use, and disclosure of information including responding to subpoenas or court orders. Quality control practices should address the tracking and monitoring of requests from receipt through final disposition; priority and efficiency of processing requests; and managing productivity, turnaround times, and backlogs (Bock et al. 2008). Tracking and monitoring requests should include recordkeeping that includes the date on which a request was made or received, who made the request, the date on which the request was honored (and if not honored, why not), what was disclosed, and to whom. Information of this nature may also be encompassed in the process for adhering to the HIPAA accounting of disclosures requirements discussed in chapter 9 and in more detail below. There are many concepts and practices to consider when managing the ROI, which are discussed below.

Definition of LHR and DRS

In managing the ROI process, it is important for the healthcare organization or provider to define its legal health record (LHR) and its designated record set (DRS) as discussed in chapter 8. Remember, the LHR serves as the organization's business record and is the record that is released upon request (AHIMA 2011). The DRS is broader than the LHR because it includes not only the health record, but also records involved in billing and insurance enrollment and coverage and other documents "used, in whole or in part to make decisions about individuals" (45 CFR 164.501). The DRS inherently includes information in any format and may include videotapes, photographs, cassettes, and other reproductions and duplicates. Knowledge of what constitutes the LHR and DRS helps set parameters for what patient information may be disclosed.

The health record often contains a variety of documents that are not directly related to patient treatment and, therefore, are not considered part of the LHR or included in disclosures. Such documents include correspondence, information about other family members, copies of insurance cards and records from other providers, authorizations for disclosure of information, internal memoranda about the disclosure of information, and correspondence from and records of requesters. Although not subject to disclosure, such documents may be maintained with the patient record. Information received from other providers or brought by the patient to the health organization should not automatically be included in the patient's health record. Only information that is pertinent and needed for patient care and treatment decisions should be physically incorporated into the health record to be released in response to authorizations, subpoenas, and court orders.

Determining Who Will Disclose/Release Information

A determination must be made regarding which departments will disclose/release information when it is requested, since PHI and electronic PHI (ePHI) can be stored in multiple forms and multiple systems. Departments may be responsible for processing a request for the records that are under their control. For example, radiology may be responsible for directly releasing x-rays or the laboratory for releasing lab results in response. Another alternative is that all requests be handled through the health information management (HIM) department. In this situation, HIM personnel would be responsible for gathering all requested documents, such as health records, billing office records, and x-rays, and releasing them to the requester.

Many HIM departments have moved toward a shared services model with commercial copy service vendors that function as HIHs and business associates. This arrangement allows the healthcare organization to perform front-end functions such as logging ROI requests, confirming validity, identifying what information is to be disclosed, and checking the record for completeness. The copy service vendor usually assumes responsibility for back-office processes such as releasing the record to the requester, communicating with customers, maintaining compliance, invoicing and billing, applying fees to specific types of records, handling postage, and dealing with telephone and walk-in inquiries. Under the shared services model, fees are usually shared between the vendor and the HIM department. Turnaround time for complying with the request tends to decrease with this model, as do customer complaints. When information is disclosed through a copy service vendor, policies and procedures must be clear as to the responsibilities of the vendor versus the responsibilities of the HIM department.

Types of Requests for Access, Use, and Disclosure/Release of PHI

Requests for access, use, and disclosure/release of patient information commonly occur via mail, telephone, or physical presence of the requester, either unannounced (a "walk-in") or by a prearranged on-site review. Requests may also be received electronically via fax or e-mail. In addition, a requester may ask that information be faxed or e-mailed to a given location or sent electronically via a given website. Requests are made directly by the patient or personal representative for the purpose of inspecting and copying the patient's PHI or disclosing the information to a third party. Requests are also commonly made by third parties such as other healthcare entities, insurance companies, attorneys, health oversight agencies (for example, public health agencies, the SSA, state disability determination services, coroners, RACs, and MACs), and other government-related agencies (AHIMA 2013b).

Regardless of the type of request made, if the request is from the patient, a formal authorization form is not required per the HIPAA Privacy Rule; however, many healthcare providers will ask the patient to complete an authorization form for the patient's own protection. An authorization is not required for a number of public interest and benefit situations (45 CFR 164.512) but is required if the requester is a third party to the patient, such as an attorney. If the authorization form is required, then it should include the elements of a valid authorization as defined by the HIPAA Privacy Rule (see figure 9.5 in chapter 9) (45 CFR 164.508).

Verification of Requester

Because providers are not always aware of family situations or other relationships, proof of the requester's relationship to the patient must be verified before health information is disclosed, as required by the HIPAA Privacy Rule (45 CFR 164.514(h)(1)). Such verification generally applies to in-person disclosures in which information is not being released to a destination specified and authorized by the patient. For example, contracted reviewers and representatives of insurance companies or other payers should be required to present documentation of their relationship with the company they represent. A patient's personal representative should also be required to present documentation to appropriate personnel in order to verify that the requester has the legitimate right to access the information. Whoever the requester is, the HIPAA Privacy and Security Rules require the verification of the identity and authority of the person making the request, if not known, before any information is disclosed (45 CFR 164.514(h) (1); 45 CFR 164.312(d)). If the patient is deceased, policy relating to who can legitimately access the record is followed, as discussed previously.

The validity of the authorization should be verified before information is released. Specifically, the following should be done:

- Check to be sure that all applicable parts of the form have been completed.

- Make sure that the information does not appear to be falsified.

- Check the date of the authorization to be certain it has not expired.

- Compare the patient's signature to one in the actual health record to ensure validity.

- Exercise good judgment to ensure that there is no suggestion in the authorization or circumstances surrounding it that the authorization was not given freely, that releasing the information will damage the relationship between the patient and the facility in which he or she sought treatment, or that disclosing the information will be harmful to the patient.

In addition, all responses to requests should be noted in the organization's procedure for managing requests. It is important for those managing ROI functions to understand each type of request and clearly establish policies and procedures to respond to requests in a time frame set forth by organizational policy and federal and state regulations.

Mail Requests

The most typical request to access, use, or disclose patient information is received through the mail. A letter or a form is received that requests health information to be copied and mailed or sent electronically to the requester. The healthcare organization reviews the authorization, determines if it is valid, and either processes the request or asks for additional information. For example, an insurance company may send a paper authorization requesting a copy of a patient's discharge summary and operation report. Similarly, many payment integrity review contractors such as RACs and MACs will send a written letter requesting medical documentation from patient records. These are just a few examples. The types of requests received via mail are virtually limitless.

Telephone Requests

Requests by phone tend to come from physician offices, insurance companies, or patients. The healthcare employee who receives a telephone request should request the name, address, telephone number, and, if applicable, the company of the caller to identify the requesting party and verify that the party is entitled to receive the information requested. Once the party is identified and verified, the employee should return the call to disclose the information, if appropriate. In emergencies, the employee should request the calling party to furnish additional pertinent information about the patient that might not be generally known but could be verified by the medical history or some other information found within the patient record. A telephone request can be honored without an authorization if it is for purposes of treatment, payment, or healthcare operations such as transferring the patient to another facility for continuity of care purposes. If the healthcare organization uses a voice mail message system, the voice mail message should request callers to leave their name and callback number or to return the call during working office hours. Patient-identifying information should not be left on the voice mail system as it might not be secure.

Electronic Requests and Requests to Electronically Send Information via Fax or Internet (E-Mail or Web Portal)

Requests may be received via fax or e-mail. A process of identifying and verifying the requester must occur before the information is disclosed. There may be a request to fax or e-mail patient information to a given location. If requests of this nature are received, security safeguards should be implemented to ensure the validity of the fax numbers and/or e-mail addresses to which information will be sent; to ensure that the receiving fax machine or e-mail is attended when information is sent; to ensure that a cover sheet containing a confidentiality statement (and a telephone number that an unintended recipient can call to report a transmission error) is used; and to ask the recipient to verify receipt of the transmitted documents (Davis et al. 2006). Guidance for handling fax and e-mail requests was discussed in detail in chapter 11. Figure 11.4 (p. 314) and figure 11.5 (p. 316) offer further recommendations for disclosing PHI by fax and e-mail.

Some requesters are now offering providers the option of sending patient information to a secure website. For example, the SSA and state disability determination services, as discussed previously, have implemented the Electronic Records Express program, which enables providers to submit records related to disability claims to a secure website (SSA 2010). In addition, the CMS pilot program, esMD, enables providers to electronically submit requested PHI to participating review contractors and HIEs.

Walk-In Requests

Most unannounced walk-in requests are from patients who wish to inspect or obtain copies of their records; however, third parties may also present themselves unannounced. Once the request is determined to be legitimate, if possible, the requested information should be provided. Space must be provided for individuals to wait and to review the information requested. Personnel should be present at all times during an on-site review to assist the requester with the record, to assure the record is not altered or documents removed or destroyed, and to answer questions where appropriate. Because of the resources involved with walk-in requests, advance notice by requesters should be encouraged and a scheduled appointment process implemented, such as the one discussed in the next section.

On-Site Record Review Requests

On-site record reviews differ from walk-in requests in that an on-site review is prearranged for a specific day and time when patient information will be made available to the requester. The organization must follow the Privacy Rule time frames when responding to requests, so the setting of appointments must adhere to these time frames. The requesters of on-site reviews are usually attorneys, insurance companies, Quality Improvement Organization representatives, or researchers. Prior to the on-site review, a request should be received and the type of information requested should be specified. If the requester and the authorization for use and disclosure of the information are determined to be legitimate, a time and place for the review is established along with the information requested. As discussed with walk-ins, personnel should be present at all times during on-site reviews to assist the requester with the record, to assure the record is not altered or documents removed or destroyed (if a paper health record) or deleted (if in a EHR system), and to answer questions where appropriate.

Determining If Disclosure Is Appropriate

Once it has been determined that a request is HIPAA- and state-compliant, an organization must determine whether the information can be disclosed. State and federal laws should be consulted to ensure no conflicts exist between the two. In addition, records related to adopted children, mental health, substance abuse, HIV/AIDS, potential lawsuits, genetic testing, or minors receiving treatment not requiring parental consent warrant special protections when disclosure or access has been requested.

If there is no conflict, the next step is to determine what content is requested. Dunn (2010) states that requests are often written for "any and all records," which can be problematic to address since there may be multiple records stored in a variety of ways and in a variety of places. Requests for "any and all records" should be compared to the HIPAA minimum necessary requirement (exceptions are provided in chapter 9). If the request does not meet the requirement, it should be sent back to the sender for clarification (Dunn 2010). Copying documents in a health record or from multiple sites can be costly; thus, verification of the requester's needs should be sought before the request is honored if there is any question or concern regarding what the requester is asking for.

If the request is appropriate and patient information is disclosed, the signed authorization form should be retained with a notation of the specific information disclosed, the reason for disclosure, the date of disclosure, and the signature of the employee who disclosed the information. The actual authorization form does not become part of the LHR or the DRS and should not automatically be disclosed when information from the patient's record is disclosed in the future. For convenience, however, the authorization form may be maintained with the patient record, as noted above.

Subpoena or Court Order

There are times when a health record is required for litigation such as malpractice cases, car accidents, criminal cases, and divorce proceedings. The health record is produced for discovery and litigation purposes through the use of subpoenas and court orders. As discussed in chapter 3, a **subpoena** is a legal tool used to compel one's appearance at a certain time and place to testify or produce documents or other tangible items (*subpoena duces tecum*—"bring with") either during the discovery process or at trial. A subpoena can be issued by a court, a grand jury, a lawyer representing a party in a civil or criminal lawsuit, or a government agency. A **court order** is a document issued by a judge that compels certain action, such as testimony or the production of documents such as health records.

A healthcare provider or organization must have policies and procedures in place that enable it to respond as directed by the subpoena or court order. The process for responding will vary based on state and federal regulations, including HIPAA requirements. Legal counsel should be notified immediately if the provider is party to the litigation. The subpoena or court order may ask for the original health record; however, whenever possible the court should be contacted to request that a copy be placed into evidence rather than the original record. Whether a copy of the record can be provided rather than the original is determined by state or federal regulation. For example, in Ohio a certified copy of the health record can be offered into evidence without the custodian needing to appear in court if attorneys for both parties stipulate that the records can be offered as evidence (OH Rev. Code 2317.422). If the original record must be submitted, then a process for return of the record must be in place. Whether the record is in paper or electronic form, the facility should have policies and procedures in place for disclosing PHI for discovery (e-discovery) and litigation purposes. Appendix 12.A provides a list of steps involved in responding to a subpoena.

ROI Reimbursement and Fee Structure

The release of health information is a function of doing business and thus has a cost associated with it. Many federal and state laws address the reimbursement of costs for disclosing/releasing health information. The HIPAA Privacy Rule permits reasonable, cost-based charges for labor, postage, and supplies involved in photocopying health information for the patient or his or her personal representative. However, the fee limitations do not apply to other permissible disclosures (45 CFR 164.524(c)(4)). Fees related to providing copies of accounting of disclosures to a patient are defined in Section 164.528(c)(2) of the Privacy Rule. The rule states:

> . . . the covered entity must provide the first accounting to an individual in any 12-month period without charge. The covered entity may impose a reasonable, cost-based fee for each subsequent request for an accounting by the same individual within the 12-month period, provided that the covered entity informs the individual in advance of the fee and provides the individual with an opportunity to withdraw or modify the request for a subsequent accounting in order to avoid or reduce the fee.

Other federal programs either reimburse healthcare organizations for providing copies or allow healthcare organizations to set fees such as the following (Hjort 2004):

> The Centers for Medicare and Medicaid Services reimburses hospitals at a rate of 12 cents per page for information released to the Quality Improvement Organizations (QIOs). The State Operations Manual for Long Term Care (LTC) Facilities, regulation F153(2)(ii), directs LTC facilities to allow an individual to purchase copies of his/her own records "at a cost not to exceed the community standard." The correspondent interpretive guideline 483.10(b)(2)

further instructs an organization to follow the state standard, if defined, or if not, a rate such as one used by the public library, the Post Office, or a commercial copy center.

In 29 CFR 1910.1020(e), the Occupational Safety and Health Administration (OSHA) provides for related records requested by an employee or designated representative to be supplied without cost the first time and allows reasonable charges for additional copies of the same information. "Reasonable" is defined as "non-discriminatory administrative costs (that is search and copying expenses but not including overhead expenses)."

Most states have enacted statutes that control the amount of reimbursement that a healthcare facility or provider can charge for copying health records and electronically stored information (ESI). A state-by-state reference guide to health record copying charges can be found online at http://LambLawOffice.com (Law Offices of Thomas J. Lamb, P.A. 2010). Copy cost and fee schedules for ROI tend to vary depending on who is requesting the information: workers' compensation, state disability, insurance company, patient, or attorney/patient (Hjort 2004). For example, workers' compensation services usually have state-established charges for copying records. Some states do not allow providers to charge the injured person for copies, while other states pay a flat fee. State disability determination services often pay a flat rate with no additional fees for postage. Indigent patients who request health record copies to support a claim or to appeal a denial under any provision of the SSA should not be charged for copies. Reasonable proof of indigence and/or a copy of the denial may be required by the provider, although this may differ by state. Physicians, as providers, are required not to withhold copies of health records due to an unpaid bill for services by many state statutes as well as their ethical code of conduct (American Medical Association 2001).

Providers should determine reasonable cost-based fees for their operations, taking into consideration state laws on ROI cost guidelines, federal program guidelines deemed appropriate, and other federal initiatives such as the SSA Electronic Records Express initiative, CMS's esMD project, SSA and HIE initiatives for disability claims, and the meaningful use incentive program (Hjort 2004; Dunn 2010). Costs that should be factored into making a copy are provided in figure 12.3. In addition, HITECH provisions allow an individual to obtain an electronic copy of their health record from providers with EHRs and it allows providers to charge a fee for the labor associated with fulfilling the request.

The calculation of fees should also consider the costs associated with e-discovery activity (Dunn 2007). Steps that should be assessed in arriving at a cost for processing e-discovery requests are presented in figure 12.4. Part of that process should include creating an inventory of where patient information is stored in the organization, including the type of media, its format, and how it is retrieved (Dunn 2007). See table 12.1 for an example of an inventory of information for disclosure costs.

Copy cost and fee schedules vary by state, with some identifying an initial flat fee followed by a per-page fee that usually decreases as the number of pages goes up. For example, per Ohio Revised

Figure 12.3.   Costs factored into ROI costs

- Systems and hardware (such as additional workstations) to accommodate the ROI function
- Applications such as ROI tracking systems
- Peripherals such as copiers, printers, and fax machines
- Forms such as ROI authorization forms and fax cover sheets
- Routine supplies including staples, pens, paper, envelopes, toner, DVDs for scanned documents, and other media
- Postage and labor for handling
- Fees for off-site storage and retrieval
- Overhead such as utilities, space, furnishings, maintenance fees for machines, housekeeping, human resources, and payroll

Source: Dunn 2010.

Figure 12.4.   Steps in assessing costs for e-discovery

1. **Identify all places that could store patient information**, both patient-identifiable and non-identifiable. These include data stored in electronic form in equipment (e.g., echocardiogram, EKG, fetal monitoring equipment) and information transmission systems (e-mail, primarily). Electronically stored information was probably catalogued during the facility's efforts to define its designated record set.

2. **Determine how patient-specific data can be extracted** from these other locations. In the case of cancer registry or core measures reporting, these databases often have report generation functions that allow patient-specific data to be printed or exported to an electronic file. However, data in quality assurance or performance improvement and infection control databases may be more difficult to extract

3. **Determine the time and other resources required to extract data** from these files and how long data are stored in them. You will need assistance from your IT department to capture data stored electronically in both equipment and transmission vehicles. Many organizations have established retention techniques that pool or store e-mail and other digital data for a period of time to protect against spoliation.

4. **Inventory this information** to address disclosure costs. An example of an inventory is given in Table 12.1.

5. **Document inventorying effort**. Completely document the initial and ongoing efforts to maintain a current inventory, including the time involved, memoranda used, educational efforts, et cetera. This will help demonstrate that the organization has performed its due diligence in relation to the Federal Rules of Civil Procedure, which applies primarily to data maintained in an electronic format. Outlining files maintained electronically will be important in appealing unreasonable demands in front of the judge.

6. **Apply labor and supply factors**. In the example above, assume that the plaintiff's attorney requires all information from any electronic system and wants it on a CD. The labor cost would be multiplied by 0.5 hours (0.25 for each of the two electronic systems). Supplies include the CD, the current cost of which is easily determined. The time to save the files to a CD would be minimal; however, if multiple documents must be saved, it may be worth inventorying the approximate time to write a document to a CD and then applying that factor to the number of documents requested.

Source: Dunn 2007.

Code 3701.741, the Ohio Department of Health sets the amount hospitals and companies can charge for copying health records based on the Consumer Price Index, which may increase or decrease depending on the year. For example, in 2011 the fee schedule for Ohio was increased by 1.64 percent from the 2010 fees. The fee schedule for 2011 is as follows:

For requests made by *patients or their representatives*, hospitals may charge:

- No record search fee is allowed
- $2.88 per page for the first 10 pages
- 60 cents per page for pages 11–50
- 24 cents per page for pages numbering more than 50
- $1.97 per page for data resulting from x-ray, MRI, or CAT scan, recorded on paper or film
- Actual cost of postage may be charged

For requests made by *someone other than the patient or patient's representative*, hospitals may charge:

- Initial fee of $17.70 to compensate for the records search
- $1.17 per page for the first 10 pages
- 60 cents per page for pages 11–50

- 24 cents per page for pages numbering more than 50

- $1.97 per page for data resulting from x-ray, MRI, or CAT scan, recorded on paper or film

- Actual cost of postage may be charged

If a fee is assessed for a request, the fee schedule must be consulted and an invoice prepared. The fee schedule should be regularly reviewed for compliance with the HIPAA Privacy Rule and applicable state laws. A system should be developed to determine situations in which fees are not assessed, to determine when prepayment is required, and to implement collection procedures for delinquent payments following record disclosure. If a copy service company is used to handle the tasks of responding to requests for information, the company directly bills requesters (patients, attorneys, insurance company representatives, disability determination services, and others) for copying the information. A sales tax may be assessed when information is sent to states where sales tax applies.

Accounting of Disclosures and Tracking Releases

Many facilities maintain manual or electronic tracking systems to account for requesters and recipients of patient information (Dougherty 2001). Health record copying services also offer tracking

Table 12.1.   Example inventory of information for disclosure costs

Data Location	Media	Format	Retention Info	How Info Obtained	Time/Cost to Obtain
Social services	Paper	Alpha order by month patient was discharged; stored in boxes	Two years; other years stored at XYZ Storage	Identify dates of service, retrieve box, pull data from boxes	1.25 hours on site; $8 retrieval fee charged by XYZ
Performance improvement (core measures database)	Midas data system	Electronic	Currently permanent	Access Midas database, enter medical record number, search by date of service, print out or save to Word file	0.25 hours
Respiratory therapy	Paper	Services during month; no order	One year in cabinets; other years stored by month of charge at XYZ Storage	Identify dates of service for the patient, pull from file cabinet or recall box(es), sort through box to find documents for patient	2 hours on site; $8 retrieval fee charged by XYZ
Open record review data (in HIM)	Paper	Monthly; no order	Stored until next Joint Commission visit; destroyed after visit	Identify dates of service for the patient, pull from cabinet, review all open record review submissions	2 hours
Cancer registry	Electronic record system	Electronic	Currently permanent	Access system database, enter medical record number, search by date of service, print out or save to text file	0.25 hours

Source: Dunn 2007.

systems for ROI. Prior to the HIPAA Privacy Rule, the Federal Privacy Act of 1974 required federal facilities to keep a record of patient information disclosures. The Privacy Rule requires the tracking and accounting of disclosures of PHI, as discussed in chapter 9. The accounting requirement currently includes disclosures made in writing, electronically, by telephone, orally, and includes all disclosures except those:

- Needed to carry out treatment, payment, and healthcare operations

- To the individual to whom the information pertains

- Incidental to an otherwise permitted or required use or disclosure

- Pursuant to an authorization

- For use in the facility's directory, to persons involved in the individual's care, or for other notification purposes

- To meet national security or intelligence requirements

- To correctional institutions or law enforcement officials

- That are part of a limited data set

- That occurred before the compliance date for the CE

HITECH, as originally written, would have required covered entities using or maintaining an EHR to include, in an accounting of disclosures, any TPO (treatment, payment and operations) disclosures. The effective date would depend on when the entity acquired its EHR. A subsequent proposed rule issued in 2011, but still pending, however, proposes to exclude both uses and TPO from an accounting for both paper records and EHRs. Instead, individuals (upon request) would be able to receive an access report from covered entities with EHRs. This report would allow an individual to see a record of every person who viewed the individual's designated record set during the previous three years. TPO disclosures would therefore be displayed in the access report rather than in the accounting of disclosures(HHS 2011). A covered entity may either account for the disclosures of its business associate (BA) or provide for the BA to make its own accounting. A BA will have to respond to an accounting for disclosure request that is made directly to it (AHIMA 2009).

Overall, requests for information, whether received by paper or electronically, should be responded to in the same manner. While HIPAA's authorization requirements and organizational policy must continue to be followed, documents authorizing the disclosure of information may be retained electronically, along with any notations about the disclosure such as the date information was disclosed and to whom. It is important for providers responsible for releasing information to enter disclosures into a central tracking system. Care should be given to ensure that the process is consistent throughout the organization, since more than one functional area may disclose patient information. One consideration is to have accounting of disclosures and requests for accounting handled by the HIM department.

Right to Request Restrictions

As described in chapter 9, the Privacy Rule gives patients the right to request that covered entities restrict uses and disclosures of their PHI for carrying out TPO (45 CFR 164.522(a)). Covered entities were not required to agree to these requests in the past, although they must abide by requests they agree to; HITECH, however, enables an individual to restrict an organization's ability to disclose information to health plans for payment or operations purposes if the service provided was paid for completely out of the individual's pocket.

Refusal to Disclose Information

In certain circumstances, it may be necessary to refuse to disclose patient information or require additional information or documentation before information is disclosed to the requester. Reasons for refusing to disclose information or requiring additional information are as follows (Reynolds 2010):

- The identity of the person presenting the authorization is in question or the authorization appears to have been completed without the patient's knowledge or after the patient signed the form.

- There is reason to doubt that the person requesting the information is the person named in the authorization.

- The person who signed the authorization is not of legal age.

- There is a question as to the competency of the person who signed the authorization.

- There is a question as to the legal guardian of a minor or incompetent patient or there is documentation of abuse noted in the record.

- The patient has stated that the authorization should not be honored or has revoked the authorization, or the healthcare organization knows that the authorization has been revoked.

- Expiration date or event has passed.

- There is any question as to the authenticity of the patient's signature after comparison of the patient's signature on the authorization with the signature in the medical record.

- There is a question about the patient's ability to understand the authorization.

- There is false information in the form or the form is incomplete.

- There is a question about whether the patient signed the authorization under duress.

Whenever possible and appropriate, requesters should be assisted in completing proper authorizations so that requests can be honored in a timely manner.

Check Your Understanding 12.5

Instructions: Indicate whether the following statements are true or false (T or F).

1. Documents not considered part of the LHR—for example, correspondence, incident reports, and information about other family members—should be released as part of the LHR.

2. Proof of a requester's relationship to a patient must be verified before health information is released to the requester.

3. A request for any and all information on a patient should be honored without question as long as the authorization form is signed by the patient.

4. Health organizations and providers may charge a reasonable fee as set by state law for copying health records in response to a request for patient information.

5. HIPAA requires that for the purpose of accounting of disclosures, only PHI that has been released electronically or in writing must be accounted for.

Summary

Protecting the privacy and confidentiality of health information is a major priority for healthcare organizations and providers as more and more consumers become keenly aware of their rights regarding privacy. It is essential that federal and state laws are followed, statutes are enforced, and policies and procedures are developed to ensure that patients' rights are protected. This chapter discussed the many practical situations that exist regarding the access, use, and disclosure of patient information with or without patient authorization. The chapter discussed health information ownership and the right to access one's health information as a competent adult, incompetent adult, or minor. The chapter continued with an overview of workforce members who have access rights to patient information and for what reason. Issues surrounding the handling of highly sensitive information related to behavioral health, substance abuse, HIV/AIDS, genetic information, and adoption and how these issues relate to the HIPAA Privacy Rule were discussed. In addition, a number of special access, request, and disclosure situations were discussed, along with comments related to managing these situations. The chapter closed with a discussion of items for consideration in managing the ROI process, including types of requests commonly received, disclosure issues, health record copying charges for ROI purposes, and accounting and tracking disclosures.

References

Adoption.com. 2007. Glossary. http://www.glossary.adoption.com.

AHIMA. 1987. Guidelines for handling health data on individuals tested or treated for the HIV virus. *Journal of AHIMA* 58(10):26–33.

AHIMA. 2009. LTC Health Information Practice & Documentation Guidelines. http://www.ahima.org.

AHIMA. 2010. Homeland Security Act, Patriot Act, Freedom of Information Act, and HIM. http://www.ahima.org.

AHIMA. 2011. Fundamentals of the legal health record and designated record set. *Journal of AHIMA* 82(2):44–49.

AHIMA. 2013a (January 25). Analysis of Modifications to the HIPAA Privacy, Security, Enforcement, and Breach Notification Rules under the HITECH and Genetic Information Nondiscrimination Act: Other Modifications to the HIPAA Rules. Chicago: AHIMA.

AHIMA. 2013b. Release of information toolkit. Chicago: AHIMA. http://www.ahima.org.

AHIMA e-HIM Work Group on Security of Personal Health Information. 2008. Ensuring security of high-risk information in EHRs. *Journal of AHIMA* 79(9):67–71.

AHIMA Homeland Security Work Group. 2004. Practice brief: Homeland security and HIM. *Journal of AHIMA* 75(6):56A–56D.

Amatayakul, M. 2003. Practical advice for effective policies and procedures. *Journal of AHIMA* 74(4):16A–16D.

American Medical Association. 2001. Code of Medical Ethics. Chicago: AMA. http://www.ama-assn.org.

American Medical Informatics Association. 2007a. *Toward a National Framework for the Secondary Use of Health Data. Journal of AMIA* 14(1):109. . .

American Medical Informatics Association. 2007b. Secondary Uses and Reuses of Healthcare Data: Taxonomy for Policy Formulation and Planning. https://www.amia.org.

Asmonga, D. 2008. Getting to know GINA: An overview of the Genetic Information Nondiscrimination Act. *Journal of AHIMA* 79(7):18, 20, 22.

Avery, R., P. Calem, G. Canner, and R. Bostic. 2003. An overview of consumer data and credit reporting. *Federal Reserve Bulletin*, February:48–73. http://www.federalreserve.gov.

Bock, L., B. Demster, A. Dinh, E. Gorton, and J. Lanti. 2008. Management practices for the release of information. *Journal of AHIMA* 79(11):77–80.

Bowman, B. 2012. Secondary records and healthcare databases. Chapter 12 in *Health Information Management: Concepts, Principles, and Practice*, 4th ed. Edited by LaTour, K. and S. Eichenwald-Maki. Chicago: AHIMA.

Burrington-Brown, J., B. Hjort, and L. Washington. 2007. Practice brief: Health data access, use, and control. *Journal of AHIMA* 78(5):63–66.

Carpenter, J. 1999. Practice brief: Managing health information relating to infection with human immunodeficiency virus. Web extra. Chicago: AHIMA.

Centers for Medicare and Medicaid Services. n.d.a. Which HIHS plan to offer esMD gateway services to providers? https://www.cms.gov.

Centers for Medicare and Medicaid Services. n.d.b. Electronic Submission of Medical Documentation Overview. https://www.cms.gov.

Centers for Medicare and Medicaid Services. n.d.c. Gateways. https://www.cms.gov.

Davis, N., et al. 2006. Practice brief: Facsimile transmission of health information. Web extra. Chicago: AHIMA.

Demster, B. 2012. Data Ownership Evolves with Technology. *Journal of AHIMA* 83(9):52-53.

Department of Health and Human Services. n.d. Office of National Coordinator. Advancing Privacy and Security in Health Information Exchange. http://www.healthit.gov.

Department of Health and Human Services. 2008. Office of National Coordinator. National privacy and security framework for electronic exchange of individual identified health information. http://www.healthit.gov.

Department of Health and Human Services. 2009a. Office of National Coordinator, National Alliance for Health Information Technology. Defining key health information technology terms. http://www.nacua.org.

Department of Health and Human Services. 2009b. Office for Human Research Protections. Guidance on the Genetic Information Nondiscrimination Act: Implications for investigators and institutional review boards. http://www.hhs.gov/ohrp/policy/gina.html.

Department of Health and Human Services. 2009c. Child welfare information gateway. State statutes search. https://www.childwelfare.gov/.

Department of Health and Human Services. 2009d. Child welfare information gateway. Access to adoption records: Summary of state laws. http://www.childwelfare.gov.

Department of Health and Human Services. 2011. HIPAA Privacy Rule Accounting of Disclosures Under the Health Information Technology for Economic and Clinical Health Act. 45 CFR Part 164. *Federal Register* 76 (104): 31426–31449.

Dimick, C. 2009. Who has rights to a deceased patient's records? AHIMA blog post. August 4.

Dougherty, M. 2001. Practice brief: Accounting and tracking disclosures of protected health information. *Journal of AHIMA* 72(10):72E–72H.

Drociuk, D., J. Gibson, and J. Hodge. 2004. Health information privacy and syndromic surveillance systems. *MMWR Weekly* 53(Suppl.):221–225.

Dunn, R. 2007. Calculating the costs of e-discovery. *Journal of AHIMA* 78(10):64–65, 72.

Dunn, R. 2010. Release of information: Costs remain high in a hybrid, highly regulated environment. *Journal of AHIMA* 81(11):34–37.

Equal Employment Opportunity Commission. n.d. Genetic information discrimination. http://www.eeoc.gov.

Fuller, B., and K. Hudson. 2006. Genetic information. Chapter 18 in *Ethical Challenges in the Management of Health Information*, 2nd ed. Edited by Harman, L. Sudbury, MA: Jones and Bartlett.

Hall, M., and K. Schulman. 2009. Ownership of medical information. *JAMA* 301(12):1282–1284.

Healthcare Information and Management Systems Society. 2007. Sending records efficiently and securely to the Social Security Administration's disability claims system. http://www.himss.org/content/files/CPRIToolkit/version6/v7/D82_SSA_Case_Study.pdf.

Healthcare Information and Management Systems Society. 2009. HIE dramatically reduces processing time for SSA patients. http://www.himss.org.

Herrin, B. 2007. Identity proofing: Just a fancy name for verification? *Journal of AHIMA* 78(5):54–55, 60.

Hjort, B. 2004. Practice brief: Release of information reimbursement laws and regulations. Chicago: AHIMA. Web extra.

Hofman, J. 2013. Privacy after death. *Journal of AHIMA* 84(4):32-35.

Hughes, G. 2000. The ins and outs of adoption information provision. *In Confidence* 8(1):6–7.

Jones, M. 2006. Adoption information. Chapter 19 in *Ethical Challenges in the Management of Health Information*, 2nd ed. Edited by Harman, L. Sudbury, MA: Jones and Bartlett.

Law Offices of Thomas J. Lamb, P.A. 2010. Medical records copying charges. http://www.lamblawoffice.com.

Medical Information Bureau. 2011. Consumer guide. http://www.mib.com.

National Conference of State Legislatures. 2008. Genetic privacy laws. http://www.ncsl.org.

National Conference of State Legislatures. 2010. State legislatures Internet links. http://www.ncsl.org.

National Human Genome Research Institute. 2007. Health issues in genetics. http://www.genome.gov.

National Human Genome Research Institute. 2009. Title I of the Genetic Information Nondiscrimination Act of 2008 (GINA). http://www.genome.gov.

Ohio Department of Health. 2010. Adoption information. http://www.odh.ohio.gov.

Ohio Hospital Association. 2005. Media Guide for Ohio Hospitals. http://www.ohanet.org.

Privacy Rights Clearinghouse. 2011. Fact sheet 6a: Facts on FACTA, the Fair and Accurate Credit Transaction Act. http://www.privacyrights.org.

Randolph, S., and L. Rinehart-Thompson. 2006. Drug, alcohol, sexual and behavioral information. Chapter 20 in *Ethical Challenges in the Management of Health Information*, 2nd ed. Edited by Harman, L. Sudbury, MA: Jones and Bartlett.

Reporters Committee for Freedom of the Press. 2006. *Open Government Guide*, 5th ed. Arlington, VA: RCFP. http://www.rcfp.org.

Research Triangle Institute. 2009. Privacy and security solutions for interoperable health exchange: Report on state medical record access laws. Chicago: RTI International.

Reynolds, R., ed. 2010. *Tennessee Health Information Management Association Legal Handbook*, 11th ed. Winchester, TN: THIMA.

Roach, W., R. Hoban, B. Broccolo, A. Roth, and T. Blanchard. 2006. *Medical Records and the Law*, 4th ed. Sudbury, MA: Jones and Bartlett.

Russell, L., and R. Bowen. 2012. Legal issues in health information management. Chapter 10 in *Health Information Management: Concepts, Principles, and Practice*, 4th ed. Edited by LaTour, K., and S. Eichenwald-Maki. Chicago: AHIMA.

Schlossberger, E., and L. Hecker. 1996. HIV and family therapists' duty to warn: A legal and ethical analysis. *Journal of Marital and Family Therapy* 22(1):27–40.

Social Security Administration. 2010. Electronic Record Express.

Substance Abuse and Mental Health Services Administration. 2004. The confidentiality of alcohol and drug abuse patient records regulation and the HIPAA Privacy Rule: Implications for alcohol and substance abuse programs. http://www.samhsa.gov.

Substance Abuse and Mental Health Services Administration. 2007. Model plan for a comprehensive drug-free workplace program. http://www.samhsa.gov.

Substance Abuse and Mental Health Services Administration. 2010. Frequently asked questions: Applying the substance abuse confidentiality regulations to health information exchange (HIE). http://www.samhsa.gov.

Thomson Reuters. 2012. State medical records laws. FindLaw. http://law.findlaw.com/state-laws/medical-records/.

Uniform Law Commission. 2010. Health-Care Decisions Act summary. Chicago: National Conference of Commissioners on Uniform State Laws. http://uniformlaws.org.

Waller, A., and O. Alcantara. 1998. Ownership of health information in the information age. *Journal of AHIMA* 69(3):28–38.

Wiedemann, L. 2011. Correcting lab results in an EHR. *Journal of AHIMA* 81(5):38–39.

Cases, Statutes, and Regulations Cited

Tarasoff v. the Regents of the University of California, 17 CA 3d 425, 551 P.2d 334, 131 CA Rptr. 14 (1976).

16 CFR 604(g)(2): Fair Credit Reporting Act. 2006.

16 CFR 605(a)(6): Fair Credit Reporting Act. 2006.

28 CFR Part 35, 36: Americans with Disabilities Act (ADA). 1990.

29 CFR 1910.20: Access to employee exposure and medical records. 2003.

29 CFR Part 1635: Genetic Information Nondiscrimination Act. 2008.

42 CFR 2.11 Part 2: Definitions. 1987.

42 CFR 2.14(c)(2): Minor patients. 1987.

42 CFR 493.3(a)(2): Clinical Laboratory Improvements Act. 1988.

45 CFR 160.103: Definitions. 2006.

45 CFR 164.310(a)(1): Facility access controls. 2006.

45 CFR 164.312(d): Device and medic controls. 2006.

45 CFR 164.501: Definitions. 2006.

45 CFR 164.502(b): Minimum necessary. 2006.

45 CFR 164.506: Uses and disclosures to carry out treatment, payment, or health care operations. 2006.

45 CFR 164.508: Uses and disclosures for which authorization is required. 2006.

45 CFR 164.510(a): Use and disclosure for facility directories. 2006.

45 CFR 164.512: Uses and disclosures for which an authorization or opportunity to agree or object is not required. 2006.

45 CFR 164.512(g)(1): Uses and disclosures about decedents. 2006.

45 CFR 164.514(h)(1): Verification requirements. 2006.

45 CFR 164.522(a): Rights to request privacy protection for protected health information. 2006.

45 CFR 164.524: Access of individuals to protected health information. 2006.

45 CFR 164.524(c)(4): Fees. 2006.

45 CFR 164.526: Amendment of protected health information. 2006.

45 CFR 164.528(c)(2): Provisions of the accounting. 2006.

5 USC 552: Freedom of Information Act. Amended 1996.

5 USC 552(b)(6): Exemption: Personal and medical files. 2004.

15 USC 1681: Fair Credit Reporting Act. 2004.

OH Rev. Code 149.011: Ohio public records law. 2004.

OH Rev. Code 2317.422: Authentication of nursing, rest, community alternative home and adult care facilities records. 2010.

OH Rev. Code 3701.24.3, 3701.243: Disclosure of HIV test results or diagnosis. 2000.

OH Rev. Code 3701.741: Fees for providing copies of medical records. 2011.

TN Code Ann. 33-8-202: Outpatient mental health treatment. 2002.

TN Code Ann. 36-6-103: Rights of noncustodial parents. 1987, 1989.

TN Code Ann. 68-10-115: Immunity from liability for informing person of potential HIV infection. 1993.

Fair and Accurate Credit Transaction Act of 2003. Public Law 108-159.

Genetic Information Nondiscrimination Act of 2008. Public Law 110-233.

Homeland Security Act of 2002. Public Law 107-296.

Patriot Act of 2001. Public Law 107-06.

Appendix 12.A

Process for Responding to a Subpoena

The following are steps to consider when responding to a subpoena that requests paper or electronic health records.

- Check the subpoena to make sure that it names the correct facility and/or provider, that it meets state and federal requirements, that it is signed by a representative of the court (usually the clerk of court), and that the subject of the subpoena is a patient of the facility or provider in question.

- Check to see if the records being subpoenaed exist, and if not, offer certification that the requested material has been destroyed according to record retention law and/or policy.

- Notify facility administration and legal counsel according to facility policy upon receipt of the subpoena.

- Review what is requested to make sure that all documents are present. If the record is a paper record, number the pages of the original record (including shingled copies), verify that the records all belong to the correct patient, and check that the patient's name and record number are on all pages, including both sides of forms. If the record is an electronic record, access all portions of the record following site policy for what constitutes the legal health record to determine that all documents are available. Create a copy of the paper record; copy the electronic record onto the medium of choice.

- Place the paper record in a secure area to prevent anyone from altering the record. Use the concept of legal hold for electronic records.

- Prepare a document that stipulates the record was made in the normal course of business.

- Ascertain whether copies can be delivered to the location listed on the subpoena. If the original record is requested, contact the parties involved to determine whether a copy is acceptable. Remember, a copy may be used in lieu of the original record if both parties agree to use of the copy as defined by state or federal law.

- If the original record is required for court, create a receipt for health records; keep one copy for the facility and one for the person accepting the record on behalf of the court. Include on the receipt an inventory of the record content. For example: nurses notes—20 pages, physician orders—10 pages, total pages—30.

- Place the original record in a folder with the receipt and label it as the original health record.

- Deliver both the original record and the copy to the location listed on the subpoena.

- Remain with the original record at all times until you are sworn in.

- Ask the court official to review the copy to see if they will accept the copy in place of the original record. If the judge, hearing officer, or participating attorney refuses to accept the copy in place of the original record, leave the original record. Request that the original paper

Source: Adapted from AHIMA 2009.

record and/or the medium that holds the electronic health record be returned to the facility when the case is completed.

- Obtain a signature on the original copy of the receipt for health records from the clerk of court. Keep the original copy of the receipt.

- Leave the copy of the receipt with the record held by the court.

- Upon return from court, write a note on the subpoena identifying who answered the subpoena, the date and time, the attorney's name, and that the original medical record was left with the court.

- File the subpoena and the signed receipt in the record file folder or electronic system.

- After the record is returned, check the record against the receipt to make sure that all pages are present. Reassemble the record in proper order if in paper format, if necessary. Note the date returned on the receipt/subpoena and file the original record in the permanent file.

Chapter 13

Required Reporting and Mandatory Disclosure Laws

Elizabeth D. Bowman, MPA, RHIA

Learning Objectives

- Describe the four elements of the HIPAA Privacy Rule that relate to required reporting laws

- Identify the HIPAA exceptions that allow the release of health information without patient authorization

- Discuss confidentiality issues for secondary data sources not covered by HIPAA

- Discuss the common state reporting requirements related to abuse and neglect of children, the elderly, and the disabled

- Describe state responsibility for reporting vital statistics including births, deaths, and fetal deaths

- Explain a state's responsibility for reporting communicable diseases

- Discuss state reporting requirements related to abortion, birth defects, reportable deaths, wounds, workers' compensation, and unusual events

- Discuss federal and volunteer reporting requirements that do not require patient authorization

- Describe the purpose of maintaining clinical, disease, and outcome-based registries

- Identify what state reporting requirements are allowed under the HIPAA Privacy Rule

Key Terms

Birth certificate
Birth defects registry
Cancer registry
Communicable disease
Coroner
Death certificate
Diabetes registry
Fetal death
Healthcare Integrity and
 Protection Data Bank
 (HIPDB)

Health Care Quality
 Improvement Act
Histocompatibility
Immunization registry
Implant registry
Medical device reporting
Medical examiner
National Practitioner Data
 Bank (NPDB)
Notifiable disease
Preemption

Prescription drug monitoring
 program
Registry
Safe Medical Devices Act
 (SMDA)
Transplant registry
Trauma registry
Traumatic injury
Unusual event
Vital record
Workers' compensation

Introduction

In order to protect the health and safety of a community, state and federal reporting laws require certain healthcare organizations and providers to report specific information, including protected health information (PHI), to government and quasigovernment agencies. The Health Insurance Portability and Accountability Act (HIPAA) identifies 12 exceptions to the Privacy Rule that permit the use or disclosure of PHI without patient authorization. In general, the mandatory disclosure laws address issues related to disease prevention and control and community health and safety. These laws require the disclosure of PHI without patient authorization and offer protection from civil liability to those who disclose the information as a matter of law. The reporting laws usually stipulate that the information collected is not considered public information and that patient privacy and confidential information are also protected. The laws vary from state to state, most of which fall under the auspices of state public health departments, while federal reporting laws fall under various departments at the federal level. This chapter addresses common reporting requirements mandated by state laws, such as abuse and neglect of children, the elderly, and the disabled; communicable diseases; suspicious or unattended deaths; vital statistics; and registries. It also addresses some of the common federal mandatory and volunteer reporting systems related to Medicare and Medicaid programs, quality measures and oversight, medical devices, registries, and national health statistics. Before a discussion of the various reporting requirements ensues, the four elements of the Privacy Rule related to reporting laws are reviewed: disclosure without patient authorization or agreement, preemption, Notice of Privacy Practices, and accounting of disclosures.

Disclosure without Patient Authorization or Agreement for Public Health and Benefit Activities

The HIPAA Privacy Rule provides that no PHI is to be used or disclosed without authorization unless the Privacy Rule provides an exception to the authorization requirement. The Privacy Rule provides 12 public interest and benefit activities exceptions as discussed in chapter 9 (pp. 235–237). These 12 exceptions relate to legal, public health, law enforcement, research, and other public interest and benefit activities that serve society and national priority purposes (see figure 13.1). The Privacy Rule permits disclosure without patient authorization, but it does not compel or require such disclosure. Most states have statutory requirements that parallel the exceptions, and other federal reporting requirements call for PHI without patient authorization. For these 12 exceptions, an individual is not given the opportunity to agree or object to the disclosure of his or her information, nor is an authorization required. The amount of information disclosed is usually defined by law or statute; however, in the absence of such provisions, a healthcare organization or provider should limit the information disclosed to that which is the minimum necessary, under HIPAA guidance. Remember, patients have a limited right to determine who has access to their primary data. This right is limited by laws and regulations allowing access to data by governments, researchers, and other legitimate users of the data (Burrington-Brown et al. 2007, 63).

Preemption

In general, the doctrine of **preemption** provides that federal law must be followed when federal and state laws conflict, unless the state law is more stringent on the matter than federal law. In addition, state law will prevail if there are provisions of state law, including state procedures for the reporting of disease or injury, child abuse, birth, or death, or for the conduct of public health surveillance, investigation,

Figure 13.1. Public interest and benefit exceptions permitting use or disclosure of PHI without patient authorization

1. Required by law (45 CFR 164.512(a))

2. Public health activities (45 CFR 164.512(b))

3. Victims of abuse, neglect, domestic violence (45 CFR 164.512(c))

4. Health oversight activities (45 CFR 164.512(d))

5. Judicial and administrative proceedings (45 CFR 164.512(e))

6. Law enforcement purposes (45 CFR 164.512(f))

7. Decedents (45 CFR 164.512(g))

8. Cadaveric organ, eye, or tissue donation (45 CFR 164.512(h))

9. Research (45 CFR 164.512(i))

10. Prevent or lessen serious threat to health or safety (45 CFR 164.512(j))

11. Specialized government functions (45 CFR 164.512(k))

12. Workers' compensation (45 CFR 164.512(l))

or intervention (45 CFR 160.203). State reporting requirements that collect and store PHI can, therefore, be followed as exceptions to the doctrine of preemption.

Notice of Privacy Practices

Under HIPAA, generally ". . . an individual has a right to adequate notice of the uses and disclosures of protected health information that may be made by the covered entity. . ." (45 CFR 164.520). The fact that information is reported under state and federal laws or statutes without patient authorization should be included in the Notice of Privacy Practices. An example of wording from a Notice of Privacy Practices is provided in appendix 9.A (pp. 261–263).

Accounting of Disclosures

The Privacy Rule requires the tracking of disclosures of PHI, as discussed in chapter 9. The accounting requirement includes disclosures that are made in writing, electronically, by telephone, or orally. HIPAA requires that instances of reporting required by law or regulation must be included in an accounting of disclosures. It is important that healthcare organizations and providers track disclosures in a central tracking system that enables departments or areas responsible for disclosing information under mandatory reporting laws to record disclosures. A healthcare organization or provider should make a list of these departments and the types of required disclosures made by each department so that when a patient requests an accounting of disclosures, the list can be referenced for items to be included in the accounting. See table 13.1 for an example of such a list.

Common State Reporting Requirements

All states have laws, codes, statutes, and/or regulations that require the reporting of certain diseases or events. Reported data provide information on the incidence and prevalence of diseases, possible high-risk populations, survival statistics, and trends over time. Data may be collected using a variety of methods including interviews, physical examination of individuals, and review of health records.

Table 13.1. Reporting of disclosures by responsible department

Item to be Reported	Responsible Hospital Department
Births, fetal deaths	Labor and Delivery
Deaths	HIM Department
Child or elder abuse	Social Services
Notifiable diseases	Infectious Disease
Statewide cancer registry	Cancer Registry
Trauma	Trauma Registry
Medical examiners cases	Risk Management

Abuse and Neglect of Children

Reporting abuse and neglect of children is routinely required by state laws and is reportable to local or county law enforcement or county children's services boards in the county where the incident occurred. According to the federal Child Abuse Prevention and Treatment Act of 1996 (CAPTA) (42 USC 5106g), as amended by the Keeping Children and Families Safe Act of 2003, child abuse and neglect are:

> . . . at minimum, any recent act or failure to act on the part of a parent or caretaker which results in death, serious physical or emotional harm, sexual abuse or exploitation; or an act or failure to act which presents an imminent risk of serious harm. (42 USC 5106g)

Each state has its own child abuse and neglect statutes based on this federal law. In general, four types of maltreatment are defined in state law: neglect, physical abuse, sexual abuse, and emotional abuse (Child Welfare Information Gateway 2010). The state statutes tend to define a child for reporting purposes as any person under the age of 18 or any physically or mentally handicapped person up to the age of 21.

State laws identify who must report child abuse and neglect, the time frame for reporting, and the kind of information reported. Healthcare practitioners, police officers, educators, human service workers, and others who are aware of the abuse or neglect of a child are the most common individuals required to report. These individuals are afforded protection from civil or criminal liability through state statutes for reporting abuse and neglect made in good faith (Pozgar 2012). In addition, most states have incorporated waivers into their rules that preempt state physician-patient privilege and Federal Alcohol and Drug Abuse Act restrictions on disclosure of patient information if the person whose information is being requested is under prosecution for abuse (Roach et al. 2006).

Most states require that known or suspected abuse and neglect must be orally reported immediately with written reports to follow in a prescribed time frame. The information typically required in these reports includes:

- Name of child and parents, or other custodial person
- Address of child and parents, or other custodial person
- Age of child
- Nature and extent of current or previous known or suspected injuries, abuse, or neglect
- Any other information that would be useful in establishing cause of injuries, abuse, or neglect (Pozgar 2012)

The health records of the abused or neglected child may be subject to disclosure without authorization. Such state laws do not conflict with the HIPAA Privacy Rule because such disclosures are permissible without authorization, either under the public interest and benefit exceptions of "required by law," "public health activities," or "disclosures about victims of abuse, neglect, or domestic violence," or as provided by the preemption exception. If a state law permits, but does not require, disclosure of this information, steps must be taken to ensure that the individual agrees to the disclosure or the healthcare organization believes disclosure is necessary to prevent serious harm to the individual or others. If the individual is not capable of agreeing, it must be confirmed by a public authority authorized to receive the information that the information will not be used against the individual and that delay in disclosing the information will likely have an adverse effect (45 CFR 164.512(c)).

Abuse and Neglect of the Elderly and Disabled

According to the Older Americans Act (42 USC 3002), the terms "elderly" and "older individual" include individuals 60 years of age and older. The term "disability" is defined in the law as meaning (42 USC 3002):

> . . . a disability attributable to mental or physical impairment, or a combination of mental and physical impairments, that results in substantial functional limitations in 1 or more of the following areas of major life activity:

1. Self-care
2. Receptive and expressive language
3. Learning
4. Mobility
5. Self-direction
6. Capacity for independent living
7. Economic self-sufficiency
8. Cognitive functioning
9. Emotional adjustment

Abuse of the elderly generally includes physical, emotional, financial, and sexual abuse; exploitation; neglect; and abandonment. State laws vary on the definitions of elderly and disabled as well as the definitions of abuse, neglect, and exploitation. There may be separate laws covering abuse in the home setting (domestic abuse) versus abuse in an institutional setting such as a nursing home (ABA 2007, 3). These laws are commonly grouped under the term "adult protective services."

State laws also vary regarding the required reporting of abuse of the elderly and disabled. Alabama law, for example, requires physicians, practitioners of the healing arts, and caregivers to report physical abuse, neglect, exploitation, sexual abuse, or emotional abuse (AL Code 38-9-8). Florida law, on the other hand, requires any person to report abuse, neglect, or exploitation of vulnerable persons (FL Stat. Ann. 415.101 et seq.).

Such state laws do not conflict with HIPAA because under either the public interest and benefit exceptions of "required by law" or "regarding victims of abuse, neglect, domestic violence," or as provided by the preemption exception, such disclosures are permissible without authorization. If a state law permits, but does not require, disclosure of this information, steps must be taken to ensure that the individual agrees to the disclosure or the healthcare organization or provider believes disclosure is necessary to prevent serious harm to the individual or others. If the individual is not capable of agreeing, it must be confirmed by a public authority authorized to receive the information that the information will not be used against the individual and that delay in disclosing the information will likely have an adverse effect (45 CFR 164.512(c)).

Check Your Understanding 13.1

Instructions: Indicate whether the following statements are true or false (T or F).

1. State required reporting laws are an exception to the doctrine of preemption.

2. When information is released to meet state required reporting laws, the release does not have to be included in the facility's accounting of disclosures.

3. Central registries are covered by and must adhere to the requirements of HIPAA.

4. Abuse of the elderly is limited to financial exploitation of an elder person's assets.

5. Physical abuse is usually the only type of maltreatment that must be reported under child abuse reporting laws.

Vital Records

Vital records are those concerned with births, deaths, marriages, divorces, abortions, and fetal deaths. In the United States, the National Center for Health Statistics (NCHS) of the Department of Health and Human Services (HHS) is responsible for working with state vital statistics laws and regulations for the reporting of vital statistics. At the federal level, the Model State Vital Statistics Act and Regulations (currently under revision) provide uniform guidance to states related to the definitions, registration practices, disclosure procedures, and other processes that comprise states' vital statistics functions (NCHS 1992; 2009). The information is used to generate statistics such as birth and death rates as well as to identify trends in areas such as causes of death and types of birth defects. The NCHS creates standard certificates of live birth and death that contain the minimum data required for the certificates to serve as models for the states. Each state can then modify the standard forms to meet their specific data collection needs.

Vital record information from the states is shared with the NCHS. Using this information, the states and the federal government provide statistics on the vital events within their jurisdiction. The information required commonly includes demographic information as well as medical information. Cases are sometimes reported without PHI; however, most of the time PHI is included in the data since there must be a way to connect the certificate with the actual case, if required. State laws requiring the reporting of vital statistics do not conflict with the HIPAA Privacy Rule because, under the public interest and benefit exception of "public health activities" or as provided by the preemption exception, such disclosures are permissible without authorization.

Birth Certificates

A **birth certificate** must be filed for every live birth regardless of where it occurred. Information needed to complete the birth certificate may be obtained from the mother and/or father, mother's and child's attending physician, and hospital or physician records. If the birth occurred within a hospital, it is generally the hospital's responsibility to file the birth certificate with the health department's office of vital statistics. The birth certificate form has two parts. The first part includes identifying information about the parents and the child. In the second part, there is information about the mother's pregnancy and any birth defects in the newborn. The second part serves a statistical purpose only and is not a part of the official birth certificate. Regarding paternity, most state laws delineate how a father may be acknowledged on the birth certificate if the father is not married to the mother at the time of the birth. State law also defines what surname for the child is entered on the certificate.

Death Certificates

When someone dies, state law requires that a **death certificate** be completed. The funeral director or other person responsible for internment or cremation of remains generally has responsibility for filing the death certificate within a prescribed time frame as defined by state law. The death certificate includes identifying information about the deceased as well as information about the cause of death. The physician must provide the cause of death and sign the death certificate within a certain amount of time as defined by state law. The original death certificate must be filed with the local health department's department of vital statistics in the county where the death occurred.

Communicable Diseases

A **communicable disease** is one that can be transmitted from an infected person, animal, or inanimate reservoir to a susceptible person or host by either direct or indirect contact. States require the reporting of "notifiable" communicable diseases through state laws for the purpose of tracking outbreaks and preventing the spread of the disease. State health departments or agencies serve as the state entities responsible for administering communicable disease reporting requirements. State laws define what diseases are reportable, by whom, and how they should be reported. Lists of diseases vary from state to state and may include certain quarantine diseases such as cholera, plague, Ebola, and yellow fever as required by the World Health Organization.

Notifiable diseases may be classified according to their potential for endemic or epidemic spread and danger to public health. How a disease is reported will depend on its classification. The more dangerous or problematic the disease, the more quickly it must be reported. Twenty-four hours is the usual reporting time for a confirmed case or for a suspected case once it is known. However, in certain cases dealing with newborns, such as inflammation of the eyes, the reporting time may be six hours. Figure 13.2 lists the nationally notifiable infectious diseases as specified by the Centers for Disease Control and Prevention (CDC 2011).

Laws require that diseases be reported in writing, verbally, or through other rapid means of communication. Laws also identify what specific information must be reported, such as the patient's name, age, gender, and address; details of the illness; and other pertinent information. In some cases, such as sexually transmitted diseases like syphilis, HIV, and AIDS or diseases such as hepatitis or tuberculosis, information is required pertaining to contacts the infected person under investigation has had with other individuals to limit further spread of the disease. Responsibility for notifying individuals who have had contact with the infected person is defined by state law.

State laws define who must report communicable diseases. In most cases, the reporting individual is the attending physician or a person (or delegated representative) in charge of a hospital, emergency room, clinic, diagnostic laboratory, or other entity providing care or treatment and having knowledge of the case. State laws may also grant the appropriate state health director or representative the right to access and copy the patient's health record without the patient's authorization. Most state laws include regulations that, despite required reporting, keep information confidential and indicate that it will not be released or made public upon subpoena, court order, discovery, search warrant, or otherwise except in special situations as further defined by state law (TN Code Ann. 68-10-113). In addition, some state laws specify that the public health authorities must be provided access to records of patients with notifiable diseases during the investigation of the disease. Under such laws, patient authorization is not required for such access (OH Admin. Code 3701-3-08).

State laws requiring the reporting of communicable diseases do not conflict with HIPAA because, under the public interest and benefit exception of "public health activities" or as provided by the preemption exception, such disclosures are permissible without authorization. The HIPAA Privacy Rule, under the public health activities exception, further permits a covered entity (CE) to disclose PHI to persons who may have been exposed to a communicable disease or may be at risk of contracting or spreading a disease or condition, provided that the CE is authorized by law to make such notification as part of a public health intervention (45 CFR 164.512 (b)).

Figure 13.2. National reportable infectious diseases

Anthrax

Arboviral neuroinvasive and non-neuroinvasive diseases

- California serogroup virus disease
- Eastern equine encephalitis virus disease
- Powassan virus disease
- St. Louis encephalitis virus disease
- West Nile virus disease
- Western equine encephalitis virus disease

Babesiosis

Botulism (foodborne, wound, infant)

Brucellosis

Chancroid

Chlamydia trachomatis infection

Cholera

Coccidiodomyscosis

Cryptosporidiosis

Cyclosporiasis

Dengue (fever, hemorrhagic fever, shock syndrome)

Diphtheria

Ehrlichiosis/Anaplasmosis

- *Ehrlichia chaffeensis*
- *Ehrlichia ewingii*
- *Anaplasma phagocytophilum*
- Undetermined

Giardiasis

Gonorrhea

Haemophilus influenzae, invasive disease

Hansen disease (leprosy)

Hantavirus pulmonary syndrome

Hemolytic uremic syndrome, post-diarrheal

Hepatitis

- Hepatitis A, acute
- Hepatitis B, acute
- Hepatitis B, chronic
- Hepatitis B virus, perinatal infection
- Hepatitis C, acute
- Hepatitis C, chronic

HIV infection*

- HIV infection, adult/adolescent (age ≥ 13 years)
- HIV infection, child (age ≥ 18 months and < 13 years)
- HIV infection, pediatric (age < 18 months)

Influenza-associated pediatric mortality

Legionellosis

Listeriosis

Lyme disease

Malaria

Measles

Meningococcal disease

Mumps

Novel influenza A virus infections

Pertussis

Plague

Poliomyelitis, paralytic

Poliovirus infection, nonparalytic

Psittacosis

Q Fever (acute, chronic, rabies)

Rabies, animal

Rabies, human

Rubella

Rubella, congenital syndrome

Salmonellosis

Severe Acute Respiratory Syndrome–associated Coronavirus (SARS-CoV) disease

Shiga toxin-producing *Escherichia coli* (STEC)

Shigellosis

Smallpox

Spotted Fever Rickettsiosis

Streptococcal toxic-shock syndrome

Streptococcus pneumoniae, invasive disease

Syphilis

- Primary
- Secondary
- Latent
- Early latent
- Late latent
- Latent, unknown duration
- Neurosyphilis
- Late, non-neurological
- Stillbirth
- Congenital

Tetanus

Toxic-shock syndrome (other than Streptococcal)

Trichinellosis (Trichinosis)

Tuberculosis

Tularemia

Typhoid fever

Vancomycin-intermediate *Staphylococcus aureus* (VISA)

Vancomycin-resistant *Staphylococcus aureus* (VRSA)

Varicella (morbidity)

Varicella (deaths only)

Vibriosis

Viral Hemorrhagic Fevers, due to:

- Ebola virus
- Marburg virus
- Arenavirus
- Crimean-Congo Hemorrhagic Fever virus
- Lassa virus
- Lujo virus
- New world arenaviruses (Gunarito, Machupo, Junin, and Sabia viruses)

Yellow fever

Source: CDC 2011.

*AIDS has been reclassified as HIV stage III.

Induced Termination of Pregnancy (Abortion)

Most state laws require the healthcare organization where an induced termination of pregnancy was performed to file a report on the termination of pregnancy. If the induced termination of pregnancy did not occur in a healthcare facility such as a clinic or hospital, then the attending physician who administered care to the patient after the induced termination is responsible for filing a report. Usually, information identifying the individual patient or physician is not required in the reporting of induced abortions. However, some means of identifying the patient should exist in case further information is needed (Reynolds 2010). Information that is typically reported pertains to the patient's date of birth, race, marital status, and county and state of residence; the type of procedure performed; and resulting complications, if any. In some states, physicians and facilities are required to report injuries or death to a mother due to an induced abortion.

Birth Defects

Birth defect information may be obtained from birth certificates filed with the state. Such information is used to determine trends in birth defects and to look for ways to prevent them. State laws requiring the reporting of birth defects do not conflict with HIPAA because, under the public interest and benefit exception of "public health activities" or as provided by the preemption exception, such disclosures are permissible without authorization.

Reportable Deaths

State laws have developed requirements for certain deaths—such as accidental, homicidal, suicidal, sudden, and those suspicious in nature—to be reported, usually to the medical examiner or coroner. In addition, deaths resulting from abortion or induced termination of pregnancy are reportable. A **medical examiner** is typically a physician with pathology training given the responsibility by a government, such as a county or state, for investigating suspicious deaths. A **coroner** is typically an appointed or elected official, who may or may not be a physician, with the responsibility for investigating suspicious deaths. Physicians, squad members, or law enforcement members acting in their duties are required to notify the medical examiner or coroner of any death that may fit one of the categories mentioned above. Healthcare entities such as hospitals must have clearly defined policies and procedures for reporting such deaths, especially since individuals may be brought to the emergency room dead on arrival (DOA) or may expire shortly thereafter from what might be any of the types of death noted above.

Suspicious deaths are of particular interest to state law enforcement. For example, Mississippi defines a suspicious death as a "'death affecting the public interest' [which] means any death of a human being where the circumstances are sudden, unexpected, violent, suspicious or unattended" (MS Code 41-61-53). These deaths affect the public interest because they may be indicative of a crime or they may identify a cause of death that needs to be remedied, such as a death from carbon monoxide poisoning due to a faulty furnace. The information commonly reportable to the coroner or medical examiner includes:

- Name and address of the deceased
- Age of the deceased, if known
- Marital status of the deceased
- Ethnicity of the deceased
- Time of accident or onset of cause of death
- Place, mode, and manner of injury
- Place of death

- Time of death

- Location of body

- Other pertinent data

- Name of person reporting the case, including date and time

- Name of physician who pronounced person dead

Medical examiners and coroners have the right to receive medical information needed to investigate the case without authorization and may have subpoena powers to collect such information. State laws requiring the reporting of suspicious deaths do not conflict with HIPAA because such disclosures are permissible without authorization, either under the public interest and benefit exceptions of "public health activities," "disclosures for law enforcement purposes," or "about decedents," or as provided by the preemption exception.

Wounds: Knife, Gunshot, Burns

Like suspicious deaths, wounds such as knife wounds, gunshot wounds, and burns are commonly indicative of crimes and must be reported to legal authorities. State laws requiring the reporting of knife and gunshot wounds as well as burns do not conflict with HIPAA because such disclosures are permissible without authorization, either under the public interest and benefit exceptions of "public health activities," "disclosures for law enforcement purposes," or (if applicable) "about decedents," or as provided by the preemption exception.

Fetal Deaths

Fetal deaths must also be reported. A **fetal death** refers to the death of a fetus of a particular weight or gestation, frequently 500 grams or more or 22 or more completed weeks of gestation, though the weight and week gestation may vary from state to state. The definition of a fetal death is generally as found in the Vermont statute:

> . . . the complete expulsion or extraction from the mother of a product of conception; the death is indicated by the fact that after such separation, the fetus does not breathe or show any other evidence of life such as beating of the heart, pulsation of the umbilical cord, or definite movement of voluntary muscles. (VT Stat. 18-6-107 5221)

In most states, the remains of a fetal death cannot be interred until a certificate of fetal death is completed. Depending on state law, the responsibility for completing the fetal death certificate may lie with the designated person in the institution where the fetal death occurred, the funeral director or other person responsible for internment or cremation of remains, or, if the fetal death occurred outside an institution, the physician in attendance at or immediately after the delivery. If no one was in attendance and the dead fetus is brought to the hospital, the hospital should notify the medical examiner, who will file the fetal death certificate. The information requested in a fetal death certificate includes information about the parents as well as information about the pregnancy and the fetus.

Unusual Events and Other State Reporting Requirements

States sometimes require the reporting of certain **unusual events** for other public health prevention and control programs. Examples include medication errors, transfusion reactions, falls resulting in fractures, wrong patient/wrong site surgical procedures, and operative complications. Such laws have resulted from recent concerns about patient safety and may apply to any type of healthcare facility.

Most states have implemented **prescription drug monitoring programs** (PDMPs) in an effort to identify inappropriate and illegal activities involving controlled prescription drugs. States define which controlled drugs they wish to monitor and require pharmacies to report on the dispensing of these drugs. The information collected, at minimum, includes the physician name, Drug Enforcement Administration (DEA) registration number, the individual the drug was dispensed to, and the name of the drug. The information is submitted to a state data bank, which is used to monitor the dispensing of drugs. The information collected may be shared with healthcare providers or law enforcement agencies as defined by state law.

The Nuclear Regulatory Commission (NRC) has oversight responsibility for the medical use of ionizing radiation. The NRC has entered into licensing agreements with the majority of states to oversee the possession and use of radiation byproduct, source, and special nuclear material by the medical community. A listing of state radiation regulations and legislation is posted on the NRC website (NRC n.d.). Medical centers must report information on their use of radioactive materials and any misadministration of the material. If a medical event occurs, it must be reported to the state agency and the NRC (10 CFR 35.3045). The event notification information is public record and is posted daily on the commission's website (NRC 2013). Identifiable PHI is eliminated from the reports, but location and reporting individuals are not.

Other state agencies such as Medicaid and maternal and child health programs that provide state assistance to individuals who qualify for services have access to PHI by virtue of state regulation. The type and amount of PHI collected and maintained depends on the program.

In all situations discussed above, the reporting of PHI does not conflict with the Privacy Rule because, under the public interest and benefit exception of "required by law" or "to prevent or lessen a serious threat to health or safety," such disclosures are permissible without authorization.

Workers' Compensation for Occupational Illness, Injury, and Death

All states have enacted **workers' compensation** legislation to ensure that employees who are injured on the job or become ill as a result of a job are provided with some means of support while recovering from their illness or injury. The laws also provide benefits to the surviving spouse and dependents if the worker dies as a result of work-related illness or injury while working (Cornell University Law School 2010). Employers must have workers' compensation insurance or group insurance or be self-insured.

When an employee becomes ill or injured as a result of a work-related situation, the employee or employee representative may file a workers' compensation claim as defined by the state. In doing so, the employee usually signs an authorization to release his or her medical information to the workers' compensation entity. See figure 13.3 for Ohio's Bureau of Workers' Compensation Authorization for Release of Medical Information form. State workers' compensation laws require employers to collect and maintain information on the employee's illness, injury, or death, which may include medical information requested from healthcare facilities in which the individual received care. The information may be disclosed to other entities in the state or to the federal government for reporting purposes without the patient's or family's authorization. The information is used to determine if the individual or family should receive compensation for the injury, illness, or death. The information collected usually includes the following:

- Injured worker's name
- SSN, address, home and work phone
- Date of birth
- Gender
- Date of injury, disease, or death

Figure 13.3. Workers' compensation authorization to release medical information

Ohio | **Bureau of Workers' Compensation**   **Authorization to Release Medical Information**

Instructions
- Please print or type.
- List the provider(s) you are authorizing to release medical records in the space indicated on this form.
- Please sign and date the form, and send it to the customer service office where your claim is located or to your self-insured employer.

*You can obtain this form online at **ohiobwc.com***

Injured worker name (first, M.I., last)		Date of injury	Claim number
Address	City	State	Nine-digit ZIP code
Employer name		Employer MCO or QHP	

I, the above-named injured worker, understand I am allowing the Ohio Rehabilitation Services Commission and the

providers (persons or facilities) named here (_____

_____) that attend or examine
me to release the following medical, psychological and/or psychiatric information (excluding psychotherapy notes)
that are related causally or historically to physical or mental injuries relevant to my workers' compensation claim:

- Pathology slides and immunohistochemical staining results, if applicable;
- Hospital admission history and physical; emergency room reports; hospital discharge summaries; physician office notes; physical therapist, occupational therapist or athletic trainer assessments and progress notes; consultation reports; lab results; medical reports; surgical reports; diagnostic reports; procedure reports; nursing home and skilled nursing facilities documentation; home nursing progress notes; or other listed below.

_____.

I understand I am authorizing the release of this information to the following: the Ohio Bureau of Workers' Compensation (BWC), the Industrial Commission of Ohio, the above-named employer, the employer's managed care organization or qualified health plan and any authorized representatives.

I understand this information is being released to the above-referenced persons and/or entities for use in administering my workers' compensation claim.

This authorization to release medical, psychological and/or psychiatric information shall remain in effect for as long as my workers' compensation claim remains open under Ohio law. I understand I have the right to revoke this authorization at any time. However, I must submit my revocation in writing and file it with BWC or my self-insured employer. My decision to revoke this authorization will be effective, except in the case that any provider referenced above already has relied on my authorization and released information.

I understand the provider(s) referenced above may not make my completing and signing this authorization a condition of my treatment.

I understand the parties I am authorizing the release of information to are exempted from the federal privacy requirements of the Health Insurance Portability and Accountability Act of 1996 as they administer workers' compensation programs. Information disclosed pursuant to this authorization may be redisclosed by them and may no longer be protected by the federal privacy requirements. I understand such redisclosures may include but are not limited to the following:
- A copy of the medical information the employer receives may be forwarded to BWC by the employer;
- A copy of the medical information will be available to me or my physician of record upon request to BWC or to the employer.

Injured worker (or guardian or personal representative) signature	Date

If signed by the injured worker's guardian or personal representative, provide a description of the guardian

or personal representative's authority to sign on behalf of the injured worker. _____

_____.

BWC-1224 (Rev. 1/14/2011)
C-101

Source: Ohio Bureau of Workers' Compensation 2011.

- Occupation or job title

- Description of accident

- Type of injury/disease and parts of body affected

- Place of accident or exposure on employer premises

- Date hired

- Date employer notified of injury, illness, or death

State laws requiring employers and healthcare providers to report occupational illnesses, injuries, and deaths for the purpose of establishing workers' compensation do not conflict with HIPAA under the public interest and benefit exception of workers' compensation. The employer or healthcare provider is permitted to disclose PHI as necessary to comply with a state's compensation laws (45 CFR 164.512(a); CFR 164.502(b)(2)(iv)). The patient or family does not have the right to restrict the healthcare provider from this disclosure if the disclosure is required by state compensation laws. If a healthcare organization is asked for information related to a worker's previous condition not related to the claim for compensation, the organization must seek the worker's authorization before disclosing the information (45 CFR 164.508).

WorkersCompensation.com provides a workers' compensation guide to compensation law, information, and resources by state (WorkersCompensation.com 2010).

National Reporting Requirements

In addition to state laws requiring reporting of conditions and circumstances, there are federal mandatory reporting requirements, along with volunteer reporting systems hosted by agencies such as the CDC.

Reporting of Serious Occurrences or Deaths Related to Restraint or Seclusion

There are several federal regulations that require reporting to appropriate authorities any deaths or serious occurrences related to patients who have been restrained or placed in seclusion. The Conditions of Participation (CoP) regarding patient rights applies to all Medicare- and Medicaid-participating hospitals, including short-term, psychiatric, rehabilitation, long-term, children's, and alcohol and drug facilities. The CoP contains six standards requiring facilities to notify patients of their rights in regard to their care and addressing privacy and safety, confidentiality of health records, and freedom from seclusion and restraints used in behavior management unless clinically necessary. There are specific documentation requirements for orders to be written, time limitations, and notes regarding ongoing observation and monitoring and continuing assessments of the need for restraints.

In December 2006 the CoP Patient Rights final rule (42 CFR 482.13(g)) was published and specified that a hospital accredited by the Joint Commission or the American Osteopathic Association is deemed to meet all Medicare requirements and thus must report the following information:

- Each death that occurs while a patient is in restraint or seclusion.

- Each death that occurs within 24 hours after the patient has been removed from restraint or seclusion.

- Each death known to the hospital that occurs within one week after restraint or seclusion where it is reasonable to assume that use of restraint or placement in seclusion contributed directly or indirectly to a patient's death. "Reasonable to assume" in this context includes, but is not limited to, deaths related to restrictions of movement for prolonged periods of time, chest compression, restriction of breathing, or asphyxiation.

The hospital must report the death to CMS by telephone no later than the close of business the next CMS business day following knowledge of the patient's death. Hospital staff must also document in the patient's health record the date and time the death was reported (CMS 2012). In all of the above situations, the death would also be reported to a state agency as determined by state law.

The Children's Health Act of 2000, signed into law on October 17, 2000, establishes national standards that restrict the use of restraints and seclusion in all psychiatric facilities that receive federal funds and in "non-medical community-based facilities for children and youth." In those settings, the use of restraints and seclusion is restricted to emergency safety situations. In the case of a minor, the parent or legal guardian must be notified no later than 24 hours after the occurrence (42 CFR 483.374). The information must include the patient's name, a description of the occurrence, and contact information for the facility.

These requirements do not conflict with the HIPAA Privacy Rule because such reporting meets the public interest and benefit exception of either "required by law" or "to prevent or lessen a serious threat to health or safety," and patient authorization is not required.

National Reporting of Quality Measures

Medicare, in collaboration with the Joint Commission and other private organizations, has developed a number of quality measures for hospitals, physician's offices, nursing homes, and other provider entities for the purpose of improving the quality and safety of patient care. The PHI collected is used for retrospective analysis and real-time reporting that enables healthcare organizations to comprehensively evaluate and manage quality improvement efforts. Some of the reporting activities are mandatory and some are voluntary (see table 13.2). Data may be submitted to federally supported Quality Improvement Organizations (QIOs) and Clinical Data Abstraction Centers (CDACs), the CDC, or other reporting organizations.

Table 13.2. Examples of national quality reporting initiatives

Initiative	Who	Purpose
Hospital Consumer Assessment of Healthcare Providers and Systems (HCAHPS)	Hospitals	Samples discharged patients on their experience in hospital related to communication, cleanliness of facility, pain management, discharge information, overall satisfaction with hospital
Hospital Quality Alliance (HQA)	Hospitals	Reporting on 22 clinical process and two 30-day mortality (outcome) measures on: • Acute myocardial infarction (AMI) • Heart failure (HF) • Pneumonia (PN) • Surgical Care Improvement Project (SCIP)
National Healthcare Safety Network (NHSN)	Hospitals, dialysis centers, ambulatory surgical centers, long-term care facilities	Surveillance system that collects data on healthcare-associated infections, adherence to clinical practices known to prevent healthcare-associated infections, incidence or prevalence of multidrug-resistant organisms within their organizations, trends and coverage of healthcare personnel safety and vaccination, and adverse events related to the transfusion of blood and blood products
Nursing Home Improvement Feedback Tool (NHIFT)	Nursing homes	Free, computer-based, process-of-care data collection tool that assists nursing homes in collecting data and viewing process measure scores for four clinical topics: depression, pain, physical restraints, and pressure ulcers
Physician Quality Reporting Initiative (PQRI)	Physician practices	Voluntary reporting of specified quality measures, which will earn participating physician a payment bonus, subject to a cap

Source: CMS 2011.

The CMS has a number of mandatory quality reporting initiatives in place that require hospitals and other healthcare organizations to report data. In all cases the confidentiality of patient information is maintained. The reported data are shared through websites that enable comparison among all doctors, hospitals, and other healthcare organizations. Recent regulations such as Section 3004 of the 2010 Affordable Care Act establish mandatory quality reporting requirements for long-term care hospitals, inpatient rehabilitation facilities, and hospice programs, which will go into effect in 2014. Previous legislation has already made reporting mandatory for hospitals. A Medicare provider that fails to comply with the data reporting requirements is subject to a 2 percent reduction of reimbursement. Chapter 14 provides additional information on CMS quality reporting programs.

Other national mandatory reporting requirements relate to programs designed to prevent fraud and abuse. Healthcare organizations must provide copies of health records to Recovery Audit Contractors (RACs), Medicare Administrative Contractors (MACs), and Medicaid Integrity Contractors (MICs), whose responsibilities include but are not limited to measuring, preventing, identifying, and correcting incorrect payments under the Tax Relief and Health Care Act of 2006 and other federal healthcare reform legislations (Premier Advisor Live 2011).

In all of the above programs, the reporting of data is permissible under the Privacy Rule as "required by law," "for the purpose of research," or "to prevent or lessen a serious threat to health or safety."

National Practitioner Data Banks

The Division of Practitioner Data Banks located in HHS is responsible for managing the **National Practitioner Data Bank** (NPDB) and the **Healthcare Integrity and Protection Data Bank** (HIPDB). The **Health Care Quality Improvement Act** of 1986 created the NPDB, which began operations in 1990 (42 USC 11133(a)(1)). In 2010 the information contained in the NPDB was expanded by Section 1921 of the Social Security Act, as amended by Section 5(b) of the Medicare and Medicaid Patient and Program Protection Act of 1987 to (HHS n.d.):

> . . . improve the quality of healthcare by encouraging State licensing boards, hospitals and other healthcare entities, and professional societies to identify and discipline those who engage in unprofessional behavior; and to restrict the ability of incompetent physicians, dentists, and other healthcare practitioners to move from State to State without disclosure or discovery of previous medical malpractice payment and adverse action history. Adverse actions can involve licensure, clinical privileges, professional society membership, and exclusions from Medicare and Medicaid.

The HIPDB was established under Section 1128E of the Social Security Act and became operational in 2000. The purpose of the HIPDB is to establish a national healthcare fraud and abuse data collection program for the reporting of final adverse actions (not including settlements in which no findings of liability have been made) against healthcare providers, suppliers, or practitioners and to maintain a database of the information collected (42 USC 1301, 1128E).

The data banks are responsible for receiving adverse action information on healthcare providers, practitioners, or suppliers from federal and state government agencies, health plans, malpractice payers, and others and disclosing the information to those who have access rights to the information. See figure 13.4 for a listing of who is required to report, what information is available in the data banks, and to whom the information may be disclosed. For example, a hospital must report to the NPDB adverse actions against a physician on staff (such as suspension of privileges) lasting more than 30 days, medical malpractice payments, and settlement reports. When evaluating a provider's application for privileges, the facility must query the NPDB. Data bank information provides additional details regarding an applicant but does not supersede the normal investigation practices. Hospitals must query the NPDBs about staff members every two years.

Information reported to the data banks is considered confidential and is not disclosed except as specified by regulation. For example, a practitioner or physician may access the information reported

Figure 13.4. National data bank reporting requirements

Healthcare Integrity and Protection Data Bank	Expanded National Practitioner Data Bank
Who Reports? • Federal and state government agencies • Health plans	**Who Reports?** • Medical malpractice payers • State health care practitioner licensing and certification authorities (including medical and dental boards) • Hospitals • Other health care entities with formal peer review (HMOs, group practices, managed care organizations) • Professional societies with formal peer review • State entity licensing and certification authorities • Peer review organizations • Private accreditation organizations • DEA • HHS OIG
What Information Is Available? • Licensing and certification actions (practitioners, providers, and suppliers), revocation, reprimand, suspension (including length), censure, probation, voluntary surrender, any other negative action or finding by a federal or state licensing or certification agency that is publicly available information • Health care-related civil judgments (practitioners, providers, and suppliers) • Health care-related criminal convictions (practitioners, providers, and suppliers) • Exclusions from federal or state health care programs (practitioners, providers, and suppliers) • Other adjudicated actions or decisions (practitioners, providers, and suppliers)	**What Information Is Available?** • Medical malpractice payments (all health care practitioners) • Any adverse licensure (all practitioners or entities) —revocation, reprimand, censure, suspension, probation —any dismissal or closure of the proceedings by reason of the practitioner or entity surrendering the license or leaving the state or jurisdiction —any other loss of license • Adverse clinical privileging actions • Adverse professional society membership actions • Any negative action or finding by a state licensing or certification authority • Peer review organization negative actions or findings against a health care practitioner • Private accreditation organization negative actions or findings against a healthcare or entity • Adverse actions against DEA certification • Medicare exclusions
Who Can Query? • Federal and state government agencies • Health plans • Health care practitioners, providers, suppliers (self-query) • Researchers (statistical data only)	**Who Can Query?** • Hospitals • Other health care entities with formal peer review • Professional societies with formal peer review • State health care practitioner licensing and certification authorities (including medical and dental boards) • State entity licensing and certification authorities* • Agencies or contractors administering federal health care programs* • State agencies administering Federal health care programs* • State Medicaid Fraud Control Units* • U.S. Comptroller General* • U.S. Attorney General and other law enforcement* • Health care practitioners and entities (self-query) • Plaintiff's attorney/pro se plaintiffs (under limited circumstances)* • Quality Improvement Organizations* • Researchers (statistical data only) • DEA • HHS OIG

Source: FR 75(18), January 18, 2010.
*Eligible to receive only those reports authorized by section 1921.
**Eligible to receive only those reports authorized by HCQIA.

on them and entities engaged in professional review activity. The receipt, access, use, and disclosure of information from the data banks do not conflict with the HIPAA Privacy Rule because they meet the public interest and benefit "required by law" exception.

Medical Device Reporting

The **Safe Medical Devices Act** (SMDA) (21 USC 360i(b)) is a federal program that requires reporting to the Food and Drug Administration (FDA) and the product manufacturer of medical device occurrences that have or may have contributed to serious illness, serious injury, or death, including occurrences attributed to user error. The Medical Device Amendments of 1992 clarified terms and established a single reporting standard for device user facilities, manufacturers, importers, and distributors.

A serious injury or illness is identified as one that:

- Is life-threatening

- Results in permanent impairment of a body function or permanent damage to a body structure

- Necessitates medical or surgical intervention to preclude permanent impairment of a body function or permanent damage to a body structure

A medical device is anything that is used in treatment or diagnosis that is not a drug. A medical device is defined as an instrument, apparatus, or other article that is used to prevent, diagnose, mitigate, or treat a disease or to affect the structure or function of the body, with the exception of drugs. Examples of medical devices are x-ray machines, sutures, defibrillators, vascular grafts, syringes, surgical lasers, heating pads, bone screws, gauze pads, patient restraints, wheelchairs, infusion pumps, and hospital beds. The FDA requires that all reportable events involving medical devices are reported and should include the following information (FDA 2013):

- User facility report number

- Name and address of the device manufacturer

- Device brand name and common name

- Product model, catalog, serial, and lot numbers

- Brief description of the event reported to the manufacturer and/or the FDA

- Where the report was submitted (for example, to the FDA, manufacturer, or distributor)

The HIPAA Privacy Rule specifically allows **medical device reporting** (45 CFR 164.512(b)) without patient authorization as follows:

1. To collect or report adverse events (or similar activities with respect to food or dietary supplements), product defects or problems (including problems with the use or labeling of a product), or biological product deviations

2. To track FDA-regulated products

3. To enable product recalls, repairs, replacements, or lookback (including locating and notifying individuals who have received products that have been recalled or withdrawn or are the subject of lookback)

4. To conduct post-marketing surveillance

Under the Freedom of Information and Privacy Acts, however, prior to any public disclosure, the FDA is required to delete any personal, medical, and similar information that would constitute a clear unwarranted invasion of personal privacy, in addition to trade secrets and confidential commercial or financial information related to the manufacturer or identifying information of the reporter of the event. Any device that is used in the treatment of a patient that causes serious injury, illness, or death must be reported within 10 days of the occurrence to the manufacturer and the FDA. Requirements for reporting and reporting forms can be found on the website of the FDA's Center for Devices and Radiological Health.

Reporting of Occurrences with Electronic Health Record Systems

The FDA has also been studying the issue of regulating electronic health record (EHR) systems because of potential safety risks. Schulte and Schwartz report:

> Over the past two years, the FDA's voluntary notification system logged a total of 260 reports of "malfunctions with the potential for patient harm," including 44 injuries and the six deaths. Among other things the systems have mixed up patients, put test results in the wrong person's file and lost vital medical information. In one example cited in the FDA testimony, an operating room management system frequently "locked up" during surgery. Lost data had to be re-entered manually "in some cases from a nurse's recollection." Another system failed to display a patient's allergies properly because of software errors. In another case, results from lab testing done in a hospital emergency room were returned for the wrong patient. (Schulte and Schwartz 2010)

In an effort to reinforce patient safety with the use of EHRs, the Office of the National Coordinator for Health Information Technology (ONC) Certification/Adoption Workgroup recommended that ONC work with the FDA and representatives of patient, clinician, vendor, and healthcare organizations to determine the role that the FDA should play to improve the safe use of certified EHR technology (ONC 2010). While the FDA and ONC work together on this issue, users of digital medical systems such as EHRs may continue to voluntarily report problems that may include PHI without patient authorization.

Federal Registry on Implantable Cardiac Defibrillators

In January 2005, Medicare expanded its coverage of implantable cardiac defibrillators (ICDs) to eligible Medicare beneficiaries. As a requirement for covering the cost of ICDs, hospitals are required to submit data to the Medicare ICD registry. A more detailed discussion of registries is found later in the chapter. On April 1, 2006, Medicare contracted with the American College of Cardiologists (ACC) National Cardiovascular Data Registry (NCDR) to assume responsibility for the ICD registry. Every hospital that seeks reimbursement for ICDs must participate in the registry (CMS n.d.). This requirement does not conflict with the HIPAA Privacy Rule because it meets the public interest and benefit exception of "required by law," "for the purpose of research," or "to prevent or lessen a serious threat to health or safety." The NCDR also coordinates other national registries for cardiac interventions that are not government-mandated related to carotid artery stenting and endarterectomy procedures, cardiac catherizations, and quality improvement products. The PHI collected in these registries also do not conflict with the HIPAA Privacy Rule because they meet the exception related to "for the purpose of research" (NCDR 2010).

Organ Procurement Reporting

Federal law requires that a hospital notify the designated organ procurement organization (OPO) in a timely manner regarding specified organ donors who die in the hospital or for whom death is imminent (42 CFR 482.45). Hospitals must also work with the OPO to do annual death record reviews (42 CFR

482.45). A hospital is not violating confidentiality by calling the OPO and providing information about an individual who has died or whose death is imminent. Although the statute and regulations are not explicit in establishing that such notification does not violate patient confidentiality, it is implicit in the law. There is no requirement in the statute or regulations that the family be informed about the hospital's notification of the OPO before the OPO can be contacted (Reynolds 2010). Further, this federal law does not conflict with HIPAA because, under the public interest and benefit exception of "for cadaveric organ, eye or tissue donation," such disclosures are permissible without authorization.

Occupational Fatalities, Injuries, and Illnesses

Federal occupational safety and health regulation requires employers to report work-related fatalities, injuries, and illnesses (29 CFR 1904.0). According to the regulation, such events must be reported if they result in (29 CFR 1904.7(a)):

> . . . death, days away from work, restricted work or transfer to another job, medical treatment beyond first aid, or loss of consciousness. You must also consider a case to meet the general recording criteria if it involves a significant injury or illness diagnosed by a physician or other licensed health care professional, even if it does not result in death, days away from work, restricted work or job transfer, medical treatment beyond first aid, or loss of consciousness.

Federal law requiring the reporting of occupational fatalities, injuries, and illnesses does not conflict with HIPAA because, under the public interest and benefit exception of "public health activities" or as provided by the preemption exception, such disclosures are permissible without authorization. Healthcare facilities may be required to release medical information relevant to the fatality, injury, or illness to appropriate authorities.

Regarding workers' compensation for federal employees, the federal government offers federal employees a compensation program similar to state programs. The federal government's program is administered through the Office of Workers' Compensation Programs of the US Department of Labor. The federal workers' compensation program falls under the same HIPAA Privacy Rule provision as that of the state workers' compensation programs.

Check Your Understanding 13.2

Instructions: Indicate whether the following statements are true or false (T or F).

1. The attending physician usually has responsibility for filing the death certificate.

2. Reporting of notifiable diseases without the patient's authorization is allowed under the public interest and benefit exception under HIPAA.

3. National hospital quality data may only be released to the QIO or the CDAC with a signed authorization from the patient.

4. Every hospital receiving reimbursement from Medicare for implantable cardiac defibrillators must submit data to the American College of Cardiologists National Cardiovascular Data Registry.

5. Federal law requires that a hospital notify the designated organ procurement organization (OPO) in a timely manner regarding specified organ donors who die in the hospital or for whom death is imminent.

Registries

The term **registry** refers to a program that collects and stores data and the records that are created through this process. Registries are designed and used for a broad range of purposes in public health and medicine, from evaluating patient care to monitoring defective devices; examples include:

- Assessing natural history, including estimating magnitude of a problem; determining underlying incidence or prevalence rate; examining trends of disease over time; conducting surveillance; assessing service delivery and identifying groups of high risk; documenting types of patients served by a healthcare provider; and describing and estimating survival

- Determining clinical effectiveness, cost-effectiveness, or comparative effectiveness of a test or treatment, including evaluating the acceptability of drugs, devices, or procedures for reimbursement

- Measuring or monitoring safety and harm of specific products and treatments, including conducting comparative evaluation of safety and effectiveness

- Measuring or improving quality of care, including conducting programs to measure and/or improve the practice of medicine and/or public health (Gliklich and Dreyer 2010, 54)

The National Committee on Vital and Health Statistics states that a registry is an organized system for the collection, storage, retrieval, analysis, and dissemination of information on individuals who have a particular disease or condition or prior exposure to a substance or circumstance that may cause an adverse health effect (Gliklich and Dreyer 2010). Registries are maintained by healthcare organizations for a variety of purposes and are often known as clinical, disease, and/or outcome registries. States often maintain a variety of registries for the purpose of collecting extensive information on particular diseases used for setting health policy, disease prevention and control, and other reporting purposes. The types of registries required vary from state to state, as does the information collected by the registries.

Common among the registries required by state law are the requirements that the data submitted to the registry be maintained in a confidential manner and that the identity of the patient be protected from disclosure. Because these registries are maintained by state entities, the healthcare organizations releasing the data do so under the HIPAA Privacy Rule's public interest and benefit exception of "public health activities." Registries maintained by healthcare organizations and providers typically use data from patient health records under the healthcare operations provision, so individual patient authorization is not required in order for the data to be included in the registry. If the registry is maintained by a private organization for research purposes, however, the registry is subject to the research requirements of the Privacy Rule. Some common types of registries are described below.

Cancer Registries

State-based **cancer registries** are data systems that collect, manage, and analyze data about cancer cases and cancer deaths. In each state, medical facilities (including hospitals, physician's offices, therapeutic radiation facilities, freestanding surgical centers, and pathology laboratories) are required to report data to a central cancer registry as defined by state law. The data reported to a central statewide registry or incidence surveillance program are in turn reported to the CDC. In 1992 the Cancer Registries Act established the National Program of Cancer Registries (NPCR), which is administered by the CDC. State cancer surveillance programs, assisted by the NPCR, collect data on the occurrence of cancer, type, extent, location, and type of initial treatment, which are then used to determine trends, allocate resources, and advance research. For example, according to Ohio law:

> . . . each physician, dentist, hospital or person providing diagnostic or treatment services to patients with cancer shall report each case of cancer to the Ohio Cancer Incidence Surveillance

System (OCISS) at the Ohio Department of Health (ODH). . .. A reportable case is defined as: any primary malignant neoplasm with the exception of basal and squamous cell carcinoma of the skin and carcinoma in-situ of the cervix diagnosed and/or treated in any person in Ohio on or after Jan. 1, 1992, as well as cases of benign and borderline intracranial and nervous system (CNS) tumors diagnosed on or after Jan. 1, 2004. (Ohio Department of Health 2010)

Confidentiality of the data reported by healthcare facilities to state registries is protected as defined by state law. In addition, the NPCR requires that all registries that submit data to the program have a security policy in place.

Trauma Registries

Trauma registries maintain databases on patients with severe traumatic injuries. A **traumatic injury** is a wound or other injury caused by an external physical force such as an automobile accident, a shooting, a stabbing, or a fall. Information collected by the trauma registry may be used for performance improvement and research in the area of trauma care. Trauma registries may be facility-based or may include data for a region or state.

The information collected by trauma registries may include patient demographics, injury location, injury date and time, cause of injury, safety equipment used, prehospital assessment/treatment, emergency department or admission assessment/treatment, hospital assessment/treatment, disposition and diagnosis (including injury severity scores), and patient outcome. The entities usually required to report trauma are healthcare facilities of all types, other state agencies as required by state regulation, and medical examiners or coroners. Not every patient who is injured qualifies for inclusion in a trauma registry, so state regulations must be reviewed to determine what constitutes a trauma patient. For example, the New York State Trauma Registry defines a trauma patient as having at least one injury that falls within the ICD-9 diagnosis code range of 800–959.9, which includes burns, hypothermia, smoke inhalation, hanging, drowning, abuse, and DOAs (dead on arrival) (New York State Department of Health 2009). Tennessee has a registry specific to traumatic brain and spinal cord injuries as well as a general trauma registry (TN Code Ann. 68-55-101; TN Code Ann. 68-11-259). Ultimately, the information from a trauma registry might be used to assess the need for a state public health law, such as a motorcycle helmet law, or for other public safety concerns.

Immunization Registries

Immunization registries have been implemented in many states as a way to collect and maintain vaccination records on children and in some cases adults in an effort to promote disease prevention and control. These registries are different in that while they require the reporting of PHI, they also allow access to this information by the individual whose data is recorded in the registry or his or her representative. The reasons some state immunization registries have moved in this direction can be summed up as outlined by the Georgia Immunization Registry:

- Assure that all persons in Georgia receive appropriate, timely immunizations to lead healthy, disease-free lives

  — Assist providers and public health officials in reminding individuals when they or their children need or are past due for vaccination(s)

  — Assist public health officials in assessing and improving community immunization status

- Assure access to up-to-date immunization records of Georgians

  — Assist providers in evaluating the immunization status of their patients

  — Avoid duplicate immunizations

- Meet the needs of Georgia's Immunization Registry mandate

- Provide a Registry that is cost-effective, user friendly, and efficient (Georgia Department of Community Health 2010)

The party responsible for reporting immunizations is the healthcare entity (or its designee) that administers a vaccine licensed by the US Food and Drug Administration (e.g., physicians, public health departments or agencies, hospitals, and clinics). Registries usually collect patient identification information, immunization received, date administered, by whom, and where. The registry records and tracks this information, which is then made available to healthcare providers, parents, and legal guardians. Access to the information through the Internet or in some other format is usually delineated by state regulation or guidelines. The state of Wisconsin's immunization program offers a public immunization record access hyperlink that gives people the ability to look up their immunization record in the Wisconsin Immunization Registry (Wisconsin Department of Health Services n.d.).

Birth Defects Registries

Birth defects registries collect information on newborns with birth defects. Usually maintained by the state, these registries serve a variety of purposes. For example, they provide information on the incidence of birth defects to study causes and prevention of birth defects, to monitor trends in birth defects, to improve medical care for children with birth defects, and to target interventions for preventable birth defects, such as folic acid to prevent neural tube defects. Information for birth defects registries may come from reporting by healthcare facilities and providers as well as from birth, fetal death, and death certificates. In Florida, for example:

> The Florida Birth Defects Registry (FBDR) uses passive surveillance methodology to identify infants with birth defects. The FBDR uses data from the Bureau of Vital Statistics, the Department of Health Regional Perinatal Intensive Care Centers, Children's Medical Services, and Early Intervention Program/Early Steps, along with information from the Agency for Health Care Administration Inpatient Discharge Data and Ambulatory Hospital Data. If any of these identifies an infant with a birth defect before one year of age and the infant was born alive to a Florida resident, then the infant is part of the FBDR. (FBDR 2010)

The type of data collected in birth defects registries includes demographic information; birth weight; status at birth, including live-born, stillborn, or aborted; autopsies; cytogenetics results; whether the infant was a single or multiple birth; mother's use of alcohol, tobacco, or illicit drugs; father's use of drugs and alcohol; and family history of birth defects.

Diabetes Registries

Since diabetes is such a serious public health problem, **diabetes registries** have been developed to follow diabetic patients. Diabetes registries include cases of patients with diabetes for the purpose of assistance in managing care as well as for research. Patients whose diabetes is not kept under good control frequently have numerous complications. The diabetes registry can track whether a patient has been seen by a physician in an effort to prevent complications.

Diabetes registries have typically been kept in ambulatory care settings, since this is where the majority of diabetic care is provided. Illinois recently instituted the first statewide diabetes registry (University of Chicago Medical Center 2010). In addition to demographic information, other data collected may include laboratory values such as HBA1c. This test is used to determine the patient's blood glucose for a period of approximately 60 days prior to the time of the test. Moreover, facility registries may track patient visits in order to follow up with patients who have not been seen in the past year.

Implant Registries

An implant is a material or substance inserted into the body, such as breast implants, heart valves, and pacemakers. **Implant registries** have been developed for the purpose of tracking the performance of implants, including complications, deaths, and defects resulting from implants, as well as implant longevity.

The safety of implants has been questioned recently in a number of highly publicized cases. For example, there have been questions about the safety of silicone breast implants and temporomandibular joint implants. In such cases, it is often difficult to ensure that all patients with the implants have been notified of the safety questions. Some implant registries were developed in response to these types of situations. A number of federal laws have been enacted to regulate medical devices, including implants as previously mentioned. Breast implants were first covered under Section 15 of the Food, Drug and Cosmetic Act and then under the Safe Medical Devices Act of 1990 as amended through the Medical Device Amendments of 1992. Implant registries can help healthcare providers in complying with the legal requirement for reporting. Demographic data on patients receiving implants are included in the registry as well as the other data items mentioned above to facilitate reporting.

Transplant Registries

Transplant registries may have varied purposes. Some organ transplant registries maintain databases of patients who need organs. When an organ becomes available, a fair way may then be used to allocate the organ to the patient with the highest priority. In other cases, the purpose of the registry is to provide a database of potential donors for transplants using live donors, such as bone marrow transplants. Post-transplant information also is kept on organ recipients and donors.

Because transplant registries are used to try to match donor organs with recipients, they are often national or even international in scope. Examples of national registries include the UNet of the United Network for Organ Sharing (UNOS) and the registry of the National Marrow Donor Program (NMDP).

Data collected in the transplant registry may also be used for research, policy analysis, and quality control. The type of information collected varies according to the type of registry. Pretransplant data about the recipient include demographic data, patient's diagnosis, patient's status codes regarding medical urgency, patient's functional status, whether the patient is on life support, previous transplantations, and **histocompatibility** (compatibility of donor and recipient tissues). For donor registries, information on donors varies according to whether or not the donor is living. For organs harvested from patients who have died, information is collected on the cause and circumstances of the death, organ procurement and consent process, medications the donor was taking, and other donor history. For a living donor, information collected includes the relationship of the donor to the recipient (if any), clinical information, information on organ recovery, and histocompatibility.

Disclosures to Public Health Authorities Not Required by Law

Covered entities may disclose PHI to public health entities even if law does not specifically require the disclosure, if the disclosure is for the purpose of:

> . . . preventing or controlling disease, injury, or disability, including, but not limited to, the reporting of disease, injury, vital events such as birth or death, and the conduct of public health surveillance, public health investigations, and public health interventions; or, at the direction of a public health authority, to an official of a foreign government agency that is acting in collaboration with a public health authority. (45 CFR 164.512(b))

For example, information about an individual with a disease might be disclosed in order to determine the cause of the disease and prevent it from spreading (CDC 2003). In such cases, it is necessary for the facility to verify the identity of the person requesting the information if the request is made in person or to determine the authority for the request using methods such as requiring a statement on official letterhead from the public health entity (CDC 2003).

Check Your Understanding 13.3

Instructions: Indicate whether the following statements are true or false (T or F).

1. Information included in state registries is considered public information.

2. Immunization registries are different from other state registries because they allow access by the individuals included in the registry or their representatives, such as parents.

3. Transplant registries may include data about organ donors as well as organ recipients.

4. Implant registries are frequently developed in response to highly publicized cases of harm resulting from implants to provide for easier notification of individuals affected.

5. Statewide cancer registries are frequently required to report data to the National Center for Health Statistics.

Summary

Both state and federal governments have laws requiring that certain diseases, conditions, and circumstances be reported. These include communicable diseases, vital records, and registries. The statutes and regulations that require such reporting usually include a section indicating that the information may be reported without obtaining authorization from the patient and that such information collected by the government is not considered public record. The HIPAA Privacy Rule also includes regulations applicable to required reporting. These regulations indicate that such reporting is exempt from the HIPAA Privacy Rule. There is a requirement, however, that the Notice of Privacy Practices given to patients include a statement that such reporting is done without patient authorization. The HIPAA Privacy Rule also requires that such disclosures be included in the accounting of disclosures that a patient may request. Facilities must have a policy and procedure that ensure that such disclosures are included in the accounting of disclosures log or database.

References

American Bar Association Commission on Law and Aging. 2007. Information about laws related to elder abuse. http://www.americanbar.org/aba.html.

Burrington-Brown, J., B. Hjort, and L. Washington. 2007. Health data access, use, and control. *Journal of AHIMA* 78(5):63–66.

Centers for Disease Control and Prevention. 2003. HIPAA Privacy Rule and public health: Guidance from CDC and the US Department of Health and Human Services. http://www.cdc.gov.

Centers for Disease Control and Prevention. 2011. Nationally notifiable infectious diseases, United States 2011. http://www.cdc.gov.

Centers for Medicare and Medicaid Services. 2012. Survey & Certification - Certification and Compliance: Hospitals. https://www.cms.gov.

Centers for Medicare and Medicaid Services. 2011. Quality Initiatives General Information. http://www.cms.gov.

Centers for Medicare and Medicaid Services. n.d. Fact sheet: ICD registry transitions. http://www.cms.hhs.gov.

Child Welfare Information Gateway. 2010. State Definitions of Child Abuse and Neglect. http://www.childwelfare.gov.

Cornell University Law School. 2010. Workers' compensation: An overview. http://www.law.cornell.edu/.

Department of Health and Human Services. n.d. The Data Bank: National Practitioner Healthcare Integrity & Protection. http://www.npdb-hipdb.hrsa.gov.

Florida Birth Defects Registry. 2011. http://www.fbdr.org/.

Food and Drug Administration. 2013. Medical device reporting. http://www.fda.gov.

Georgia Department of Community Health. 2010. Georgia immunization registry (GRITS). http://www.health.state.ga.us.

Gliklich, R., and N. Dreyer, eds. 2010. *Registries for Evaluating Patient Outcomes: A User's Guide*, 2nd ed. Rockville, MD: Agency for Healthcare Research and Quality.

National Cardiovascular Data Registry. 2010. About NCDR. http://www.ncdr.com.

National Center for Health Statistics. 1992. Model State Vital Statistics Act and Regulations. http://www.cdc.gov.

National Center for Health Statistics. 2009. 2011 Model Law Revision. http://www.cdc.gov.

New York State Department of Health. 2009. New York State Trauma Registry Data Dictionary. http://www.health.state.ny.us.

Nuclear Regulatory Commission. 2013. Event notification reports. http://www.nrc.gov.

Nuclear Regulatory Commission. n.d. State Regulations and Legislation. http://www.nrc.gov.

Office of the National Coordinator for Health Information Technology, Health IT Policy Committee. 2010. Adoption-Certification Workgroup HIT Safety Recommendations April 22, 2010. http://www.healthit.gov.

Ohio Bureau of Workers' Compensation. 2011. Authorization to release medical information. BWC-1224 (Rev. 1/14/2011). http://www.ohiobwc.com.

Ohio Department of Health. 2010. Reporting of Ohio cancer incidence data. http://www.odh.ohio.gov.

Pozgar, G. 2012. *Legal Aspects of Health Care Administration*, 11th ed. Sudbury, MA: Jones and Bartlett.

Premier Advisor Live. 2011. Compliance with revenue audits: RACS, MACS, MICS and ZPICs. http://www.premierinc.com/advisorlive/Presentations/rac011211.pdf.

Reynolds, R., ed. 2010. *Tennessee Health Information Management Association Legal Handbook*, 10th ed. Winchester, TN: THIMA.

Roach, W., R. Hoban, B. Broccolo, A. Roth, and T. Blanchard. 2006. *Medical Records and the Law*, 4th ed. Sudbury, MA: Jones and Bartlett.

Schulte, F., and E. Schwartz. 2010 (February 23). FDA considers regulating safety of electronic health systems. *The Huffington Post*. http://www.huffingtonpost.com.

University of Chicago Medical Center. 2009. Lilly's Law: A diabetes registry for Illinois. Science Life blog. http://sciencelife.uchospitals.edu.

Wisconsin Department of Health Services. 2011. Wisconsin Immunization Program: Public immunization record access. http://www.dhs.wisconsin.gov.

WorkersCompensation.com. 2010.Workers' compensation: The workers' comp service center. http://www.workers compensation.com.

Cases, Statutes, and Regulations Cited

10 CFR 35.3045: Report and notification of a medical event. 2003.

29 CFR 1904.0: Purpose. 2001.

29 CFR 1904.7(a): Recording and Reporting Occupational Injuries and Illness; Recordkeeping Forms and Recording Criteria, Basic requirements. 2001.

42 CFR 482.13(g): Standard: Death Reporting Requirements. 2006.

42 CFR 482.45: Organ, tissue, and eye. 1998.

42 CFR 483.374: Facility reporting. 2001.

45 CFR 160.203: General rules and exceptions. 2002.

45 CFR 164.502(b)(2)(iv): Uses and disclosures of protected health information. 2002.

45 CFR 164.508: Uses and disclosures for which an authorization is required. 2002.

45 CFR 164.512(a): Uses and disclosures required by law. 2002.

45 CFR 164.512(b): Uses and disclosures for public health activity. 2002.

45 CFR 164.512(c): Abuse, neglect, and domestic violence. 2002.

45 CFR 164.520: Notice of privacy practices for protected health information. 2002.

21 USC 360i(b): Records and Reports on Devices; General Rule.

42 USC 1301,1128E: Health Care and Abuse Data Collection Program.

42 USC 11133(a)(1): Reporting of certain professional review actions by healthcare entities. 1986.

42 USC 3002: The Older Americans Act. 2006.

42 USC 5106g: Child Abuse Prevention and Treatment Act. 1996.

AL Code 38-9-8: Reports by physicians of physical, sexual, or emotional abuse, neglect or exploitation. 2000.

FL Stat. Ann. 415.101 et seq.: Adult protective services act. 2004.

MS Code 41-61-53: Reporting cases of disease. 1986.

OH Admin. Code 3701-3-08: Release of patient's records. 2009.

TN Code Ann. 68-10-113: Sexually transmitted diseases, confidentiality of information. 1992.

TN Code Ann. 68-11-259: Establishing a trauma registry, compliance, confidentiality. 2005.

TN Code Ann. 68-55-101: Brain trauma registry. 1993.

VT Stat. 18-6-107 5221: Fetal deaths. 1973.

Children's Health Act of 2000. Public Law 106-310.

Chapter 14

Risk Management and Quality Improvement

Jill Callahan Klaver, JD, RHIA

Learning Objectives

- Identify stakeholders in healthcare quality

- Define and distinguish between risk management and quality improvement processes

- Discuss how quality is measured

- Summarize the common sources of patient rights

- Describe the role of QIOs in healthcare quality

- Discuss private quality improvement initiatives

Key Terms

Adverse patient occurrences (APOs)
Against medical advice (AMA)
Charitable immunity
Darling case
Emergency Medical Treatment and Active Labor Act (EMTALA)
Failure Mode Effect and Criticality Assessment (FMECA)
Hill-Burton Act
Incident reporting
Institute for Healthcare Improvement (IHI)

Institute of Medicine (IOM)
Leapfrog Group
National Patient Safety Goals
National Practitioner Data Bank (NPDB)
Occurrence screening
Patient Care Partnership (patient rights)
Pay for performance
Quality
Quality improvement
Quality Improvement Organizations (QIOs)
Report cards
Restraints and seclusion

Risk analysis
Risk control techniques
Risk evaluation
Risk exposure or identification
Risk financing
Risk management
Risk treatment
Root cause analysis
Sentinel events

Introduction

No matter whom you ask—patients, providers, administrators, employers, scientists, or policymakers—everyone shares an interest in healthcare quality. But depending on whom you ask, quality can mean different things to different people. From a patient's perspective, quality can mean, "Did I get better after I went to the doctor?" whereas a provider might ask, "Did the patient get the right intervention at the right time?" An administrator may want to know, "Has our facility met all the required quality standards for accreditation?" while an employer may wonder, "Have I provided my employees with health plans that will provide preventive care and reduce sick days?" A scientist may want to know, "How does this new technology produce better results than the existing technology?" while a policymaker might ask, "How do we make sure that everyone has access to quality care?"

Despite the support of many different stakeholders for healthcare quality, the United States struggles with significant quality-related issues.

- 54 million people living in rural areas are often forced to travel great distances to receive specialty care.

- 18,000 people die each year because they do not receive effective interventions.

- Each year, millions of Americans receive healthcare services that are unnecessary, increase costs, and may even endanger their health.

- Between 44,000 and 98,000 lives per year are lost due to preventable medical errors, and "hospital errors rank between the fifth and eighth leading cause of death, killing more Americans than breast cancer, traffic accidents, or AIDS" (KaiserEDU.org 2007).

Healthcare quality issues not only affect lives, but they also directly and indirectly impact healthcare costs. In 2003, Medicare paid an additional $300 million for five types of adverse events in hospitals. The additional payments covered less than one third of the additional costs that hospitals incurred in treating those adverse events (*Journal of Healthcare Risk Management* 2007). Overall, medical errors cost the United States approximately $37.6 billion each year (AHRQ 2000). The cost of liability insurance, used by organizations to protect against financial loss related to medical errors and other types of negligence, is increasing rapidly. In 2002, one third of hospitals experienced an increase of 100 percent or more in liability insurance premiums. Over one fourth of hospitals reported a reduction or complete discontinuation of a service as a result of increasing liability premiums (*Journal of Healthcare Risk Management* 2007).

At the heart of advancing good medical outcomes and reducing the costs associated with poor quality care are two interrelated disciplines: quality improvement and risk management. This chapter will explore both of these concepts in detail.

Differences Between Risk Management and Quality Improvement

Before addressing quality improvement, it is important to understand the meaning of healthcare **quality**. In short, "quality healthcare means doing the right thing, at the right time, in the right way, for the right person—and having the best possible results" (AHRQ n.d.a). **Quality improvement** refers to the overall processes a facility has in place to make sure healthcare is safe, effective, patient-centered, timely, efficient, and equitable. In comparison, healthcare **risk management** refers to the processes in place to identify, evaluate, and control risk (Spath 2001). In this context, risk refers to an organization's risk of financial liability associated with accidents (Russell 1992). The risk of financial liability can be found in many situations: a nurse may administer the incorrect dose of a medication, a hospital visitor may slip and fall on a freshly mopped surface, or a natural disaster may destroy patient records. If an organization is ordered to pay damages in a negligence case or fines in an agency enforcement action, it has incurred this kind of financial liability. In other words, its financial liability has arisen from unplanned, accidental events.

According to the American Society for Healthcare Risk Management (ASHRM 2003), risk management is defined as:

> A systematic and scientific approach . . . to identify, evaluate, reduce or eliminate the possibility of an unfavorable deviation from expectation and thus, to prevent the loss of financial assets, resulting from injury to patients, visitors, employees, independent medical staff, or from damage, theft or loss of property belonging to the healthcare entity or persons mentioned.

From a clinical standpoint, there is an interrelationship between quality improvement and risk management that stems from similarities in their underlying processes. By implementing effective quality improvement processes, an organization increases its chances of improved clinical outcomes and decreases its chances of unexpected financial loss (for example, lawsuits) associated with poor outcomes. Additionally, by implementing effective risk management processes, an organization reduces its chances of financial loss from unplanned or unexpected events and promotes good clinical outcomes.

Risk Management

Quality and risk management programs have evolved concurrently over the past 40 years. An effective quality/risk management program is focused on improving the quality and safety of patient care. It incorporates the identification, analysis, evaluation, and elimination or reduction of possible risks to the institution's patients, visitors, and employees. The quality improvement department may have responsibility for the risk management program or the in-house legal department may handle risk management. In larger organizations, quality and risk management function as separate departments. The health information management (HIM) department may perform occurrence screening (analyzing records for evidence of these unplanned or unexpected events), analyze and display occurrence screening data, and assist the quality and risk management departments or various quality or risk management committees with follow-up activities. Utilization review professionals and case managers may also serve roles in the risk identification and/or management process.

Background

Historically, hospitals did not have to be concerned with financial loss occasioned by negligence. As charitable institutions, early hospitals were shielded from liability for negligence by the doctrine of **charitable immunity**. The rationale for charitable immunity was grounded in the belief that donors would not make contributions to hospitals if they thought their donation would be used to litigate claims, combined with concern that a few lawsuits could bankrupt a hospital. Hospitals were also protected by early "captain of the ship" case law holding physicians solely responsible for all aspects of the patient's care, including care provided by hospital staff. The role of the hospital was simply to provide a place for the physician to conduct his treatment—any negligence associated with that treatment was the responsibility of the physician.

Over the years, the doctrine of charitable immunity was eliminated by state legislatures and case law, and the door to hospital liability was opened. The 1965 **Darling case**—*Darling vs. Charleston Community Memorial Hospital*—is often credited as the landmark case for extending liability for negligence to hospitals. In that case, the plaintiff's broken leg had to be amputated after the hospital failed to notice that it had become gangrenous underneath the cast. In reviewing the case, the Illinois Supreme Court recognized that hospitals had evolved beyond simply furnishing facilities for treatment. Specifically, the court acknowledged that hospitals "regularly employ on a salary basis a large staff of physicians, nurses and interns, as well as administrative and manual workers, and they charge patients for medical care and treatment, collecting for such services, if necessary, by legal action." The court also noted, "The Standards for Hospital Accreditation, the state licensing regulations and the defendant's bylaws demonstrate that the medical profession and other responsible authorities regard it as both desirable and feasible that a hospital assume certain responsibilities for the care of the patient." The court ultimately determined that it was reasonable to conclude that the hospital itself was negligent when it failed to have adequate nursing staff capable of recognizing the progressive gangrenous condition of the plaintiff's leg and when it failed to require consultation of the plaintiff's condition by members of the hospital's surgical staff with expertise in the plaintiff's condition.

After the *Darling* case and other "pro-plaintiff" changes in the law, the frequency and severity of malpractice claims increased dramatically in the early 1970s (Danzon 1982). At the same time, many major malpractice insurers left the insurance market and insurance rates for physicians and hospitals significantly increased (Mello et al. 2003). Physicians and hospitals found it difficult, if not impossible, to obtain malpractice insurance (Mello et al. 2003). The resulting financial pressure led hospitals to explore the need to develop and implement risk management programs in order to control their risk of financial loss (ASHRM 2005). In 1980, the field of risk management gained momentum with the formation of the American Society for Healthcare Risk Management (ASHRM) (*Journal of Healthcare Risk Management* 1992). ASHRM provided a national voice for risk managers and guidance for organizing risk management programs, identifying risk, and gaining provider involvement in risk management programs, and continues to do so today (ASHRM 2005). In the mid-1980s, a second "malpractice crisis" occurred as lawsuits against hospitals for corporate negligence continued to become more common (*Journal of Healthcare Risk Management* 1992). Around the same time, state legislatures began passing laws requiring hospitals to implement risk management programs. During the late 1980s, the Joint Commission established its first standards for the loss control and prevention components of risk management programs (*Journal of Healthcare Risk Management* 1992).

Since the early years, the field of risk management has continued to evolve with the changing healthcare environment. Laws and standards now exist related to patient dumping, patient rights under the Conditions of Participation, corporate compliance, employment practices, medical errors, and many other healthcare-related issues (ASHRM 2005). The 1999 **Institute of Medicine** report *To Err Is Human: Building a Safer Health Care System* stated that there were many preventable errors causing patient deaths in hospitals. There is much national attention focused on issues of patient safety and the development of recommendations to improve quality, reduce errors in healthcare, and improve patient safety. All of these mandates have had a profound impact on risk management and quality efforts and will continue to sustain the continuous growth of the risk management field in the future, as discussed later in this chapter.

Check Your Understanding 14.1

Instructions: Indicate whether the following statements are true or false (T or F).

1. Risk management focuses on an organization's financial liability.

2. Quality and risk management programs have evolved concurrently.

3. A hospital's strongest legal defense is the doctrine of charitable immunity.

4. *Darling vs. Charleston Community Memorial Hospital* is a landmark case that extended negligence liability to hospitals.

5. A 1999 report by the Institute of Medicine concluded that very few preventable errors lead to patient deaths in hospitals.

Organization and Operation of Risk Management

Although standards for patient quality are found in both federal and state law and accreditation standards, risk management programs are most commonly governed by state law. State law defines the minimum scope and components of a risk management program, as well as any applicable certification standards for risk management professionals. Most of these laws identify risk in terms of incidents of actual harm or reasonable likelihood of harm to a patient resulting from substandard care, medical errors, or impaired providers. States generally require risk management programs to include a system for the investigation and analysis of the frequency and causes of incidents, measures to minimize the occurrence of incidents and their resulting injuries, and a formalized reporting system for reporting incidents to a designated individual (for example, risk manager, chief of staff, or chief administrator) (KS Stat. Ann. 65-4922).

Many healthcare facilities have risk management programs that encompass more than the baseline patient-safety aspects required by state law and include areas such as billing compliance, privacy compliance, and workplace safety. Regardless of its scope, any risk management program must be integrated throughout the organization and have support from top executives (figure 14.1).

Steps

The steps of risk management can vary depending on the type of risk being addressed. For example, the specific steps taken to monitor, investigate, and prevent medication errors will be different than those steps taken to monitor, investigate, and prevent patient falls. However, from a broader perspective, ASHRM (2000) identifies the following four key components and specific steps for a risk management program.

Risk Exposure or Identification

Risk exposure or identification refers to a systematic means of identifying potential losses and requires an understanding of the facility's business, legal, organizational, and clinical components. For example, from a clinical service standpoint, a risk manager should at least gather the following information:

- General description of each service
- Detailed description of how each service is rendered

Figure 14.1. The integrated risk management system

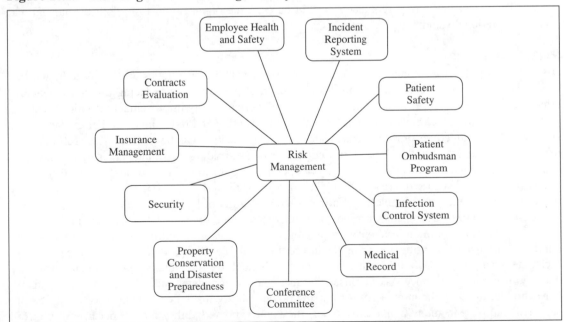

Source: ASHRM 2000, 78.

- List of personnel and tasks performed

- Required and necessary qualifications of personnel

- Supplies and products

- Processes used to select equipment

- Processes used for product failures that occur within and outside of the organization

- Types of equipment maintenance schedules established and records thereof

Certain types of data can also help identify risk:

- The organization's claims experience

- Databases compiled from local and national claims experience

- Incident reports and patient complaints

An additional method for identifying risk is **occurrence screening**, defined in the Joint Commission Sentinel Event Glossary of Terms (Joint Commission 2006a) as:

A system for concurrent or retrospective identification of **adverse patient occurrences** (APOs) through medical chart-based review according to objective screening criteria. Examples of criteria include admission for adverse results of outpatient management, readmission for complications, incomplete management of problems on previous hospitalization, or unplanned removal, injury, or repair of an organ or structure during surgery.

Risk Analysis

Risk analysis involves the process of identifying which risks should be proactively addressed and which risks are lower in priority. In making this judgment, a risk manager should consider:

- The probable frequency of the occurrence of the loss

- The possible severity of the loss

- The effect that any potential loss would have on the organization from both a financial and operational standpoint

Risk Treatment

Risk treatment involves applying risk control and risk financing techniques to determine how a risk should be treated. **Risk control techniques** are aimed at preventing or reducing the chances and/or effects of a loss occurrence. Often, data gathered from internal quality improvement activities can assist in determining what techniques are most effective in preventing and reducing risks. For example, data about accidental punctures or lacerations during surgical procedures can be used to reduce future occurrences of such events. Another type of risk control involves avoiding a risk altogether by intentionally choosing not to engage in a particular activity or operation. For example, if a hospital closes its neonatal intensive care unit because the risk is too high, risk avoidance has occurred. Risk avoidance is the only risk treatment activity that completely eliminates the possibility of loss.

    Risk financing refers to the methods used to pay for the costs associated with claims and other expenses. The most common form of risk financing is the purchase of liability insurance. Simply stated, liability insurance is a contract requiring the insurer to pay for certain losses sustained by the insured in exchange for a premium. In today's market, it can be difficult for individuals and organizations to use liability insurance to finance risk because insurance may be completely unavailable or too expensive. For example, in 1999, the annual cost of nursing home liability insurance in Ohio was about $50 per bed. That same year, many major carriers left the nursing home liability market because of concern about increased losses related to nursing home liability. The next year, remaining insurers charged about $80–$160 per bed. In 2001, "rates increased to about $270 per bed; in 2002, about $500 per bed, and in 2003, to about $800 per bed. Thus, between 1999 and 2003, the cost of professional liability insurance [for nursing homes] in Ohio increased by about 16-fold" (Burwell et al. 2006). Nationally, trends regarding rate increases have been similar for both organization and individual providers. If an organization cannot finance a risk through insurance, then it may be forced to avoid the risk altogether (for example, close a service) or assume the financial burden of the risk itself (risk assumption).

Risk Evaluation

Risk evaluation is the final step in the risk management process, which involves evaluating each piece of the process in order to determine whether objectives are being met. For example, in evaluating the risk identification step, ASHRM recommends that the following questions be asked: Have exposures been missed in the identification activity? If so, why? What adjustments are necessary to improve this phase? Is useful data being gathered? Are exposures being updated with other current data input?

In evaluating risk management, the following questions are suggested: Does the analysis capture important quantitative data and consider important qualitative issues? Is the analysis being used to make decisions on risk treatment? With respect to the evaluation of risk treatment, suggested questions are: Are risk control and financing methods used for each exposure type? Are exposures actually evaluated to determine which treatment methods are appropriate? What are the current insurance market conditions concerning the availability and cost of insurance coverage?

Tools

Any time an adverse event occurs at a facility, the potential exists for financial loss as well as damage to the facility's reputation. When designed and implemented effectively, a claims management program can help prevent or reduce financial loss in the occurrence of an adverse event. Claims management generally requires knowledge about a facility's insurance polices, a system to identify potential loss quickly, and the ability to accurately estimate potential liability. More specifically, ASHRM (2000) recommends that claims management programs contain at least the following elements:

- Retention of all insurance policies

- Understanding of insurance policies (such as lines of coverage, limits, and exclusions)

- Drafting insurance coverage policy language to avoid later coverage-adjusting problems

- Following all loss provision notices carefully (loss provision notices require the insured to give the insurer notice of any loss within a certain timeframe) (Cox 2002)

- Investigation of potential loss quickly

- Preservation of evidence

- Estimation of potential liability

- Estimation of judgment value

- Resolution of claim, if appropriate

Incident reporting is an important tool that assists risk managers with identifying and responding to adverse events and other occurrences that are inconsistent with the standard of care (figure 14.2). More specifically, incident reporting serves to:

- Describe occurrences that are unexpected, unusual, or out of the ordinary routine of a health-care facility's operations, whether or not they cause injury

- Provide the basis for a timely and comprehensive investigation of an incident, if necessary

Figure 14.2.   Incident reporting process

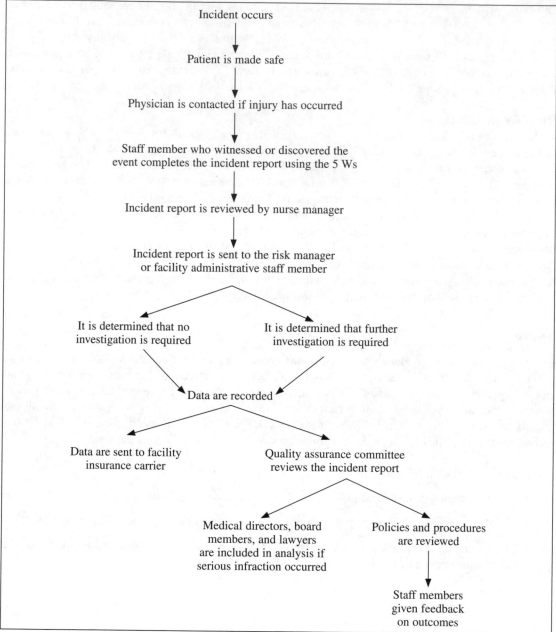

Incident occurs

Patient is made safe

Physician is contacted if injury has occurred

Staff member who witnessed or discovered the
event completes the incident report using the 5 Ws

Incident report is reviewed by nurse manager

Incident report is sent to the risk manager
or facility administrative staff member

It is determined that no
investigation is required

It is determined that further
investigation is required

Data are recorded

Data are sent to facility
insurance carrier

Quality assurance committee
reviews the incident report

Medical directors, board
members, and lawyers
are included in analysis if
serious infraction occurred

Policies and procedures
are reviewed

Staff members
given feedback
on outcomes

Source: Dunn 2003.

- Provide information with which corrective or remedial action may be planned

- Provide raw data to identify risk trends for recurring issues and patient safety risks and to institute procedural changes or in-service training

- Provide the information necessary to defend staff members or healthcare facilities (Dunn 2003)

When an adverse event has occurred, it can be intimidating for individuals with knowledge about that event to come forward or fully disclose all of the facts surrounding the incident (figure 14.3). They may not want to get a colleague in trouble or they may be worried about their own reputation

Figure 14.3. Data to be included in incident reports

Patient data	• Monitors in use
• Age	• Patient diagnosis and condition
• Medical record number	• Physician's examination data, if appropriate, and signature with date
• Patient name	• Physiological consequences
Event data	• Reason for hospitalization, if appropriate
• Bed rail status	• Signature of person completing report with date
• Condition of individuals involved	• Manager of department
• Date and time of event	• Person completing report
• Description of occurrence by observer	• Physician
• Equipment in use	• Witnesses
• Exact location of event	• Follow-up data
• Identification of causative and contributing factors (for example, staffing patterns, experience level of staff members, fatigue, complexity of patient management)	• Classification section for retrieval, trend analysis, and future outcomes and recommendations for prevention
• Medical and nursing personnel present	• Section for evaluation and follow-up of patient harm

Source: Dunn 2003.

or liability. Administrators may be concerned about lawsuits and fearful that internal investigation documents could be used against the facility in court. In order to address these concerns, state and federal law (to varying degrees) protects incident reporting from disclosure for litigation purposes because the reports are working documents investigating the event. Under the HIPAA Privacy Rule, individuals do not have a right of access to information compiled in reasonable anticipation of, or for use in, a civil, criminal, or administrative action or proceeding (HHS 2002). For these reasons, incident reports should not be placed in the patient's medical record, nor should the record refer to incident reporting documents. However, the facts of the incident itself should be documented in the record.

Despite the protections provided by state and federal law, documents related to incident reporting can sometimes still be admitted as evidence in a legal proceeding. This usually occurs when a party has inadvertently released those documents or handled that information in a way that does not adhere to the laws granting protection of the information from discovery (that is, waived the privilege) or a court has issued an order specifically commanding the release of those documents. Therefore, it is important that employees understand when to fill out incident reports and what information should be included in those reports.

A facility should have policies identifying which errors should be reported and to whom as well as the steps required to complete incident reporting (Dunn 2003). Generally, incidents should be documented by the individual(s) who witnessed the event or who were involved in the occurrence as soon as reasonably possible after an event (Dunn 2003). Documentation of incidents should be objective and concise and only present the facts of a situation. Helpful questions to ask include "the five Ws":

1. What? Describe what happened in detail.

2. When? Give the date and time of the incident.

3. Where? Describe the incident's location.

4. Who? Tell who did what to whom and who witnessed the incident.

5. Why? Did equipment fail? Did someone fail to perform a certain test? (Dunn 2003)

Some organizations choose to restrict incident reporting to the first four questions, and to leave the "why" question to the subsequent investigation of the incident. This often occurs in states where incident reports are not well protected from discovery.

Many states have laws requiring reporting of events. The Tennessee Health Data Reporting Act of 2002 (Unusual Events Reporting) requires that the affected patient and the patient's family, as appropriate, be notified of the incident (TN Code Ann. 68-11-211). The law requires hospitals and other healthcare facilities to report unusual events within seven days to the Department of Health and provide a correction notice report. Tennessee law defines an unusual event as follows, "An unusual event is an unexpected occurrence or accident resulting in death, life-threatening or serious injury to a patient that is not related to a natural course of the patient's illness or underlying condition. An unusual event also includes an incident resulting in the abuse of a patient." According to the Tennessee law, the information received in event reports and corrective action plans is considered confidential and is not subject to subpoenas or discovery or admissible in any civil or administrative proceeding other than disciplinary proceedings by the Department of Health or regulatory board (TN Code Ann 68-11-211).

Check Your Understanding 14.2

Instructions: Indicate whether the following statements are true or false (T or F).

1. A review of patient complaints can assist in the risk identification process.

2. Establishing the frequency or severity of a particular loss occurring is part of the risk treatment process.

3. A claims management program should include the retention of all insurance policies.

4. An incident report should be completed by an individual who investigated a situation and determined its cause.

5. Incident reports are protected from discovery in all states.

Role of the Health Record in Risk Management

The health record plays a key role in many different types of proceedings. In negligence cases or licensure actions, information in the record is relied upon to determine whether there has been a deviation from the standard of care. Health record information may also be used to determine the extent of a party's injuries and to determine what caused those injuries.

After an adverse event, some individuals may be tempted to access a patient's records for wrongful reasons such as altering documentation or stealing or deleting the record itself. Other individuals may have well-intentioned desires to "clarify" their documentation, especially if they are concerned that their original documentation could be misconstrued. Alterations or clarifications of medical records can cast a shadow of fault over a facility and should be prevented. Most often, this is accomplished through sequestering the record in a secure place and monitoring access to that record. In the case of electronic records, user rights to edit a record could be suspended and user access audits could be conducted.

No matter how high the quality of care actually provided, poor medical record documentation practices can give the appearance of poor quality care. Therefore, it is important for all staff (including providers, risk managers, and HIM and informatics professionals) to recognize good and poor documentation practices. Figure 14.4 lists 12 indicators that signal a possible problem or area of inconsistency in the record.

Figure 14.4. Twelve indicators of problems in medical records

1. *Illegibility.* Illegible notes and orders may be misinterpreted by other members of the healthcare team to the detriment of the patient. Juries may assume that care was haphazard from the scribbled entries, unintelligible handwriting, misplaced decimals, or misspelled names of drugs. Illegibility is a focus of the Joint Commission and other groups trying to improve patient safety, particularly reducing the number of medication errors.

2. *Vague terminology.* Vague or relative terminology fails to communicate the patient's condition. A more detailed record allows a better defense by the facility.

3. *Criticism.* The health record should not contain any remarks that are critical of treatment rendered by another professional or facility. If remarks are made by the patient or patient's family, they should be referenced as such.

4. *Omissions of date or time.* The note may appear to have been made either before or after treatment.

5. *Countersignatures.* Certain entries require countersignatures as determined by various regulations and the medical staff rules and regulations.

6. *Abbreviations.* Physicians and medical personnel use a number of abbreviations in order to save time. Abbreviations may, however, be misinterpreted if they are ambiguous or illegible. Acceptable abbreviations should be defined by the healthcare organization and maintained in an official abbreviation list. The Joint Commission has an official "Do Not Use" list for certain abbreviations listing the potential problems and what to write instead. These are "red flags" for those looking at consistency and looking for problems in quality care.

7. *Opinions.* The opinion must be based on the provider's observation of fact, and such observation must be documented.

8. *Delayed entries.* Delays in dictating or transcribing reports may result in harm to the patient. Late signatures on reports may signal that the information was not seen or used in a timely manner.

9. *Inconsistencies.* An internal inconsistency should be questioned.

10. *Corrections.* If a correction needs to be made in a paper health record, one line should be neatly drawn through the error, leaving the incorrect material legible, and then it should be initialed and dated so it will be obvious that it was a corrected mistake. Note: Documentation with such language as "error," "wrong patient's chart," and so forth. should be discouraged. For a computer record, a new entry should be identified as a new entry without deleting the original entry. A brief explanation of any error should be included if appropriate. Any changes to the health record could be viewed as trying to cover up errors by persons looking at the record in the future, so corrections must be noted as explained above.

11. *Lack of evidence of informed consent.* The physician should document in the progress notes the circumstances surrounding the patient's consent to any surgical, diagnostic, or therapeutic activity that involves significant risk.

12. *Improper alteration of records.* Various record-altering practices, such as improper revisions, contradictions, omissions, or removal or obscuring of important information, can, in cases involving litigation, create a suspicion of intent to conceal information. It is better legally to acknowledge the error and offer a settlement rather than having altered records submitted as evidence. Inaccurate, false, or incomplete entries may be interpreted by a court as deliberate tampering with the medical record. A jury may be persuaded that if the records were erroneous in one respect, they were erroneous in other respects. Falsification of medical records is both a civil and a criminal offense. Entering in a medical record a diagnosis or other information which is known to be erroneous, for the purpose of inducing a third party to pay for the patient's care, can be considered as fraud. Fraud is defined as "willful and intended misrepresentation that could cause harm or loss to personal property." Altering records which are, or are likely to be, subpoenaed is considered an attempt to withhold evidence and obstruct justice, and is a criminal offense.

Source: Adapted from McCain and Bowman 2006.

Some additional commonsense documentation suggestions follow:

- Document all examinations, even if the findings are normal

- Have a system to follow up on abnormal results and document all related information, including tests ordered and treatment(s) or action(s) instituted

- Document all elements of the informed consent process

- Use approved abbreviations only

- Keep the record legible, if documenting in writing

- Pay special attention to medication dosages (especially decimals) as errors may have life-and-death implications. Place a leading zero in front of all dosages starting with a decimal (e.g., 0.25 mg instead of .25 mg)

- Record all patient noncompliance with medical advice

- Record the substance of every pertinent conversation and how you evaluated patient/family understanding of that conversation

- Describe your thought processes and list the various clinical factors you have considered

- Stick to recording objective facts related to patient care given

- Refrain from opinionated discourse and judgmental comments

- Do not argue with colleagues in the record. Talk to them in person, come to a mutually agreeable understanding, and let the chart reflect that understanding

The Joint Commission and Sentinel Events

The Joint Commission has a variety of accreditation programs designed to continuously improve the safety and quality of care provided to the public. Currently, the Joint Commission evaluates and accredits more than 17,000 healthcare organizations and programs in the United States, including:

- General, psychiatric, children's, and rehabilitation hospitals

- Critical access hospitals

- Medical equipment services, hospice services, and other home care organizations

- Nursing homes and other long-term care facilities

- Behavioral healthcare organizations and addiction services

- Rehabilitation centers, group practices, office-based surgeries, and other ambulatory care providers

- Independent or freestanding laboratories (Joint Commission 2010a)

The accreditation standards used by the Joint Commission are designed to address an organization's level of performance in specific functional areas, such as patient rights, patient treatment, and infection control (Joint Commission 2010a). According to the *Journal of Healthcare Risk Management* (1992):

> During the late 1980s, the Joint Commission established its first standards for the loss control and prevention components of risk management programs. the Joint Commission has not developed standards for risk financing, which falls outside the Joint Commission's focus on factors that directly affect healthcare safety and quality; standards for clinical services, quality management, plant safety and many other areas have existed for years.

One important aspect of the Joint Commission's focus on quality is its standards related to **sentinel events**, defined as:

> . . . an unexpected occurrence involving death or serious physical or psychological injury, or the risk thereof. Serious injury specifically includes loss of limb or function. The phrase, "or the risk thereof" includes any process variation for which a recurrence would carry a significant chance of a serious adverse outcome. Such events are called "sentinel" because they signal the need for immediate investigation and response. (Joint Commission 2007)

It is important to note that sentinel events and medical errors are not the same thing. Not all sentinel events occur because of a medical error and not all medical errors result in sentinel events (Joint Commission 2006a). the Joint Commission website contains a sentinel events glossary of terms that should be referenced to avoid confusion and potential miscommunication about these terms. The goals of the Joint Commission policy are to have a positive impact in improving patient care by focusing the attention of an organization that has experienced a sentinel event on understanding the causes that underlie the event and on making changes in the organization's systems and processes to reduce the probability of such an event in the future as well as to increase the general knowledge about sentinel events, their causes, and strategies for prevention.

The Joint Commission organizes sentinel events into reviewable and nonreviewable categories. Reviewable events include the following:

- The event has resulted in an unanticipated death or major permanent loss of function, not related to the natural course of the patient's illness or underlying condition

- The event was one of the following (even if the outcome was not death or major permanent loss of function unrelated to the patient's illness or underlying condition):

    — Suicide of any patient receiving care, treatment, and services in a staffed around-the-clock care setting or within 72 hours of discharge

    — Unanticipated death of a full-term infant

    — Abduction of any patient receiving care, treatment, and services

    — Discharge of an infant to the wrong family

    — Rape

    — Hemolytic transfusion reaction involving the administration of blood or blood products having major blood group incompatibilities

    — Surgery on the wrong patient or body part

    — Unintended retention of a foreign object in a patient after surgery or other procedure

    — Severe neonatal hyperbilirubinemia

    — Prolonged fluoroscopy with cumulative dose >1500 rads to a single field or any delivery of radiotherapy to the wrong body region or >25 percent above the planned radiotherapy dose (Joint Commission 2007).

The Joint Commission categorizes "near misses" and other specific events as nonreviewable. Even if an event is nonreviewable, an organization may well still intensively evaluate that event as part of its performance improvement activities.

The Joint Commission has standards that specifically relate to the management of sentinel events. First, each organization must develop its own definition of a sentinel event for purposes of establishing procedures for identifying, reporting, and managing these events. While the organization's overall definition of *sentinel event* must be consistent with that of the Joint Commission, it can tailor specific terms such as *unexpected*, *serious*, and *the risk thereof* to its own needs (Joint Commission 2007).

Second, organizations are expected to identify and respond appropriately to all sentinel events. This involves conducting a **root cause analysis** (RCA), developing an action plan, implementing improvements, and monitoring the effectiveness of those improvements (Joint Commission 2007). For additional information, see the Joint Commission's "A Framework for a Root Cause Analysis and Action Plan in Response to a Sentinel Event" online (Joint Commission 2009).

An RCA is a tool designed to identify the basic underlying factors that contributed to the sentinel event. It involves a series of questions designed to identify issues related to both clinical and organizational systems and processes, not individual performance (Joint Commission 2007). For example, an

RCA might ask, "How did equipment performance affect the outcome?" or "How did actual staffing levels compare with ideal levels?"

An action plan is the product of an RCA and identifies actions that the organization will implement in order to prevent the same or similar sentinel events from occurring again. Action plans should identify who is responsible for implementing and overseeing actions, as well as timelines for implementation, any necessary pilot testing, and plans for measuring the effectiveness of the actions (Joint Commission 2007).

Another methodology to determine the cause of sentinel events is the **Failure Mode Effect and Criticality Assessment** (FMECA), often also described as a failure mode and effect analysis, which is defined by the Joint Commission (2007) as:

> A systematic way of examining a design prospectively for possible ways in which failure can occur. It assumes that no matter how knowledgeable or careful people are, errors will occur in some situations and may even be likely to occur.

As part of the ongoing process to assist organizations in identifying and preventing sentinel events, the Joint Commission publishes a patient safety newsletter called the *Sentinel Event Alert*. The *Alert* identifies specific sentinel events, describes their common underlying causes, and suggests prevention steps related to those events (Joint Commission n.d.). Organizations should incorporate information provided by the *Alert* into their processes for evaluating and preventing sentinel events.

The Joint Commission Safety Goals

Each year, the Joint Commission publishes **National Patient Safety Goals** designed to improve patient safety in specific healthcare areas identified as problematic. These goals and corresponding requirements for meeting those goals are primarily based on informal recommendations made in the *Sentinel Event Alert* and information from the Joint Commission's sentinel event database. Specific goals and requirements are developed by the Sentinel Event Advisory Group. As part of the accreditation process, organizations are evaluated for their compliance with specific requirements related to patient safety goals applicable to their setting (Joint Commission 2010b). The National Patient Safety Goals for various organizations can be found on the Joint Commission website. The 2010 National Patient Safety Goals for hospitals includes many requirements that support proper documentation, including the following (Joint Commission 2010c):

- Use at least two patient identifiers (neither to be the patient's room number) whenever administering medications or blood products, taking blood samples and other specimens for clinical testing, or providing any other treatments or procedures

- Prior to the start of any invasive procedure, conduct a final verification process (such as a "time out") to confirm the correct patient, procedure, and site using active—not passive—communication techniques

- Improve the effectiveness of communication among caregivers. For verbal or telephone orders or for telephonic reporting of critical test results, verify the complete order or test result by having the person receiving the order or test result "read-back" the complete order or test result

- Standardize a list of abbreviations, acronyms, and symbols that are not to be used throughout the organization

- Measure, assess and, if appropriate, take action to improve the timeliness of reporting, and the timeliness of receipt by the responsible licensed caregiver, of critical test results and values

Check Your Understanding 14.3

Instructions: Indicate whether the following statements are true or false (T or F).

1. Patient noncompliance with medical advice should not be documented in the health record because it might upset the patient.

2. A sentinel event is an unexpected occurrence involving death or serious physical or psychological injury, or the risk thereof.

3. All medical errors are sentinel events.

4. Joint Commission–accredited organizations are expected to complete a root cause analysis following a sentinel event.

5. National Patient Safety Goals are optional standards that an organization may choose to meet in order to receive a special designation from the Joint Commission.

Quality Improvement

The Joint Commission's current quality improvement activities for health record documentation include a process for the identification, testing, specification, and implementation of core performance measures for hospitals:

- Acute myocardial infarction

- Heart failure

- Community-acquired pneumonia

- Perinatal care and pregnancy and related conditions

- Children's asthma care

- Hospital-based inpatient psychiatric services

- Venous Thromboembolism (VTE) Core Measure Set

- Stroke (STK) Core Measure Set

The Joint Commission is using this information to focus activities for the onsite accreditation survey and is publishing measurement data on its website at QualityCheck.org. Consumers can search for an organization, check on its performance on the Joint Commission performance measures, and determine the organization's accreditation status. HIM professionals are key players in the collection of data and development of processes to ensure that data is collected properly and that records reflect documentation.

After its 1999 *To Err Is Human* report, the Institute of Medicine published a second report titled *Crossing the Quality Chasm—A New Health System for the 21st Century* in 2001. This report identified six broad objectives that should be central to the US healthcare system. Specifically, the report stated that healthcare should be safe, patient-centered, efficient, effective, equitable, and timely.

- *Safety*—With respect to safety, the IOM report stated, "Patients should not be harmed by the care that is intended to help them, nor should harm come to those who work in health care." Today, many resources for monitoring and improving safety exist in the healthcare industry. As

413

discussed above, annual Patient Safety Goals are published by the Joint Commission. Another resource is the Agency for Healthcare and Quality (AHRQ) Patient Safety Network (PSNet). PSNet provides a national Web-based resource that includes weekly updates of patient safety literature, news, tools, and meetings, as well as links to research and other information on patient safety (AHRQ n.d.b). AHRQ also publishes patient safety indicators and resources specifically aimed at consumers.

- *Patient-Centered Care*—The objective regarding patient-centered care focuses "on the patient's experience of illness and healthcare and on the systems that work or fail to work to meet individual patients' needs." In this area, AHRQ has conducted quality studies that specifically focus on patient perceptions regarding their care. Measures are built around topics such as patient-provider communication, patient-provider relationship, cultural competency (for example, how well patients feel that providers understand their cultural backgrounds), and health information (for example, how well patients understand information that has been provided to them) (AHRQ 2003).

- *Efficiency*—Efficiency of healthcare refers to eliminating the overuse of "those services where a 'health care service is provided when the potential risks outweigh the benefits' and medical errors.'" Administrative costs can be reduced through the elimination of duplicative paperwork, redundant testing, and multiple reentries of various types of practitioner orders (AHA 2006).

- *Effectiveness*—According to the IOM report, effectiveness is defined as "care that is based on the use of systematically acquired evidence to determine whether an intervention, such as a preventive service, diagnostic test, or therapy, produces better outcomes than alternatives—including the alternative of doing nothing." Quality improvement organizations, discussed below, play a key role in identifying interventions that have been proven effective.

- *Equitable*—The aim for equitable healthcare focuses on eliminating disparities in healthcare services based on factors such as race, ethnicity, or gender. In 1999, Congress mandated that AHRQ produce an annual report on healthcare disparities in the Unitied States (Pub. L. 106-129). Each year, AHRQ publishes the National Healthcare Disparities Report, which includes a broad set of performance measures that can be used to monitor progress toward improved healthcare quality for all groups.

- *Timely*—Timely healthcare refers to the availability of healthcare services or information about the results of those healthcare services within an appropriate time. For example, it is not uncommon for people to have long waits for appointments or in waiting rooms. According to a recent Consumer Assessment of Healthcare Providers and Systems (CAHPS) survey, only 58 percent of Medicare enrollees surveyed reported that it was "not a problem" to get care quickly (AHRQ 2006).

Today, quality improvement processes are guided by the federal agencies such as CMS and AHRQ. At the federal level, the Affordable Care Act established the National Strategy for Quality Improvement in Health Care, known as the National Quality Strategy. The priorities of the strategy are discussed later in the chapter (HHS 2011a, AHRQ n.d.c.).

Patients' Rights as a Condition of Quality Healthcare

Central to providing quality healthcare is ensuring that patients are aware that they have rights related not only to clinical quality of care but also to other aspects of their healthcare, such as communication about their care and protection of their privacy. Specific patient rights are externally driven by both government and private standards and internally driven by organizational policies. Summarized below are some of the common sources of patient rights.

American Hospital Association Patient Care Partnership

The American Hospital Association has developed a **Patient Care Partnership** (originally called Patient Bill of Rights) that helps patients understand their expectations, rights, and responsibilities when receiving hospital services (AHA 2003). Under the partnership, patients can expect quality care in a clean and safe environment. They can also expect to be informed about their care and to have active involvement in their treatment decisions. During and after their stay, patients can expect their medical information to be safeguarded. Once discharged, patients can expect a hospital to help with identifying sources of follow-up care and help with understanding hospital bills, filing insurance claims, or making other financial arrangements to pay hospital bills.

Medicare Conditions of Participation

In order to participate in the Medicare and Medicaid programs, healthcare facilities must meet certain minimum requirements related to health and safety. These requirements are found in the Medicare Conditions of Participation (CoP), which are located in Title 42 of the Code of Federal Regulations. Patient rights are an important piece of the Medicare CoP and the following are generally required:

- Patients must be given notice of their rights and a process for bringing grievances.

- Patients must be allowed to exercise rights related to participating in their care plans, making informed decisions, establishing advance directives, and notifying family and physicians of a hospitalization.

- Patients have the right to personal privacy, care in a safe setting, and freedom from abuse and harassment.

- Patients have the right to confidentiality of their records.

- Patients have the right to be free from non-medically necessary **restraints and seclusion** (used to manage behavior) (HHS 1999).

HIPAA Privacy Rule Revisited

As detailed in chapter 9, the HIPAA Privacy Rule provides individuals with rights related to the access and control of their protected health information (PHI). Specifically, individuals have the right to:

- Access their PHI (with certain exceptions)

- Request amendments to their PHI

- Request an accounting of certain disclosures that a covered entity has made of their PHI

- Request certain restrictions regarding how their PHI is used or disclosed to carry out treatment, payment, or operations

- Request that communications of PHI be routed to an alternative location or by an alternative method.

Additionally, individuals may lodge a complaint about a covered entity's alleged noncompliance with its policies and procedures or the Privacy Rule. They also have the right to receive a Notice of Privacy Practices on or before their first visit at a covered entity.

The Joint Commission Standards

As with the Medicare CoP, the Joint Commission accreditation standards have specific requirements pertaining to patient rights. Like the CoP patient rights, the Joint Commission patient rights center on patient autonomy and self-determination. For example, the Joint Commission standards for patient rights in hospital settings generally involve:

- Providing patients with adequate information

- Allowing patients to have meaningful participation in their own care, including end-of-life decisions

- Protecting patients from abuse

- Protecting patients' privacy (Joint Commission 2006b)

Facility Policy Regarding Patient Rights

Every facility should have policies in place that identify patient rights. At a minimum, the rights should meet applicable CoP and Joint Commission requirements but may also include other rights deemed appropriate by the facilities. Processes must be in place to ensure that both patients and staff are aware of these rights. Patients should be given notice of their rights at their first encounter or admission or as soon as reasonably possible afterward.

Right to Admission/Duty to Treat

The rights discussed above are all triggered from an actual encounter or admission. From a patient perspective, one of the most important rights is the simple right to receive healthcare services at all. Various laws outline the circumstances where individuals have the right to receive medical treatment or hospitalization.

Impact of Hill-Burton

In 1946, Congress passed the **Hill-Burton Act**, which provided hospitals and certain other healthcare facilities money for construction and modernization. As a condition of receiving Hill-Burton financial assistance, facilities had to agree to provide a reasonable volume of services to those unable to pay and make their services available to all persons residing in the facilities' area. More specifically, Hill-Burton facilities must comply with the following:

- A person residing in the Hill-Burton facility's service area has the right to medical treatment at the facility without regard to race, color, national origin, or creed.

- Hill-Burton facilities must participate in the Medicare and Medicaid programs unless they are ineligible to participate.

- Hill-Burton facilities must make arrangements for reimbursement for services with principal state and local third-party payers that provide reimbursement that is not less than the actual cost of the services.

- A Hill-Burton facility must post notices informing the public of its community service obligations in English and Spanish. If ten percent or more of the households in the service area usually speak a language other than English or Spanish, the facility must translate the notice into that language and post it as well.

- A Hill-Burton facility may not deny emergency services to any person residing in the facility's service area on the grounds that the person is unable to pay for those services.

- A Hill-Burton facility may not adopt patient admissions policies that have the effect of excluding persons on grounds of race, color, national origin, creed, or any other ground unrelated to the patient's need for the service or the availability of the needed service (HHS 2006).

The Hill-Burton program stopped providing funds in 1997, leaving about 200 facilities nationwide that are still obligated to provide free or reduced-cost care under Hill-Burton obligations (HHS n.d.).

EMTALA/Anti-Dumping

In 1986, Congress enacted the **Emergency Medical Treatment and Active Labor Act** (EMTALA) as part of the Consolidated Omnibus Reconciliation Act. EMTALA was passed largely in response to some hospitals' engaging in "patient-dumping"—transferring, discharging, or refusing to treat indigent emergency department patients because of their inability to pay. Under the EMTALA regulations, hospitals must comply with the following:

- An appropriate "medical screening exam" must be provided to anyone coming to the emergency department seeking medical care;

- If an emergency medical condition is found, the hospital must treat and stabilize the emergency medical condition, or the hospital must transfer the individual; and

- Transfers of nonstabilized patients are not allowed unless several specific conditions are met (AAEM n.d.).

EMTALA protections are applicable to any patient seeking care in a Medicare-participating hospital. Penalties for EMTALA violations include fines and possible exclusion from the Medicare program (AAEM n.d.).

Right to Discharge

Except in limited circumstances, competent adults have the right to discharge themselves from a hospital at any time. If a provider fails to discharge a patient, it might be considered battery or false imprisonment. When a patient discharges himself or herself before a physician has determined it to be medically appropriate, a discharge **against medical advice** (AMA) has occurred. Each year, about 0.8 percent to 2.2 percent of discharges from acute care hospitals are AMA discharges (AHRQ 2005). Since AMA discharges are associated with poor outcomes, hospitals should have a discharge AMA protocol in place. This protocol could include attempting to arrange outpatient services or other follow-up care for the patient, filling prescriptions in an in-house pharmacy, communication with other providers involved in the patient's care, and providing a patient with a written summary of his or her stay (AHRQ 2005).

The circumstances surrounding a patient's AMA discharge as well as actions taken in response to the discharge should be documented in the patient's record. Patients leaving against medical advice should be asked to sign a form acknowledging that they understand the potential consequences of the discharge to their health and agreeing not to hold the healthcare facility liable for any poor outcome they experience as a result. Having the patient sign such a form may strengthen protections from legal liability associated with poor outcomes related to AMA discharges but may not be a total shield to liability. In addition, many patients refuse to sign such a form, or leave before staff can present them with the form.

Safekeeping of Property

Hospitals, nursing homes, and other institutional providers have a general duty to respect and protect patients' property. Patients should have access to their personal belongings, and those belongings should be returned to the patient upon discharge.

Patient Obligations

Most hospitals and physicians, along with organizations such as the American Medical Association (AMA), have adopted codes of patient responsibilities. These codes are meant to recognize the collaborative nature of the relationship between providers and patients. Generally speaking, patients have the responsibility to:

- Provide full and honest information to providers

- Ask questions regarding information that they do not understand

- Work with providers in carrying out agreed-upon treatment plan

- Show respect for providers and other patients

- Make good-faith efforts to meet their financial obligations

Check Your Understanding 14.4

Instructions: Indicate whether the following statements are true or false (T or F).

1. Patient-centered care is one of 10 objectives recommended by the Institute of Medicine in 2001 as central to the US healthcare system.

2. The American Hospital Association's Patient Bill of Rights is now the Patient Care Partnership, which focuses on patient expectations, rights, and responsibilities.

3. The Hill-Burton Act is federal legislation, passed in 1946, that provided hospitals money for construction and modernization.

4. EMTALA was passed by Congress to combat transfer and discharge of patients, and refusal to treat, based on inability to pay.

5. In addition to recognizing patient rights, many hospitals have adopted codes of patient responsibility.

Peer Review and the National Practitioner Data Bank

Another area of concern for risk management and quality improvement is the credentialing and peer review process. The 1986 Health Care Quality Improvement Act (42 USC 11101) created the **National Practitioner Data Bank**, which began operating in 1990. The data bank collects malpractice, disciplinary, and credentialing information on physicians, dentists, and other facility-based practitioners.

Facilities must report to the data bank adverse actions (such as suspensions of privileges) lasting more than 30 days, medical malpractice payments, and settlement reports. When evaluating a provider's application for privileges, the facility must query the data bank. Data bank information provides additional details regarding an applicant but does not supersede the normal investigation practices. Hospitals must query the data bank about staff members every two years. A discussion of the data bank also appears in chapter 13.

Americans with Disabilities Act (ADA)

The Americans with Disabilities Act (ADA) (Pub. L. 101-336) prohibits discrimination based on disability in employment, state and local government, public accommodations, commercial facilities, transportation, and telecommunications. It also applies to the United States Congress.

To be protected by the ADA, one must have a disability or have a relationship or association with an individual with a disability. An individual with a disability is defined by the ADA as a person who has a physical or mental impairment that substantially limits one or more major life activities, a person who has a history or record of such impairment, or a person who is perceived by others as having such impairment. The ADA does not specifically name all of the impairments that are covered. The ADA compels risk managers to ensure the safety of patients, visitors, and staff and ensure that the facility is complying with the law.

Restraints and Seclusion

The CoP regarding patient rights applies to all Medicare and Medicaid participating hospitals, including short-term, psychiatric, rehabilitation, long-term, children's, and alcohol and drug facilities. The CoP contains six standards requiring facilities to notify patients of their rights in regard to their care and addressing privacy and safety, confidentiality of medical records, freedom from restraints unless clinically necessary, and freedom from seclusion and restraints used in behavior management unless clinically necessary. There are specific documentation requirements for orders to be written, time limitations, and notes regarding ongoing observation and monitoring and continuing assessments of the need for restraints (CFR 482.13).

The Children's Health Act of 2000 (Pub. L. 106-310), signed into law on October 17, 2000, establishes national standards that restrict the use of restraints and seclusion in all psychiatric facilities that receive federal funds and in "non-medical community-based facilities for children and youth." In those settings, the use of restraints and seclusion is restricted to emergency safety situations.

Regarding restraint devices, FDA guidelines state that the facility must obtain informed consent from the patient/resident or guardian prior to use. Patients have the right to be free from restraints. However, if it is determined that a restraint is necessary, the facility must explain the reason for the device to the patient/resident and/or guardian to prevent misinterpretation and to ensure cooperation.

Quality Improvement Organizations (QIOs)

Quality Improvement Organizations (QIOs) are community-based organizations selected by CMS to conduct activities designed to:

- Improve the quality of care for beneficiaries;

- Protect the integrity of the Medicare Trust Fund by ensuring that Medicare pays only for services and goods that are reasonable and medically necessary, and that are provided in the most appropriate setting; and

- Protect beneficiaries by addressing issues such as beneficiary complaints, provider-issued notices of non-coverage, Notice of Discharge and Medicare Appeal Rights, EMTALA violations, and other related responsibilities (CMS 2010a.).

Specific QIO activities are governed by a three-year contract cycle with CMS called the Statement of Work (SOW). Currently, CMS contracts with one quality improvement organization in each state as well as the District of Columbia, Puerto Rico, and the US Virgin Islands (CMS 2010a).

History

With the passage of Medicare and Medicaid in 1964, the federal government became a major player in the financing of healthcare services for the elderly, disabled, and poor. In order to make sure that only medically necessary care for these groups was being funded, Congress amended the Social Security Act to establish Professional Standards Review Organizations (PSROs) in 1972. Among other activities, PSROs were responsible for conducting hospital utilization review in order to ensure that only necessary and appropriate services were being provided. At one time, there were as many as 300 PSROs, and their case-review activities often involved policing providers and punishing those who were deemed not to be in compliance with applicable standards (Sprague 2002). Under the PSRO system, reviewing physicians were allowed to review cases involving their own colleagues and competitors.

In 1982, under the Medicare Utilization and Quality Control Peer Review Program, Congress replaced PSROs with 54 Peer Review Organizations (PROs). This program introduced the statement of work system and prospective PROs had to competitively bid for contracts. It also restricted reviewing physicians' ability to review their local colleagues and competitors. PROs conducted case-review activities centered on utilization review, coding, and medical necessity. Despite the differences between PSROs and PROs, providers still regarded PROs as adversarial and punitive in nature (Sprague 2002).

In 1992, the peer review system was again restructured to provide greater emphasis on helping providers improve the mainstream of care rather than dealing with individual clinical errors. Specifically, the Healthcare Quality Improvement Program (HCQIP) was implemented. Under this program, PROs adopted a more collaborative approach with providers to:

- Develop quality indicators firmly based in science

- Identify opportunities to improve care through careful measurement of care patterns

- Communicate with professional and provider communities about these patterns of care

- Intervene to foster quality improvement through system improvements

- Remeasure to evaluate success and redirect efforts (KFMC 2010)

In 2001, the United States Department of Health and Human Services (HHS) announced a new program called the Quality Initiative, with a focus on ensuring quality healthcare through accountability and public disclosure. At the launch of the Nursing Home Quality Initiative in 2002, the term PRO was replaced by QIO in order to better reflect the overall mission to improve quality (Sprague 2002). The Quality Initiative is discussed in more detail under the report cards section below.

Role in Improving Quality

In fulfilling their role in federal quality improvement efforts, QIOs provide specific consultation and quality improvement resources to a wide range of providers, including hospitals, physician practices, managed care organizations, and others. For example, QIOs provide resources regarding:

- Widely accepted quality indicators and data collection instruments

- Analysis and feedback of state and facility-level data about patterns of care

- Effective quality improvement strategies and expertise

- Pretested educational materials for providers and patients

- A forum for collaboration among providers, payers, and others to improve care and increase the value of healthcare expenditures (KFMC 2010)

Tools, toolkits, presentations, links, and other resources are provided on the Medicare Quality Improvement Community (MedQIC) that functions as a repository for resources created or endorsed by the QIOs (QualityNet n.d.).

Tenth Statement of Work

The QIO's SOW contract cycle requires change every three years. Each QIO's performance is evaluated at 18 months and also at the end of the contract term against contract requirements. The QIO program is in its fourth phase. The first two phases included review of hospital utilization of individual beneficiaries, followed by measure-based quality improvement. The third phase focused on transformational change via QIO collaboration with providers to substantially improve quality of healthcare on all major fronts. Each QIO works intensively with a group of providers and practitioners in their state, known as identified participants, to improve quality of care to Medicare beneficiaries (CMS 2010b).

The tenth SOW began August 1, 2011, and reflects the six priorities outlined in the National Quality Strategy (HHS 2011b):

- Ensuring that each person and family is engaged as partners in their care

- Promoting effective communication and coordination of care

- Promoting the most effective prevention and treatment practices for the leading causes of mortality, starting with cardiovascular disease

- Working with communities to promote wide use of best practices to enable healthy living

- Making quality care more affordable for individuals, families, employers, and governments by developing and spreading new health care delivery models

- Making care safer by reducing harm caused in the delivery of care

The tenth SOW has four major aims requiring QIOs to use their expertise at the state level to promote change. In the Pharmacy Quality Alliance (PQA) bimonthly briefings the aims are described as follows:

Beneficiary and Family-Centered Care: QIOs will provide case review and quality of care review for Medicare beneficiaries. This aim focuses on mandated case review activities while encouraging patient and family engagement in their own healthcare.

Improving Individual Patient Care: This aim includes four specific topics that address the National Quality Strategy to make care safer and more affordable. QIOs will 1) work to reduce healthcare-associated infections such as central line–associated blood stream infections, catheter-associated urinary tract infections, *Clostridium difficile* infections and surgical site infections in hospitals; 2) reduce healthcare-acquired conditions such as pressure ulcers, injuries related to physical restraints, falls and catheter-associated urinary tract infection in nursing homes; 3) reduce adverse drug events through community teams using the model and information from the Patient Safety and Clinical Pharmacy Services Collaborative (PSPC); and 4) provide technical assistance to hospitals to improve their inpatient and outpatient quality reporting.

Integrating Care for Populations and Communities: QIOs will work to improve the quality of care for patients as they transition among care settings. QIOs will coordinate with community-based organizations and healthcare stakeholders to improve care transitions and reduce hospital readmissions, emergency room visits, and mortality.

Improving Health for Populations and Communities: QIOs will promote influenza and pneumococcal immunization and colorectal and breast cancer screening in physician offices via EHRs. The QIOs will also strive to improve participation in the Physician Quality Reporting System. In collaboration with other stakeholders, QIOs will improve cardiovascular health of the community through promotion of appropriate aspirin therapy, cholesterol and blood pressure control, and smoking cessation.

The four aims of the 10th Statement of Work will be accomplished using three mechanisms. QIOs will convene and support learning and action networks to achieve large scale improvement around a specific aim. These networks will include key stakeholders and leaders that can rapidly spread successful knowledge and skills. QIOs will provide technical assistance on quality improvement, onsite mentoring, and data collection and analysis. The third driver of change is *care reinvention through innovation spread project* or "CRISP." This driver will spread successful strategies of all aims through a variety of communication tools. (PQA Quality Connection 2011)

Public Reporting of Quality Measures

Many voluntary and government programs report quality measures through comparison sites or what some term as **report cards**. For example, HealthGrades, an independent organization, provides profiles and ratings for numerous hospitals, nursing homes, and physicians in the United States (Health-Grades 2010). Another example is the National Committee for Quality Assurance (NCQA), which reports information on health plans on its Website (NCQA 2011). Hospitals use favorable ratings as marketing tools, but it is generally thought that consumers have not used the information for choosing providers.

Another example of a quality initiative under the oversight of the QIO is the Nursing Home Quality Initiative (NHQI), which was launched in 2002 and typifies the report card systems. The overall goals of the initiative were to provide consumers with quality information about nursing homes and to help providers give better care in nursing homes. To accomplish both of these goals, specific quality measures were developed in collaboration with multiple stakeholders. Through the NHQI, consumers can view how specific nursing homes compared with one another on these measures through Medicare's Nursing Home Compare.

In 2003, the Home Health Quality Initiatives (HHQI) and Hospital Quality Initiatives (HQI) were launched. Similar to the NHQI, the HHQI and HQI both included collaboration with stakeholders to identify specific quality measures for home health and hospital settings. Consumer information related to these initiatives is available through Medicare's Home Health Compare and Hospital Compare websites.

In 2004, the Physician Focused Quality Initiative was developed. The focus of this initiative revolves around assessing quality of care measures for key illnesses and clinical conditions, supporting physicians treating those illnesses and conditions, preventing avoidable health problems, and investigating the concept of payment for performance. Several specific quality projects are conducted under the Physician Focused Quality Initiative. One such project is the Physician Quality Reporting Initiative (PQRI) that started in 2006. The PQRI provides eligible healthcare professionals with incentives for reporting defined quality measures. Each year the reporting requirements are updated (CMS 2010c). In 2010 an electronic health record (EHR)-based reporting mechanism was introduced that provides incentives to eligible professionals who submit their data using a PQRI-qualified EHR system (CMS, 2010d).

In 2005 the Deficit Reduction Act provided new requirements for the Hospital Inpatient Quality Reporting Program (HIQRP), which was originally built on the CMS voluntary hospital quality initiative. Hospitals who receive Medicare funding must now submit data for specific quality measures for health conditions that commonly result in hospitalization for Medicare patients. Another federally sponsored quality reporting program is the Hospital Consumer Assessment of Healthcare Providers and Systems (HCAHPS) survey which is the first national, standardized publicly reported survey of patients' perspectives of hospital care. This program is administered by the Hospital Quality Alliance (HQA), a public/private partnership among hospitals, medical associations, consumer groups, government, and others. A sample of patients are surveyed post-discharge and queried on a number of questions that relate to their experience while hospitalized on matters such as communication, cleanliness of facility, pain management, discharge information, and overall satisfaction (CMS 2010e). If hospitals fail to report data for either of these programs their will receive a 2 percent reduction in annual Medicare reimbursement. Data collected through these program are available on the Hospitals Compare website (HHS 2012).

Private Quality Watchdogs

In addition to federally sponsored and state-sponsored oversight of healthcare quality, several private consumer, academic, business, and think-tank groups also monitor and conduct research related to quality and safety. Some of these groups are politically active and advocate for laws that support greater patient safety and empower consumers to have more access to quality information.

The Leapfrog Group

The **Leapfrog Group** (Leapfrog) is a voluntary program that was founded in 2000 by the Business Roundtable and receives support from the Robert Wood Johnson Foundation as well as other supporters. The group is composed of a consortium of major companies and other entities that are responsible for purchasing healthcare coverage for employees. Leapfrog is comprised of private and public-sector purchasers representing more than 34 million Americans and more than $62 billion in healthcare expenditures. The goals are to "reduce preventable medical mistakes and improve the quality and affordability of health care."

The group hopes that the public will report outcomes so that everyone can make more knowledgeable choices through the publishing of hospital quality ratings. A hospital rewards program has been developed to reward providers for improving quality, safety, and affordability. Leapfrog works with medical experts throughout the United States to identify problems and propose solutions for improvement. The Leapfrog organization believes that medical errors are caused by broken systems that do not support the providers. Prevention of death, permanent disabilities, extended hospital stays, longer recovery periods, and additional treatment is the ultimate goal. Consumers will have information to make choices, and the medical purchasing power of the Leapfrog companies and organizations will accelerate the rate of systems. Leapfrog members agree to purchase their healthcare on the basis of quality care and consumer involvement. The group has identified "leaps" in hospital quality, safety, and affordability, such as computer physician order entry, evidence-based hospital referral, ICU physician staffing, and a Leapfrog "safe practices" score. Each of these is described on Leapfrog's website as follows:

- Computer Physician Order Entry (CPOE): With CPOE systems, hospital staff enters medication orders via [a] computer linked to prescribing error prevention software. CPOE has been shown to reduce serious prescribing errors in hospitals by more than 50 percent.

- Evidence-Based Hospital Referral (EHR): Consumers and healthcare purchasers should choose hospitals with extensive experience and the best results with certain high-risk surgeries and conditions. By referring patients needing certain complex medical procedures to hospitals offering the best survival odds based on scientifically valid criteria—such as the number of times a hospital performs these procedures each year or other process or outcomes data—research indicates that a patient's risk of dying could be reduced by 40 percent.

- ICU Physician Staffing (IPS): Staffing ICUs with doctors who have special training in critical care medicine, called "intensivists," has been shown to reduce the risk of patients dying in the ICU by 40 percent.

- The Leapfrog Safe Practices Score: The National Quality Forum's Safe Practices cover a range of practices that, if utilized, would reduce the risk of harm in certain processes, systems, or environments of care. Included in the 30 practices are the original three Leapfrog leaps. For this new leap, added in April 2004, hospitals' progress on the remaining 27 safe practices will be assessed.

Other Organizations

Another group of importance in improving quality and safety is the **Institute for Healthcare Improvement** (IHI) (IHI n.d.). IHI is:

> . . . a reliable source of energy, knowledge, and support for a never-ending campaign to improve healthcare worldwide . . . [that] helps accelerate change in health care by cultivating promising concepts for improving patient care and turning those ideas into action.

Its mission is to improve the lives of patients, the health of communities, and the joy of the health care workforce. IHI also strives to accelerate the measurable and continual progress of health care systems throughout the world toward safety, effectiveness, patient-centeredness, timeliness, efficiency, and equity. Its goals are:

- No needless deaths
- No needless pain or suffering
- No helplessness in those served or serving
- No unwanted waiting
- No waste (IHI n.d.)

The federal government is promoting electronic exchange of health information as a way of improving the quality and safety of patient care so that records are immediately available to providers. There is much interest in this, as well as privacy and security, and concerns about proper patient identification. Health information exchange, the development of electronic health records, and quality organizations such as Leapfrog and the Institute for Healthcare Improvement are all initiatives that require the attention and participation of health information management and informatics professionals. Information must be protected and must be correct if it is to be of use in documenting improvement efforts.

There are many groups trying to improve patient safety. A number of organizations—governmental, private, and/or not-for-profit—are engaged in patient safety initiatives. All of these groups have websites with excellent information.

- Agency for Healthcare Research and Quality (AHRQ)
- National Center for Patient Safety (NCPS)
- National Patient Safety Foundation (NPSF)
- Commonwealth Fund (CMWF)
- National Quality Forum (NQF)
- The Joint Commission on Accreditation of Healthcare Organizations
- The Institute for Safe Medication Practices (ISMP)
- American Association of Retired Persons (AARP) Research Center
- Leapfrog Group
- Center for Quality Assessment and Improvement in Mental Health
- National Initiative for Children's Healthcare Quality

Pay for Performance

The Institute of Medicine (IOM) report of September 2006, *Rewarding Provider Performance: Aligning Incentives in Medicare,* focuses on planned changes in Medicare that will help ensure that patients receive the highest quality of care. According to the IOM, under the **Pay for Performance** (P4P) system, reimbursement to providers will ". . . encourage coordinated, preventive, and primary care that could save money and produce better health outcomes." Providers will be given incentives to deliver care that ". . . meets professionally recommended quality standards, is centered on individual patients' needs, and is delivered efficiently" (IOM 2006, 1). The recently passed Patient Protection Affordable Care Act of 2010 provides for P4P pilot programs to be implemented by January 1, 2016, in support of efforts to improve quality of care and reduce spending (Pub. L. 111-148, sec. 10326). The development and progress of P4P initiatives should be monitored as this methodology is adopted by Medicare, since it will fundamentally change the way that Medicare reimbursement is handled. Quality reporting will be tied to the income of individual providers and healthcare facilities. Legal issues will evolve in the areas of quality standards, coordination of care among providers, methods of quality reporting, and comparisons on the amount of reimbursement received by providers.

Check Your Understanding 14.5

Instructions: Indicate whether the following statements are true or false (T or F).

1. The National Practitioner Data Bank collects malpractice and disciplinary action information on physicians.

2. The Medicare Conditions of Participation encourage restraints in the interest of patient safety.

3. Quality Improvement Organizations provide consultation and quality improvement resources to a wide range of providers.

4. The Leapfrog Group consists of organizations that are responsible for purchasing healthcare coverage for employees.

5. Pay for performance provides incentives to healthcare providers to deliver high-quality care.

Summary

State and federal governments and many private organizations are committed to reducing medical errors, improving patient safety, and increasing public awareness. The objectives of all of these efforts concern learning, collaboration, and providing public access to healthcare information. There will be more electronic reporting of information, more consumer and provider education on error prevention and error reporting, and annual safety reports. Information on patient safety and healthcare errors will be reported and professional educational institutions encouraged to include patient safety training programs in professional curricula. The public interest in these activities should increase with the rise in the elderly population and with increased expectations of the healthcare system.

References

Agency for Healthcare Research and Quality. 2000. Medical errors: The scope of the problem. Fact sheet. http://www.ahrq.gov.

Agency for Healthcare Research and Quality. 2003. National healthcare disparities report. http://www.ahrq.gov.

Agency for Healthcare Research and Quality. 2005. Morbidity and mortality rounds on the Web: Case and commentary: Discharge against medical advice. http://www.webmm.ahrq.gov.

Agency for Healthcare Research and Quality. 2006. What consumers say about the quality of their health plans and medical care? 2006 CAHPS Health Plan Survey Chartbook. September. http://www.cahps.ahrq.gov.

Agency for Healthcare Research and Quality. n.d.a. Your guide to choosing quality health care: A quick look at quality. http://www.ahrq.gov.

Agency for Healthcare Research and Quality. n.d.b. About AHRQ Patient Safety Network (PSNet). http://www.psnet.ahrq.gov.

Agency for Healthcare Research and Quality. n.d.c. Working for Quality. http://www.ahrq.gov

American Academy of Emergency Medicine. n.d. Emergency Medical Treatment and Active Labor Act (EMTALA). http://www.aaem.org.

American Hospital Association. 2003. The Patient Care Partnership. http://www.aha.org.

American Hospital Association. 2006. Resources. http://www.aha.org.

American Society for Healthcare Risk Management of the American Hospital Association. 2000. Risk management program development tool kit, sample excerpt.

American Society for Healthcare Risk Management of the American Hospital Association. 2003. Barton Certificate in Healthcare Risk Management program glossary.

American Society for Healthcare Risk Management of the American Hospital Association. 2005. Celebrating 25 years, 1980–2005: A brief history of ASHRM. http://www.ashr.org.

Burwell, B., K. Gerst, and E. Tell. 2006. The nursing home liability insurance market: A case study of Ohio. Report prepared under contract between the US Department of Health and Human Services (HHS), Office of Disability, Aging and Long-Term Care Policy (DALTCP), and Medstat. http://www.aspe.hhs.gov.

Centers for Medicare and Medicaid Services. 2010a. Quality Improvement Organizations Overview. http://www.cms.gov.

Centers for Medicare and Medicaid Services. 2010b. Quality Improvement Organizations Statement of Work: What's New Under the 9th SOW? http://www.cms.gov.

Centers for Medicare and Medicaid Services. 2010c (January). What's new for the 2010 Physician Quality Reporting Initiative (PQRI). https://www.cms.gov.

Centers for Medicare and Medicaid Services. 2010d (January). 2010 PQRI Electronic Health Record (EHR) Reporting Made Simple. https://www.cms.gov.

Centers for Medicare and Medicaid Services. 2010e (October). HCAHPS: Patients' Perspectives of Care Survey. https://www.cms.gov.

Cox, C.H. 2002 (June). Notice of loss requirements—Risk primer. *Risk & Insurance* 13(7):12.

Danzon, P.M. 1982. *The Frequency and Severity of Malpractice Claims.* Santa Monica, CA: Rand. http://www.rand.org.

Department of Health and Human Services. 1999. Medicare and Medicaid programs; Hospital conditions of participation: Patients' rights; interim final rule. 42 CFR 482.13 *Federal Register* 64 (127): 36069–89.

Department of Health and Human Services. 2002. Standards for privacy of individually identifiable health information; Final rule. 45 CFR 164.524(a)(1)(ii). *Federal Register* 67 (157):53181–273.

Department of Health and Human Services. 2006. Your rights under the community service assurance provision of the Hill-Burton Act. June. http://archive.hhs.gov

Department of Health and Humans Services. 2011a. National Quality Strategy will promote better health, quality care for Americans. http://www.hhs.gov.

Department of Health and Human Services. 2011b. Report to Congress National Strategy for Quality Improvement in Health Care. http://www.healthcare.gov.

Department of Health and Human Services. 2012. Hospital Compare. http://www.hospitalcompare.hhs.gov.

Department of Health and Human Services. n.d. Hill-Burton free and reduced cost health care.

Dunn, D. 2003 (June). Incident reports: Their purpose and scope. *AORN Journal* 78(1):46, 49–61, 65–66, 67–70.

HealthGrades, 2010. How do your local healthcare providers rate? http://www.healthgrades.com.

Institute for Healthcare Improvement. n.d. About. http://www.ihi.org.

Institute of Medicine. 1999. *To Err Is Human*. Washington: National Academies Press.

Institute of Medicine. 2001. *Crossing the Quality Chasm—A New Health System for the 21st Century*. Washington, DC: National Academies Press.

Institute of Medicine. 2006 (September). Report Brief: *Rewarding Provider Performance: Aligning Incentives in Medicare*. Washington, DC: National Academies Press.

Joint Commission. 2006a. Sentinel event glossary of terms. http://www.jointcommission.org.

Joint Commission. 2006b (September). Individual Rights. *Comprehensive Accreditation Manual for Hospitals, The Official Handbook*, CAMH Update 2 RI-10. Oakbrook Terrace, IL: Joint Commission.

Joint Commission. 2006c. Introduction to the National Patient Safety Goals. http://www.jointcommission.org.

Joint Commission. 2007. Joint Commission sentinel event policy and procedures. http://www.jointcommission.org.

Joint Commission. 2009. A framework for a root cause analysis and action plan in response to a sentinel event. http://www.jointcommission.org.

Joint Commission. 2010a. Facts about the Joint Commission. http://www.jointcommission.org.

Joint Commission. 2010b. 2010 National Patient Safety Goals. PowerPoint presentation.

Joint Commission. 2010c. National Patient Safety Goals. http://www.jointcommission.org.

Joint Commission. n.d. Sentinel Event Alert. http://www.jointcommission.org.

Journal of Healthcare Risk Management. 1992 (September 1). The emergence of health care risk management. Academic OneFile. http://www.gale.cengage.com

Journal of Healthcare Risk Management. 2007 (Jan. 1). Cost of adverse events borne by provider. Academic OneFile. http://www.gale.cengage.com

KaiserEDU.org. 2007. Reducing medical errors: Background brief. http://www.kaiseredu.org.

Kansas Foundation for Medical Care (KFMC). 2010. Healthcare Provider and Professionals. http://www.kfmc.org.

The Leapfrog Group. http://www.leapfroggroup.org.

McCain, M., and E. Bowman, editors. 2006. *Tennessee Health Information Management Association Legal Handbook*, 10th ed. Winchester, TN: THIMA.

Mello, M.M., D.M. Studdert, and T.A. Brennan. 2003. The new medical malpractice crisis. *New England Journal of Medicine* 348(23):2281–84.

National Committee for Quality Assurance. 2011. Report cards. http://www.ncqa.org.

PQA Quality Connection. 2011. New CMS QIO 10th "Statement of Work" Sets Ambitious Quality Goals for Medicare. http://www.pqaalliance.org.

QualityNet. n.d. QIO Listings. https://www.qualitynet.org.

Russell, L. 1992. The emergence of health care risk management. *Risk Management* 39(9):25.

Spath, P.L. 2001. Risk management: An art or a science? *The Quality Resource* 20(3).

Sprague, L. 2002. Contracting for quality: Medicare's Quality Improvement Organizations. *NHPF Issue Brief* 774.

Cases, Statutes, and Regulations Cited

Darling v. Charleston Community Memorial Hospital, 33 IL 2d 326, 211 N.E.2d 253, 14 A.L.R.3d 860. 1965.

42 USC 1395dd et seq.: Emergency Medical Treatment and Active Labor Act of 1986.

42 USC 11101 01/26/98: Title IV: Health Care Quality Improvement Act of 1986.

45 CFR 164.524(a)(1)(ii): Access of individuals to protected health information. 2006.

CFR 482.13: Conditions of Participation Patients' Rights. 1999.

KS Stat. Ann. 65-4922: Kansas Risk Management Statute, healthcare providers.

Pub. L. 106-129: Healthcare Research and Quality Act of 1999.

Pub. L. 106-310: Children's Health Act. 2000.

Pub. L. 106-336: Americans with Disabilities Act of 1990.

Pub. L. 109-41: Patient Safety and Quality Improvement Act of 2005.

Pub. L. 107-204: Sarbanes-Oxley Act of 2002.

Pub. L. 111-148 (Sec. 10326): Patient Protection and Affordable Act of 2010.

TN Code Ann. 68-11-211: Health Data Reporting Act: Unusual Events Reporting. 2002.

Chapter 15

Corporate Compliance

Sue Bowman, RHIA, CCS

Learning Objectives

- Differentiate between the concepts of fraud and abuse

- Identify the major statutes, rules, and regulations that relate to compliance and fraud and abuse issues

- List examples of policies and procedures to ensure the accuracy of coding

- Explain the role of the Office of Inspector General and the Department of Justice

- Describe the coordinated federal fraud and abuse programs

- Describe the Recovery Audit Contractor Program and state efforts to enforce fraud laws

- Explain corporate compliance programs

Key Terms

Abuse
Civil Monetary Penalties
   (CMP) law
Compliance officer
Corporate code of conduct
Corporate compliance
   program
Corporate integrity
   agreement (CIA)
Correct Coding
   Initiative (CCI)
Deficit Reduction Act of
   2005 (DRA)
Designated health services
Duplicate billing
Evaluation and management
   (E/M) coding

False Claims Act (FCA)
False cost reports
Federal Anti-Kickback Statute
Federal Physician Self-
   Referral Statute
Fraud
Fraud Enforcement and
   Recovery Act of 2009
   (FERA)
Knowing standard
Local Coverage
   Determinations
Medical necessity
National Coverage
   Determinations
Office of Inspector
   General (OIG)

Overcoding
Patient Protection and
   Affordable Care Act
   (PPACA)
Qui tam
Recovery Audit Contractor
   (RAC)
Relator
Revenue cycle management
Safe harbor
Sherman Antitrust Act
Stark Law I, II
Unbundling
Upcoding
Whistleblower

Introduction

Compliance is defined as conforming or acquiescing. In healthcare, compliance generally refers to adherence to federal statutes and regulations designed to prevent unjust financial enrichment and patient privacy breaches by healthcare providers or organizations. The federal government is involved in aggressive efforts to combat fraud and abuse as well as privacy and security violations. As a result of the government's initiatives, the development of formal corporate compliance programs has become a core function in healthcare organizations. This chapter focuses on fraud and abuse and the importance of correct documentation to prevent fraud and abuse from occurring. An overview of the major laws, such as the False Claims Act and the Stark Law, and their relationship to coding and billing processes is discussed. Fraudulent billing practices that represent major compliance risks are presented, along with a discussion of the federal agencies involved in healthcare compliance activities. The chapter concludes with a discussion of the role of corporate compliance programs and the standards, policies, and procedures that healthcare organizations should have in place to assure they are in compliance with government-funded healthcare programs. As the federal government's enforcement efforts and penalties evolve, staying abreast of compliance requirements continues to be a challenge for those responsible for the management and integrity of healthcare information.

Fraud and Abuse

Fraud significantly impacts the US health economy. In 2007, $2.26 trillion was spent on healthcare and more than four billion health insurance claims were processed in the United States (NHCAA n.d.). The National Health Care Anti-Fraud Association (NHCAA) estimates that "of the nation's annual healthcare outlay at least 3 percent was lost to outright fraud" (NHCAA n.d.). Other estimates by government and law enforcement agencies place the loss as high as 10 percent of annual expenditures, or $170 billion. Healthcare fraud is a serious and growing crime nationwide, linked directly to the nation's increasing healthcare outlay (Bowman 2007).

Fraud in healthcare is defined independently by a number of legal authorities, but all definitions share common elements:

- A false representation of fact

- A failure to disclose a fact that is material (relevant) to a healthcare transaction

- Damage to another party that reasonably relies on the misrepresentation or failure to disclose

The NHCAA (n.d.) defines healthcare fraud as an intentional deception or misrepresentation that the individual or entity makes knowing that the misrepresentation could result in some unauthorized benefit to the individual, the entity, or some other party.

Healthcare **abuse** is commonly associated with fraud but specifically refers to provider, supplier, and practitioner practices that are inconsistent with accepted sound fiscal, business, or medical practices, which directly or indirectly may result in:

- Unnecessary costs to the program

- Improper payment

- Services that fail to meet professionally recognized standards of care or are medically unnecessary

- Services that directly or indirectly result in adverse patient outcomes or delays in appropriate diagnosis or treatment

According to the NHCAA, the most common types of fraud include:

- Billing for services that were never rendered (either by using actual patient information to fabricate entire claims or by padding claims with charges for services that were not provided)

- Billing for more expensive services or procedures than were actually provided or performed, also known as "upcoding" (this practice often includes falsifying the patient's diagnosis so that it supports the fraudulent service or procedure)

- Performing medically unnecessary services in order to increase revenue

- Misrepresenting noncovered treatments as medically necessary covered treatments

- Falsifying a patient's diagnosis to justify tests or procedures that aren't medically necessary

- Unbundling (billing individual components of a complete procedure or service separately)

- Billing patients more than the co-pay amount for services that were prepaid or paid in full by the benefit plan under the terms of a managed care contract

- Accepting kickbacks for patient referrals

- Waiving patient co-pays or deductibles and overbilling the health plan (NHCAA n.d.)

Only a small percentage of the estimated four billion healthcare claims submitted each year are fraudulent. Taken in total, however, the resulting cost is high, and the scope of activity is wide. Fraud takes many different forms, such as incorrect reporting of diagnoses or procedures to maximize payments, fraudulent diagnosis, and billing for services not rendered. The federal government is looking at quality of care as an indicator of false claims and is seeking recovery of payment for care that does not meet defined standards of care.

Now more than ever, it is important for a healthcare provider to engage in **revenue cycle management**, which is the supervision of all administrative and clinical functions that contribute to the capture, management, and collection of patient service revenues (Casto and Forrestal 2013). This includes claims reports to ensure that charges are captured and properly claimed in accordance with coding and billing regulations to avoid errors, compliance violations, and investigations of potential fraud and abuse.

There are stiff penalties for healthcare entities that are targeted for enforcement action. According to the **Office of Inspector General** (OIG) for the US Department of Health and Human Services (HHS), a national home healthcare staffing business paid an $8 million penalty for submitting false claims to Medicare, Medicaid, and other government payers. Documentation issues included lack of physician orders and care plans, homebound status, and improper coding, and in some cases care was provided by unqualified individuals.

The OIG reported to Congress that $72 million in improper claims resulted from incorrect coding of discharges by hospitals where patients were coded as "discharged home" rather than "transferred." In a case involving inflation of the cost-to-charge ratio, which increased the diagnosis-related group (DRG) outlier payments, a hospital chain had to pay a $265 million penalty and enter a six-year corporate integrity agreement (CIA). A CIA is a compliance program imposed by the government on a healthcare provider (CIAs are discussed in more detail later in the chapter). Providers often choose to settle or pay the monetary penalties levied by the government because it is so difficult, time-consuming, and expensive for them to defend themselves against the findings of an investigation.

Role of Documentation

The importance of correct documentation to support billing and claims filed cannot be overstated. Constant and consistent education is critical, and it is imperative that attention be given to the changes in regulations that occur. Documentation must support the billing. Documentation of all physician and other professional services should be proper (i.e., in accordance with regulatory standards and generally accepted documentation practices), complete, and timely to ensure that only accurate and properly documented services are billed (Bowman 2007). The OIG states in its program guidance that all claims and requests for reimbursement from federal healthcare programs, and all supporting documentation, must be complete and accurate and reflect reasonable and necessary services ordered by an appropriately licensed medical professional who is a participating provider in the healthcare program from which the individual or entity is seeking reimbursement (HHS OIG 1998). The principles and standards for complete and accurate documentation are equally applicable to paper-based and electronic health records, although the processes may be different (Bowman 2007). At a minimum, health records should be retained according to Medicare requirements so they are available to support the organization's compliance efforts.

Check Your Understanding 15.1

Instructions: Indicate whether the following statements are true or false (T or F).

1. Healthcare abuse relates to a false representation of fact.

2. Billing for services never rendered is one of the most common types of healthcare fraud.

3. Unbundling is a billing practice preferred by payers.

4. A corporate integrity agreement is a voluntary compliance program adopted by a healthcare organization.

5. Although desirable, correct documentation in the health record is not necessary to support billing.

Major Statutes, Rules, and Regulations

Health information management and informatics professionals should be aware of the major statutes, rules, and regulations related to compliance. Because they change quickly, it is imperative to monitor them regularly to ensure that an organization or provider is following the most current version of the laws. Federal and state statutes, rules, and regulations must be understood since a claim of ignorance will not excuse the organization or provider from penalties. Significant federal laws related to compliance and discussed below are the False Claims Act, the Fraud Enforcement and Recovery Act, the Federal Anti-Kickback Statute, the Civil Monetary Penalties law, the Health Insurance Portability and Accountability Act, the Federal Physician Self-Referral Statute (the Stark Law), the Sherman Antitrust Act, and the Deficit Reduction Act of 2005.

False Claims Act

The **False Claims Act** (FCA) (31 USC 3729) is the government's primary litigation tool for combating fraud. It provides that anyone who "knowingly" submits false claims to the government is liable for penalties. This includes not only those with actual knowledge of the false claim, but also those who act in deliberate ignorance of the truth or falsity of the information and those who act in reckless disregard of the truth or falsity of the information. The FCA contains both criminal and civil provisions.

Violations of the FCA result in damages up to three times the amount of the erroneous payment plus mandatory penalties between $5,500 and $11,000 for each false claim submitted. In addition to bringing about civil penalties, submitting false claims is a criminal offense. An organization can be fined either $500,000 or twice the false claim amount, whichever is greater, and an individual can be fined either $250,000 or twice the false claim amount, whichever is the larger sum, and can be imprisoned for up to five years. The burden of proof is higher in criminal prosecutions than in civil cases. In a civil FCA action, the standard is a "preponderance of the evidence," whereas in a criminal FCA case, the government must prove beyond a reasonable doubt that the defendant knew the claim was false.

The FCA empowers both the attorney general and private persons to institute civil actions to enforce the FCA. Under the *qui tam* or **whistleblower** provisions of the FCA, private persons known as **relators** may enforce the FCA by filing a complaint, under seal, alleging fraud committed against the government. The government investigates the allegations while maintaining the complaint under seal. If the government determines that the allegations have merit, the Department of Justice intervenes in the action, unseals the complaint, and assumes responsibility for prosecuting the claim. When the government intervenes, the relator generally receives 15 to 25 percent of the government's recovery, the relator's contribution to the action, and reimbursement of legal fees and expenses. If the government believes the claim lacks merit and declines to intervene, the *qui tam* plaintiff may elect to prosecute the action without the government. If the government does not intervene in the action, the relator's statutory recovery is between 25 and 30 percent of the government's recovery plus reimbursement of reasonable legal fees and expenses.

The FCA provides protection to *qui tam* relators who are discharged, demoted, suspended, threatened, harassed, or in any other way discriminated against in the terms or conditions of their employment as a result of their furtherance of an action under the FCA. Remedies include reinstatement with seniority comparable to what the qui tam relator would have had if not for the discrimination, two times the amount of any back pay, interest on any back pay, and compensation for any special damages sustained as a result of the discrimination, including litigation costs and reasonable attorney's fees.

What Constitutes a False Claim?

To establish liability under the FCA, the government or whistleblower must establish that the claim was false or fraudulent. Since the FCA does not specifically define what constitutes a false claim, the standard has been developed through case law. There are two general types of healthcare claims that the government considers false: (1) furnishing inaccurate or misleading information to the government to obtain payment or approval of a claim, such as upcoding or submitting claims for services not rendered; and (2) omission of information from a claim or implicitly certifying compliance with rules, without actually complying with the rules.

The FCA has been extended to cover quality of care cases. In *United States v. NHC Healthcare Corp.*, the government alleged that two residents at the defendant nursing home did not receive care that satisfied Medicare and Medicaid program standards because the residents developed pressure sores, incurred unusual weight loss, were in what was deemed to be unnecessary pain, and ultimately died. The court ruled that as a condition of receiving reimbursement from federal healthcare programs, the facility agrees in principle to provide care in such a manner and in such an environment as will promote the maintenance or enhancement of patients' quality of life.

Most providers believe that the FCA was not intended to reach so far. They believe that quality of care issues should be addressed through private malpractice actions or loss of provider status under Medicare or Medicaid, rather than through expanded application of the FCA. They question how a provider can know when it may be liable for submitting false information by omission. Providers are concerned that noncompliance with a minor requirement unrelated to billing may create FCA exposure. Most, but not all, cases reject the theory that claims can be tainted or implicitly false based on noncompliance with a minor regulatory rule, requiring instead that the falsity appear on the face of the claim or statement.

The Knowing Standard

Falsity alone is not enough to impose FCA liability. The **knowing standard** refers to the fact that the provider must have knowingly submitted the false claim. The FCA defines "knowing" and "knowingly" to mean that a person:

- Has actual knowledge of the falsity of the information,

- Acts in deliberate ignorance of the truth or falsity of the information, or

- Acts in reckless disregard of the truth or falsity of the information.

No proof of specific intent to defraud is required. Therefore, submission of claims in a sloppy, unsupervised fashion without due care regarding the accuracy of the claim can constitute reckless disregard and create an FCA violation.

Interpreting the law is sometimes difficult for providers. When a provider acts in accordance with one interpretation of the law, even if the government has another interpretation, the FCA action should not succeed. If a provider's actions are based on the advice of legal counsel, it may also be difficult to prove intent to violate the FCA. However, as a practical matter, many providers settle such cases rather than proceeding to trial to defend the action, which makes the FCA a powerful government enforcement tool.

Fraud Enforcement and Recovery Act of 2009: Revisions to the FCA

The **Fraud Enforcement and Recovery Act of 2009** (FERA) amended the FCA. It expanded the potential for liability under the FCA and also expanded the government's investigative powers. The FERA eliminated the requirement that a person must present a false claim to a US government officer or employee or a member of the US armed services in order to be liable under the FCA. With the passage of this legislation, the FCA penalties apply to "any person who knowingly presents, or causes to be presented, a false or fraudulent claim for payment or approval," regardless of to whom the claim was made. The statutory definition of a "claim" has been expanded to include claims submitted "to a contractor, grantee, or other recipient, if the money or property is to be spent or used on the Government's behalf, or to advance a Government program or interest" (31 USC 3729). This revision substantially broadens the types of payments that fall within the scope of the FCA, such as claims submitted to Medicare and Medicaid managed care plans and other federally funded healthcare payers. These amendments to the FCA are intended to ensure that those who submit false or fraudulent claims or make false statements related to a claim—to any contractor, subcontractor, or entity to which payment is made by the government—are liable to the same extent that they would be if they made such claims or provided such information to the government itself.

Further, the FERA established that FCA penalties apply to "any person who knowingly makes, uses, or causes to be made or used, a false record or statement material to a false or fraudulent claim." A violation of the FCA also occurs when any person "knowingly makes, uses, or causes to be made or used, a false record or statement material to an obligation to pay or transmit money or property to the Government, or knowingly conceals or knowingly and improperly avoids or decreases an obligation to pay or transmit money or property to the Government."

"Material" is defined as "having a natural tendency to influence, or be capable of influencing, the payment or receipt of money or property." These revisions allow the government and whistleblowers to pursue violations of regulatory statutes with penalty provisions as FCA cases and to pursue false documents that are "material to an obligation to pay or to transmit money ... to the Government," regardless of whether a false claim has been submitted. For example, a physician who creates backdated health records to support a claim already submitted could be liable under this provision. Also, since the definition of "obligation" expressly includes retention of overpayments, the FERA makes it clear that providers have an affirmative duty to notify the applicable entity and repay the overpayment.

The FERA also expanded anti-retaliation protections for whistleblowers by allowing nonemployees, including contractors and agents, to sue for retaliation. In addition, the FERA expanded the US Attorney General's authority to issue civil investigative demands and broadened the government's authority to share documents obtained through subpoena with *qui tam* relators and other parties.

Patient Protection and Affordable Care Act: Revisions to the FCA

The **Patient Protection and Affordable Care Act** (PPACA), widely known as the health reform bill, was signed into law by President Obama in March 2010. Its purpose was to further amend the FCA by allowing private individuals to be more successful in filing false claims lawsuits. Previously, cases based on information the individual had obtained from other legal proceedings or the news media ("public disclosure") were grounds for dismissal by the court. Now, the federal government ultimately determines whether dismissal is appropriate. Further, the PPACA broadened the definition of "original source" to allow the public disclosure defense to be overcome if the individual bringing suit possesses knowledge that adds to publicly disclosed information. Prior to the PPACA, knowledge had to be independent of publicly disclosed information. Finally, the PPACA clarified "retention of overpayments." This further clarified both FCA and FERA amendments to FCA by requiring reporting and return of overpayments within 60 days of discovery (31 USC 3730(e)(4)(A) and (B)).

Federal Anti-Kickback Statute

The **Federal Anti-Kickback Statute** (42 USC 1320a-7b) establishes criminal penalties for individuals and entities that knowingly and willfully offer, pay, solicit, or receive remuneration in order to induce business for which payment may be made under any federal healthcare program. Remuneration covered by the Anti-Kickback Statute includes, but is not limited to, kickbacks, bribes, and rebates. "Remuneration" is defined broadly to include the transfer of anything of value, directly or indirectly, overtly or covertly, in cash or in kind. Prohibited conduct includes not only remuneration intended to induce referrals, but also remuneration intended to induce the purchasing, leasing, ordering, or arranging for any good, facility, service, or item paid for by a federal healthcare program.

Violation of the Federal Anti-Kickback Statute constitutes a felony punishable by a fine of up to $25,000, imprisonment for up to five years, or both. Criminal conviction constitutes automatic exclusion from federal healthcare programs, although the Secretary of HHS may seek exclusion from federal healthcare programs through an administrative proceeding whether or not a criminal conviction is obtained.

The Federal Anti-Kickback Statute is expansive in scope and clearly prohibits payments for patient referrals. However, application of the statute becomes less clear when applied to arrangements that do not simply involve a payment for patient referral, but instead embody business or investment relationships between two or more individuals or organizations. The courts have broadly interpreted the prohibition to encompass many business arrangements. In addition, the PPACA provides that claims submitted in violation of the Federal Anti-Kickback Statute are automatically false claims under the FCA.

Statutory Exceptions

Because of the broad sweep of the Federal Anti-Kickback Statute, exceptions were created to protect legitimate business arrangements. There are many exceptions, including the following:

- Discounts that are properly disclosed and reflected in the costs claimed or charges made by the provider

- Payments by an employer to an employee for provision of covered items and services

- Amounts paid by providers to a group purchasing organization where there is a written agreement that discloses the amount of the administrative fee to providers purchasing from the group purchasing organization

- Waivers of coinsurance amounts in connection with certain federally qualified healthcare centers

- Activities protected by the safe harbor regulations, which provide protection from civil or criminal penalties

- Certain risk-sharing arrangements

- The waiver or reduction by pharmacies of cost-sharing obligations under Medicare Part D

- Remuneration between a federally qualified health center and any individual or entity providing goods, services, items, donations, or loans to the federally qualified health center

- Exceptions related to hardware, software, information technology, and training services used to receive and transmit electronic prescription information

Safe Harbors

Congress authorized HHS to establish additional safe harbors by regulation. These **safe harbors** are activities that are not subject to prosecution and protect the organization from civil or criminal penalties. The OIG (HHS OIG 1999) has created a number of regulatory safe harbors covering such arrangements as:

- Investments in certain large or small entities

- Investments in entities in underserved areas

- Space and equipment rentals

- Sales of physician practices in health professional shortage areas to hospitals or other entities

- Sales of practices by one practitioner or another

- Bona fide employment arrangements

- Group purchasing organizations

- Coinsurance and deductible waivers

- Practitioner recruitment activities in underserved areas

- Investments in group practices

- Referral arrangements for specialty services

- Investments in ambulatory surgical centers

- Electronic prescribing and electronic health records arrangements

A common theme that runs through these safe harbors is the intent to protect certain arrangements in which commercially reasonable items or services are exchanged for fair market value compensation. The statute does not define the term "fair market value" but makes it clear that fair market values cannot vary based on referrals or the additional value that one party would attribute to property as a result of its proximity or convenience to sources of Medicare or Medicaid business or referrals.

Special Fraud Alerts are issued periodically by the OIG to provide insight into the OIG's views on the application of the Federal Anti-Kickback Statute to various types of arrangements. The Special Fraud Alerts often contain descriptions of specific features that the OIG considers suspect. Arrangements that contain such features are more likely to be subject to further government scrutiny.

The OIG also issues Advisory Opinions regarding whether specific arrangements violate the Federal Anti-Kickback Statute. Advisory Opinions may address what constitutes prohibited remuneration, whether an arrangement fits an exception or safe harbor, what constitutes inducement to reduce or limit services, and whether the activity described would constitute grounds for the imposition of sanctions. Advisory Opinions have been issued on a variety of topics including percentage compensation arrangements, joint ventures, beneficiary inducement, discounts, and waivers of deductibles and copayments. There have also been numerous informal letters issued by the OIG relating to subjects such as discounts and the provision of free items or services. Most of these and other federal government documents related to healthcare fraud and abuse are included on the OIG's website (HHS OIG n.d.a).

Civil Monetary Penalties Law

In order to combat an increase in healthcare fraud and abuse, Congress enacted the **Civil Monetary Penalties (CMP) law** under section 1128A of the Social Security Act (42 USC 1320a-7a) in 1981. As one of several administrative remedies, the CMP law authorized the Secretary and Inspector General of HHS to impose CMPs, assessment, and program exclusions on individuals and entities whose wrongdoing caused injury to HHS programs or their beneficiaries. The statutory penalty and assessment amounts under section 1128A generally provided for a penalty of no more than $2,000 for each item or service at issue and an assessment in lieu of damages of not more than twice the amount claimed. Since 1981, Congress has expanded the CMP provisions to apply to numerous types of fraudulent and abusive activities related to Medicare and state healthcare programs.

Health Insurance Portability and Accountability Act

HIPAA significantly expanded the OIG's sanction authorities. It extended the application of CMP provisions beyond those funded by HHS to include all federal healthcare programs (such as Tricare, Veterans Affairs, and the Public Health Service). HIPAA also significantly revised and strengthened the OIG's CMP authorities pertaining to violations under Medicare and state healthcare programs. The maximum penalty amount per false claim was increased from $2,000 to $10,000, and the amount of authorized assessments was raised from double to triple the amount claimed. HIPAA allowed CMPs to be assessed for incorrect coding, medically unnecessary services, and persons offering remuneration to induce a beneficiary to order from a particular provider or supplier receiving Medicare or state healthcare funds. A new CMP was established for the false certification of eligibility for Medicare-covered home health services (HHS OIG 2000, 24400).

Check Your Understanding 15.2

Instructions: Indicate whether the following statements are true or false (T or F).

1. The False Claims Act targets anyone who knowingly submits false claims to a private insurance company.

2. A *qui tam* action involves whistleblowers who file a complaint alleging fraud against the government.

3. The False Claims Act utilizes a knowing standard, which includes acting in deliberate ignorance.

4. The Federal Anti-Kickback Statute targets those who pay, solicit, or receive payment in exchange for business that will be reimbursed by a federal healthcare program.

5. Under the CMP law, a hospital may be excluded from the Medicare program if its wrongdoing caused harm to an HHS program.

Federal Physician Self-Referral Statute (the Stark Law)

The **Federal Physician Self-Referral Statute** (Social Security Act 1877; 42 USC 1395nn) prohibits physicians from ordering **designated health services** for Medicare (and to some extent Medicaid) patients from entities with which the physician, or an immediate family member, has a financial relationship. This statute is commonly referred to as the "**Stark Law**" after Congressman Pete Stark, who introduced and supported the statute. The original statute, referred to as "Stark I," only prohibited physicians from ordering clinical laboratory services for Medicare patients from an entity with which the physician had a financial relationship. The expansion of the Stark Law to the other designated health services is typically referred to as Stark II (see figure 15.1). The application of the Stark Law to traditional fee-for-service Medicaid and other issues are included in Phase III of the Stark Regulations (42 CFR 411 and 424).

Exclusions

Excluded from the definition of "designated health services" are services that are reimbursed by Medicare as part of a composite rate (such as services performed in an ambulatory surgery center), except for the services listed in figure 15.1 that are themselves payable through a composite rate (such as home health and outpatient hospital services).

"Financial relationship" is defined in the Stark Law to include both compensation arrangements and investment and ownership interests. "Referral" under the Stark Law is defined more broadly than merely recommending a vendor of designated health services to a patient. Instead, "referral" means, for Medicare Part B services, "the request by a physician for the item or service" and, for all other Medicare and Medicaid services, "the request or establishment of a plan of care by a physician which includes the provision of the designated health service" (42 USC 1395(h)(5)(A)). Under the Stark Law, certain referral relationships are deemed not to constitute a referral if the services are furnished by (or under the supervision of) a specialist pursuant to a consultation. Specifically, the Stark Law excludes from the term "referral":

- A request by a pathologist for clinical diagnostic laboratory tests and pathological examination services

- A request by a radiologist for diagnostic radiology services

- A request by a radiation oncologist for radiation therapy, if such services are furnished by or under the supervision of the pathologist, radiologist, or radiation oncologist

Penalties for violating the Stark Law include denial of payment, refunds of amounts collected in violation of the statute, a civil monetary penalty of up to $15,000 for each bill or claim a person knew or should have known was for a service for which payment may not be made, three times the amount of the improper payment the designated health service entity received from the Medicare program, and a civil monetary penalty of up to $100,000 for each arrangement or scheme that the physician or entity knew or should have known had a principal purpose of ensuring referrals that, if directly made, were in violation of the Stark Law.

Figure 15.1. Designated health services as defined by the Stark Law

• Clinical laboratory services	• Parenteral and enteral nutrients, equipment, and supplies
• Physical therapy, occupational therapy, and speech language pathology services	
• Radiology and certain other imaging services	• Prosthetics, orthotics, and prosthetic devices
	• Home health services and supplies
• Radiation therapy services and supplies	• Outpatient prescription drugs
• Durable medical equipment and supplies	• Inpatient and outpatient hospital service

The Stark Law does, however, provide a number of exceptions to the general prohibition. The exceptions are complex and beyond the scope of the brief examples provided in this chapter. Some exceptions protect only compensation arrangements, some protect only ownership interest, and some protect compensation and ownership arrangements. One example is the Physician Services Exception, which provides an exception for physician services provided:

- Personally by or under the personal supervision of another physician in the same group practice as the referring physician, or

- Under the supervision of another physician who is a member of the referring physician's group practice or is a physician in the same group practice

Another example is the In-Office Ancillary Services Exception, a highly technical and complicated exception that protects designated health services furnished by a physician in the physician's office setting except for parenteral and enteral nutrients, equipment, and supplies and some durable medical equipment. The exception is intended to protect only services that are ancillary to physician services and contains specific requirements regarding the location, supervision, and billing of the services.

Yet another exception was created to address the unique financial arrangements between academic institutions and their affiliated hospitals and physicians. A crucial element of this exception is that the compensation paid by all medical center components to the referring physician is set in advance, does not exceed fair market value, is not determined in a manner that takes into account the volume or value of any referrals or other business generated by the physician, and does not violate the Federal Anti-Kickback Statute or any federal or state law or regulation governing billing or claims submission.

Sherman Antitrust Act

The **Sherman Antitrust Act** (15 USC 1-7), passed in 1890, is one of several antitrust laws, including the Clayton Act of 1914. They collectively make it illegal to restrain trade through contracts or conspiracies, and they prohibit price fixing and mergers that lessen competition. There are civil and criminal sanctions. The Federal Trade Commission (FTC) and the Department of Justice enforce these laws. Their respective websites contain information about healthcare issues. Healthcare mergers and joint ventures among providers for the purchase of equipment are examples of arrangements that must be carefully reviewed to ensure that competition is not hindered and that consumers are not harmed. Credentialing and peer review processes also may be scrutinized to ensure that privileges are not denied or restricted to limit competition. Physicians and hospitals cannot set different prices for services for one group of consumers, such as members of a particular health plan.

Deficit Reduction Act of 2005

The **Deficit Reduction Act of 2005** (DRA) was enacted in 2006. The DRA is particularly significant to compliance because it has transformed compliance programs from voluntary to mandatory. This act contains the Employee Education about False Claims Recovery provision, which requires any entity that annually receives or makes at least $5 million in Medicaid payments to establish written policies for all employees of the entity (including management) and for any contractor or agent of the entity. This written policy must provide detailed information about the FCA, administrative remedies for false claims and statements, any state laws pertaining to civil or criminal penalties for false claims and statements, and whistleblower protections under such laws, with respect to the role of such laws in preventing and detecting fraud, waste, and abuse in federal healthcare programs. The entity's written policies must include detailed provisions regarding the entity's policies and procedures for detecting and preventing fraud, waste, and abuse. The entity's employee handbook must include a specific discussion of the federal and state laws pertaining to false claims and statements, the rights of employees to be protected as whistleblowers, and the entity's policies and procedures for detecting and preventing fraud, waste, and abuse.

Compliance with the DRA provisions became effective January 1, 2007. Failure to comply may result in the affected entity being ineligible to receive Medicaid payments. Also, any affected entity that knowingly violates these requirements may be penalized for submitting false claims under the FCA.

Nonfederal Healthcare Fraud Laws

Many states also have enacted laws that address healthcare fraud and abuse. These state laws apply to all payers, not just federal healthcare programs. Some states have enacted laws that prohibit self-referral, which is the referral of patients for healthcare services by a physician or other healthcare professional to healthcare facilities in which that healthcare professional has an investment or other financial interest. Some state laws are similar to the Stark Law, while other states only require the referring physician or other healthcare professional to disclose their financial interests in a healthcare facility prior to the referral.

Many states have enacted laws that prohibit certain financial arrangements between healthcare practitioners that constitute illegal remuneration in return for the referral of patients, such as kickbacks or bribes. States also may have laws prohibiting fee-splitting among healthcare professionals and others in return for patient referrals. Private insurers also have taken measures to control healthcare fraud and may work with state or federal agencies to report or detect healthcare fraud.

Interaction Among the Laws

The interaction among the laws can be convoluted. For example, neither the Federal Anti-Kickback Statute nor the Stark Law contains a private right of action allowing a private plaintiff to file a lawsuit. Nevertheless, the government and *qui tam* plaintiffs have successfully argued that violations of the Federal Anti-Kickback Statute and Stark Law can serve as the basis for a claim under the FCA. According to this theory, a claim to the government is rendered "false" for the purposes of the FCA if the medical services or items were furnished in violation of the Federal Anti-Kickback Statute or Stark Law, even though the services or items provided were themselves appropriate and proper. Despite vigorous opposition by the healthcare industry and defense attorneys, a number of courts have accepted these theories. It is important that competent legal counsel be consulted on these matters as the laws, regulations, and case law change frequently.

Check Your Understanding 15.3

Instructions: Indicate whether the following statements are true or false (T or F).

1. The Stark Law prohibits physicians from ordering certain health services for Medicare patients from entities with which the physician or an immediate family member has a financial relationship.

2. A purpose of antitrust laws is to discourage marketplace competition.

3. In its definition of "referral," the Stark Law excludes a request by a radiologist for diagnostic radiology services.

4. State healthcare fraud and abuse laws apply to all payers.

5. The Deficit Reduction Act of 2005 made compliance programs voluntary rather than mandatory.

High-Risk Areas

Fraudulent billing practices represent a major compliance risk area for healthcare organizations. Some reasons why incorrect claims are submitted include:

- Physicians may graduate from medical school without an understanding of the Medicare rules, including the **evaluation and management (E/M) coding** and documentation guidelines, and limited knowledge of CPT and ICD-9-CM coding. Many physicians are unaware that they are coding and billing inappropriately and that their documentation in the health record does not adequately justify the diagnosis and/or treatment.

- Healthcare facilities, especially those with outpatient centers, may not have invested enough time and resources in training staff, including physicians, on proper coding, documentation, and billing requirements.

- Medicare rules are vast and ever-changing, as are payment system changes such as Medicare severity diagnosis related groups (MS-DRGs).

- Information may be missing from the record during code assignment.

- Electronic records may include information that was pasted incorrectly from another health record.

The best in-depth resource for learning how Medicare and other payers monitor and deal with fraudulent billing practices is the OIG website. The website includes "compliance guidance" for various healthcare entities (HHS OIG n.d.b). These compliance guidance documents contain specific risk areas pertinent to each entity. Three of these risk areas are vitally important to the accuracy of the claims submission process: coding and billing, documentation, and medical necessity for tests and procedures. Several of these are discussed below in the context of providers billing Medicare.

Billing for Noncovered Services

There are three categories of services to be considered when billing to Medicare: services Medicare considers medically necessary, services that are statutorily noncovered, and services that are covered under certain conditions—for example, only for certain diagnoses or at a certain frequency.

It is certainly legitimate to bill for noncovered services, as Medicare understands that there are times when a healthcare provider, or the patient, wants a test or procedure performed that Medicare does not cover. The services that are statutorily noncovered by Medicare are listed on Medicare's Notice of Exclusions from Medicare Benefits (NEMB) form. Medicare does not require that this form be presented to a patient who is to receive a noncovered service, but it is highly recommended because it is important that patients know when Medicare will not reimburse for the service, since the patient will then be held responsible for the bill.

Altered Claim Forms

The provider is ultimately responsible for the filing of accurate claims. The FCA differentiates between errors that are made intentionally and those that are honest mistakes. For example, if the OIG or a Medicare auditor had identified what appeared to be a pattern of false claims, their full investigation would determine whether the mistakes were innocent ones or whether there was intent to commit fraud. The difference might be return of overpayments versus jail time.

In the physician's office setting, the claim should be submitted in keeping with the individual payer's requirements and as reflected on the bill submitted by the physician or other healthcare provider. No changes should be made to what the provider has entered without permission and correction by that provider.

The coding and billing must be based on the provider's documentation, and a claim that was submitted correctly should never be resubmitted as a result of a patient's complaint about owing money. Coding is based on the original intent of the encounter as documented in the health record. A claim that is resubmitted incorrectly to appease a disgruntled patient who does not want to pay is a false claim.

Health plans and countless other entities make judgments about how physicians and other providers care for patients and utilize resources based on claims data. This information is now being used in the credentialing process for many health plans. All parties involved in the claims submission process should work together to refine the claims submission process so that it is as accurate as possible.

Duplicate Billing

Duplicate billing is the practice of submitting more than one claim for the same item or service. Duplicate billing occurs when a claim for an item or service is submitted more than once to a payer, either by the same or different providers. Duplicate billing may be the result of an unintentional billing error, but systematic or repeated duplicate billing generally may be viewed as a false claim, especially if any overpayments are not refunded promptly. The OIG has identified duplicate billing as a significant risk area for hospitals, nursing facilities, third-party medical billing companies, durable medical equipment vendors, hospices, home health agencies, and physician practices.

Many physician practices send duplicate claims by submitting a claim every month until they receive reimbursement, similar to the way they bill their patients who have not paid. Medicare will pay the first correctly submitted claim and deny all the others, which causes extra work for everyone concerned.

Contending with duplicate billing for Medicare is not only labor-intensive, it is also one of the major reasons for denied claims. Every denial should be thoroughly investigated and resubmitted only if appropriate. Payments received as a result of duplicate billing must be promptly refunded. In December 2006, Jackson Memorial Hospital, Florida's largest Medicaid provider, agreed to pay $14.2 million to the federal government to settle a whistleblower lawsuit accusing the Miami hospital of keeping millions of dollars in Medicare and Medicaid overpayments that it knew should be returned to the federal and state programs.

Misrepresentation of Facts on Claim Form

This risk area is very similar to the issue of altered claim forms. Some examples of misrepresenting facts on a claim form are as follows:

- A new physician partner joins a practice and the credentialing process has not been completed for his Medicare claim submission. The biller submits all his claims using the Medicare number of another partner to circumvent the credentialing process and obtain speedy reimbursement.

- A patient presents for an annual exam, but the physician knows her health plan does not reimburse for annual exams. Since the patient happens to have hypertension, the physician bills for an office visit for hypertension, even though that is not the reason for this encounter. This results in a noncovered service being incorrectly billed as a covered service.

- The hospital services of a nurse practitioner are intentionally billed under the Medicare number of the supervising physician as "incident to" in order to receive 100 percent reimbursement. The nurse practitioner is billing subsequent hospital visit E/M services under the physician's Medicare number when the notes contain only the nurse practitioner's documentation not supplemented by the supervising physician. This is a false claim, because Medicare does not allow for "incident to" billing in the hospital setting.

The bottom line is that misrepresenting facts on a claim to obtain Medicare payment that the healthcare entity is not legally entitled to is a false claim.

Failing to Return Overpayments

Failure to return overpayments is always perceived as an action designed to keep money that is not rightfully the provider's money, even though it could result from honest oversight. Overpayments should be promptly returned with an explanation to either the health plan or the patient as appropriate.

In January 2007, a cardiology group agreed to enter into a criminal pretrial diversion agreement, separate civil settlements with the federal and state governments, and a five-year CIA with the OIG for failing to return overpayments. The government alleged that the group had a number of credit balance practices that, taken together, amounted to a "policy" to avoid repaying credit balances. The group's policy was to retain overpayments unless they were specifically requested by a payer or patient, and at times the group took actions to delay or obstruct the return or refund of such overpayments. Under the terms of the settlement, the group agreed to pay more than $2.9 million in civil penalties and restitution to private payers and 11,220 patients. This case is significant because it was the first enforcement action against providers for failing to repay overpayments and because it broke new ground in the use of government fraud authorities related to provider conduct affecting private payers and patients, not just Medicare and Medicaid programs.

Unbundling

Unbundling is a billing practice in which providers use multiple procedure codes for a group of procedures instead of the appropriate comprehensive code in order to inappropriately maximize reimbursement. Separate billing for pre- and post-surgery physician services that normally are provided as part of a larger surgical procedure is one form of unbundling. All diagnostic tests that are furnished by a hospital, directly or under arrangement, to a registered hospital outpatient during an encounter at a hospital are subject to the bundling requirements. For durable medical equipment suppliers, unbundling items or supplies involves billing for individual components when a specific billing code provides for the components to be billed as a unit—for example, billing the individual parts of a wheelchair rather than the wheelchair as a whole. The OIG has identified unbundling as a high-risk area for hospitals, laboratories, nursing facilities, physicians, durable medical equipment vendors, and third-party billing companies (HHS OIG 2005).

A single, comprehensive Current Procedural Terminology (CPT) code may be "unbundled" into separate CPT codes representing individual components of the complete procedure. Reporting separate CPT codes for the components of a procedure instead of the code representing the entire procedure often results in higher reimbursement than if the claim was coded correctly. Even if this is an innocent mistake, it is perceived as an attempt to game the system and receive reimbursement that is not rightfully the provider's. Medicare's **Correct Coding Initiative** (CCI) lists pairs of CPT codes that should not be billed together because Medicare will only pay for one of the codes in the pair and considers the other bundled into it. The CCI is updated on a quarterly basis and is available free on the Centers for Medicare and Medicaid Services (CMS) website (CMS n.d.a).

Correct coding is imperative in order to avoid unbundling. If one code describes all the services rendered, then that one code is all that should be used.

Billing for Medically Unnecessary Services

There are two areas that are consistently identified by the OIG as being responsible for 70 percent of erroneous claims. One is insufficient or missing documentation, and the other is the failure to document **medical necessity** appropriately.

"Medical necessity" is a confusing term, especially to patients. Patients generally believe that any tests or treatments their doctor recommends should be considered medically necessary from a clinical perspective. Medicare and other payers disagree. The exact Medicare definition of "medically necessary" is listed on the patient/public section of the HHS website as: "Services or supplies that are needed for the diagnosis or treatment of your medical condition, meet the standards of good medical practice in the local area, and aren't mainly for the convenience of you or your doctor" (HHS 2008).

Medicare has designed a system that allows providers to identify which services have coverage restrictions (at the state level, called **Local Coverage Determinations**, and at the national level, **National Coverage Determinations**) and to determine how to correctly submit their claims and receive rightful reimbursement. Since not all services have restrictions, the best way to know which ones do is to go to the Medicare carrier's website and review the current Local Coverage Determinations (LCDs, earlier called LMRPs for Local Medical Review Policies). When a patient is going to receive a service that does not meet Medicare's coverage criteria, the provider should present the patient with an Advance Beneficiary Notice (ABN) describing the service and explaining why Medicare will deny payment. Providers are not required to provide beneficiaries with advance notice of charges for services that are excluded from Medicare by statute. See the CMS website for Medicare's specific requirements for issuing an ABN (CMS n.d.b.).

This process is problematic because most physicians and other providers are not thinking about billing issues at the beginning of an encounter with a patient; they are concentrating on the patient's complaints and their evaluation. Unfortunately, after the service is rendered and the patient has left the premises, it is too late. Once a denial for medical necessity is received, the patient cannot be billed unless there is an ABN. A diagnosis cannot be added for the purpose of appealing a denial.

Every test and procedure ordered and submitted on the claim should be documented in the health record along with the reason justifying medical necessity. Even if the correct codes are submitted to Medicare, if Medicare requests a copy of a note to substantiate medical necessity for a test such as bone density measurement (Dexascan) and the physician's note does not state why the Dexascan was ordered, Medicare will ask for overpayment recovery for that Dexascan. Acceptable documentation would be: "Mrs. Jones is 65 and at risk for bone loss due to post-menopausal status, therefore today we are ordering a Dexascan."

Adherence to payer rules regarding medical necessity should always be included in the monitoring component of the compliance program.

Overcoding or Upcoding

Upcoding, or **overcoding**, refers to the practice of using a billing code that provides a higher reimbursement rate than the code applicable to the service actually furnished to the patient. This is one of the riskiest of all fraudulent billing practices. Upcoding is one of the risk areas identified in the OIG's compliance guidance for most industries, including hospitals, physician practices, nursing homes, home health agencies, hospices, durable medical equipment vendors, clinical laboratory services, and third-party billing services. It is a particularly high-risk area for E/M coding. One of the most important compliance activities is auditing and monitoring E/M coding and documentation. If the provider does not have the resources or expertise to do this within the practice, these activities should be outsourced to a reliable consultant.

Overcoding by physicians and other providers is not necessarily intentional. In many cases, healthcare providers are not sufficiently familiar with applicable reimbursement rules to know what documentation is needed to support proper code assignment. And when it comes to reporting E/M codes, it is not only *what* is said but *how* it is said that is important. The provider's E/M coding should reflect the documentation in the record, not the provider's opinion of how sick the patient is. In some cases "underdocumenting" occurs, whereby the documentation doesn't adequately support the patient's severity of illness or care provided. Unfortunately, underdocumenting will result in having to pay back what could be a huge sum of money if it represents a pattern and is detected through post-payment reviews or other OIG audit methods. The old adage, "if it wasn't documented, it wasn't done," still applies.

Billing for Items or Services Not Rendered

One of the most common types of Medicare fraud involves billing for items not provided or services not rendered as claimed. Variations of this practice include billing for nonexistent items or services and misrepresenting noncovered services as covered services to obtain reimbursement.

Sometime the fraudulent billing is intentional, such as billing for nonexistent services, supplies, or patients, supported by fraudulently obtained beneficiary numbers or fictitious or forged health records.

In other cases, the fraudulent billing may be due to "reckless disregard" for the truth or falsity of the information, such as billing from an appointment schedule without confirming that the patient arrived for the appointment and that services were rendered.

False Cost Reports

Institutional providers of Medicare-covered services, as well as some other providers, must file annual cost reports with their Medicare contractors. For those providers who are paid on the basis of reasonable costs, interim payments are made throughout the year, and cost reports then are used to provide a final determination of the payments for the year. Therefore, Medicare payments can be increased inappropriately through **false cost reports**.

Originally, Medicare paid hospitals on a reasonable cost payment system. Most institutional providers are now paid under a prospective payment system, but they are still required to keep cost records and submit cost reports. Hospitals continue to file cost reports, in part to provide CMS with data to help the agency set prospective payment rates and because most hospitals have some portions of their operations that are still reimbursed on a reasonable cost basis.

The Social Security Act defines reasonable cost as "the cost actually incurred, excluding there from any part of incurred cost found to be unnecessary in the efficient delivery of needed health services." The act stipulates that a provider will be paid the lesser of its reasonable costs or customary charges for Medicare-covered services. Certain costs cannot be included in annual cost reports, even though they are related to patient care. Cost reporting procedures are complex and tedious. In addition, Medicare reimburses teaching hospitals directly and indirectly for graduate medical education.

Check Your Understanding 15.4

Instructions: Indicate whether the following statements are true or false (T or F).

1. Fraudulent billing practices are a major compliance risk area for healthcare organizations.

2. A claim that is resubmitted based on a patient complaint is not a false claim because it was not initiated by the healthcare provider.

3. Sending a duplicate claim each month to a payer until the claim is paid is an acceptable billing practice.

4. CPT codes that should not be billed together are listed in Medicare's Correct Coding Initiative.

5. Medicare deems all services to be medically necessary if they are ordered by a patient's attending physician.

Role of the Office of Inspector General

The mission of the OIG for HHS is to protect the integrity of HHS programs as well as the health and welfare of the beneficiaries of those programs. The OIG has a responsibility to report program and management problems to both the HHS Secretary and Congress, along with recommendations to correct them. The OIG's duties are carried out through a nationwide network of audits, investigations, inspections, and other mission-related functions performed by OIG components.

The OIG sets forth an annual Work Plan with various projects to be addressed during the next fiscal year by the OIG's Office of Audit Services, Office of Evaluation and Inspections, Office of Investigations, and Office of Counsel to the Inspector General (HHS OIG 2011). The Work Plan includes projects planned in each of HHS's major entities: the CMS; the public health agencies; and the Administrations for Children, Families, and Aging. Information is also provided on projects related to issues that cut across departmental programs, including state and local government use of federal funds as well as the functional areas of the Office of the Secretary.

Examples of initiatives included in the OIG's 2011 Work Plan are hospital admissions with conditions coded "present on admission," hospital readmissions, payments for diagnostic x-rays in hospital emergency departments, accurately coding claims for Medicare home health resource groups, quality of care in skilled nursing facilities, physician coding of place of service, laboratory test unbundling by clinical laboratories, and Medicare billings with the modifier "GY."

OIG reviews have identified payments for noncovered services, improper coding, and other types of improper payments for various inpatient and outpatient services. Improper payments range from reimbursement for services provided to inadequately documented and inadvertent mistakes to outright fraud and abuse. The OIG work has uncovered problems with hospitals taking advantage of enhanced payments by manipulating billing; hospitals reporting inaccurate wage data, which affects future Medicare payments; and inpatient facilities that may be gaming prospective payment reimbursement systems by discharging patients or transferring them to other facilities for financial rather than clinical reasons. The OIG also has identified vulnerabilities related to certain types of services provided by physicians and other health professionals, including services related to advanced imaging, pain management, and mental health.

Office of Audit Services

The Office of Audit Services (OAS) provides auditing services for HHS, either by conducting audits with its own audit resources or by overseeing audit work done by others. Audits examine the performance of HHS programs and/or its grantees and contractors in carrying out their respective responsibilities and are intended to provide independent assessments of HHS programs and operations. These assessments help reduce waste, abuse, and mismanagement and promote economy and efficiency throughout HHS.

For example, an OAS audit of the billing of oxaliplatin at several facilities found that these facilities had received overpayments because they had billed the incorrect number of units of oxaliplatin on some claims.

Office of Evaluation and Inspections

The Office of Evaluation and Inspections (OEI) conducts national evaluations to provide HHS, Congress, and the public with timely, useful, and reliable information on significant issues. These evaluations focus on preventing fraud, waste, and abuse and promoting economy, efficiency, and effectiveness in departmental programs. OEI reports also present practical recommendations for improving program operations.

For example, in 2006 the OEI found that 63 percent of Medicare-allowed claims for facet joint injections did not meet program requirements, resulting in $129 million in improper payments. Thirty-eight percent of facet joint injection services had a documentation error and 31 percent had a coding error. For services that had a coding error, just over 60 percent were overpaid because physicians incorrectly billed additional add-on codes to represent bilateral facet joint injections instead of using modifier 50. Eight percent of services had a medical necessity error. Fourteen percent of services had one or more overlapping errors.

Office of Investigations

The Office of Investigations (OI) conducts criminal, civil, and administrative investigations of fraud and misconduct related to HHS programs, operations, and beneficiaries. With investigators working in all 50 states and the District of Columbia, OI utilizes its resources by actively coordinating with the

Department of Justice and other federal, state, and local law enforcement authorities. The investigative efforts of OI often lead to criminal convictions, administrative sanctions, and/or civil monetary penalties.

For fiscal year (FY) 2009, the OIG reported savings and expected recoveries of $20.97 billion. Also for FY 2009, OIG reported exclusions of 2,556 individuals and entities from participation in federal healthcare programs; 671 criminal actions against individuals or entities that engaged in crimes against HHS programs; and 394 civil actions, which included FCA and unjust enrichment lawsuits filed in federal district court, CMP law settlements, and administrative recoveries related to provider self-disclosure matters.

OIG investigators are implementing state-of-the-art, cutting-edge technology to identify and analyze potential fraud with unprecedented speed and efficiency. Using this technology, federal law enforcement officials are receiving an unprecedented amount of data, helping them to more quickly detect potential patterns of healthcare fraud.

Top Management Challenges Facing HHS

In a memorandum outlining the OIG's list of top management and performance challenges facing HHS in FY 2009, promoting compliance with federal healthcare program requirements is listed as one of the top management challenges (HHS OIG 2009). The OIG notes that helping healthcare providers and suppliers adopt practices that promote compliance with program coverage, payment, and quality requirements must be an integral part of the HHS's program integrity strategy.

The OIG (2009) identifies the following five principles that it believes should guide HHS's integrity strategy for Medicare, Medicaid, and the Children's Health Insurance Program (CHIP):

- **Enrollment**—Scrutinize individuals and entities that seek to participate as providers and suppliers prior to their enrollment in healthcare programs.

- **Payment**—Establish payment methodologies that are reasonable and responsive to changes in the marketplace.

- **Compliance**—Assist healthcare providers and suppliers in adopting practices that promote compliance with program requirements, including quality and safety standards.

- **Oversight**—Vigilantly monitor programs for evidence of fraud, waste, and abuse.

- **Response**—Respond swiftly to detected fraud, impose appropriate punishment to deter others, and promptly remedy program vulnerabilities.

Role of the Department of Justice

The role of the Department of Justice (DOJ) is to root out fraud and safeguard taxpayers from illegal conduct. DOJ works in collaboration with a number of other federal agencies, as discussed below, who investigate and prosecute fraudulent activities. In fiscal year 2010, DOJ convicted 726 defendants of crimes related to healthcare fraud, opened 942 new civil healthcare fraud investigations, and had 1,290 civil healthcare fraud matters pending at the end of the year (HHS OIG 2010). The DOJ reported that antifraud efforts have yielded about a $4.90 return to the Medicare trust fund for every $1 spent. The United States secured $2.5 billion in settlements and judgments in cases involving fraud against the government in the fiscal year ending September 30, 2010. This represents the second largest annual recovery of civil fraud claims in history. It brings total recoveries since 1986, when Congress substantially strengthened the civil False Claims Act, to more than $24 billion. In FY 2009, healthcare fraud recoveries reached $1.6 billion, two-thirds of the year's total. The largest healthcare recoveries came from the pharmaceutical and medical device industries, which accounted for $866.7 million in settlements (HHS OIG 2010).

Coordinated Federal Fraud and Abuse Programs

In 1996, as part of the HIPAA legislation, Congress mandated the establishment of a nationwide Coordinated Fraud and Abuse Control Program as a joint effort between the Attorney General and HHS through the Inspector General to coordinate federal, state, and local enforcement efforts against healthcare fraud and abuse. The program is in its 14th year. It works to identify, prosecute, and prevent healthcare fraud and abuse. The program's activities also include the coordination and sharing of data with private health insurers (HHS OIG 2010).

The joint DOJ–HHS Medicare Fraud Strike Force is a multiagency team of federal, state, and local investigators designed to combat Medicare fraud through the use of Medicare data analysis techniques and an increased focus on community policing. The Medicare Fraud Strike Force supplements the criminal healthcare fraud enforcement activities of the US Attorneys' Offices by targeting chronic fraud as well as emerging or migrating schemes perpetrated by criminals operating as healthcare providers or suppliers.

As a part of further department collaboration, in 2009 a new interagency task force, the Health Care Fraud Prevention and Enforcement Team (HEAT), was created to increase coordination and optimize criminal and civil enforcement. The HEAT team consists of senior DOJ and HHS employees. They are charged with strengthening existing fraud prevention tools and investigating new ways to detect and prevent fraud. The Medicare Fraud Strike Force is part of HEAT.

Recovery Audit Contractor (RAC) Program

Section 302 of the Tax Relief and Health Care Act of 2006 required the Secretary of HHS to utilize **Recovery Audit Contractors** (RACs) under the Medicare Integrity Program to identify underpayments and overpayments and recoup overpayments associated with services for which payment is made under part A or B of title XVIII (the Medicare program) of the Social Security Act. The mission of the RAC program is to reduce improper Medicare payments through efficient detection and collection of overpayments, identification of underpayments, and implementation of actions to prevent future improper payments.

Unless otherwise prohibited, the RAC may attempt to identify improper payments that result from any of the following:

* Incorrect payment amounts (except in cases where CMS has issued instructions directing contractors not to pursue certain incorrect payments)
* Noncovered services
* Incorrectly coded services
* Duplicate services

The RAC may not attempt to identify improper payments arising from any of the following:

* Services provided under a program other than Medicare Fee-for-Service
* Cost report settlement process
* Claims more than three years past the date of initial determination
* Claim paid earlier than October 1, 2007
* Claims where the beneficiary is liable for the overpayment because the provider is without fault with respect to the overpayment
* Random selection of cases
* Claims identified with a Special Processing Number
* Prepayment review

The RACs review claims on a postpayment basis, utilizing data analysis techniques to identify claims most likely to contain overpayments (a process known as "targeted review"). They conduct two types of review: automated and complex. In an automated review, the RAC makes a claim determination at the system level without human review of the health record. In a complex review, a claim determination is based on human review of the health record. RACs are paid contingency fees based on the amount of over- and underpayments they identify. Any potential fraud is reported to CMS and potential quality issues are reported to quality improvement organizations. Contracts for RACs are regionally awarded and may change over contract periods. For information about the current RAC auditors please refer to the CMS website (CMS n.d.c). This site contains links to the federal regulations that created the RAC program as well as the jurisdiction of each contractor.

Other Medicare Program Review Contractors

In addition to RACs, CMS employs a number of other types of contractors to process and review Medicare claims submitted by hospitals, physicians, and other healthcare providers. Program Safeguard Contractors (PSCs) and Zone Program Integrity Contractors (ZPICs) conduct medical reviews of claims either prepayment or postpayment. They identify claims suspected of fraud and take corrective action. Medicare Administrative Contractors (MACs), which serve as Medicare claims payment processors, also have responsibility for detecting fraud and abuse. At the state level, Medicaid Integrity Contractors (MICs) are responsible for detecting fraud and abuse, but they are limited in their ability to suspend, deny, or recoup payments until the specific state Medicare program has reviewed their findings (Keohane 2011).

State Enforcement Efforts

Since the early 1990s, many states have strengthened their insurance fraud laws and penalties and have also required health insurers to meet certain standards of fraud detection. At least 32 states and the District of Columbia have implemented versions of the FCA. These acts have been effective in helping fight fraud in Medicaid and other state-related programs and funds (Phillips & Cohen 2011). Currently, if a state prosecutes an entity for defrauding Medicaid, the state is required to forward the federal government its share of the recovered funds. However, if a state's FCA meets federal requirements under section 1909(b) of the Social Security Act, 42 USC 1396(h)(b), the state is allowed to retain 10 percent of the federal share that would normally be forward to the federal government. This law was passed to incentivize states to partner with the federal government in its efforts to fight Medicaid fraud (Kaiser Foundation 2009). See Table 15.1 for examples of state healthcare fraud activity and monetary recovery.

Table 15.1.   Examples of state Medicaid fraud and monetary recovery

State	Company	Industry	Type of Fraud	Recovery (Year)
CA	City of Angels Medical Center	Hospital	False claims kickback	$4.1m*
FL	WellCare	Managed Care	False claims conspiracy	$80m (2009)
IL	Condell Health Network	Hospital	False claims	$2.88m (2008)
MI	OmniCare	Pharmaceutical	False claims, racketeering	$52.5m (2006)
NY	HealthFirst	Managed Care	False claims, scheme to defraud, falsifying business records	$35m (2008)

*m = millions

Source: Rosenbaum, Lopez, and Stifler 2009.

Corporate Compliance Programs

Corporate compliance programs became common after Federal Sentencing Guidelines were adopted by the US Sentencing Commission (USSC) in 1991. The guidelines reduce fines and penalties to organizations found guilty of healthcare fraud if the organization has a fraud prevention and detection program in place. Thus, healthcare entities had an incentive to develop compliance programs and the field of healthcare compliance was born.

In addition to reducing criminal fines and penalties, corporate compliance programs help organizations identify problems and improve performance. The adoption of a compliance program may help an organization avoid the imposition of a **corporate integrity agreement** (CIA), which is a compliance program imposed by the government, with substantial government oversight and outside expert involvement in the organization's compliance activities (HHS OIG n.d.c). The OIG generally requires a CIA as a condition of settling a fraud and abuse investigation, but if a healthcare organization can demonstrate that it has an "effective" compliance program in place, the OIG may not require the execution of a CIA. If a CIA is required, it may not be as intrusive and may allow the organization to perform its own compliance functions, such as auditing, rather than requiring a more expensive third-party auditor, referred to as an independent review organization.

The Federal Sentencing Guidelines outline seven steps as the hallmark of an effective program to prevent and detect violations of law (USSC 2009). These seven steps have become the blueprint for an effective compliance program for healthcare organizations (see figure 15.2).

Both the Federal Sentencing Guidelines and subsequent compliance guidance from the OIG emphasize that a compliance program must be tailored to meet the specific needs of the organization, taking into account the size of the organization, the likelihood that certain offenses may occur because of the nature of the business, and the prior history of the organization. The OIG guidance provides specific examples of what the OIG expects to be included in an effective compliance program, such as policy and procedures on high-risk areas and the structure and characteristics of the compliance officer and compliance committee. A **compliance officer** is responsible for overseeing the processes

Figure 15.2. Seven steps for an effective compliance program

1. Establish compliance standards and procedures that are reasonably capable of reducing the prospect of criminal conduct to be followed by employees and other agents.

2. Assign responsibility to oversee compliance with the standards and procedures to specific individual(s) within high-level personnel of the organization.

3. Use due care to avoid delegation of substantial discretionary authority to an individual who the organization knows, or should know, through the exercise of due diligence, has a propensity to engage in illegal activities.

4. Communicate the standards and procedures to all employees and other agents by developing effective training programs.

5. Achieve compliance with the standards through monitoring and auditing reasonably designed to detect criminal conduct by employees and other agents and by adopting a reporting system where employees and other agents can report criminal conduct within the organization without fear of retribution.

6. Enforce standards through appropriate disciplinary mechanisms, including, as appropriate, discipline of individuals responsible for the failure to detect an offense.

7. Respond appropriately to any offense detected to prevent similar offenses in the future, including any necessary modifications to the compliance program.

Source: Adapted from 2009 Federal Sentencing Guidelines, US Sentencing Commission.

that promote an organization's ethical business practices and its conformity to federal, state, and private payer program requirements.

The OIG has issued specific compliance guidance for the following entities (HHS OIG 1998; HHS OIG 2005):

- Hospitals

- Clinical laboratories

- Home health agencies

- Third-party medical billing companies

- Durable medical equipment providers

- Hospices

- Medicare+Choice organizations

- Nursing facilities

- Ambulance suppliers

- Individual and small group physician practices

- Pharmaceutical manufacturers

- Recipients of US Public Health Service (PHS) research awards

- Part D plan sponsors (included in the Medicare Prescription Drug, Improvement and Modernization Act of 2003)

Although a compliance program is a basic document tailored specifically to the individual organization, the OIG guidance considers the following minimum elements to be essential to an effective compliance program (HHS OIG 1998):

- Development and distribution of written standards of conduct and policies and procedures

- Designation of compliance officer and other appropriate bodies (such a corporate compliance committee) charged with responsibility for developing, operating, and monitoring the compliance program

- Development and implementation of regular, effective education and training programs

- Creation and maintenance of effective line of communication between compliance officer and employees

- Use of audits and/or other risk evaluation techniques to monitor compliance, identify problem areas, and assist in reduction of identified problems

- Development of policies and procedures addressing non-employment or retention of individuals or entities excluded from participation in federal healthcare programs and enforcement of appropriate disciplinary action against employees or contractors who have violated institutional policies/procedures or federal requirements

- Development of policies and procedures for investigation of noncompliance or misconduct

These minimum elements are similar to those covered in the next section.

Elements of a Corporate Compliance Program

Compliance programs were first discussed in 1966, early in the implementation of Medicare, when a study determined that incorrect claims represented 14 percent of claims and resulted in $23 billion in overpayments.

Over the years, the 14 percent of expenditures for incorrect claims has decreased substantially through the efforts of providers to become more aware of Medicare's rules regarding claims submission, but billions of dollars are still paid out for incorrect claims. For 2009, CMS significantly revised and restructured the way it calculates the Medicare Fee-for-Service error rate based on both the recommendations contained in recent OIG audit reports and those of CMS's advisory medical staff. As a result of refining their procedures, the error rate calculation for 2009 was 7.8 percent. While this is an increase over the 2008 level of 3.6 percent, CMS indicated that the use of new methodology and stricter review criteria makes it difficult to compare error rates between the two years.

The creation of compliance program guidances has become a major initiative of the OIG in its efforts to engage the private healthcare community in combating fraud and abuse. The OIG's compliance program guidance is intended to help organizations develop effective internal controls that promote adherence to applicable federal and state law and the program requirements of federal, state, and private health plans. It should be noted that following OIG's compliance guidance documents is voluntary, not mandatory.

An effective corporate compliance program is one of the most effective tools to minimize a healthcare organization's fraud and abuse exposure. The adoption and implementation of compliance programs significantly advance the prevention of fraud, abuse, and waste while at the same time furthering the fundamental mission of all hospitals, which is to provide quality care to patients. Any entity engaged in submitting claims to Medicare cannot afford to be without a compliance program in these times of shrinking Medicare reimbursement and ever-increasing regulatory requirements that impact healthcare providers, particularly physicians.

A successful compliance program addresses the public and private sectors' mutual goals of reducing fraud and abuse, enhancing healthcare providers' operations, improving the quality of healthcare services, and reducing the overall cost of healthcare services (HHS OIG 1998; HHS OIG 2005). Additional benefits include:

- Demonstration of an organization's commitment to honest and responsible corporate conduct;

- Increased likelihood of preventing, identifying, and correcting unlawful and unethical behavior at an early stage;

- Encouragement of employees to report potential problems to allow for appropriate internal inquiry and corrective action; and

- Through early detection and reporting, minimization of any financial loss to government and taxpayers, as well as any corresponding financial loss to the hospital.

A sincere effort by healthcare providers to comply with federal and state laws and regulations through an effective compliance program is a mitigating factor in reducing a provider's liability. It is not enough to have a compliance program—the organization must be able to demonstrate that its program is effective. To demonstrate that its compliance program is effective, every healthcare organization must include an evaluation and measurement of effectiveness as a component of its program (Bowman 2007).

A good compliance program and plan should include the elements explained as follows.

Code of Conduct

The compliance plan should include the organization's corporate code of conduct. The **corporate code of conduct** expresses the organization's commitment to ethical behavior. The code should be the organization's constitution, detailing the fundamental principles, values, and framework for action within the organization. The code of conduct helps to define the organization's culture. All relevant operating policies are a derivative of its principles. The code of conduct must be communicated and accepted throughout the organization. Corporate codes of conduct, which can be quite lengthy, may be included on an organization's website. See figure 15.3 for an excerpt from a corporate code of conduct.

Designation of a Compliance Officer or Contact

In order for a corporate compliance program to be effective, there must be appropriate oversight. OIG compliance guidance calls for someone to be responsible for the overall administration of the compliance activities in an organization. Oversight may be provided completely within the organization, or some portion of it may be outsourced to another party. If compliance activities are outsourced to consultants, it is recommended that such consultants be reliable, well acquainted with the organization, and in reasonable proximity to its location. In order to be effective, the compliance officer should be a good leader and educator and possess good organizational and record-keeping skills. Attention to follow-up action is also required.

A compliance officer must have the appropriate authority and power to carry out the duties of the position in relationship to the laws and regulations governing compliance. Some of these duties are included in figure 15.4.

Consideration might be given to instituting a corporate compliance committee, which would include the compliance officer and key members of the organization representing all practice areas. The OIG compliance guidance does not state that such a committee is necessary, only that appropriate oversight and responsibility should be assigned in the organizational compliance program and plan.

Policies and Procedures (Practice Standards)

The compliance plan must include policies and procedures that define the process for compliance and claims submission in the organization. The policies and procedures should be concise and easy to read and understand. These documents become a teaching tool for staff education and training. Policies and procedures should be reviewed and revised accordingly as part of the annual review of the compliance program. All staff members should have a current copy of the compliance plan containing the current policies and procedures.

Figure 15.3. Excerpt from HCA's Corporate Code of Conduct

Coding and Billing for Services

We have implemented policies, procedures, and systems to facilitate accurate billing to government payers, commercial insurance payers, and patients. These policies, procedures, and systems conform to pertinent Federal and state laws and regulations. We prohibit any colleague or agent of HCA from knowingly presenting or causing to be presented claims for payment or approval which are false, fictitious, or fraudulent.

In support of accurate billing, medical records must provide reliable documentation of the services we render. It is important that all individuals who contribute to medical records provide accurate information and do not destroy any information considered part of the official medical record.

Accurate and timely documentation also depends on the diligence and attention of physicians who treat patients in our facilities. We expect those physicians to provide us with complete and accurate information in a timely manner.

Any subcontractors engaged to perform billing or coding services are expected to have the necessary skills, quality control processes, systems, and appropriate procedures to ensure all billings for government and commercial insurance programs are accurate and complete. HCA expects such entities to have their own ethics and compliance programs and code of conduct. In addition, third-party billing entities, contractors, and preferred vendors under contract consideration must be approved consistent with the corporate policy on this subject.

Source: HCA 2009, 14–15.

Figure 15.4. General duties of a compliance officer

- Overseeing and monitoring the implementation of the compliance program
- Establishing methods, such as periodic audits, to improve the efficiency and quality of services and to reduce the entity's vulnerability to fraud and abuse
- Revising the compliance program in light of changes in organizational need, laws and regulations and private payer health plans
- Developing, coordinating, and participating in compliance program training and ensuring that training materials are appropriate
- Ensuring that the OIG's List of Excluded Individuals and Entities, and the General Services Administration (GSA) List of Parties Debarred from the Federal Programs have been checked with respect to all employees, medical staff, and independent contractors
- Investigating any report or allegation concerning possible unethical or improper business practices and monitoring subsequent corrective action and/or compliance
- Auditing and monitoring billing activity and following up to ensure that corrections as noted have been made and staff have been trained to prevent future submission of inaccurate claims
- Keeping accurate records and/or minutes of all compliance activities

The policies and procedures should address the risks identified in the OIG compliance guidance that are pertinent to the organization. Here are some examples:

- Coding and billing issues, including billing Medicare or Medicaid in excess of usual charges

- Documentation of reasonable and necessary services

- Consistent reporting of all compliance activities, including any potential instances of violation of Medicare laws and regulations (such as the Stark Laws)

- Accuracy of claims submission; payments to limit or reduce services

- Compliance with the Emergency Medical Treatment and Active Labor Act (EMTALA; see chapter 14)

- HIPAA Privacy and Security Rules and transaction standards

Education and Training

Education and training are essential elements of a compliance plan and should occur as part of a new employee's orientation to the organization and as an ongoing continuing education activity for staff. Compliance orientation should be provided to all new staff members, including physicians. The training should focus on compliance policies and procedures, with each staff member receiving a copy of the organizational compliance plan. Staff and physicians should understand their role in the compliance program and how to report compliance concerns, in an anonymous manner if they so choose. Compliance orientation should also include an overview of the various laws and regulations, such as the FCA and the Stark Laws, which mandate compliance by healthcare entities. Attendance records should be kept, along with detailed records of new hire compliance orientation and training as well as records of ongoing education and training of staff. The modalities used for education and training may include in-service sessions, teleconferences, reading material, and videoconferencing, to name a few.

See figure 15.5 for suggested content areas that should be addressed in education and training activities. This is not an all-inclusive list. Compliance education and training must be as detailed and as frequent as required by the size of the organization and the frequency of changes in laws and regulations.

Open Lines of Communication

Open lines of communication are an important element of compliance activity. Key to this element of a compliance program is a mechanism for staff members to report compliance violations or suspected

Figure 15.5. Examples of content for coding and billing compliance education and training activities

- **Coding, billing, and claims submission:** Yearly updates on ICD-9-CM and CPT changes with emphasis on appropriate use of modifiers, global surgery package rules, add-on codes, E&M coding and documentation, and coding conventions in general.
- **Medicare billing rules:** Emphasis on areas that have been problematic, such as billing of consultations, billing of annual exams, billing services "incident to," appropriate assignment of DRGs, and billing for consolidated services in skilled nursing facilities.
- **Documentation guidelines and accessing personal health information:** Includes required elements of the patient record, accessing patient information and records, maintenance and retention of patient records, and release of information. Included in this section would be what is expected to be documented in the health record (who can make entries, how entries may be revised, who should authenticate, and so on).
- **Medicare bulletins, seminars, and other related compliance resources:** Ongoing and yearly updates, revisions, and new resources related to compliance that should be shared throughout the organization.

violations. Every healthcare provider should develop a procedure for reporting violations and ensure that all staff members understand how to report compliance concerns.

It is important that the procedure for reporting allow staff members to report anonymously if they choose to do so. This may be accomplished by a dedicated phone line to the compliance officer or a report form that can either be placed in a specified secure location (similar to a suggestion box) accessible only to the compliance officer or mailed to the compliance officer through the US mail.

In smaller organizations, an open-door policy is encouraged. Ideally, a staff member would have no fear of reporting a compliance concern. Built into the compliance plan should be a clear statement of disciplinary action taken against anyone in authority who punishes or causes any measure of retribution to a staff person who reports a compliance concern in good faith. Similarly, all staff members should be made aware that it is their responsibility to report compliance concerns and that they could face disciplinary action if they were aware of a compliance violation and did not report it.

Open communication means that everyone in the organization is mutually committed to maintaining compliance with the appropriate laws and regulations and ultimately committed to doing the right thing.

Auditing and Monitoring

Two important elements of a compliance program deal with the auditing and monitoring of compliance activities. The compliance program should be flexible enough to accommodate responding to current areas of priority with Medicare and other payers. If Medicare announces a new focus on E/M billings for subsequent visits in the hospital, auditing in this area should be increased. The auditing and monitoring activities should be pertinent, focused, and ongoing while recognizing that it is not possible to monitor everything that is done all the time. However, consideration should be given to monitoring activities related to the following:

- What is high-risk? E/M coding is always a high-risk area in claims submission. Any entity submitting E/M codes on claims to Medicare needs to have ongoing auditing and monitoring of the accuracy of E/M coding and documentation. Insufficient documentation creates many noncompliance complaints. An OIG auditor is not going to "read between the lines." If residents are the care providers, there should be assurance that the Teaching Physician Rules related to the participation and physical presence of the attending physician are followed and that the documentation is entered by the attending physician.

- What is high-volume? For example, a diagnostic center with a recently purchased ultrasound machine and a great number of echocardiograms (in most states, echocardiograms are subject to a Local Coverage Determination policy that limits Medicare coverage), should be monitored for appropriate usage. If the organization frequently bills "99211" to Medicare, the billing and documentation of these encounters should be audited.

- What is problem-prone in the facility? Denials of laboratory services due to medical necessity may suggest that providers are not aware of the lab tests that have limited coverage or that providers are not obtaining ABNs when appropriate. Billing Medicare for outpatient tests performed in the hospital may be problem-prone because a physician may order an outpatient test or procedure that has coverage restrictions, or the physician may not include a clinical reason for the test on the order. This is an area that will need ongoing auditing and monitoring and should be clearly defined in the compliance plan.

Offense Detection and Corrective Action Initiatives

Responding to detected offenses and engaging in corrective action initiatives are core principles in determining whether the compliance program is effective or not. Effective action must be taken when problems are identified, and future monitoring must be done to ensure the problems stay solved.

All suspected or confirmed violations of the compliance plan, or of laws and regulations described in the plan, should be immediately investigated. The compliance officer should be the designated individual informed of such a violation or suspected violation and should be responsible for initiating the investigation. The outcome of the investigation may be any one of the following: no problem was found; a problem was found but is believed to be isolated and not likely to occur again; or a problem was found and needs corrective action—for example, not a violation of a law but an aberrant billing practice by one provider. If a problem is verified, then the corrective action plan should be appropriate to the seriousness of the offense. The following are sample actions that could be taken on confirmed compliance violations or errors:

- In-service education or retraining
- Fine or penalty
- Discipline
- Termination

If the investigation shows that overpayments have been received, restitution should be made. For potential criminal violations, the entity, in collaboration with legal counsel, should self-disclose the violation to the appropriate government and/or law enforcement agency. As mentioned before, all actions conducted during the investigation of compliance issues and actions taken should be carefully documented and maintained in the files of the compliance officer.

Enforcing Disciplinary Standards through Well-Publicized Guidelines

Enforcement and disciplinary provisions are necessary to add credibility and integrity to a compliance program. As with failure to investigate compliance violations and develop corrective action plans, if appropriate discipline is withheld, the compliance program is rendered ineffective and is not taken seriously by the staff.

Disciplinary actions should be appropriate to the compliance violation and, in some cases, they should reflect whether the violation is part of a pattern of behavior or a first offense. Discipline should be fair and consistent. Following is an example of inconsistent discipline:

A large hospital employs five coders in the HIM Department. In the spring of the year, one of the coders is found to be upcoding all pneumonia cases in order to maximize the DRG and reimbursement. She is terminated. The next year, a new coder is found to be coding all urinary tract infections as septicemia in order to maximize reimbursement. This employee is suspended for two weeks without pay and brought back to full employment.

Where appropriate, peer review should be part of the investigative process for physicians under disciplinary review. Obviously, in the case of a criminal offense, discipline would ultimately be determined by the court system.

Disciplinary actions might include, but are not limited to, the following:

- Oral warnings
- Written reprimands
- Probation
- Demotion
- Temporary suspension
- Termination
- Restitution of damages
- Referral for criminal prosecution

Check Your Understanding 15.5

Instructions: Indicate whether the following statements are true or false (T or F).

1. A corporate code of conduct expresses an organization's commitment to ethical behavior.

2. The corporate compliance officer position is ideally suited to a clerical staff person.

3. Federal Sentencing Guidelines encourage organizations to have fraud prevention and detection programs in place.

4. Anonymous reporting of compliance violations should be prohibited because it inhibits open communication.

5. The mission of the Office of the Inspector General is to protect the integrity of HHS programs and the health and welfare of those programs' beneficiaries.

Summary

Compliance requires significant attention from healthcare providers. Although complex, compliance with federal and state requirements is essential. On an organizational level, proper documentation and adherence to applicable statutes and regulations reduces the possibility of audits and subsequent penalties. Industrywide, compliance ultimately prevents fraud and abuse as well as billing and payment errors. Further, it promotes efficiency, high-quality care, and an ethical culture that fosters public confidence. Effective compliance programs support an ongoing commitment to system integrity. A compliance plan supported by the entire staff shows an organization's good faith in creating an environment where compliance is expected. The risks associated with failing to create a culture of compliance and the costs of noncompliance are both significant. Looking forward, the benefits of promoting compliance—and the costs of noncompliance—will grow as beneficiary populations and healthcare costs increase.

References

Bowman, S. 2007. *Health Information Management Compliance: Guidelines for Preventing Fraud and Abuse.* Chicago: AHIMA.

Casto, A., and E. Forrestal. 2013. *Principles of Healthcare Reimbursement*, 4th ed. Chicago: AHIMA.

Centers for Medicare and Medicaid Services. n.d.a. National Correct Coding Initiatives edits. https://www.cms.gov.

Centers for Medicare and Medicaid Services. n.d.b. http://www.cms.gov.

Centers for Medicare and Medicaid Services. n.d.c. Recovery Audit Contractor overview. http://www.cms.gov.

Department of Health and Human Services. 2008. Glossary. http://www.medicare.gov.

Department of Health and Human Services Office of Inspector General. 1998. Compliance program guidance for hospitals. *Federal Register* 63(35):8987–8998. http://oig.hhs.gov.

Department of Health and Human Services Office of Inspector General. 1999. Federal anti-kickback and regulatory safe harbors fact sheet. http://oig.hhs.gov.

Department of Health and Human Services Office of Inspector General. 2000. Health care program: Fraud and abuse; Revised OIG civil money penalties resulting from Public Law 104-191. *Federal Register* 65(81):24400–24419.

Department of Health and Human Services Office of Inspector General. 2005. Supplemental compliance program guidance for hospitals. *Federal Register* 70(19):4858–4856. http://oig.hhs.gov.

Department of Health and Human Services Office of Inspector General. 2009. Top management and performance challenges. http://oig.hhs.gov.

Department of Health and Human Services Office of Inspector General. 2010. Health care fraud and abuse control program annual report for fiscal year 2010. http://oig.hhs.gov.

Department of Health and Human Services Office of Inspector General. 2011. Work plan. http://oig.hhs.gov.

Department of Health and Human Services Office of Inspector General. n.d.a. Fraud alerts. http://oig.hhs.gov.

Department of Health and Human Services Office of Inspector General. n.d.b. Compliance guidance. http://oig.hhs.gov.

Department of Health and Human Services Office of Inspector General n.d.c. Corporate integrity agreements. http://oig.hhs.gov.

Hospital Corporation of America (HCA). 2009. Code of conduct. http://www.hcahealthcare.com.

Kaiser Foundation. 2009. States that have enacted a false claims act. http://www.statehealthfacts.org.

Keohane, P. 2011. MICs: What Makes Them Different? *RACMonitor.enews*. http://www.micmonitor.com.

National Health Care Anti-Fraud Association. n.d. The problem of health care fraud. http://www.nhcaa.org.

Phillips & Cohen, LLP. 2011. State false claims statutes. http://www.phillipsandcohen.com.

Rosenbaum, S., N. Lopez, and S. Stifler. 2009. Health care fraud. Department of Health Policy, George Washington University School of Public Health and Health Services. http://www.gwumc.edu.

US Sentencing Commission. 2009. Federal sentencing guidelines, section 8B2.1: Effective compliance and ethics program. http://ftp.ussc.gov.

Cases, Statutes, and Regulations Cited

United States v. NHC Healthcare Corporation, 163 F. Supp.2d. 1051, 1056 n. 4 (w.d. MO 2001).

42 CFR 411 and 424: Physician Referral to Health Care Entities with Which They Have Financial Relationships (Phase III). 2007.

15 USC 1-7: Sherman Antitrust Act. 1890.

31 USC 3729: False Claims Act. 1986. Amended 2009, 2010.

31 USC 3730(e)(4)(A)(B): Patient Protection and Affordable Care Act. 2010.

42 USC 1320a-7a: Civil Monetary Penalties 1128A. 1981.

42 USC 1320a-7b: Federal Anti-Kickback Statute. 1972.

42 USC 1395nn 42 CFR 411.350 et seq.: Physician Self-Referral (Stark Law). 1989.

42 USC 1395nn(h)(5)(A): Limitation on Certain Physician Referrals. 2010.42

USC 1396a(a)(68): Deficit Reduction Act. 2006.

42 USC 1396(h)(b): State False Claims Act. 2010.

Fraud Enforcement and Recovery Act of 2009. Public Law 111-21.

Patient Protection and Affordable Care Act of 2010. Public Law 111-148.

Chapter 16

Medical Staff

**Rebecca B. Reynolds, EdD, MHA, RHIA, FAHIMA, and
Melanie S. Brodnik, PhD, RHIA, FAHIMA**

Learning Objectives

- Discuss the relationship of a healthcare organization's governing board to its medical staff

- Describe the components of medical staff bylaws as required by The Joint Commission accreditation standards for medical staff

- Identify the various categories of medical staff membership

- Explain the significance of the medical staff credentialing process

- Describe the process of applying for medical staff privileges, including primary source verification, and how privileges are determined

- Discuss the duties and rights of a medical staff and issues related to disciplinary action, suspension of privileges, and due process under the law

Key Terms

Accreditation Council
  for Graduate Medical
  Education (ACGME)
American Board of Medical
  Specialties (ABMS)
Board of directors
Bylaws
Comprehensive Accreditation
  Manual for Hospitals
Credentialing
Credentials verification
  organization (CVO)
Deemed status

Due process
Economic credentialing
Focused professional practice
  evaluation
Governing board
The Joint Commission
Medical staff
Medical staff bylaws
Medical staff executive
  committee
National Committee for
  Quality Assurance
  (NCQA)

National Practitioner Data
  Bank (NPDB)
Office of the Inspector
  General (OIG)
Ongoing professional practice
  evaluation
Primary source verification
Procedural due process
State action
Substantive due process

Introduction

The **medical staff** of a healthcare organization is comprised of physicians and healthcare providers such as dentists, optometrists, pharmacists, podiatrists, and psychologists who may be employed by a healthcare organization or who may function as independent contractors. In either situation, the practitioner is governed by medical staff bylaws that define the responsibilities and obligations of the practitioner to provide quality patient care and to document care rendered. To practice in a healthcare organization, a physician or care provider such as those listed previously must apply for and be admitted to the medical staff. The application process includes a credentialing procedure that verifies the background of the care provider and assists in defining the type of appointment granted to the practitioner (full staff privileges, partial privileges, and so forth). The credentialing process requires continuing review of credentials and renewal of staff appointments on a regular basis. Since a major responsibility of a medical staff member is accurate and timely documentation in a patient record, a collaborative working relationship exists between the medical staff and health information management (HIM) department to ensure that bylaws, regulations, and laws related to proper documentation of patient care are followed.

This chapter focuses on medical staff organization and the **bylaws** that govern the performance of the staff. It discusses the elements of medical staff bylaws and the application process for granting medical staff privileges. It covers the process of medical staff credentialing and the duties and rights of the medical staff with regard to patient record documentation requirements. The chapter concludes with a discussion of consequences for not carrying out these duties, issues related to granting or denial of medical staff privileges, and the legal concept of **due process**.

Governing Board

The business model for healthcare organizations and particularly hospitals is unique. The healthcare organization relies on the medical staff to admit and treat patients, which ultimately generates business for the organization. In order for a patient to receive care a physician or other authorized care provider as designated by state licensing law must order the treatment or service delivered to the patient. The **governing board** (also called the **board of directors** or board of trustees) of a healthcare organization must ensure that its medical staff members are qualified, competent, and up-to-date on the education and training required to provide appropriate medical care and avoid legal risk.

The governing board as discussed in chapter 6 has the ultimate responsibility for the quality of care and financial well-being of the healthcare organization. It is the controlling authority for the hospital or other healthcare organization and is responsible for providing adequate staff. See figure 16.1 for a list of typical responsibilities of a hospital board. The composition of the board for a hospital may include physicians, community leaders, church leaders, businesspeople, and attorneys. Members of the board are usually

Figure 16.1.   Responsibilities of the governing board

- Define the mission and purpose of the organization
- Select (hire) the chief executive officer (CEO)
- Review and support the CEO
- Ensure adequate organization planning
- Ensure the financial health of the organization (fiduciary duty)
- Ensure the quality of patient care
- Enhance the public image of the organization
- Serve as a court of appeals (for due process of the medical staff)
- Assess the performance of the board of directors (BOD)

appointed, but the structure may allow for elected positions as well. The board delegates power to the organized medical staff to provide patient care and to ensure quality of care for the patients in the facility.

The board hires the healthcare administrator or chief executive officer (CEO), who reports directly to the board and works with the organized medical staff to provide patient care services. The CEO is responsible for the overall management of the healthcare facility while the organized medical staff is responsible for oversight of the quality of patient care and is also directly accountable to the governing board. To fulfill its responsibilities, the medical staff is governed by bylaws that are voted upon by the medical staff and approved by the governing board of the organization. A sample organizational chart for a healthcare organization is shown in figure 16.2.

Medical Staff Bylaws

Medical staff bylaws outline medical staff obligations to the board; operation of the medical staff organization to accomplish required functions; safeguards that protect the rights and privileges of individual staff members; and the organizational structure of divisions, committees, departments, officers, and department chairs. Medical staff bylaws are considered a contract and are legally binding in most states. Neither the medical staff nor the governing body can unilaterally modify medical staff bylaws or the rules and regulations of the medical staff without a vote of the medical staff and ultimate approval by the governing body.

The requirement for an organized medical staff is found in hospital licensure standards as well as the accrediting standards of **The Joint Commission** and other standard-setting organizations.

Figure 16.2. Organization chart

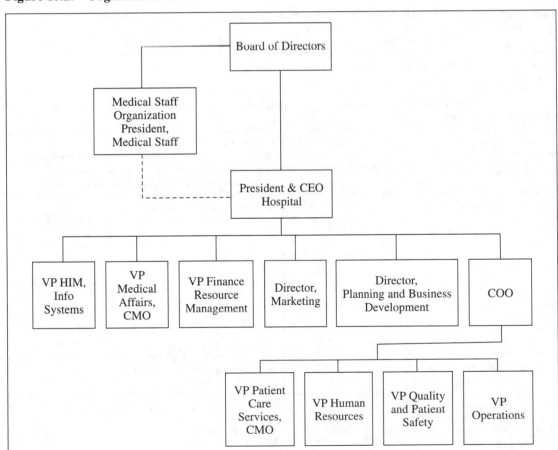

See table 16.1 for a list of standards organizations that govern medical staff quality. Because The Joint Commission is the dominant accrediting organization in the United States, it is important to understand The Joint Commission medical staff standards and the liabilities for noncompliance of these standards.

Joint Commission hospital standards require that the medical staff bylaws address self-governance and accountability of the medical staff to the governing body. The required content areas for the medical staff bylaws standards are as follow (The Joint Commission 2010, MS.01.01.01):

1. The definition of the medical staff structure

2. The definition of the criteria and qualifications for appointment to the medical staff

3. The definition of the qualifications and roles and responsibilities of department chairs if the organization functions with departments

4. Credentialing, privileging, and appointment processes

5. Related medical staff governance documents

Included in the standards are the following:

*   The definition of the criteria and qualifications for appointment to the medical staff

*   The qualifications and roles and responsibilities of the department chair

Table 16.1.   Useful links for medical staff quality and standards organizations

Organization	Web site
Accreditation Association for Ambulatory Health Care (AAAHC)	http://www.aaahc.org
Accreditation Council for Graduate Medical Education (ACGME)	http://www.acgme.org/acWebsite/home/home.asp
American Board of Medical Specialties (ABMS)	http://www.abms.org/
American Medical Association Masterfile request	http://www.ama-assn.org/ama/pub/about-ama/ physician-data-resources/physician-masterfile.page
American Osteopathic Association (AOA)	http://www.osteopathic.org
College of American Pathologists (CAP)	http://www.cap.org
Commission on Accreditation of Rehabilitation Facilities (CARF)	http://www.carf.org
Federation of State Medical Boards	http://www.fsmb.org
The Joint Commission	http://www.jointcommision.org
National Committee for Quality Assurance (NCQA)	http://www.ncqa.org
National Practitioner Data Bank and the Healthcare Integrity and Protection Data Bank	http://www.npdb-hipdb.hrsa.gov
National Quality Forum (NQF)	http://www.qualityforum.org/about/home.htm
URAC/American Accreditation Healthcare Commission	http://www.urac.org

- A description of the **medical staff executive committee** including the function, size, composition, and methods for selecting and removing its members and the medical staff officers

- A statement empowering the medical staff executive committee to act for the organized medical staff between meetings of the medical staff

- A description of indications for automatic suspension or summary suspension of a practitioner's medical staff membership and clinical privileges

- A description of when automatic suspension or summary suspension procedures are implemented

- A description of the mechanism to recommend medical staff membership or terminations, suspensions, or reductions in privileges

- A description of the mechanism for a fair hearing and appeal process

- A description of the credentialing and privileging processes

- A description of the process of appointment to membership of the medical staff

The standards require that the organized medical staff operate under the direction of the medical staff officers and a committee structure. The medical staff officers typically consist of a president, president-elect, chief of staff, and vice chief of staff, with the president-elect transitioning to president and the vice chief of staff transitioning to the chief of staff position. Depending on the size and organization of the medical staff, there might be an associate chief of staff for each department. In the case of multisite facilities with a common organized medical staff, there might be an associate chief of staff for each department from each facility that shares a common medical staff. This provides greater representation for the medical staff in larger facilities.

Often the president of the medical staff serves as the chair of the medical staff executive committee and presides over meetings of the general medical staff. By virtue of position, the president of the medical staff is typically a member of the hospital board and serves as a spokesperson for the medical staff in its public relations and external professional capacities. Additionally, the leadership of the medical staff consists of a chair of each clinical department and chairs of major medical staff committees. See figure 16.3 for a list of typical medical staff committees. The chair of each clinical department is usually an appointed position to minimize the pressures on this individual to enforce rules. The chair typically serves a term greater than one year and tends to be an established, experienced, and respected member of the medical staff.

Executive Committee

The Joint Commission requires that the medical staff executive committee be comprised of elected members of the medical staff who are authorized to act on behalf of the medical staff. Only those physicians who are medical doctors (MD), clinical psychologists, doctors of osteopathy (DO), or

Figure 16.3.   List of typical medical staff committees

• Medical staff executive committee	• Clinical oversight committee
• Credentials committee	• Health information and informatics management (HIM services) committee
• Bylaws committee	
• Continuing medical education (CME) committee	• Quality improvement committee
• Nominating committee	• Infection Control committee
• Professional affairs committee	• Pharmacy and therapeutics (P&T) committee

Note: These are hospitalwide medical staff committees. Each department typically has a medical staff department committee that conducts the business of the specific department.

oral surgeons and dentists (DDS) approved by the board for medical staff membership may serve as members of the medical staff executive committee and have voting rights. Others may belong to the committee as ex officio members without voting rights. An example of an ex officio member would be the organization CEO. The Joint Commission requires that hospitals who use Joint Commission accreditation for **deemed status** have a medical staff executive committee (The Joint Commission 2010, MS.02.01.01). Deemed status enables a healthcare organization that is Joint Commission accredited to use its accreditation status in lieu of a separate Medicare or Medicaid Conditions of Participation healthcare organization certification process. In small hospitals the entire medical staff may serve as the executive committee. Regardless of the size of the medical staff, the medical staff executive committee must follow the function and structure as described in the medical staff bylaws for the organization.

Categories of Medical Staff Membership

The medical staff bylaws describe the classifications or categories of medical staff membership. Table 16.2 details several typical categories. The distinction between categories of members of the medical staff is important since this defines the responsibilities and privileges of each member. Multiple categories of membership provide flexibility and allow for a larger pool of staff to assist with patient care needs. The organized medical staff defines the scope of practice via the privileges that are extended to practitioners.

The medical staff is comprised of those medical staff members who are granted permission or clinical privileges to provide care to patients in the hospital. The medical staff may be comprised of physicians, dentists, optometrists, pharmacists, podiatrists, and psychologists. There may be licensed independent practitioners such as physician assistants or nurse practitioners who are allowed by state laws and licensing regulations to practice without direction of a physician and may also be granted medical staff membership.

Table 16.2.   Classification (categories) of medical staff membership

Active (regular)	This category has all the responsibilities of medical staff membership and all the privileges. They can serve as medical staff officers and chair medical staff committees.
Associate	This category has all the responsibilities of medical staff membership and all the privileges. However, they cannot serve as medical staff officers or chair medical staff committees.
Courtesy	This category is reserved for those medical staff who have a primary clinical practice at another facility. It allows for a limited number of hospital admissions without the responsibilities of membership.
Consulting	This category is intended for those medical staff who do not admit patients but who serve as consultants to other members of the medical staff. They typically do not have to attend committee meetings and cannot serve as medical staff officers.
Honorary	This category is intended for those medical staff who practice very little and may not admit patients, but their reputation and previous service to the hospital is such that the hospital wishes to recognize their contribution.
Affiliate	This category is designated for those nonphysicians who are allowed to join the staff. There may be restrictions on what role these members have on committees and what, if any, voting privileges they have.

Medical Staff Credentialing

The landmark case *Darling v. Charleston Community Memorial Hospital* (as discussed in chapter 14) resulted in healthcare governing boards assuming responsibility for reviewing the qualifications of their medical staff through the processes of medical staff credentialing. **Credentialing** refers to the process of reviewing and validating the qualifications (degrees, licenses, and other credentials) of physicians and other licensed practitioners for granting medical staff membership to provide patient services. It provides a mechanism to:

1. Protect the public from professional incompetence

2. Protect the medical staff from working with incompetent professionals

3. Protect the facility from liability due to providing inadequate care

4. Protect the rights of the medical staff from unfair restrictions on their practice

A functional credentialing process results in the granting of privileges to practice at a site based on the practitioner's credentials. It protects the self-governance of the professional community and allows a medical staff to regulate its practices within a healthcare organization. Anyone who applies for medical staff privileges must go through the credentialing process maintained by the healthcare organization where they wish to practice. All healthcare providers are subject to the same credentialing process as defined by the organization's medical staff bylaws and employment criteria.

Other nonphysician allied health professionals (such as nurse anesthetists, occupational therapists, and physical therapists) who are not considered part of the medical staff may also go through the credentialing process depending on the policy of the healthcare organization. These individuals may be licensed through a state licensing board and in some cases professional certifications before they are allowed to practice in a given discipline. For the most part these individuals work under the direction and supervision of a physician. However, in some states nonphysician healthcare providers such as physical therapists are allowed to offer services without a physician's order. The ability to practice without physician oversight for some disciplines is seen as one way of lowering healthcare costs and addressing physician workforce shortages.

Check Your Understanding 16.1

Instructions: Indicate whether the following statements are true or false (T or F).

1. The medical staff has the ultimate responsibility for the quality and financial well-being of the health organization.

2. Medical staff bylaws are considered a contract and are legally binding in most states.

3. Joint Commission standards require that the medical staff bylaws address issues of self-governance and accountability to the governing board.

4. Credentialing is the process of reviewing and validating qualifications of practitioners for granting medical staff membership.

5. If a practitioner is assigned a medical staff category of "associate," he or she can chair the medical staff executive committee.

Joining the Medical Staff

Healthcare organizations must have rigorous processes in place to ensure that only competent, qualified physicians and other licensed independent practitioners are providing patient care. Hospitals and other healthcare organizations typically have a dedicated medical staff office or individual (medical staff coordinator) responsible for oversight of the credentialing and privileging processes. Joining the medical staff begins with a written application. The application for appointment and reappointment to the medical staff is usually a lengthy and detailed document that attempts to gather information about the medical education, training, and professional experiences of the practitioner. Common categories of information found on an application are listed in figure 16.4.

Primary Source Verification

Once the application is received, the process of verifying all the information begins. The practitioner is responsible for the accuracy, truthfulness, and completeness of the information on any medical staff credentialing or privileging application. Therefore, all practitioners are required to sign an attestation statement attesting to the accuracy, truthfulness, and completeness of the information they have provided on the application. Verification of practitioners' credentials is known as **primary source verification**. Credentialing standards of The Joint Commission and the **National Committee for Quality Assurance** (NCQA) require verification from the primary source of information on the medical staff application. An example would be obtaining an official certified transcript directly from the medical school, the primary source, rather than accepting an unofficial copy from the applicant.

Methods for conducting primary source verification of credentials may include direct correspondence, telephone verification, secure electronic verification from the original qualification source, and obtaining reports from a **credentials verification organization** (CVO). A CVO gathers and verifies the background, licensing, schooling, continuing education, and other performance measures of an applicant for a healthcare organization. However, the responsibility for ultimately granting privileges to a practitioner still rests with the medical staff and governing board of the healthcare organization.

Healthcare organizations also have a duty to share information on practitioners upon a legitimate request. In *Kadlec Medical Center v. Lakeview Anesthesia Associates*, the Louisiana Federal Court found that hospitals have a duty to disclose information about their current or former medical staff members to other healthcare providers in order to protect future patients when a physician moves on. This case has a significant impact on primary source verification because it is no longer sufficient to state that a physician once served on the medical staff; information regarding disciplinary action should include the same information as that reported to the National Practitioner Data Bank.

Figure 16.4.   Common categories of information on a medical staff application

• Personal information (including residence status)	• Licensure (active)
• Medical education	• Medical society memberships
• Formal medical training	• Board certification
—residency	• Other certifications
—fellowship	• Peer references
• Practice information	• Professional liability insurance
• Hospital affiliations	• Disclosure of conflicts of interest*
• Fellowship/teaching appointments	• Privileges requested and specialty

*The American Medical Association's policy, "Conflict of Interest Guidelines for Organized Medical Staffs," is available on their website.

Source: AMA 2005.

National Practitioner Data Bank

Title IV of Public Law 99-660, the Health Care Quality Act of 1986, as amended in 1998, created the **National Practitioner Data Bank** (NPDB) (42 USC 11101). As discussed in chapter 13, the NPDB is an information clearinghouse created by Congress to improve healthcare quality and reduce healthcare fraud and abuse. The NPDB receives and discloses information related to the professional competence, final adverse actions taken, and conduct of physicians, dentists, and other healthcare practitioners. When a facility evaluates a provider for privileges, it must query the data bank for adverse actions taken against practitioners including the revocation, suspension, or surrender of a license; payments made on behalf of physicians in connection with medical malpractice settlements or judgments; and adverse peer review decisions against licenses, clinical privileges, and professional society memberships. In addition, it must query the data bank every two years for all providers on staff (42 USC 11135(a)(1)(2)).

Office of the Inspector General

The medical staff office should also check the **Office of the Inspector General** (OIG) list of individuals and organizations that have been excluded from participation in Medicare, Medicaid, and all federal healthcare programs. A healthcare organization that knowingly hires an excluded provider may face civil monetary penalties. Some states also publish a list of providers excluded from state programs. This list should be referenced also.

Review of Credentials Documents

All credentialing documents are presented to the credentialing committee for review and recommendation. The recommendation is then presented to the medical staff executive committee, who recommends approval or disapproval to the board. The board has ultimate authority for the selection of medical staff members.

Determination of Clinical Privileges

The determination or delineation of clinical privileges is the process whereby the medical staff determines what clinical treatment and clinical procedures a practitioner is authorized to perform. The privileging decision is made by comparing the qualifications of the applicant with predetermined criteria deemed necessary to perform the privileges being requested. The processes for medical staff appointment and clinical privileges are typically the same, and a practitioner may apply for them simultaneously. In the 2010 Joint Commission *Comprehensive Accreditation Manual for Hospitals* (CAMH), there are six areas of "general competencies" developed by the **Accreditation Council for Graduate Medical Education** (ACGME) and the **American Board of Medical Specialties** (ABMS), which should be incorporated into the comprehensive evaluation of a practitioner's professional practice. These "general competencies" include patient care, medical/clinical knowledge, practice-based learning and improvement, interpersonal and communication skills, professionalism and systems-based practice (The Joint Commission 2010, MS.06.01.01).

The 2010 CAMH also includes concepts of **focused professional practice evaluation** and **ongoing professional practice evaluation**. Focused evaluation is defined as a time-limited period during which an organization evaluates and determines a practitioner's professional performance of privileges. It will occur in all requests for new privileges and when there are concerns regarding the provision of safe, high-quality care by a current medical staff member. Ongoing evaluation refers to documenting data on credentialed staff on an ongoing basis rather than at the two-year reappointment process. These two evaluations encourage the medical staff to create continuous evaluations of performance. The board is ultimately responsible for ensuring that medical staff members are qualified, and it may be held liable for the negligent acts of its practitioners. Healthcare facilities have a duty to select competent practitioners and to protect patients from the negligent acts of practitioners.

Medical Staff Duties and Rights

One of the responsibilities of medical staff membership is the duty or obligation to provide patient care, treatment, and service as needed to patients. Physicians are allowed access to hospital facilities to admit and render treatment to their patients. As a result, the physician must respond to calls from the emergency department regarding patients and provide consultation services, when appropriate, for patients regardless of their payer source. This means that a physician must treat patients with whom he or she does not have an established relationship and who may or may not have the capacity to pay the hospital or the physician. This is a potential area for sanctions if members of the medical staff refuse to take calls or do not provide the appropriate level of care to patients. Facilities that use Joint Commission accreditation for deemed status are required to have a doctor of medicine or osteopathy on duty at all times (The Joint Commission 2010, MS.03.01.03).

The frequency of physician or other healthcare provider on-call time is typically established by clinical department rules and may vary based on the categories of the medical staff. For example, a physician classified as an active member of the medical staff may be required to be on call on a regular schedule, whereas a physician classified as courtesy may not be required to take call. The trade-off for these categories is that physicians with greater rights also have greater responsibilities, and vice versa. The physician classified as courtesy may be able to admit only five patients per year while the physician classified as an active member of the medical staff may have an unlimited ability to admit patients.

Additional responsibilities of active members of the medical staff include service on medical staff committees. There may be standing committees such as the credentials committee, performance improvement committee, infection committee, critical care committee, and other functional committees to improve patient care quality and safety. Attendance is required at medical staff meetings, and a member of the medical staff office typically coordinates and records attendance at these meetings. A physician who misses too many meetings, as delineated in the medical staff bylaws, is reported to the department chair along with the chair of the committee. The medical staff bylaws typically include a progressive discipline plan for physicians who either do not attend meetings or do not meet other obligations as specified in the medical staff bylaws.

In teaching facilities members of the medical staff are required to supervise fellows, residents, and interns. The medical staff must define the responsibility of the licensed independent provider who has responsibility for the professional graduate education program. Medical staff rules, policies, procedures, or bylaws must designate participants in professional graduate education programs who may write patient care orders, and what entries require countersignature by the supervising licensed independent practitioner (The Joint Commission 2010, MS.04.01.01).

Health Record Integrity and Documentation Requirements

There is generally a medical staff committee responsible for patient record issues, including electronic health records (EHRs). Individual medical staff members must adhere to bylaws related to timely completion of health records as well as documentation guidelines and requirements. This also supports an organization's patient safety and quality efforts and helps to minimize legal risk and vulnerability to lawsuits. Overall, the concern is that failure to document may compromise patient care.

Typical medical staff bylaws provide for timely completion of health records, including legibility requirements (or, alternatively, use of the institution's EHR or health information system to record patient notes); communication and coordination of care with other members of the staff; and completion of reports of history and physical examinations, operative notes, and other required documents based on best practices and facility policies. Failure to comply with any of the provisions of health record documentation may result in progressive discipline up to and including suspension of medical staff membership. Information about incomplete and delinquent records is typically reported by the HIM department during committee meetings. Because of this, it is important to acknowledge the medical staff bylaws, Joint Commission standards, Medicare and Medicaid Conditions of Participation, state statutes, and other facility licensure requirements regarding the documentation requirements and timely completion of health records.

Disciplinary Actions and Suspension

Physicians and other healthcare providers agree to adhere to the bylaws in order to have access to healthcare facility resources including the operating room, emergency department, cardiac catheterization lab, radiology services, and other equipment and personnel that assist him or her in the diagnosis and treatment of patients. Physicians who have patient performance issues and noncompliant documentation practices (for example, incomplete documentation or inappropriate references in the health record to patients and staff in the health record) may face disciplinary action.

Hospitals typically have procedures to notify the admissions department, surgical care department, and other key hospital departments when a practitioner's privileges are suspended. Depending on their staff privileges, suspension limits or restricts the ability of healthcare providers to admit patients or schedule time in the operating room. Hospital bylaws should prohibit the practice of partners admitting patients on behalf of the suspended physician. Admission patterns should be reviewed to ensure that suspended physicians are following the suspension regulations set forth in the bylaws. Any adverse action against a practitioner's medical staff membership or clinical privileges is a reportable event to the NPDB. The medical staff services office typically communicates this action to the NPDB.

Due Process

In healthcare employment and medical staff privileges, the right to liberty and property may be applied to one's ability to make a living. Thus, due process is required in hiring, disciplinary process, or other actions that affect a practitioner's medical staff privileges or employment. Due process of law is inherent in the US Constitution and Bill of Rights. There are two elements of due process (Showalter 2008).

1. **Substantive due process**—guarantees that laws are fair, reasonable, and not arbitrary; allows for challenges to a law's content and substance.

2. **Procedural due process**—applies due process to the federal and state governments; provides that the government shall not take a person's life, liberty, or property without due process of law. Procedural due process intends fair processes and procedures.

Due process places restrictions on governments and public facilities (for example, Veterans Administration hospitals), and it also may apply to private organizations that perform public functions or have significant government involvement. Such organizations are involved in **state action**.

Government funding of healthcare organizations has not traditionally constituted state action, but courts are broadening the scope to apply due process requirements to private organizations. Further, statutes and regulations hold private organizations to governmental due process standards. Examples of this are Title VII of the Civil Rights Act, which prohibits discrimination of certain federally protected classes in employment, and the Medicare Conditions of Participation. Although not law, Joint Commission standards also compel procedural due process among private healthcare facilities.

While due process is a hallmark of the US court system, the legal system as a whole is increasingly requiring that it be exercised outside of the court system by companies and other entities. In many cases, both public and private entities must apply due process through various sources of law: the Constitution, statutory law, administrative regulations, or judicial precedent.

In healthcare organizations, conflicts related to employment and medical staff privileges (for example, termination of employment or adverse credentialing) are resolved through internal procedures that exercise due process. Such procedures allow for notice and the opportunity to be heard through a fair hearing in which the individual can voice objections to the organization's proposed actions. Due process should be evident in the facility's policies and procedures and the medical staff bylaws.

In addition to due process, consideration must be given to antitrust laws in the granting or denial of medical staff privileges in order to avoid anticompetitive conduct that violates antitrust laws. As addressed in chapter 6, activities such as favoring or excluding entire categories of practitioners and drafting excessively restrictive noncompete agreements may draw legal scrutiny. Organizations must also consider the appropriateness of **economic credentialing** (also discussed in chapter 6), where medical staff privileges are granted or denied based on financial indicators rather than factors related to clinical performance.

Check Your Understanding 16.2

Instructions: Indicate whether the following statements are true or false (T or F).

1. The process for verifying the credentials of a physician who wishes to join a medical staff is referred to as primary source verification.

2. A healthcare organization does not have a duty to share information on a practitioner upon legitimate request.

3. The National Practitioner Data Bank enables a healthcare facility to check on the background of a practitioner to determine if the practitioner has had his or her license to practice suspended for any reason.

4. An adverse action against a physician is not reportable to the National Practitioner Data Bank.

5. Due process is required in the hiring and disciplinary process that affects a practitioner's medical staff privileges or employment.

Summary

The medical staff is comprised of those medical staff members who are granted clinical privileges to provide care to patients in the hospital. The medical staff may be comprised of physicians and others such as dentists, optometrists, pharmacists, podiatrists, and psychologists. It may also include licensed independent practitioners (LIPs) such as physician assistants or nurse practitioners who are allowed by state licensing laws to practice without the direction of a physician. The requirements for an organized medical staff are found in hospital licensure standards as well as in The Joint Commission accreditation standards. The medical staff is governed by bylaws, which are typically voted upon by the medical staff and approved by the healthcare organization's governing board, which must ensure that the medical staff is competent to treat patients. The bylaws explain the application process for admission to a medical staff, which includes a credentialing process whereby the education and background of the applicant is verified as true. The bylaws describe the categories of medical staff, membership that may be granted to an individual who has successfully passed the credentialing process. The bylaws also define the duties and responsibilities of the medical staff, which includes delivering quality patient care and documenting care rendered. Issues arising from poor patient performance, inaccurate or incomplete documentation, or noncompliance with bylaws may subject the medical staff member to disciplinary action. However, due process of the law must be taken into consideration regarding the denial of medical staff privileges, including the denial of an individual's initial application for privileges. Health information management and informatics professionals as well as administrators and others involved in the delivery of healthcare must be cognizant of laws and standards that constitute the actions of a medical staff as defined by medical staff bylaws. An understanding of the bylaws and one's role in supporting them will help to diminish overall legal risk to an organization.

References

The Joint Commission. 2010 (September). *Comprehensive Accreditation Manual for Hospitals (CAMH)*. Oakbrook Terrace, IL: Joint Commission.

Showalter, Stuart. 2008. *The Law of Healthcare Administration*, 5th ed. Chicago: Health Administration Press.

Cases, Statutes, and Regulations Cited

Darling v. Charleston Community Memorial Hospital, 33 IL 2d 326, 211 N.E.2d 253, 14 A.L.R.3d 860 (IL Sep 29, 1965).

Kadlec Medical Center v. Lakeview Anesthesia Associates, No. Civ.A. 04-0997 (E.D.La. May 19, 2005).

42 USC 11101: Health Care Quality Improvement Act of 1986.

42 USC 11135(a)(1)(2): Duty of hospitals to obtain information.

Pub.L. 99-660. The Healthcare Quality Improvement Act of 1986, amended 1998.

Chapter 17

Workplace Law

**Rebecca Reynolds, EdD, MHA, RHIA, FAHIMA, and
Melanie S. Brodnik, PhD, RHIA, FAHIMA**

Learning Objectives

- Identify the major laws related to discrimination in the work setting

- Describe the components of the Federal Labor Standards Act and related laws in regard to wages, overtime, compensation, and benefits

- Discuss the concept of unions and their relationship to healthcare workers

- Discuss the components of the Occupational Safety and Health Act

Key Terms

Age Discrimination in
　Employment Act of 1967
Americans with Disabilities
　Act of 1990
Arbitration
Benefits
Collective bargaining
Compensation
Consolidated Omnibus Budget
　Reconciliation Act of 1986
　(COBRA)
Employee Retirement Income
　Security Act of 1974
　(ERISA)
Equal Employment
　Opportunity Act of 1972
　(EEOA)

Equal Employment
　Opportunity Commission
　(EEOC)
Equal Pay Act of 1963
Exempt employee
Fair Labor Standards Act of
　1938 (FLSA)
Genetic Information
　Nondiscrimination Act of
　2008 (GINA)
Grievance procedure
Immigration Reform and
　Control Act of 1986
Labor-Management Relations
　Act of 1947
Limited English proficiency
　(LEP)

National Labor Relations Act
　of 1935 (Wagner Act)
National Labor Relations
　Board (NLRB)
Nonexempt employee
Pregnancy Discrimination Act
　of 1973
Title VII of the Civil Rights
　Act of 1964
Uniform Guidelines on
　Employee Selection
　Procedures
Union steward

Introduction

The healthcare industry is very complex and operates within the constraints of numerous laws and standards designed to support the delivery and financing of quality healthcare while protecting the rights and responsibilities of healthcare consumers and providers. The delivery of quality healthcare depends on personnel or human resources who "do no harm" and "do the right thing." Human resources are protected in the workplace by employment laws that function to protect both employee and employer. "Laws that address the workplace are rooted in the essential value system of the United States, which includes the right to privacy, freedom from discrimination, the right to self-determination and the opportunity to live and work in a safe environment" (Fried and Fottler 2008, 100). The goal of workplace law is to strike a balance between employee and employer that protects the employee from personal injury, prejudice, duress, and unwanted sexual advances while allowing the employer to pursue desired business outcomes (Fried and Fottler 2008). Federal employment laws deal with employee-employer issues, whereas federal labor laws often refer to employer-union issues or other labor protections.

Managing department staff requires an understanding of the federal and state laws that govern employment. Most healthcare organizations have a human resources department or someone dedicated to human resources oversight who can assist managers in ensuring that proper labor practices are in place. This chapter provides an overview of common workplace laws. The civil rights of employees are discussed in terms of discrimination related to age, color, national origin, race, religion, and sex. Wage and salary regulations are introduced along with employee occupational and safety laws. The chapter closes with a discussion of fair labor practices and laws related to union activity and collective bargaining.

Discrimination and Related Laws

Discrimination laws focus on issues that protect applicants and employees from discrimination in all aspects of employment. The United States **Equal Employment Opportunity Commission** (EEOC) is responsible for enforcing federal laws that prohibit discriminating against a job applicant or employee on the basis of:

- Age
- Disability
- Equal pay/Compensation
- Genetic information
- National origin
- Pregnancy
- Race/Color
- Religion
- Retaliation
- Sex
- Sexual harassment

In addition, the EEOC oversees discrimination or retaliation against an individual who has complained about discrimination, filed a charge of discrimination, or participated in an employment discrimination investigation or lawsuit (EEOC n.d.a). The laws apply to all types of work situations, as listed in figure 17.1. The EEOC enforces laws, works to prevent discrimination, and

Figure 17.1. Illegal discriminatory workplace practices

Under Title VII of the Civil Rights Act of 1964, the Americans with Disabilities Act, and the Age Discrimination in Employment Act, it is illegal to discriminate in any aspect of employment, including:

- Hiring and firing
- Compensation, assignment, or classification of employees
- Transfer, promotion, layoff, or recall
- Job advertisements
- Recruitment
- Testing
- Use of company facilities
- Training and apprenticeship programs
- Fringe benefits
- Pay, retirement plans, and disability leave
- Other terms and conditions of employment

Discriminatory practices under these laws also include:

- Harassment on the basis of race, color, religion, sex, national origin, disability, or age
- Retaliation against an individual for filing a charge of discrimination, participating in an investigation, or opposing discriminatory practices
- Employment decisions based on stereotypes or assumptions about the abilities, traits, or performance of individuals of a certain sex, race, age, religion, or ethnic group or individuals with disabilities
- Denying employment opportunities to a person because of marriage to, or association with, an individual of a particular race, religion, or national origin or an individual with a disability. Title VII also prohibits discrimination because of participation in schools or places of worship associated with a particular racial, ethnic, or religious group

Source: EEOC Discriminatory Practices 2004.

investigates job discrimination complaints. The **Equal Employment Opportunity Act of 1972 (EEOA)** gives the EEOC authority to sue in federal courts when there is reasonable cause to believe discrimination has occurred. If a complaint cannot be settled, the EEOC can file a federal lawsuit against the employer. EEOC complaints are generally handled through field offices at the state or local agency level.

To assist employers in the hiring process and to help alleviate potential discrimination issues related to hiring, the EEOC (n.d.b) publishes **Uniform Guidelines on Employee Selection Procedures**. The overriding principle is that employee selection must be made on qualifications related to job performance.

An overview of discrimination laws follows.

Civil Rights Act and Related Acts

Title VII of the Civil Rights Act, passed in 1964, and as amended by the EEOA, prohibits discrimination based on age, race, color, national origin, sex, religion, age, disability, political beliefs, and marital or familial status. The EEOC was created and implemented as part of the Civil Rights Act for the purpose of enforcing laws against discrimination as discussed above. The Civil Rights Act prohibits not only *intentional discrimination* but also *practices* that have the effect of discriminating against individuals because of their race, color, national origin, religion, or sex. In 1991, the Civil Rights Act was expanded to authorize compensatory and punitive damages in cases of intentional discrimination (EEOC n.d.a).

Age Discrimination

Age discrimination involves treating an applicant or employee less favorably because of age. The **Age Discrimination in Employment Act of 1967** (29 USC 621-34) protects individuals 40 years and older; however, some states have laws that protect younger workers. Age discrimination applies to any aspect or terms of employment (hiring, promotion, discharge, pay, fringe **benefits**, job training, and classification referral). It also includes harassing someone (verbally or in writing) because of his or her age or condoning a hostile or offensive work environment (EEOC n.d.c).

Disability Discrimination

Disability discrimination occurs when an employer treats someone with a disability unfavorably because of the disability. The **Americans with Disabilities Act of 1990** protects individuals with disabilities, which are broadly defined to include physical conditions, psychological conditions, contagious diseases, substance abuse, and other conditions. Employees must be able to perform the necessary functions of a job with "reasonable accommodations." Reasonable accommodations include modifications to the workplace or conditions of employment so that a worker with a disability can perform the job (EEOC n.d.d). Accommodations include auxiliary aids for individuals who are deaf or hard of hearing or who are blind (HHS Office for Civil Rights 2006). See table 17.1 for examples of auxiliary aids.

Equal Pay

The **Equal Pay Act of 1963** amended the **Fair Labor Standards Act of 1938** (FLSA), which will be discussed in more detail later in the chapter. The Equal Pay Act (29 USC 206(d)) made it illegal to pay workers differently on the basis of sex. It regulates the concept of equal pay for men and women who perform similar work requiring similar skills, effort, and responsibility under similar working conditions. These four compensable factors are compared to ensure that pay is equal (EEOC n.d.e).

Genetics

Title II of the **Genetic Information Nondiscrimination Act of 2008** (GINA) prohibits health insurers and employers from discriminating against an individual or employee on the basis of genetic information in hiring, promotion, discharge, pay, fringe benefits, job training, classification, referral, and other aspects of employment. GINA restricts access and disclosure of genetic information, as discussed in chapter 12. Genetic information includes information about an individual's genetic tests, family members' genetic tests, and manifestation of diseases or disorders in family members (family medical history); requests for or receipt of genetic services; or participation in research

Table 17.1. Workplace auxiliary aids for people with hearing and sight disabilities

• Assistive listening headset	• Taped text
• Braille materials	• Telecommunications devices for the deaf
• Large-print materials	• Television captioning and decoders
• Qualified interpreter	• Videotext displays
• Readers	

Source: HHS Office for Civil Rights 2006.

that includes genetic services by an applicant, employee, or his or her family members (29 CFR 1635.3(c)(1)).

National Origin

Discrimination based on national origin refers to treating someone differently because he or she is from a certain part of the country or world. The EEOC (n.d.f) states the following regarding national origin:

> It is illegal to discriminate against an individual because of birthplace, ancestry, culture, or linguistic characteristics common to a specific ethnic group. A rule requiring that employees speak only English on the job may violate Title VII unless an employer shows that the requirement is necessary for conducting business. If the employer believes such a rule is necessary, employees must be informed when English is required and the consequences for violating the rule.
>
> The **Immigration Reform and Control Act of 1986** require employers to assure that employees hired are legally authorized to work in the U.S. However, an employer who requests employment verification only for individuals of a particular national origin, or individuals who appear to be or sound foreign, may violate both the Civil Rights Act and Immigration Reform and Control Act; verification must be obtained from all applicants and employees. Employers who impose citizenship requirements or give preferences to U.S. citizens in hiring or employment opportunities also may violate this act.

Related to discrimination and national origin, Title VI of the Civil Rights Act emphasizes that no person, because of race, color, or national origin, should be excluded from participation in or discriminated against by any program receiving federal financial assistance. While the focus of Title VI is on persons with **limited English proficiency** (LEP), aspects of the law are applicable to employees as well. Title VI applies to any healthcare organization or entity that receives federal funding. The Department of Health and Human Services (HHS) provides LEP guidance to healthcare organizations in determining how to comply with Title VI, including the obligation to translate vital materials such as informed consents for LEP persons. It suggests healthcare organizations take steps to ensure that interpreters are available upon request and that they understand issues of privacy, confidentiality, and security of patient information (HHS Office for Civil Rights 2004).

Sex and Sexual Harassment

It is unlawful to discriminate on the basis of sex (gender) in any aspect of employment. The term "sex" in the Civil Rights Act was expanded by the **Pregnancy Discrimination Act of 1973**, which prohibits discrimination against pregnancy, childbirth, or related medical conditions. These conditions must be handled like any other medical condition, and the individual must be afforded the same protections that would be granted a nonpregnant person in terms of accommodations, if necessary.

The EEOC (n.d.g) defines sexual harassment as unwelcome sexual advances, requests for sexual favors, and other verbal or physical harassment of a sexual nature. When unwanted sexual action by one individual to another interferes with work performance by creating an intimidating, hostile, or offensive work environment, a claim of sexual harassment may be made. The harasser may be a man or a woman and can be a supervisor, co-worker, or nonemployee or other agent of the organization. If sexual harassment is reported, the employer must take action in order to avoid legal risk.

Check Your Understanding 17.1

Instructions: Indicate whether the following statements are true or false (T or F).

1. The EEOC enforces laws that protect the employer from poor job applicants.

2. The Age Discrimination in Employment Act of 1967 protects individuals 40 years and older from being discriminated against in the employment setting.

3. If an employee discovers he is carrying the gene that causes colon cancer, his insurance company can deny him insurance.

4. A hospital has the right to deny employment to an applicant from another country if the applicant does not speak English.

5. Employers must handle the conditions of pregnancy and childbirth, or related medical conditions, in the same manner as they handle medical conditions afforded an individual who is not pregnant.

Labor Laws

In addition to the employment laws related to an employee's civil rights and protection against discrimination, there are labor laws designed to protect employees' rights to a safe and healthful work environment. These laws address wages and overtime, compensation and benefits, and union activity.

Wages and Overtime

The Fair Labor Standards Act (29 USC 201) has been amended a number of times since its original enactment in 1938. It addresses minimum wage and overtime pay as related to private and public employment. It also sets standards that prescribe the age limitations on hiring children. For example, it restricts the number of hours a child under the age of 16 can work and forbids children under the age of 18 to work in jobs identified as too dangerous. The act sets the minimum wage standard and defines which employees may be exempt from the standards. **Exempt employees** include individuals identified as professionals, administrators, or salespeople. Managers and supervisors are generally considered exempt employees as well. **Nonexempt employees** must be paid at least the minimum wage up to 40 hours, and time and a half for any hours worked over 40. Accurate time records must be kept. Healthcare facilities have much flexibility because of the scheduling of healthcare workers such as nurses.

According to Fottler, Hernandez, and Joiner (1998, 23):

> The laws prohibiting discrimination in employment do not require everyone to treat everyone in the same manner. Rather, an employer may treat applicants or employees differently based on factors unrelated to an individual's protected status. Examples of business reasons include experience, objective qualifications, subjective behavior, length of service and quality and quantity of work, attendance or any other factor that relates to job performance.

Compensation and Benefits

Compensation is a complex issue and includes all direct and indirect pay. In addition to wages and mandatory benefits such as unemployment insurance and workers' compensation, the types of benefits offered to employees may vary but include:

- Medical insurance

- Dental insurance

- Life insurance

- Accidental death insurance

- Short- and long-term disability

- Child care

- Elder care

- Retirement plans

- Longevity pay

These benefits are often included in a flexible benefits plan or cafeteria plan, which allows employees to choose from among the listed benefits.

Retirement plans are governed by federal law. The **Employee Retirement Income Security Act of 1974** (ERISA) (29 USC 1001 et seq.) sets minimum standards for most voluntarily established pension and health plans in private industry to provide protection for individuals in these plans.

Insurance benefits are also governed by federal laws and regulations. The **Consolidated Omnibus Budget Reconciliation Act of 1986** (COBRA 1986) provides continued health insurance for a certain period of time for those who have lost coverage because of termination (except for gross misconduct). The Department of Labor (n.d.) website states one of the major purposes of the Health Insurance Portability and Accountability Act of 1996 (HIPAA) is as follows:

HIPAA provides rights and protections for participants and beneficiaries in group health plans. HIPAA includes protections for coverage under group health plans that limit exclusions for preexisting conditions; prohibit discrimination against employees and dependents based on their health status; and allow a special opportunity to enroll in a new plan to individuals in certain circumstances. HIPAA may also give you a right to purchase individual coverage if you have no group health plan coverage available, and have exhausted COBRA or other continuation coverage.

Unions

According to the US Department of Labor's Bureau of Labor Statistics report for 2010, 11.9 percent of employed wage and salary workers were union members, down from 12.3 percent a year earlier. The total number of unionized workers in 2010 was 14.7 million, with 9.2 percent of those union members listed in the category of healthcare support occupations (Department of Labor Bureau of Labor Statistics 2011). Members include all types of healthcare workers, such as nurses, physicians, and those who work in departments such as health information management (HIM).

Unions that represent healthcare workers include the Service Employees International Union (SEIU); the American Federation of State, County and Municipal Employees (AFSCME), which represents healthcare workers in public healthcare facilities; the American Federation of Teachers (AFT) healthcare division; and the Teamsters Union healthcare division. Examples of issues for healthcare workers are minimum staffing, overtime pay, and recruitment as well as other contract issues common to all types of workers. With the increasing number of healthcare workers, the healthcare arena is a focus area for growth for unions, especially with the decline in blue-collar membership. Employees join and support unions because they feel a need to protect their jobs and want a formal method of communicating with management. Wages and benefits are commonly the primary issues for negotiation between management and unionized employees.

The **National Labor Relations Act of 1935** (NLRA; also known as the Wagner Act) (29 USC 151-169) regulates union and employer relations in the private sector. Section 7 of the act gives employees the right to self-organize and to form, join, or assist labor organizations. It allows employees to bargain collectively through whomever they choose as their representative and to engage in other activities for mutual aid protection. The law was expanded by the **Labor-Management Relations Act of 1947** (29 USC 141 et seq.), which amended the Wagner Act to prohibit unfair labor practices on the part of unions and to allow the president of the United States to stop strikes in cases that might impact national health and safety.

While the act established worker rights related to union activity and membership, it also identified behaviors considered to be unfair labor practices. For example, employers cannot keep employees from forming or joining a union, and employers must bargain with union representatives in good faith. See table 17.2 for a list of worker rights and unfair labor practices.

Table 17.2.   Worker rights and unfair labor practices

Private Sector Workers Rights
• Organize a union to negotiate with your employer concerning your wages, hours, and other terms and conditions of employment.
• Form, join or assist a union.
• Bargain collectively through representatives of employees' own choosing for a contract with your employer setting your wages, benefits, hours, and other working conditions.
• Discuss your terms and conditions of employment or union organizing with your co-workers or a union.
• Take action with one or more co-workers to improve your working conditions by, among other means, raising work-related complaints directly with your employer or with a government agency, and seeking help from a union.
• Strike and picket, depending on the purpose or means of the strike or the picketing.
• Choose not to do any of these activities, including joining or remaining a member of a union.

Unfair Labor Practices—Employer	Unfair Labor Practices—Union
• Prohibit you from soliciting for a union during non-work time, such as before or after work or during break times; or from distributing union literature during non-work time, in non-work areas, such as parking lots or break rooms.	• Threaten you that you will lose your job unless you support the union.
• Question you about your union support or activities in a manner that discourages you from engaging in that activity.	• Refuse to process a grievance because you have criticized union officials or because you are not a member of the union.
• Fire, demote, or transfer you, or reduce your hours or change your shift, or otherwise take adverse action against you, or threaten to take any of these actions, because you join or support a union, or because you engage in concerted activity for mutual aid and protection, or because you choose not to engage in any such activity.	• Use or maintain discriminatory standards or procedures in making job referrals from a hiring hall.
• Threaten to close your workplace if workers choose a union to represent them.	• Cause or attempt to cause an employer to discriminate against you because of your union-related activity.
• Promise or grant promotions, pay raises, or other benefits to discourage or encourage union support.	• Take other adverse action against you based on whether you have joined or support the union.
• Prohibit you from wearing union hats, buttons, t-shirts, and pins in the workplace except under special circumstances.	
• Spy on or videotape peaceful union activities and gatherings or pretend to do so.	

Source: Department of Labor National Labor Relations Board n.d.

National Labor Relations Board

The **National Labor Relations Board** (NLRB) is an independent federal agency that safeguards employees' rights to engage in union activity. It oversees union elections and handles unfair labor practices committed by private sector employers and unions. For many years, healthcare organizations were not included under the NLRA, because of the concern that healthcare services could be disrupted. The NLRB assumed jurisdiction over hospitals in 1974. Sometimes the union represents more people in the organization than those who actually pay dues and are members of the union.

Labor unions exist in many healthcare facilities, and the administration and unions must work together in collaboration. The person most responsible for the operation of the union contract on a day-to-day basis is the supervisor, and training of supervisors and departmental management is important to ensure good relationships between employees and management while providing effective and efficient patient care. When union organizing begins in an organization, there are regulations about what can be done. An election following NLRB regulations is conducted to determine whether a union will be authorized to bargain and negotiate a labor contract with the management, as well as which employees will be part of the bargaining unit that will be covered. The contract spells out details of the relationship between management and the employees. According to Dunn (2006), contracts deal with matters such as union recognition, management rights, union security, wages, conditions, hours of work, vacations, holidays, leaves of absence, seniority, promotions, and similar terms and conditions of employment. Pension issues and healthcare benefits are important in today's climate as employers attempt to lower their expenditures for employees and retirees.

Collective Bargaining

During **collective bargaining**, a contract is negotiated that sets forth the relationship between the employees and the healthcare organization. In a unionized facility, management must be very careful to abide by the contract in matters of discipline when employees do not follow the organization's rules and in handling employee grievances or complaints. The human resources department is available to assist, but the manager is responsible for the daily activities of the department. The manager will work closely with the union steward to handle disciplinary issues.

Every healthcare organization will have some type of **grievance procedure** to handle situations such as violation of a work rule or other condition of employment. This procedure begins with the employee and the supervisor. In a unionized environment, a **union steward** represents the employee. It is important for supervisors and management to know the grievance procedure and to be trained in how to handle disciplinary issues. Issues may relate to insubordination or refusal to obey orders, absenteeism, failure to follow work rules, and so on. Good recordkeeping will provide the information needed to back up supervisory actions. The employee has the right to due process (as discussed in chapter 16), which means that employers must be sure that procedural requirements spelled out in either the personnel procedure manual or the union contract are followed. Issues that are not settled may be submitted to **arbitration** (hearings by a third party).

Downsizing and Layoffs

Another issue that must be handled carefully is downsizing or layoffs. Seniority is protected by most union contracts and has become a problem in healthcare organizations with poorly written job descriptions. In a layoff issue, for example, a cafeteria worker with more seniority could bump a clerical employee in the HIM department. Job descriptions are important tools of management, but in a unionized system with seniority protections, qualifications including specific experience must be included in job descriptions.

State Laws

State labor laws may be fashioned after federal labor laws, or a state law may establish its own version of the law. Many states have enacted "right to work" laws that specify that a worker does not have to join a labor union to keep or land a job. Federal labor law is considered minimum law. A state may enact stricter labor laws or labor laws that go beyond the federal laws. If the state law is considered stricter than the federal law, the state law will preempt the federal law.

Employee Safety

In 1970 Congress passed the Occupational Safety and Health Act (29 CFR 1910) to help employers reduce injuries, illnesses, and deaths on the job. The act established the Occupational Safety and Health Administration (OSHA) under the auspices of the Department of Labor for the purpose of providing leadership in occupational safety and health. OSHA is responsible for setting and enforcing workplace safety standards, and providing information, training, and assistance to employers and workers, as summarized in figure 17.2 (Department of Labor Occupational Safety and Health Administration 2006). OSHA regulations enable states to seek approval from OSHA to administer their own occupational safety and health programs at the state level. At least 25 states have approved plans.

OSHA works closely with the Centers for Disease Control (CDC) in identifying best practices for the management of diseases and injuries that may affect employees in the workplace. OSHA standards and CDC guidelines for conditions or situations commonly found in healthcare settings that may affect healthcare workers include numerous hazardous chemicals, equipment, and waste products—for example, hazardous chemicals or equipment used in laboratories and radiology and waste products like body fluids and tissues related to patient treatment. The standards and guidelines spell out in detail how such products are to be handled as well as what employers must communicate to healthcare workers regarding the safety and disposal of the products.

Because of healthcare workers' increased exposure to viruses, microorganisms such as human immunodeficiency virus (HIV) and hepatitis viruses B and C, and other bloodborne pathogens, the Occupational Exposure to Bloodborne Pathogens standard (29 CFR 1910.1030) was enacted in 1991. Subsequently, in 2001 Congress passed the Needlestick Safety and Prevention Act (2001), which directed OSHA to revise the bloodborne pathogen standard to require employers to establish an exposure control plan that includes controls to eliminate or minimize employee risk as a result of a needlestick (Department of Labor Occupational Safety and Health Administration 2001).

Figure 17.2. OSHA responsibilities

- Encourages employers and employees to reduce workplace hazards and to implement new safety and health management systems or improve existing programs
- Develops mandatory job safety and health standards and enforces them through worksite inspections, and, sometimes, by imposing citations, penalties, or both
- Promotes safe and healthful work environments through cooperative programs including the Voluntary Protection Programs, OSHA Strategic Partnerships, and Alliances
- Establishes responsibilities and rights for employers and employees to achieve better safety and health conditions
- Supports the development of innovative ways of dealing with workplace hazards
- Establishes requirements for injury and illness recordkeeping by employers, and for employer monitoring of certain occupational illnesses
- Establishes training programs to increase the competence of occupational safety and health personnel
- Provides technical and compliance assistance, and training and education to help employers reduce worker accidents and injuries
- Works in partnership with states that operate their own occupational safety and health programs
- Supports the consultation programs offered by all 50 states, the District of Columbia, Puerto Rico, Guam, Northern Mariana Islands, and the Virgin Islands

Employer Responsibility and Employee Rights

Employers have a duty under OSHA standards to provide employees with a safe working environment, especially in a healthcare setting. Noncompliance with the standards puts employers at risk for violations resulting in citations and fines. Employees also have a duty to comply with OSHA standards and report problems, follow safety rules, and wear protective equipment if required to do so. Employers and employees may appeal negative decisions under certain situations. Overall, employers must (Department of Labor Occupational Safety and Health Administration 2011):

- Follow all relevant OSHA safety and health standards

- Find and correct safety and health hazards

- Inform employees about chemical hazards through training, labels, alarms, color-coded systems, chemical information sheets, and other methods

- Notify OSHA within eight hours of a workplace fatality or when three or more workers are hospitalized

- Provide required personal protective equipment at no cost to workers

- Keep accurate records of work-related injuries and illnesses

- Post OSHA citations, injury and illness summary data, and the OSHA "Job Safety and Health—It's the Law" poster in the workplace where workers will see them

- Not discriminate or retaliate against any worker for using his or her rights under the law

OSHA requires employers to keep detailed records on all safety issues. Recordkeeping requirements are defined in the 2001 Occupational Injury and Illness Recording and Reporting Requirements ("the Recordkeeping rule"). In 2005, OSHA published *OSHA Recordkeeping Handbook*, which discusses the regulations and related interpretations for recording and reporting occupational injuries and illnesses.

Under OSHA, employees have the right to (Department of Labor Occupational Safety and Health Administration 2011):

- Working conditions that do not pose a risk of serious harm

- Receive information and training (in a language workers can understand) about chemical and other hazards, methods to prevent harm, and OSHA standards that apply to their workplace

- Review records of work-related injuries and illnesses

- Get copies of test results done to find and measure hazards in the workplace

- File a complaint asking OSHA to inspect their workplace if they believe there is a serious hazard or that their employer is not following OSHA rules. When requested, OSHA will keep all identities confidential

- Use their rights under the law without retaliation or discrimination. If an employee is fired, demoted, transferred, or discriminated against in any way for using their rights under the law, they can file a complaint with OSHA. This complaint must be filed within 30 days of the alleged discrimination

OSHA Inspections

OSHA inspections are usually unannounced; however, under special circumstances, an employer may be given a 24-hour notice of a pending inspection. An employee's representative must also be informed of the advance notice by the employer or OSHA. Circumstances that warrant an advance notice include the following (Department of Labor Occupational Safety and Health Administration 2002):

- Imminent danger situations that require correction as soon as possible

- Accident investigations where the employer has notified the agency of a fatality or catastrophe

- Inspections that must take place after regular business hours or that require special preparation

- Cases where notice is required to ensure that the employer and the employee representative or other personnel will be present

- Cases where an inspection must be delayed for more than five working days when there is good cause

- Situations in which the OSHA area director determines that advance notice would produce a more thorough or effective inspection

OSHA is responsible for inspecting more than 111 million workplaces, and thus it has set inspection priorities based on worst-case situations. These priorities are listed in figure 17.3.

Figure 17.3. OSHA inspection priorities

Imminent Danger

Imminent danger situations receive top priority. An imminent danger is any condition where there is reasonable certainty that a danger exists that can be expected to cause death or serious physical harm immediately or before the danger can be eliminated through normal enforcement procedures. If a compliance officer finds an imminent danger situation, he or she will ask the employer to voluntarily abate the hazard and remove endangered employees from exposure. Should the employer fail to do this, OSHA, through the regional solicitor, may apply to the Federal District Court for an injunction prohibiting further work as long as unsafe conditions exist.

Catastrophes and Fatal Accidents

Second priority goes to the investigation of fatalities and accidents resulting in a death or hospitalization of three or more employees. The employer must report such catastrophes to OSHA within 8 hours. OSHA investigates to determine the cause of these accidents and whether existing OSHA standards were violated.

Complaints and Referrals

Third priority goes to formal employee complaints of unsafe or unhealthful working conditions and to referrals from any source about a workplace hazard. The act gives each employee the right to request an OSHA inspection when the employee believes he or she is in imminent danger from a hazard or when he or she thinks that there is a violation of an OSHA standard that threatens physical harm. OSHA will maintain confidentiality if requested, inform the employee of any action it takes regarding complaints, and, if requested, hold an informal review of any decision not to inspect.

Programmed Inspections

Programmed inspections are aimed at specific high-hazard industries, workplaces, occupations, or health substances, or other industries identified in OSHA's current inspection procedures. OSHA selects industries for inspection on the basis of factors such as the injury incidence rates, previous citation history, employee exposure to toxic substances, or random selection.

Follow-up Inspections

A follow-up inspection determines if the employer has corrected previously cited violations. If an employer has failed to abate a violation, the compliance officer informs the employer that he or she is subject to "Failure to Abate" alleged violations. This involves proposed additional daily penalties until the employer corrects the violation.

Source: Department of Labor Occupational Safety and Health Administration 2002.

In healthcare organizations, adherence to OSHA standards is absolutely required as a means to minimize legal risk from the standpoint of delivering quality patient care and protecting employees from harm. Healthcare organizations require employees to complete training on a variety of OSHA-related subjects as well as discrimination in the workplace, sexual harassment, and HIPAA privacy and security issues. HIM and informatics professionals, while not involved with patient care, are still required to participate in training activities as deemed relevant to their position in the organization.

Check Your Understanding 17.2

Instructions: Indicate whether the following statements are true or false (T or F).

1. The number of hours a child under the age of 16 may work is protected by law.

2. ERISA refers to pension plans, while COBRA refers to health insurance.

3. Employees may not self-select to join a union.

4. Labor unions exist to protect employers from demanding employees.

5. Hospital employers must provide healthcare workers with information regarding what to do if the worker is accidentally stuck with a needle that has been used on a patient.

Summary

The delivery of quality healthcare depends on personnel or human resources who "do no harm" and "do the right thing." Human resources are protected in the workplace by employment laws that function to protect both employee and employer. Discrimination laws focus on issues that protect job applicants and employees from discrimination based on person characteristics such as age, disability, race, national origin, sex, and religion in addition to issues such as sexual harassment, pay, and compensation. Title VII of the Civil Rights Act, along with other federal laws, ensures employees are fairly treated in the employment setting. The EEOC is the federal oversight body that ensures employers carry out the spirit of the laws. In addition to employment laws, labor laws related to employer-employee relations exist to further support fairness in the work setting in regard to wages, overtime, compensation, and benefits. The NLRA established the NLRB, which oversees the right of employees to participate in union activity and the overall process of union activity. To reduce employee injuries, illnesses, and deaths on the job, OSHA enforces workplace safety standards and provides information, training, and assistance to employers and workers. Overall workplace laws exist to protect the employer and the employee in achieving the business goals of the organization.

References

Department of Health and Human Services Office for Civil Rights. 2004. Guidance to federal financial assistance recipients regarding Title VI prohibition against national origin discrimination affecting limited English proficient persons. http://www.hhs.gov/

Department of Health and Human Services Office for Civil Rights. 2006. Your rights under the Americans with Disabilities Act. http://www.hhs.gov/

Dunn, R.T. 2006. *Healthcare Management*, 8th ed. Chicago: Health Administration Press.

Fottler, M.D., S.R. Hernandez, and C.L. Joiner. 1998. *Essentials of Human Resources Management in Health Services Organizations*. Albany, NY: Delmar.

Fried, B., and M. Fottler. 2008. *Human Resources in Healthcare*. Chicago: Health Administration Press.

US Department of Labor. n.d. Health plans and benefits: Portability of health coverage (HIPAA). http://www.dol.gov/.

US Department of Labor Bureau of Labor Statistics. 2011. Union members—2010. http://www.bls.gov/.

US Department of Labor National Labor Relations Board. n.d. Employee rights under the National Labor Relations Act. http://www.dol.gov/.

US Department of Labor Occupational Safety and Health Administration. 2001. Revision to OSHA's bloodborne pathogens standard. http://www.osha.gov/.

US Department of Labor Occupational Safety and Health Administration. 2002. OSHA inspections. http://www.osha.gov/.

US Department of Labor Occupational Safety and Health Administration. 2005. OSHA recordkeeping handbook. http://www.osha.gov/.

US Department of Labor Occupational Safety and Health Administration. 2006. All about OSHA. http://www.osha.gov/.

US Department of Labor Occupational Safety and Health Administration. 2011. At a glance OSHA. http://www.osha.gov/.

US Equal Employment Opportunity Commission. n.d.a. Overview. http://www.eeoc.gov/.

US Equal Employment Opportunity Commission. n.d.b. Uniform guidelines on employee selection procedures. http://www.uniformguidelines.com/.

US Equal Employment Opportunity Commission. n.d.c. Age discrimination. http://www.eeoc.gov/.

US Equal Employment Opportunity Commission. n.d.d. Disability discrimination. http://www.eeoc.gov/.

US Equal Employment Opportunity Commission. n.d.e. Equal pay/compensation discrimination. http://www.eeoc.gov/.

US Equal Employment Opportunity Commission. n.d.f. National origin discrimination. http://www.eeoc.gov/.

US Equal Employment Opportunity Commission. n.d.g. Sexual harassment. http://www.eeoc.gov/.

Cases, Statutes, and Regulations Cited

29 CFR 1635.3(c)(1): Genetic Information Nondiscrimination Act. 2008.

29 CFR 1910: Occupational Safety and Health Act. 1970.

29 CFR 1910.1030: Bloodborne pathogens. 1991.

8 USC 1101: The Immigration Reform and Control Act. 1986.

29 USC 141 et seq.: Labor-Management Relations Act. 1947.

29 USC 151-169: National Labor Relations Act. 1935.

29 USC 201: The Fair Labor Standards Act. 1938.

29 USC 206(d): Equal Pay Act. 1963.

29 USC 621-34: Age Discrimination in Employment Act. 1967.

29 USC 1001 et seq.: Employee Retirement Income Security Act. 1974.

Consolidated Omnibus Budget Reconciliation Act of 1986. Public Law 99-272.

Needlestick Safety and Prevention Act of 2000. Public Law 106-480.

Glossary

A

Abbreviation: Shortened form of a word or phrase; in healthcare, when there is more than one meaning for an approved abbreviation, either only one meaning should be used or the context in which the abbreviation is to be used should be identified

Abuse: Provider, supplier, and practitioner practices that are inconsistent with accepted sound fiscal, business, or medical practices and that may directly or indirectly result in unnecessary costs to the program, improper payment, services that fail to meet professionally recognized standards of care or are medically unnecessary, or services that directly or indirectly result in adverse patient outcomes or delays in appropriate diagnosis or treatment

Acceptance: Agreeing to an offer, reflecting a meeting of minds on terms of a contract

Access: One of the rights protected by the Privacy Rule, the right of access allows an individual to inspect and obtain a copy of his or her own protected health information that is contained in a designated record set, such as a health record; also an information security term that refers to the ability to enter an electronic system and make use of the data within it

Access report: Proposed by the Department of Health and Human Services in the May 31, 2011, Notice of Proposed Rulemaking, it would allow individuals (upon request) to receive a listing from covered entities with EHRs of every person who viewed the individuals' designated record set during the previous three years

Accounting of Disclosures: A list of all disclosures made of a patient's health information; Section 164.528 of the Privacy Rule states that an individual has the right to receive an accounting of certain disclosures made by a covered entity within the six years prior to the date on which the accounting was requested

Accreditation Council for Graduate Medical Education (ACGME): Accrediting body for medical schools that sets practice standards for graduates of medical school

Accuracy: The extent to which information reflects the true, correct, and exact description of the care that was delivered with respect to both content and timing

Act of God: Natural disaster, such as an earthquake or a flood, that is not human related

Active record: A health record of an individual who is a currently hospitalized inpatient or an outpatient

Addendum: *See* **Amendment**

Addition of entries: Changes to the health record in the form of late entries, amendments, or addenda

Addressable standards: The implementation specifications of the HIPAA Security Rule that are designated "addressable" rather than "required"; to be in compliance with the rule, the covered entity must implement the specification as written, implement an alternative, or document that the risk for which the addressable implementation specification was provided either does not exist in the organization or exists with a negligible probability of occurrence

Adhesion contract: An agreement that may be unenforceable because unequal bargaining power between the parties forces the weaker party to agree to unfavorable terms

Administrative agency: An executive branch agency; source of administrative law

Administrative agency tribunal: A form of alternative dispute resolution in which a tribunal is created by statute or the Constitution to hear a dispute arising from administrative law

Administrative data: Coded information contained in secondary records, such as billing records, describing patient identification, diagnoses, procedures, and insurance

Administrative information: Information used for administrative and healthcare operation purposes such as billing and quality oversight

Administrative law: Rules and regulations created by administrative agencies

Administrative safeguards: A set of nine standards defined by the HIPAA Security Rule: security management functions, assigned security responsibility, workforce security, information access management, security awareness and training, security incident reporting, contingency plan, evaluation, and business associate contracts and other arrangements

Administrative simplification: The original intent of HIPAA—the streamlining and standardization of the healthcare industry's nonuniform and seemingly inefficient business practices, such as billing and creating standards for the electronic transmission of data

Admissibility: Evidence that is allowed to be admitted in a court of law

Admission of facts: A discovery method in which a party elicits from the opposing party certain admissions that will diminish the amount of time and money that would otherwise be spent proving those facts

Adoption: A legal status in which the parental rights and responsibilities of one set of parents are legally terminated and a new parental relationship is established by law

Advance directive: A legal document that specifies an individual's healthcare wishes in the event that he or she has a temporary or permanent loss of competence

Adverse patient occurrence (APO):   An occurrence such as admission for adverse results of outpatient management, readmission for complications, incomplete management of problems on previous hospitalization, or unplanned removal, injury, or repair of an organ or structure during surgery; covered entities must have a system for concurrent or retrospective identification through medical chart–based review according to objective screening criteria

Affidavit of merit: A measure to deter excessive and/or frivolous litigation. It is required by some jurisdictions especially in medical malpractice claims whereby an expert witness must attest in an affidavit that in the opinion of the expert witness a standard of care has been breached

Affiliated covered entities: Legally separate covered entities, affiliated by common ownership or control; for purposes of the Privacy Rule, these legally separate entities may refer to themselves as a single covered entity

Affirmative defenses: Those defenses for which the defendant bears the burden of proving he or she is entitled to rely on them

Against medical advice (AMA): When a patient discharges himself or herself before a physician has determined it to be medically appropriate

Age Discrimination in Employment Act of 1967: A law that protects individuals 40 years or older from employment discrimination

Age of majority: In most states, the age of 18; an individual generally must have reached the age of majority in order to be considered a competent adult

AHIC: *See* **American Health Information Community**

AHIMA: *See* **American Health Information Management Association**

Allied health professional: A credentialed healthcare worker who is not a physician, nurse, psychologist, or pharmacist (for example, a physical therapist, dietitian, social worker, or occupational therapist)

Alternative dispute resolution: Ways of resolving a dispute or lawsuit other than through the court system, including arbitration, mediation, or resolution through an administrative agency

AMA: *See* **American Medical Association**

Amendment: Synonymous with addendum; a type of late entry in which information is added to support or clarify a previous entry and that often requires additional space for documentation

Amendment request: The right of individuals to ask that a covered entity amend their health records, as provided in Section 164.526 of the Privacy Rule

American Board of Medical Specialties: Not-for-profit organization that assists 24 approved medical specialty boards in the development and use of standards in the ongoing evaluation and certification of physicians

American Health Information Community (AHIC): A public-private federal advisory committee associated with the Office of the National Coordinator that makes recommendations to the secretary on how to accelerate adoption of interoperable electronic health information technology

American Health Information Management Association (AHIMA): The professional membership organization for managers of health information services and healthcare information systems as well as coding services; provides accreditation, advocacy, certification, and educational services

American Medical Association (AMA): A national professional membership organization for physicians that distributes scientific information, informs members of legislation related to health and medicine, and represents the medical profession's interests in national legislative matters

American Medical Informatics Association (AMIA): A professional organization of health informatics and information management personnel, biomedical informatics professionals, educators, and others

American National Standards Institute (ANSI): An organization that governs standards in many aspects of public and private business; developer of the Health Information Technology Standards Panel

American Recovery and Reinvestment Act of 2009 (ARRA): Federal legislation that included significant funding for health information technology and provided for significant changes to the HIPAA Privacy Rule

American Society for Testing and Materials (ASTM): A national organization whose purpose is to establish standards on materials, products, systems, and services

Americans with Disabilities Act of 1990: Law that ensures equal opportunity for, and elimination of discrimination against, persons with disabilities

AMIA: *See* **American Medical Informatics Association**

Analysis: Review of health record for proper documentation and adherence to regulatory and accreditation standards

ANSI: *See* **American National Standards Institute**

Answer: A defendant's response to a legal complaint, which may take the form of a denial, an admission, a plea of ignorance to the allegations, additional legal actions, or a request for dismissal

APO: *See* **Adverse patient occurrence**

Apology Statutes: State laws that, to varying degrees, deem apologies by healthcare providers to patients and their relatives following unanticipated medical outcomes to be inadmissible as evidence in court

Appeal: The next stage in the litigation process after a court has rendered a verdict; must be based on alleged errors or disputes of law rather than errors of fact

Appellant: The party appealing a case, also known as the petitioner

Appellate courts: Courts that hear appeals on final judgments of the state trial courts or federal trial courts

Appellee: The party against whom a case is appealed, also known as the respondent

Arbitration: A form of alternative dispute resolution in which a dispute is submitted to a third party or a panel of experts outside the judicial trial system

Assault: A form of intentional tort that involves conduct that causes *apprehension* of a harmful or offensive contact instead of actual contact

Assumption of risk: An affirmative defense that bars a plaintiff from recovering on his or her negligence claim if the defendant proves that the plaintiff: 1. had actual knowledge of a danger, 2. understood and appreciated the risks associated with the danger, and 3. voluntarily exposed himself or herself to those risks

ASTM: *See* **American Society for Testing and Materials**

Attorney in fact: Agent authorized by an individual to make certain decisions, such as healthcare determinations, according to a directive written by the individual

Audit trail: A record that shows who has accessed a computer system, when it was accessed, and what operations were performed

Authenticated evidence: Evidence that appears to be relevant and has been shown to have a baseline authenticity or trustworthiness

Authentication: Verification of a record's validity (that is, it is the record of the individual in question and it is what it purports to be) and, therefore, its reliability and truthfulness as evidence; also a security mechanism to validate the identity of a user in an electronic system

Authenticity: The genuineness of a record, that it is what it purports to be; information is authentic if proved to be immune from tampering and corruption

Authorization: A patient's permission to disclose protected health information (PHI); the form or detailed document that gives covered entities permission to use PHI for specified purposes, generally other than for treatment, payment, or health care operations, or to disclose PHI to a third party specified by the individual

Authorship: The origination or creation of recorded information attributed to a specific individual or entity acting at a particular time

Auto-authentication: A process by which the failure of an author to review and affirmatively either approve or disapprove an entry within a specified time period results in authentication

Automatic log-off: A security procedure that causes a computer session to end after a predetermined period of inactivity, such as 10 minutes

Autonomy: A core ethical principle centered on the individual's right to self-determination that includes respect for the individual; in clinical applications, the patient's right to determine what does or does not happen to him or her in terms of healthcare

Autopsy: A postmortem examination to determine cause of death

B

Bailiff: The person responsible for maintaining order and decorum in the court, as well as managing the schedule of the judge; depending on state law, the bailiff may or may not be required to also be a peace officer

Battery: Intentional and nonconsensual contact with a person

Behavioral health: A broad array of psychiatric services provided in acute, long-term, and ambulatory care settings; includes treatment of mental disorders, chemical dependency, mental retardation, and developmental disabilities as well as cognitive rehabilitation services

Behavioral healthcare information: Information related to treatment for conditions such as mental disorders, mental retardation, and other developmental disabilities

Belmont Report: A statement of ethical principles to prevent the unethical use of human subjects in research, sponsored by the Department of Health and Human Services

Bench trial: A trial without a jury

Beneficence: A legal term that means promoting good for others or providing services that benefit others, such as releasing health information that will help a patient receive care or will ensure payment for services received

Benefits: Healthcare services for which the healthcare insurance company will pay

Best evidence rule: A rule under which in order to prove the contents of a writing, recording, or photograph, the original writing, recording, or photograph is required; protects against intentional perjury or faulty memory

Biometric identification system: A security system that analyzes biological data about the user, such as a voiceprint, fingerprint, handprint, retinal scan, faceprint, or full-body scan

Birth certificate: Paperwork that must be filed for every live birth, regardless of where it occurred

Birth defects registries: Database that includes information on newborns with birth defects, usually maintained by the state

Board of directors: The elected or appointed group of officials who bear ultimate responsibility for the successful operation of a healthcare organization

Board of trustees: *See* **Board of directors**

Boilerplate: Standard contract provisions

Breach notification: An American Recovery and Reinvestment Act requirement that mandates the notification of individuals following the unauthorized use or disclosure of their protected health information, as the information's security or privacy may be compromised

Breach of confidentiality: A type of claim based on the special relationship—fiduciary in nature—between patients and healthcare providers

Breach of contract: Violation of one of more terms of a contract that can result in a lawsuit

Brief: A legal document prepared by each party's attorney for a case heard before an appellate or supreme court

Burden of proof: The task of sufficiently proving or establishing the requisite degree of belief for each element of a case; usually belongs to the plaintiff

Business associate: A person or organization other than a member of a covered entity's workforce that performs functions or activities on behalf of or affecting a covered entity that involve the use or disclosure of individually identifiable health information

Business associate agreement: A written and signed contract that allows covered entities to lawfully disclose protected health information to business associates such as consultants, billing companies, accounting firms, or others that perform services for the provider, provided that the business associate agrees to abide by the provider's requirements to protect the information's security and confidentiality

Business record: A record that is made and kept in the usual course of business, at or near the time of the event recorded

Business records exception: A rule under which a record is determined not to be hearsay if it was made at or near the time by, or from information transmitted by, a person with knowledge; it was kept in the course of a regularly conducted business activity; and it was the regular practice of that business activity to make the record

Bylaws: Internal rules of an organization or company

C

CAMH: *See* **Comprehensive Accreditation Manual for Hospitals**

Cancer registry: Records maintained by many states for the purpose of tracking the incidence (new cases) of cancer

Case law: The body of law that is created when, as the result of a dispute, a court renders a decision

Case management: 1. The ongoing, concurrent review performed by clinical professionals to ensure the necessity and effectiveness of the clinical services being provided to a patient; 2. A process that integrates and coordinates patient care over time and across multiple sites and providers, especially in complex and high-cost cases; 3. The process of developing a specific care plan for a patient that serves as a communication tool to improve quality of care and reduce cost

CCHIT: *See* **Certification Commission for Health Information Technology**

Center for Democracy & Technology: A nonprofit public interest organization that promotes privacy in communications technologies; it houses the Health Privacy Project

Centers for Medicare and Medicaid Services (CMS): Division of the Department of Health and Human Services responsible for developing healthcare policy and administering the Medicare program and federal portion of the Medicaid program

Certification Commission for Health Information Technology (CCHIT): An independent non-profit group formed and funded in 2004 to compare products submitted by vendors against current standards

CEs: *See* **Covered entities**

CFR: *See* **Code of Federal Regulations**

Charitable immunity: A doctrine that shields hospitals (as well as other institutions) from liability for negligence because of the belief that donors would not make contributions to hospitals if they thought their donation would be used to litigate claims, combined with concern that a few lawsuits could bankrupt a hospital

Chief of staff: The physician designated as leader of a healthcare organization's medical staff

CIA: *See* **Corporate Integrity Agreement**

Circuit courts: Federal appellate courts distributed throughout the United States, including the District of Columbia and US territories, so that each court represents a specific number of the district courts

Circumstantial evidence: Evidence that is not directly from an eyewitness or participant and requires some reasoning to prove a fact

Civil law: Noncriminal law

Civil Monetary Penalties Act (CMP): Section 1128A of the Social Security Act, passed in 1981 as one of several administrative remedies to combat increases in healthcare fraud and abuse, which authorizes the secretary and inspector general of Health and Human Services (HHS) to impose civil monetary penalties, assessment, and program exclusions on individuals and entities whose wrongdoing causes injury to HHS programs or their beneficiaries

Civil procedure: The rule and parameters that govern civil (noncriminal) cases

Class action: A type of lawsuit involving multiple plaintiffs, often a group of consumers filing suit against a large and generally powerful entity for alleged wrongdoing

Clayton Act: Federal antitrust statute that exempts union activities from antitrust laws and prohibits discriminatory pricing practices, tying arrangements, and mergers and acquisitions that reduce competition

Clerk of courts: A government official responsible for officially maintaining documents associated with legal actions filed in a court system

CLIA: *See* **Clinical Laboratory Improvement Act**

Clinical Laboratory Improvement Act (CLIA): A law that provides that clinical laboratories are to disclose test results or reports only to "authorized persons"—unless state law defines them otherwise, defined by the law as the person who orders the test

Closing argument: The point in a trial after both sides have presented and rested their cases when each side presents an argument that seeks to compel the jury to find in favor of its client

CME: *See* **Continuing medical education**

CMP: *See* **Civil Monetary Penalties Act**

COBRA: *See* **Consolidated Omnibus Budget Reconciliation Act of 1986**

Code of ethics: A statement of ethical principles regarding business practices and professional behavior

Code of Federal Regulations (CFR): A publication of the regulations issued by administrative agencies, or administrative laws

Collateral source payment: Payment a plaintiff in a tort case receives from a source other than the defendant(s), can be from multiple sources

Collective bargaining: A process through which a contract is negotiated, which sets forth the relationship between the employees and the healthcare organization

Common law: The body of law (that is, judicial or case law) that is created when a court renders a decision as the result of a dispute

Communicable disease: A disease that can be transmitted from an infected person, animal, or inanimate reservoir to a susceptible person or host by either direct or indirect contact

Comparative negligence: A defendant is able to demonstrate that the plaintiff's conduct contributed in part to the injury the plaintiff suffered

Compensation: All direct and indirect pay, including wages, mandatory benefits, and benefits such as medical insurance, life insurance, child care, elder care, retirement plans, and longevity pay

Compensatory damages: Damages in which the plaintiff is compensated for losses incurred; actual damages

Competent adult: An individual who has reached the age of majority and is mentally and physically competent to tend to his or her own affairs; may consent to treatment and may authorize the access or disclosure of his or her health information

Complaint: The document that is filed with a court in order to commence a lawsuit

Completeness: An element of a legally defensible health record; the health record is not complete until all its parts are assembled and the appropriate documents are authenticated according to medical staff bylaws

Compliance: 1. The process of establishing an organizational culture that promotes the prevention, detection, and resolution of instances of conduct that do not conform to federal, state, or private payer healthcare program requirements or the healthcare organization's ethical and business policies; 2. The act of adhering to official requirements

Compliance officer: An individual responsible for overseeing an organization's compliance program and ensuring that the program promotes ethical business practices and conformity to federal, state, and private payer program requirements

Compound authorization: An authorization that combines informed consent with an authorization for the use and/or disclosure of protected health information

Comprehensive Accreditation Manual for Hospitals (CAMH): Accreditation manual published by the Joint Commission

Computer key: A number unique to a specific individual for purposes of authentication

Computer virus: The most common and virulent forms of intentional computer tampering; types may include file infectors, system or boot-record infectors, and macro viruses

Conditioned authorization: Requires authorization in order to receive treatment or some other service or benefit

Conditions of Participation: The standards that govern providers receiving Medicare and Medicaid reimbursements

Confidential communications: As defined by HIPAA, a request that protected health information be routed to an alternative location or by an alternative method; must be honored by health plans under HIPAA

Confidentiality: A legal and ethical concept that establishes the healthcare provider's responsibility for protecting health records and other personal and private information from unauthorized use or disclosure

Confidentiality of Alcohol and Drug Abuse Patient Records Regulation: Regulation enacted for the purpose of encouraging individuals to seek substance abuse treatment without fear of their health information being disclosed

Conflict of laws: An inconsistency between the laws of different states arising from a legal action that involves the territory of more than one jurisdiction

Consent: 1. A patient's acknowledgment that he or she understands a proposed intervention, including that intervention's risks, benefits, and alternatives; 2. A patient's agreement that protected health information can be disclosed; the document that provides a record of the patient's consent

Consideration: An element necessary for a valid contract; what each party will receive from the other party in return for performing the obligations described in the contract

Consolidated Omnibus Budget Reconciliation Act of 1986 (COBRA): The federal law requiring every hospital that participates in Medicare and has an emergency room to treat any patient in an emergency condition or active labor, whether or not the patient is covered by Medicare and regardless of the patient's ability to pay; COBRA also requires employers to provide continuation benefits to specified workers and families who have been terminated but previously had healthcare insurance benefits

Constitution: A document that defines and lays out the powers of a government; considered the supreme law of that government

Constitutional law: Body of law that deals with the amount and types of power and authority that governments are given

Consultation: The response by one healthcare professional to another healthcare professional's request to provide recommendations or opinions regarding the care of a particular patient or resident

Consumer Coalition for Health Privacy: Affiliated with the Health Privacy Project, this organization was created to educate and empower healthcare consumers on privacy issues at the various levels of government and consists of patients and consumer advocacy organizations

Context-based access control: The most stringent type of access control, which takes into account the person attempting to access the data, the type of data being accessed, and the *context* of the transaction in which the access attempt is made

Contingency fee: A lawyer's fee that is paid based on a percentage of the money awarded to the client; this fee is commonly one-third of the total recovery

Contingency planning: A plan for recovery in the event of a power failure, disaster, or other emergency that limits or eliminates access to facilities and electronic protected health information (ePHI); an important component of protecting ePHI

Continuing medical education (CME): Activities such as accredited sponsorship, nonaccredited sponsorship, medical teaching, publications that advance medical care, and other learning experiences, proof of which is required for a physician to maintain certification

Contract: 1. A legally enforceable agreement; 2. An agreement between a union and an employer that spells out details of the relationship of management and the employees

Contract law: The body of civil law relating to agreements between parties, most often in the context of business or commercial relationships

Contributory negligence: An individual's conduct contributed in part to the injury that the individual suffered

Coroner: Typically, an appointed or elected official, who may or may not be a physician, who is responsible for investigating suspicious deaths

Corporate Code of Conduct: A part of the compliance plan that expresses the organization's commitment to ethical behavior

Corporate compliance programs: Programs that became common after the Federal Sentencing Guidelines reduced the fines and penalties to organizations found guilty of healthcare fraud if the organization has a fraud prevention and detection program in place; the programs also help organizations identify problems and improve performance

Corporate Integrity Agreement (CIA):　A compliance program imposed by the government that involves substantial government oversight and outside expert involvement in the organization's compliance activities and is generally required as a condition of settling a fraud and abuse investigation

Corporate negligence:　A doctrine under which hospitals may be held liable in their own right

Corporation:　An organization created as an artificial and legally distinct being under the authority of state statute

Correct Coding Initiative (CCI):　A national initiative designed to improve the accuracy of Part B claims processed by Medicare carriers

Counterclaim:　A claim by a defendant against a plaintiff

Countersignature:　Authentication by a second provider that signifies review and evaluation of the actions and documentation, including authentication, of a first provider

Court of Claims:　A federal or state court in which legal actions against the government are brought

Court order:　A document issued by a judge that compels certain actions, such as testimony or the production of documents such as health records

Court reporter:　An individual who is present during the entire course of a trial and is responsible for providing a verbatim transcript of the trial

Covered entities (CEs):　Persons or organizations that must comply with the HIPAA Privacy and Security Rules; include healthcare providers, health plans, and healthcare clearinghouses

Credentialing:　The process of reviewing and validating the qualifications (degrees, licenses, and other credentials) of physicians and other licensed independent practitioners for the purpose of granting medical staff membership to provide patient care services

Credentials verification organization (CVO):　An organization that verifies healthcare professionals' backgrounds, licensing, and schooling and tracks continuing education and other performance measures

Creditor:　Anyone who regularly, and in the ordinary course of business, meets one of the following criteria: 1. obtains or uses consumer reports in connection with a credit transaction; 2. furnishes information to consumer reporting agencies in connection with a credit transaction; or 3. advances funds to, or on behalf of, someone (except for funds for expenses that are incidental to a service provided by the creditor to that person)

Criminal law:　A type of law in which the government is a party prosecuting an accused who has been charged with violating a criminal statute or regulation

Criminal negligence:　Reckless disregard for another individual's safety or, stated differently, willful indifference to a harm that could result from an act

Cross appeal:　An appeal in which both the respondent and the petitioner file appeals

Cross-claim:　A claim by one party against another party who is on the same side of the main litigation

Cryptography:　The study of encryption and decryption techniques

Custodian:　*See* **Custodian of health records**

Custodian of health records:　The person designated as responsible for the operational functions of the development and maintenance of the health record and who may certify through affidavit or testimony the normal business practices used to create and maintain the record

CVO:　*See* **Credentials verification organization**

D

Damages: Monetary compensation awarded by a court to an individual injured in a civil action through the wrongful act of another party

Darling case: Often credited as the landmark case for extending liability for negligence to hospitals (*Darling v. Charleston Community Memorial Hospital*)

Data encryption: A form of technical security used to ensure that data transferred from one location on a network to another are secure from anyone eavesdropping or seeking to intercept them

Data security: The process of keeping data, both in transit and at rest, safe from unauthorized access, alteration, or destruction

Data stewardship: The responsibilities and accountabilities associated with managing, collecting, viewing, storing, sharing, disclosing, or otherwise making use of personal health information (AMIA 2007)

DDS: *See* **Disability determination services**

Death certificate: As directed by state law, paperwork that must be completed when someone dies; generally filled out by the funeral director or another person responsible for internment or cremation of remains and signed by the physician, who provides the cause of death

Deemed status: Enables a Joint Commission–accredited healthcare organization to use its accreditation status in lieu of a separate Medicare or Medicaid Conditions of Participation healthcare organization certification process

Defamation: False communication about a person to someone else that harms the person's reputation

Default judgment: An automatic judgment by the court against the defendant that is made when the defendant fails to respond to a complaint within the time frame specified by the court

Defendant: The individual or organization that is the object of the lawsuit, and against whom a lawsuit is brought; wrongdoer

Deficit Reduction Act of 2005 (DRA): A law enacted in 2006 that transformed the nature of compliance programs from voluntary to mandatory; failure to comply may result in the affected entity being ineligible to receive Medicaid payments

Deidentified information: Information from which personal characteristics have been stripped and that, as a result, neither identifies nor provides a reasonable basis to believe it could identify an individual

Deliberations: The secret conversation of a jury before it renders a decision or verdict

Demonstrative evidence: Actual objects, pictures, models, and other devices that are supposedly intended to clarify the facts for the judge and jury

Department of Health and Human Services (HHS): The federal agency that oversees Medicare, Medicaid, and other health and essential human services

Deponent: A person directed by subpoena to appear at an appointed time and place to testify under oath at a deposition

Deposition: A formal proceeding by which the oral testimonies of individuals are obtained as part of the discovery process

Designated health services: Services defined by the Federal Physician Self-Referral Statute (Stark Law), which prohibits physicians from ordering certain services for patients from entities with which the physician or an immediate family member has a financial relationship

Designated record set: A group of records maintained by or for a covered entity encompassing medical records and billing records about individuals and enrollment, payment, claims adjudication, and case or medical management record systems maintained by or for a health plan used, in whole or in part, by or for the covered entity to make decisions about individuals

Destruction of records: The act of breaking down the components of a health record into pieces that can no longer be recognized as parts of the original record; for example, paper records can be destroyed by shredding, and electronic records can be destroyed by magnetic degaussing

Diabetes registries: Database that includes cases of patients with diabetes for the purpose of assisting in the management patient care and research

Digital signature: A type of e-signature that encrypts the document (represented by a series of numbers), identifies who performed the encryption (that is, the person who is authenticating), and validates and detects whether any subsequent changes have been made to the document

Direct evidence: "Real, tangible or clear evidence of a fact, happening or thing that requires no thinking or consideration to prove its existence" (ALM Media Properties 2012)

Directed verdict: A request made by an attorney for the judge to determine that a case is over and rule favorably to the requesting party, even without the opposition presenting its case

Disability determination services (DDS): State agencies responsible for providing to the Social Security Administration medical evidence to determine whether a resident of a state is or is not disabled under the Social Security disability law

Disaster recovery planning: A plan for securing electronic protected health information (ePHI) in the event of a disaster that limits or eliminates access to facilities and ePHI

Discharge analysis: A detailed review of the health record at or following discharge

Discharge summary: A recapitulation of an individual's stay at a healthcare facility that is used along with the postdischarge plan of care to provide continuity of care upon discharge from the facility

Disclosure: The act of making information known; the release of confidential health information about an identifiable person to another person or entity; release, transfer, provision of access to, or divulging in any other manner of information outside the entity holding the information (45 CFR 160.103) (*See also* **Release of information**)

Discoverability: Limitations on the ability of parties to discover pretrial information held by another party

Discovery: The next pretrial stage after the commencement of a lawsuit, which allows all parties (generally via their legal counsel) to use various strategies to discover or obtain information held by other parties and, subsequently, to assess the strengths and weaknesses inherent in each party's case

Disposition: The removal of records from a record storage system, whether through destruction, transfer, or loss

Dismissal: Termination of a legal proceeding

District courts: The first and lowest level in the federal court system

Diversity: Differences including, but not limited to, age, ethnicity, gender, religious beliefs, sexual orientation, socioeconomic status, and physical abilities

Diversity jurisdiction: A form of court that enables parties from different states to engage in a lawsuit in federal court if the suit fulfills the following obligations: (1) *no* plaintiff can be from the same state as *any* of the defendants and (2) the amount in controversy must be at least $75,000

DNR: *See* **Do not resuscitate (DNR) order**

Do not resuscitate (DNR) order: A specific type of advance directive in which an individual states that healthcare providers should not perform CPR if the individual experiences cardiac arrest or cessation of breathing

DPOA: *See* **Durable power of attorney**

DRA: *See* **Deficit Reduction Act of 2005**

Due diligence: A legally acceptable level of care required of members of corporate boards of directors

Due process: The right of individuals to fair treatment under the law

Due process of law: The guarantee provided under the Constitution and the Bill of Rights that laws will be reasonable and not arbitrary and allow for challenges to a law's content and substance

Duplicate billing: The practice of submitting more than one claim for the same item or service

Durable power of attorney (DPOA): A power of attorney that remains in effect even after the principal is incapacitated; can be drafted to take effect only when the principal becomes incapacitated

Durable power of attorney for healthcare decisions (DPOA-HCD): A legal instrument through which a principal appoints an agent to make healthcare decisions on the principal's behalf in the event the principal become incapacitated

Duty of loyalty: A requirement of members of corporate boards of directors; placing the interests of the corporation ahead of one's own personal interests

Duty of responsibility: A requirement of members of corporate boards of directors; acting with due care in exercising their duties

Duty to warn: The legal obligation of a health professional to disclose information to warn an intended victim when a patient threatens to harm an individually identifiable victim or victims, and the psychiatrist or other mental health provider believes that the patient is likely to actually harm the individual(s)

E

Economic credentialing: Granting medical staff privileges to a provider based on volume of services rather than quality of care

e-Discovery: Pretrial legal process used to describe the methods by which parties will obtain and view electronically stored information

EEOC: *See* **Equal Employment Opportunity Commission**

eHealth Initiative: A private organization that involves many groups working on the improvement of health information through information technology and health information exchange

EHR: *See* **Electronic health record**

Electronic health record (EHR): A computerized record of health information and associated processes; an electronic record of health-related information on an individual that conforms to nationally recognized standards and that can be created, managed, and consulted by authorized clinicians and staff across more than one healthcare organization

Electronic medical record (EMR): An electronic record of health-related information on an individual that can be created, gathered, managed, and consulted by authorized clinicians and staff within a single healthcare organization

Electronic Protected Health Information (ePHI): Under HIPAA, all individually identifiable information that is created or received electronically by a healthcare provider or any other entity subject to HIPAA requirements

Electronic Records Express: A program implemented by the Social Security Agency and state Disability Determination Services that enables providers to submit records related to disability claims to a secure website

Electronic signature: Technological corollary to the handwritten signature in a paper record; any representation of a signature in digital form, including an image of a handwritten signature. Authentication of a computer entry can be completed via a digitized image of one's signature, a biometric identifier, a secret code or password, or a digital signature that is linked to the user's name, credentials, and access rights to verify the identity of the signer in the system and create an individual signature on the record.

Electronic Signatures in Global National Commerce Act (E-SIGN): An act passed in 2000 that gives e-signatures the same legality as handwritten signatures where interstate commerce is involved and that provides guidance on how records may be stored and retained electronically

Electronically stored information (ESI): Data or documents used in digital format that are created, stored, manipulated, and communicated electronically through the use of computer hardware and software

E/M codes: *See* **Evaluation and management (E/M) codes**

Emancipated minor: One who is under the age of majority and is self-supporting, and whose parents have surrendered their rights of custody, care, and support

Emergency Medical Treatment and Active Labor Act (EMTALA): A 1986 law enacted as part of the Consolidated Omnibus Reconciliation Act largely to combat "patient-dumping"—transferring, discharging, or refusing to treat indigent emergency department patients because of their inability to pay

Emotional distress: May include manifestations such as sleeplessness, anxiety, irritability, or the emotional inability to perform activities or go places that a plaintiff was capable of prior to the event for which a lawsuit has been filed

Employee health record: A record kept on an employee as part of employment that contains any and all information related to such items as medical tests, drug tests, examinations, physical abilities, immunizations, screenings required by law, biohazardous exposure, and physical limitations

Employee nondisclosure agreement: A contract between employer and employee in which the employee promises not to divulge specified information, subject to disciplinary action or termination

Employee Retirement Income Security Act of 1974 (ERISA): An act that sets minimum standards for most voluntarily established pension and health plans in private industry in order to provide protection for individuals in these plans

EMR: *See* **Electronic medical record**

EMTALA: *See* **Emergency Medical Treatment and Active Labor Act**

Encryption: A technique used to ensure that data transferred from one location on a network to another are secure from eavesdropping or interception

Enforcement rule: A rule that created standardized procedures and substantive requirements for investigating complaints and imposing civil monetary penalties (CMPs) for HIPAA violations, as well as a uniform compliance and enforcement mechanism that addresses *all* of the Administrative Simplification regulations, including privacy, security, and transactions and code sets

Entity authentication: The corroboration that an entity is the one claimed (HHS n.d.); the computer reads a predetermined set of criteria to determine whether the user is who he or she claims to be

ePHI: *See* **Electronic Protected Health Information**

Equal Employment Opportunity Act of 1972: An act that, in combination with Title VII of the Civil Rights Act, prohibits discrimination based on age, race, color, sex, religion, or national origin

Equal Employment Opportunity Commission (EEOC): Enforces the Equal Employment Opportunity Act, Title VII of the Civil Rights Act, the Immigration Reform and Control Act, the Fair Labor

Standards Act, and the Americans with Disabilities Act, among others, investigates job discrimination complaints and can bring federal lawsuits against employers

Equal Pay Act of 1963: An act that regulates the concept of equal pay for men and women who perform similar work requiring similar skills, effort, and responsibility under similar working conditions

Equity: A form of judgment in which the defendant is required to do or to refrain from doing something

ERISA: *See* **Employee Retirement Income Security Act of 1974**

ESI: *See* **Electronically stored information**

E-SIGN: *See* **Electronic Signatures in Global National Commerce Act**

Ethical principles: Set of four principles to assist healthcare professionals in addressing healthcare related dilemma (*See also* **Autonomy, Beneficence, Nonmaleficence, Justice**)

Ethics: A field of study that deals with moral principles, theories, and values; in healthcare, a formal decision-making process for dealing with the competing perspectives and obligations of the people who have an interest in a common problem

Evaluation and management (E/M) codes: *Current Procedural Terminology* codes that describe patient encounters with healthcare professionals for assessment counseling and other routine healthcare services

Evidence: The means by which the facts of a case are proved or disproved

Exculpatory contract: An agreement that may be unenforceable; seeks to excuse a party in advance from any potential liability

Executive branch: The branch of government charged with enforcing laws, including the issuance of regulations by administrative agencies, with ultimate executive-branch power vested in the chief executive (the president of the United States on the federal level and the governor of each state at the state level)

Exempt employee: An employee for whom minimum wage and overtime regulations do not apply

Expert witness: An individual with expertise in a certain subject who is called to testify in a case

Express consent: Consent that is communicated through words, regardless of whether those words are written or spoken

External security threat: A security threat caused by individuals or forces outside the organization

F

Facility: A building necessary in the provision of health services (for example, hospitals, nursing homes, and ambulatory care centers)

Facility directory: A directory of patients being treated in a healthcare facility

FACTA: *See* **Fair and Accurate Credit Transaction Act**

Failure Mode Effect and Criticality Assessment (FMECA): A methodology for determining the cause of sentinel events

Fair and Accurate Credit Transaction Act (FACTA): An act that requires advance employee (i.e., patient) authorization for a consumer reporting agency to share medical information with employers for employment or insurance purposes; it also requires financial institutions and creditors to develop and implement written identity theft programs that identify, detect, and respond to red flags that may signal the presence of identity theft

Fair Labor Standards Act of 1938 (FLSA):   An act that provides regulations for wages and overtime

False Claims Act: The government's primary litigation tool for combating fraud, which provides that anyone who "knowingly" submits false claims to the government is liable for damages up to three times the amount of the erroneous payment plus mandatory penalties between $5,500 and $11,000 for each false claim submitted

False cost reports: A way of increasing Medicare payments inappropriately

False imprisonment: The intentional confinement of another person against that person's will

Federal Anti-Kickback Statute: A statute that establishes criminal penalties for individuals and entities that knowingly and willfully offer, pay, solicit, or receive remuneration in order to induce business for which payment may be made under any federal healthcare program

Federal Physician Self-Referral Statute (Stark Law):   A law that prohibits physicians from ordering designated health services for Medicare (and to some extent Medicaid) patients from entities with which the physician or an immediate family member has a financial relationship; also known as the Stark Law

Federal Rules of Civil Procedure (FRCP):   The rules governing civil cases at the trial level in federal courts

Federal Rules of Evidence (FRE):   Rules governing evidence used in cases presented in federal court because they involve federal laws

Federal Trade Commission Act: Federal antitrust statute that gives the Federal Trade Commission broad powers to act against organizations engaging in unfair methods of competition, or unfair or deceptive acts that affect commerce

Felony: A crime such as murder, larceny, rape, or assault that is more serious in nature than a misdemeanor; under federal law and many state statutes, a felony is punishable by a minimum of imprisonment exceeding one year

Fetal death: The death of a fetus of a particular weight or gestation, frequently 500 grams or more or 22 or more completed weeks of gestation, though the weight and week gestation may vary from state to state

Fiduciary duty: Obligation to act in the best interest of another party based on a special relationship of trust, confidence, or responsibility in certain obligations

Firewall: Hardware or software devices that examine traffic entering and leaving a network and prevent some traffic from entering or leaving based on established rules; can be used to describe the software that protects computing resources or to describe the combination of the software, hardware, and policies that protect the resources

FLSA: *See* **Fair Labor Standards Act of 1938**

FMECA: *See* **Failure Mode Effect and Criticality Assessment**

Focused professional practice evaluation: A time-limited period during which an organization evaluates and determines a practitioner's professional performance of privileges; it occurs in all requests for new privileges and when there are concerns regarding the provision of safe, high-quality care by a current medical staff member

FOIA: *See* **Freedom of Information Act of 1967**

For-profit organization: The tax status assigned to business entities that are owned by one or more individuals or organizations and that earn revenues in excess of expenditures that are subsequently paid out to the owners or stockholders

Fraud: A false representation of fact or a failure to disclose a fact that is material (relevant) to a healthcare transaction that results in damage to another party that reasonably relies on the misrepresentation or failure to disclose

Fraud Enforcement and Recovery Act of 2009 (FERA): Expands both the potential for liability under the False Claims Act (FCA) and the government's investigative powers, and it eliminates the requirement that a person has to present a false claim to a US government officer or employee, or a member of the US armed services, in order to be liable under the FCA

FRCP: *See* **Federal Rules of Civil Procedure**

FRE: *See* **Federal Rules of Evidence**

Freedom of Information Act of 1967 (FOIA): A law covering the right of disclosure to and access by the public regarding federal agency records

Fundraising: Money-generating activities that benefit a HIPAA-covered entity and are subject to the HIPAA Privacy Rule

G

Garnishment: A method of collecting a monetary award in which a certain percentage of the defendant's wages are routinely set aside and paid to the plaintiff toward full satisfaction of the judgment

General consent: A form that covers routine diagnostic procedures and medical treatment by hospital staff, as well as other activities such as release of information for treatment purposes and disposal of human tissue and body fluids

General damages: Damages that naturally and necessarily flow from a tort and directly result from the tort

General jurisdiction: Courts that hear more serious criminal cases (for example, felonies) or civil cases that involve large amounts of money; may hear all matters of state law except for those cases that must be heard in courts of special jurisdiction

Genetic Information Nondiscrimination Act of 2008 (GINA): Federal legislation that prohibits discrimination by health insurers and employers based on genetic information

Good Samaritan statute: State law or statute that protects healthcare providers from liability for not obtaining informed consent before rendering care to adults or minors at the scene of an emergency or accident

Governing Board: *See* **Board of directors**

Grievance: A formal written description of a complaint or disagreement

Grievance procedures: The steps employees may follow to seek resolution of disagreements with management on job-related issues

Gross negligence: Very great or excessive negligence that implies an extreme departure from the ordinary standard of care and shows a reckless disregard for the rights of others

H

Handwritten signature: The most common method for authenticating paper health records

HCQIA: *See* **Health Care Quality Improvement Act**

Health Care Decisions Act: Legislation, usually by states, that encourages the making and enforcement of advance healthcare directives and provides a means for making healthcare decisions for those who have failed to plan

Health Care Quality Improvement Act (HCQIA): A 1986 act that requires facilities to report professional review actions on physicians, dentists, and other facility-based practitioners to the National Practitioner Data Bank (NPDB)

Health informatics and information management (HIIM): Refers to the individuals responsible for managing healthcare data and information in paper or electronic form and controlling its collection, access, use, exchange, and protection through the application of health information technology

Health information: The data generated and collected as a result of delivering care to a patient

Health information exchange (HIE): Electronic movement of health-related information among organizations within a region or community that facilitates access to and retrieval of clinical data in support of safe, timely, efficient, and effective patient-centered care; an organization or entity that forms to create an electronic framework to connect physicians to pharmacies, hospitals, and other healthcare entities

Health information handler (HIH): Organization or entity that handles information on behalf of a provider

Health information management (HIM) department: Healthcare facility department responsible for the management and safeguarding of information in paper and electronic form

Health Information Management Systems Society (HIMSS): A national membership association that provides leadership in healthcare for the management of technology, information, and change

Health Information Organization (HIO): An organization that oversees and governs the exchange of health-related information among organizations according to nationally recognized standards

Health Information Security and Privacy Collaboration (HISPC): An organization for exchanging ideas and developing solutions to promote interoperability

Health information technology (HIT): The technical aspects of processing health data and records, including classification and coding, abstracting, registry development, storage, and so on

Health Information Technology for Economic and Clinical Health (HITECH) Act: Federal legislation that was passed as a portion of the American Recovery and Reinvestment Act; contains changes to the HIPAA Privacy Rule

Health Insurance Portability and Accountability Act of 1996 (HIPAA): A law enacted by Congress on August 21, 1996, governing various aspects of health information; federal legislation enacted to provide continuity of health coverage, control fraud and abuse in healthcare, reduce healthcare costs, and guarantee the security and privacy of health information

Health Level 7 (HL7): An international organization of healthcare professionals dedicated to creating standards for the exchange, management, and integration of electronic information

Health Privacy Project: A nonprofit organization whose mission is to raise public awareness of the importance of ensuring health privacy in order to improve healthcare access and quality

Health record: Individually identifiable data, in any medium, that are collected, processed, stored, displayed, and used by healthcare professionals; documents the care rendered to the patient and the patient's healthcare status

Healthcare Information Technology Standards Panel (HITSP): An organization developed under the auspices of the American National Standards Institute (ANSI) to deal with the many issues of privacy and security as the United States Nationwide Health Information Network develops

Healthcare Integrity and Protection Data Bank (HIPDB): A database maintained by the federal government to provide information on fraud-and-abuse findings against US healthcare providers

Hearsay: A written or oral statement made outside of court that is offered in court as evidence

HHS: *See* **Department of Health and Human Services**

HIE: *See* **Health information exchange**

Highly sensitive health information: Certain types of patient information that require special handling in regard to access, requests, uses, and disclosures due to the nature of the information

HIH: *See* **Health information handler**

HIIM: *See* **Health informatics and information management**

Hill-Burton Act: A 1946 act that provided hospitals and certain other healthcare facilities money for construction and modernization as long as the facilities agreed to provide a reasonable volume of services to those unable to pay and to make their services available to all persons residing in the area of the facility

HIM: *See* **Health information management (HIM) department**

HIMSS: *See* **Health Information Management Systems Society**

HIO: *See* **Health Information Organization**

HIPAA: *See* **Health Insurance Portability and Accountability Act of 1996**

HIPAA Privacy Rule: Federal regulations created to implement the privacy requirements within the administrative simplification subtitle of the Health Insurance Portability and Accountability Act of 1996 and safeguard identifiable health information

HIPAA Security Rule: Federal regulations created to implement the security requirements within the administrative simplification subtitle of the Health Insurance Portability and Accountability Act of 1996

HISPC: *See* **Health Information Security and Privacy Collaboration**

Histocompatibility: Compatibility of donor and recipient tissues

History: Pertinent information about a patient, including chief complaint, past and present illnesses, family history, social history, and review of body systems

HITSP: *See* **Healthcare Information Technology Standards Panel**

HIV: *See* **Human immunodeficiency virus**

HL7: *See* **Health Level 7**

Hold harmless: Contract clause that either transfers liability or establishes the assumption of liability by a particular party to the contract

Homeland Security Act: A 2002 act with the goal of preventing terrorist attacks in the United States while reducing the vulnerability of terrorism, minimizing its damages, and assisting in recovery from attacks in the United States; gives government authorities the right to access information needed to investigate and deter terrorism

Horizontal restraint of trade: Situation in which competitors agree to fix prices, divide the market, and attempt to exclude others from competing in the same market

House staff: A physician in training who is continuing his or her medical education in a residency program and working with specialists to obtain higher-level skills and experience treating patients

Human Genome Project: A multiyear project that ended in 2003 in which all human DNA was identified and mapped

Human immunodeficiency virus (HIV): The virus that causes acquired immunodeficiency syndrome (AIDS)

Hybrid entity: An entity that performs both covered and noncovered functions under the Privacy Rule; for example, a university that educates students and maintains student educational records is not covered by the Privacy Rule. However, the same university that operates a medical center is covered by the Privacy Rule, as it meets the definition of "healthcare provider."

Hybrid health record: A health record that uses a combination of paper and electronic formats

I

Identity theft: A crime in which an individual's personal information is stolen, often through the ease of obtaining data in electronic environments

I'm Sorry Laws: *See* **Apology Statutes**

Immigration Reform and Control Act of 1986: A law that requires employers to ensure that employees hired are legally authorized to work in the United States

Immunization registry: Registries implemented in many states as a way to collect and maintain vaccination records on children—and in some cases, adults—in an effort to promote disease prevention and control

Implant registries: Database for tracking the performance of implants, including complications, deaths, and defects resulting from implants, as well as implant longevity

Implied consent: Consent for medical treatment that is communicated through a person's conduct or some other means besides words

In camera inspection: A form of inspection in which the judge personally reviews disputed records in his or her chambers and decides whether the records are discoverable or admissible in the case

Incidence: New cases of a particular disease or condition in a particular population

Incident report: The means through which occurrences that are inconsistent with a healthcare facility's routine patient care practices or operations are documented

Incident reporting: A process for identifying and responding to adverse events and other occurrences that are inconsistent with the standard of care

Incompetent adult: An individual who is at or above the age of majority and becomes incapacitated due to illness or injury, either permanently or temporarily; another person should be designated to make decisions for that individual, including decisions about the use and disclosure of the individual's protected health information

Indemnification clause: *See* **Hold harmless**

Individual: According to the HIPAA Privacy Rule, a person who is the subject of protected health information

Infliction of emotional distress: A common law tort for intentional conduct that results in extreme emotional distress, such as sleeplessness, anxiety, irritability, or the emotional inability to perform activities or go places that the plaintiff was capable of prior to the event

Information governance: Strategic management of enterprise electronic information, including the standards, policies, and procedures for access, use, and control of that information

Information system (IS): An automated system that uses computer hardware and software to record, manipulate, store, recover, and disseminate data (that is, a system that receives and processes input and provides output); often used interchangeably with "information technology"

Informed consent: A type of consent in which the patient should have a basic understanding of which medical procedures or tests may be performed as well as the risks, benefits, and alternatives for those tests or procedures

Initials: An authentication method for paper health records that may be permitted in lieu of a full signature as long as the initials are readily identifiable as the author's through a signature legend on the same document

Injunction: Court order where one party to a contract is ordered to do or stop doing something in order to prevent irreparable harm to the other party

Inpatient: A currently hospitalized patient

Institute for Healthcare Improvement (IHI): A quality and safety improvement group

Institute of Medicine (IOM): A branch of the National Academy of Sciences whose goal is to advance and distribute scientific knowledge with the mission of improving human health

Institutional review board (IRB): A committee of at least five members with varying backgrounds that determines the acceptability of proposed human subjects research in accordance with institutional policies, applicable law, and standards of professional practice and conduct

Integrated health record: A system of health record organization in which all paper forms are arranged in strict chronological order and forms created by different departments are intermixed

Integrity: The state of being whole or unimpaired

Intentional torts: Torts that involve a deliberate or intentional act

Internal security threat: A security threat caused by individuals or forces within an organization

Interoperability: The ability of different information systems and software applications to communicate and exchange data

Interrogatories: Discovery devices consisting of written questions given to a party, witness, or other person who has information needed in a legal case

Invasion of privacy: A form of tort based on the violation of a person's right to privacy

IOM: *See* **Institute of Medicine**

IRB: *See* **Institutional review board**

IS: *See* **Information system**

J

Joinder: Action by a defendant to bring in ("join") an outsider as a codefendant

Joint and several liability: A principle that allows each defendant in a legal action to be held responsible for the entire amount of damages that a plaintiff is awarded, regardless of the defendant's degree of fault

Joint Commission: An agency that develops standards for healthcare organizations and certifies healthcare organizations on the basis of adherence to those standards

Joint ventures: Partnerships created for a specific purpose and designed to have a limited lifespan

Judge: The person who presides over a trial and the courtroom and who makes critical decisions regarding the admissibility of evidence, which will guide the outcome of a case; in a trial without a jury, the judge also serves as the fact-finder

Judge-made law: *See* **Common law**

Judgment lien: A method of collecting judgment in which a defendant's property is encumbered and the debtor-defendant is prevented from taking any money from its sale until the judgment owed to the plaintiff has first been paid

Judicial branch: The branch of government responsible for interpreting the law and adjudicating disputes, thus creating common law

Judicial law: The body of law created as a result of court (judicial) decisions

Judicial search warrant: A judge's written order authorizing a law enforcement officer to conduct a search of a specified place and to seize evidence

Jurisdiction: The legal authority that a body possesses to make decisions

Jury: The fact-finding body that hears evidence given by the parties, if they testify, and other witnesses; observes evidence presented by both sides; hears the opening statements and closing arguments of each side; and decides facts based on the perceived credibility of the evidence, but does not decide law

Jury instructions: The legal instructions given to the jury by the judge

Justice: The impartial administration of policies or laws that takes into consideration the competing interests and limited resources of the individuals or groups involved

K

Knowing standard: A method of determining Federal Claims Act liability, requiring that the provider must have knowingly submitted the false claim

L

Labor-Management Relations Act of 1947: A law that amended the Wagner Act to prohibit unfair labor practices on the part of unions and allows the president to stop strikes in cases of national health and safety

Late entry: An addition to the health record in which a pertinent entry was missed or was not written in a timely manner

Law: Set of governing rules designed to protect citizens living in a civilized society, establish order, provide parameters for conduct, and define the rights and obligations of the government and its citizens

Lay witness: An individual's testifying based on his or her own observations of the situation(s) that prompted the case at hand

LCD: *See* **Local Coverage Decisions**

Leapfrog Group: A voluntary program founded in 2000 that is composed of a consortium of major companies and other entities that are responsible for purchasing health care coverage for employees; the program encourages the public to report outcomes and runs a Hospital Rewards program to reward providers for improving quality, safety, and affordability

Learned intermediary: A defense doctrine used most often by pharmaceutical companies and medical device manufacturers that says companies have a duty to warn physicians directly about potential adverse effects caused by their products; in doing so, the physician (or other user of the product) becomes a "learned intermediary" who interprets the information and advises patients appropriately

Legal guardian: Individual designated by the court system to assume legal responsibility for another individual

Legal health record (LHR): The form of a health record that is the legal business record of the organization and serves as evidence in lawsuits or other legal actions; what constitutes an organization's legal health record varies depending on how the organization defines it

Legal hold: A court order that suspends the processing or destruction of paper or electronic records; also known as a preservation order, preservation notice, or litigation hold

Legibility: An aspect of the quality of provider entries; if an entry cannot be read, it must be assumed that it cannot be used or was not used in the patient care process

Legislative branch: The branch of government charged with enacting laws in the form of statutes through the Senate and the House of Representatives

LEP: *See* **Limited English proficiency**

LHR: *See* **Legal health record**

Liability: 1. A legal obligation or responsibility that may have financial repercussions if not fulfilled; 2. An amount owed by an individual or organization to another individual or organization

Libel: Defamation in a written form

Licensed independent practitioner (LIP): Professionals such as physician assistants or nurse practitioners who are allowed by state laws and licensing regulations to practice without direction of a physician

Licensure: The legal authority or formal permission from authorities to carry on certain activities that by law or regulation require such permission (applicable to institutions as well as individuals)

Limited data set: Protected health information that excludes direct identifiers of the individual and the individual's relatives, employers, or household members but still does not deidentify the information

Limited English proficiency (LEP): Limited English speaking skills as identified in Title VI of the Civil Rights Act

Limited jurisdiction: Refers to courts that hear cases pertaining to a particular subject matter (for example, landlord-tenant or juvenile cases), that involve crimes of lesser severity (for example, misdemeanors), or involve civil matters of lesser dollar amounts

LIP: *See* **Licensed independent practitioner**

Litigation: The legal proceedings that accompany a lawsuit

Living will: A document executed by a competent adult that expresses that individual's wishes to limit treatment measures when specific health-related diagnoses or conditions exist

Local Coverage Decisions (LCD): Medicare coverage restrictions at the state level

Local Coverage Determination (LCD): New format for LMRPs: Coverage rules, at a fiscal intermediary (FI) or carrier level, that provide information on what diagnoses justify the medical necessity of a test; LCDs vary from state to state

Long form consent: In the context of human subjects research, a consent form that includes all of the informed consent requirements included in the Common Rule

M

Malicious software: Software whose purpose is to harm or destroy legitimate software

Malfeasance: A wrong or improper act

Marketing: Communication about a product or service that encourages the recipient to purchase or use that product or service

Master patient index (MPI): A patient-identifying directory that serves as a link to the patient record or information, facilitates patient identification, and assists in maintaining a longitudinal patient record from birth to death

Meaningful use: A requirement per the American Recovery and Reinvestment Act for healthcare providers to receive Medicare and Medicaid incentive payments; emphasizes collection of electronic data in the electronic health record (EHR) and subsequent use of EHR functionalities for tracking, reporting, and patient-care purposes

Mediation: A form of alternative dispute resolution in which a dispute is submitted to a third party and the outcome is decided by agreement of the parties

Medical device reporting: The Food and Drug Administration (FDA) requires that deaths and severe complications thought to be due to a device must be reported to the FDA and the manufacturer

Medical emergency: Severe injury or illness (including pain); definition depends on healthcare insurer

Medical examiner: Typically a physician with pathology training given the responsibility by a government, such as a county or state, for investigating suspicious deaths

Medical identity theft: A type of identity theft and financial fraud that involves the inappropriate or unauthorized misrepresentation of one's identity to obtain medical goods or services, or to obtain money by falsifying claims for medical services

Medical malpractice: A type of action in which the plaintiff must demonstrate that a physician–patient, nurse–patient, therapist–patient, or other healthcare provider–patient relationship existed at the time of the alleged wrongful act

Medical malpractice insurance: Insurance that protects a party from claims of medical negligence or other tortious injury arising out of care provided to patients

Medical necessity: As defined by Medicare, "services or supplies that are needed for the diagnosis or treatment of your medical condition, meet the standards of good medical practice in the local area, and aren't mainly for the convenience of you or your doctor" (Medicare.gov/Glossary)

Medical staff: The staff members of a healthcare organization who are governed by medical staff bylaws; may or may not be employed by the healthcare organization

Medical staff bylaws: Standards governing the practice of medical staff members that are typically voted on by the organized medical staff and the medical staff executive committee and then approved by the facility's board; medical staff members must abide by these bylaws in order to continue practicing in the healthcare facility

Medical staff executive committee: A body composed of those elected representative members of the medical staff who are authorized to act on behalf of the medical staff

Medicare: A program that provides healthcare services to qualified individuals

Mental examination: A discovery method in which an individual may request an independent mental examination, particularly if the mental condition of an individual is in question

Metadata: Data about data; generally refers to information about an electronic data element's content, including means of creation, purpose, time and date of creation, author, revisions, placement on a network, and standards used

Minor: An individual who is under the age of majority (usually 18 years of age) who has not been legally emancipated (declared an adult) by the court

Misdemeanor: A crime that is less serious than a felony and is generally punishable by a fine or imprisonment other than in a penitentiary

Misfeasance: Relating to negligence or improper performance during an otherwise correct act

Mitigation: Required by the Privacy Rule (45 CFR 164.530(f)), the lessening as much as possible of harmful effects that result from the wrongful use and disclosure of protected health information; possible courses of action may include an apology, disciplinary action against the responsible employee or employees (although such results will not be able to be shared with the wronged individual), repair of the process that resulted in the breach, payment of a bill or financial loss that resulted from the infraction, or gestures of goodwill and good public relations (such as a gift certificate) that may assuage the individual

Moral values: Principles formed through the influence of family, culture, religion, and society

Motion to quash: A document filed with the court that asks the judge to nullify a subpoena

MPI: *See* **Master patient index**

N

National Alliance for Health Information Technology (NAHIT): A partnership of government and private sector leaders from various healthcare organizations that worked toward using technology to achieve improvements in patient safety, quality of care, and operating performance; founded in 2002; ceased operations in 2009

National Cardiovascular Data Registry: A database supported by Medicare and maintained by the American College of Cardiologists that requires hospitals that are reimbursed by Medicare for implantable cardiac defibrillators to submit data on patients who receive implants to the registry

National Committee for Quality Assurance (NCQA): An organization with credentialing standards that requires verification from the primary source of information on the medical staff application; accredits managed care organizations

National Committee on Vital and Health Statistics (NCVHS): An advisory group to Congress and the Department of Health and Human Services regarding health policy

National Coverage Decisions: Medicare coverage restrictions at the national level

National Coverage Determination (NCD): An NCD sets forth the extent to which Medicare will cover specific services, procedures, or technologies on a national basis. Medicare contractors are required to follow NCDs

National Human Genome Research Institute: A division of the National Institutes of Health that discusses the issues and questions around the Human Genome Project and how the information and technology will affect standards of patient care

National Labor Relations Act of 1935 (Wagner Act): A law that established conditions for collective bargaining, listed unfair labor practices, and created the National Labor Relations Board (NLRB) to oversee union elections and handle situations of unfair labor practices; also known as the Wagner Act

National Labor Relations Board (NLRB): An organization that governs the activities between employers and unions and assumed jurisdiction over hospitals in 1974

National Patient Safety Goals: A set of goals published each year by the Joint Commission and designed to improve patient safety in specific healthcare areas identified as problematic by the Sentinel Event Advisory Group

National Practitioner Data Bank (NPDB): A data bank created by the 1986 Health Care Quality Improvement Act that collects malpractice, disciplinary, and credentialing information on physicians, dentists, and other facility-based practitioners

National Regulatory Commission: A body that has oversight responsibility for the medical use of ionizing radiation and to which medical events must be reported

National Research Act of 1974: An act that required the Department of Health, Education, and Welfare (now the Department of Health and Human Services) to codify its policy for the protection of human subjects into federal regulations and created a commission that generated the Belmont Report

Nationwide Health Information Network (NHIN): A term that refers to the building blocks or foundation for interoperability; the physical and national network components that make electronic health records interoperable

NCQA: *See* **National Committee for Quality Assurance**

NCVHS: *See* **National Committee on Vital and Health Statistics**

Negligence: A type of tort in which the defendant does not necessarily intend to cause harm but harm is a foreseeable consequence of his or her conduct

Next-of-kin: An individual who, by virtue of his or her relationship to the patient (such as a spouse, adult child, parent, or adult sibling), may make healthcare decisions on the patient's behalf

NHIN: *See* **Nationwide Health Information Network**

NLRB: *See* **National Labor Relations Board**

No-fault insurance: A term used to describe any type of insurance contract under which insured individuals are indemnified for losses by their own insurance company, regardless of fault in the incident generating losses

Nominal damages: Damages awarded simply to recognize wrongdoing by the defendant when there is no substantial injury suffered by the plaintiff that necessitates compensation or the plaintiff has failed to demonstrate a dollar amount

Noncompete agreement: A contract provision in which an employee or contractor agrees not to compete directly or work for a competitor for a certain period of time after leaving his or her employment or contracting position

Non compos mentis: Not of sound mind

Noncustodial parent: A parent who does not have custody of a child or children as designated by the court system in cases of divorce or legal separation

Nondisclosure agreement: An agreement relating to the confidentiality and privacy of patient information that employees may be required to sign as a condition of employment

Noneconomic damages: Damages that are not monetary in nature; an issue targeted by tort reforms

Nonexempt employee: An employee for whom overtime and minimum wage regulations do apply; nonexempt employees must be paid at least the minimum wage up to 40 hours and time and a half for any hours worked over 40

Nonfeasance: A type of negligence meaning failure to act

Nonmaleficence: A legal principle that means "first do no harm"

Nonrepudiation: The claim that guarantees that the source of the health record documentation cannot deny later that he or she was the author.

Not-for-profit organization: An organization that is not owned by individuals whose profits are retained by the organization and reinvested back into the organization for the benefit of the community it serves

Notice of Privacy Practices (NPP): A statement (mandated by the HIPAA Privacy Rule) issued by a healthcare organization that informs individuals of the uses and disclosures of patient-identifiable health information that may be made by the organization, as well as the individual's rights and the organization's legal duties with respect to that information

Notifiable diseases: Communicable diseases that must be reported to the state for the purpose of tracking outbreaks and preventing spread of the disease

NPDB: *See* **National Practitioner Data Bank**

O

Occupational Safety and Health Administration (OSHA): Federal Occupational Safety and Health Administration (OSHA) regulations ensure that an employee (or designated representative) is given access to his or her own medical and exposure records within 15 days of a request

Occupational safety and health record: As part of employment, a record kept on an employee that contains any and all information related to such items as medical tests, drug tests, examinations, physical abilities, immunizations, screenings required by law, biohazardous exposure, and physical limitations

Occurrence screening: A method for identifying risk through health record review according to objective screening criteria

OCR: *See* **Office for Civil Rights**

Offer: A communicated promise by a party to a contract to either do or not do something if the other party agrees to do or not do something

Office for Civil Rights (OCR): An office within the Department of Health and Human Services (HHS) that is responsible for enforcing civil rights laws that prohibit discrimination on the basis of race, color, national origin, disability, age, sex, and religion by healthcare and human services entities over which the Office for Civil Rights (OCR) has jurisdiction, such as state and local social and health services agencies, hospitals, clinics, nursing homes, or other entities receiving federal financial assistance from HHS; this office also has the authority to investigate alleged violations of the HIPAA Privacy Rule

Office of Inspector General (OIG): Branch of the Department of Health and Human Services (HHS) with responsibility for audits, investigations, inspections, and other activities to protect the integrity of HHS programs and their beneficiaries

Office of the National Coordinator for Health Information Technology (ONC): An office created in 2004 by the federal government to "provide leadership for the development and nationwide implementation of an interoperable health information technology infrastructure to improve the quality and efficiency of health care and the ability of consumers to manage their care and safety" (Office of the Secretary for HHS 2005)

OHCA: *See* **Organized Healthcare Arrangement**

OIG: *See* **Office of Inspector General**

ONC: *See* **Office of the National Coordinator for Health Information Technology**

Ongoing professional practice review: Documenting data on credentialed staff on an ongoing basis rather than at the two-year reappointment process

Open records laws: Laws that define what information is subject to public disclosure and are used to deny Freedom of Information Act (FOIA) requests that include protected health information; also known as public records, sunshine law, or freedom of information laws

Opening statement: The beginning of a trial in which each side outlines the evidence that will be heard

Opinion: A court's written determination that outlines the facts of the case and the legal theories followed in reaching an outcome

Oral argument: The form of argument used, instead of a trial, in appellate courts, state supreme courts, US circuit courts, and the US Supreme Court

Ordinary negligence: Failure to exercise ordinary care under same or similar circumstances

Organ procurement organization: A nonprofit entity that serves as the link between individuals who donate organs and tissues and the recipients who are waiting to receive organs and tissues for transplants

Organized Healthcare Arrangement (OHCA):   An agreement characterized by two or more covered entities that share protected health information to manage and benefit their common enterprise and are recognized by the public as a single entity (HHS 2003)

OSHA: *See* **Occupational Safety and Health Administration**

Outpatient: A patient currently being seen in an ambulatory care, clinic, or physician setting who is not admitted to a hospital as an inpatient

Overcoding: The practice of using a billing code that provides a higher reimbursement rate than the code applicable to the service actually furnished to the patient

Ownership: In healthcare, the person to whom the health record belongs (traditionally, the healthcare provider)

P

Parties: In a lawsuit, the plaintiff and the defendant, accompanied by their respective attorneys unless they are providing legal representation for themselves

Partnership: A legal business entity in which two or more parties agree to share the risk and rewards of the entity

Password: A sequence of characters used to verify that a computer user requesting access to a system is actually that particular user

Patient Care Partnership (patient rights):   A group developed by the American Hospital Association that helps patients understand their expectations, rights, and responsibilities when receiving hospital services

Patient Protection and Affordable Care Act (PPACA):   A federal statute that was signed into law on March 23, 2010. Along with the Health Care and Education Reconciliation Act of 2010 (signed into law on March 30, 2010), the act is the product of the healthcare reform agenda of the Democratic 111th Congress and the Obama administration

Patient rights: *See* **Patient Care Partnership**

Patient Self-Determination Act: A law that became effective in 1991 requiring healthcare institutions that bill Medicare or Medicaid for services to provide adult patients with information about the various types of advance directives

Patriot Act: A 2001 law enacted to deter and punish terrorist acts in the United States and around the world and to enhance law enforcement investigations; gives government authorities the right to access information needed to investigate and deter terrorism

Pay for performance: Programs that reward quality and safety in hospitals and by providers in an attempt to align quality and outcomes with payment

Peer review: A broad range of activities undertaken by a peer review committee to ensure that a facility provides quality care, which may include such activities as the review of quality and safety issues and determinations of medical staff credentials

Per se antitrust violation: Activities that are automatically considered to be antitrust violations

Peremptory challenge: A process through which attorneys may excuse jurors for unstated reasons

Personal health record (PHR): An electronic or paper health record maintained and updated by an individual for himself or herself

Personal identification number (PIN): A private electronic password or code

Personal representative: A person with legal authority to act on behalf of another individual and who is treated the same as the individual regarding the use and disclosure of the individual's protected health information

Persuasive authority: The principle by which courts that are not bound by precedent to follow one another may nonetheless look to one another's decisions for guidance

Petition for writ of certiorari: The process by which a party submits a request for the Supreme Court to hear a case

Petitioner: The party appealing a case, also known as the appellant

PGP: *See* **Pretty good privacy**

PHI: *See* **Protected health information**

PHR: *See* **Personal health record**

Physical examination: A discovery method in which a party may request an independent physical examination, particularly if the physical or mental condition of a party is in question; for example, a defendant may request that a physical examination be performed on the plaintiff in a personal injury lawsuit if the nature and extent of the injuries being claimed are in question

Physical safeguards: A set of four standards defined by the HIPAA Security Rule: facility access controls, workstation use, workstation security, and device and media controls

Physician order(s): A type of documentation within the health record that provides mandatory instructions regarding medical interventions such as treatments, ancillary medical services, tests and procedures, medications, or seclusion and restraint

Physician–patient privilege: The legal protection from confidential communications between physicians and patients related to diagnosis and treatment being disclosed during civil and some misdemeanor litigation

Piercing the corporate veil: An exception to corporate immunity in which the owners of a corporation may be liable for particularly bad acts such as fraud or crime

PIN: *See* **Personal identification number**

PKI: *See* **Public key infrastructure**

PL: *See* **Public law**

Plaintiff: The individual who initiates a lawsuit to enforce either his or her rights or another's obligations

Pleadings: Limited documents that emanate from parties involved in a lawsuit, such as complaints and answers, and are central to the litigation process

Power of attorney: A legal instrument used by a principal (person) to grant legal authority to one or more agents to make certain legal and financial decisions on behalf of the principal

Precedent: A legal doctrine stating that local courts within a court system are bound to follow (apply) the decisions of higher courts in the same court system in order to determine the outcome of a case, as long as the fact pattern of the case in the higher court is similar to that of the current case; also known as *stare decisis*

Preemption: A legal doctrine that requires a covered entity to comply with federal law when federal and state law conflict (that is, federal law preempts contrary state law)

Pregnancy Discrimination Act of 1973: An expansion of Title VII of the Civil Rights Act that requires that pregnancy and related conditions be handled like any other medical condition

Prescription drug monitoring program: A program implemented by most states in an effort to identify inappropriate and illegal activities involving controlled prescription drugs

Pretrial conference: A meeting between the parties, their attorneys, and the court in which the upcoming trial and potential settlement negotiations are discussed

Pretty good privacy (PGP): A type of encryption software that uses public key cryptology and digital signatures for authentication

Primary data source (in healthcare): A record developed by healthcare professionals in the process of providing patient care

Primary source verification: Verification of healthcare practitioners' (physician) credentials as part of the credentialing process for medical staff privileges

Privacy: The quality or state of being hidden from, or undisturbed by, the observation or activities of other people or freedom from unauthorized intrusion; in healthcare-related contexts, the right of a patient to control disclosure of personal information

Privacy Act of 1974: A law that requires federal agencies to safeguard personally identifiable records and provides individuals with certain privacy rights

Privacy and Security Solutions for Interoperable Health Information Exchange Project: A project sponsored by the Agency for Healthcare Research and Quality "to assess variations in organization-level business practices, policies, and state laws that affect electronic health information exchange and to identify and propose practical ways to reduce the variation to those 'good' practices that will permit interoperability while preserving the necessary privacy and security requirements set by the local community" (Dimitropoulos 2007, ES-7)

Privacy board: A group formed by a HIPAA-covered entity to review research studies in which authorization waivers are requested and to ensure the HIPAA privacy rights of research subjects

Privacy officer: A position mandated under the HIPAA Privacy Rule—covered entities must designate an individual to be responsible for developing and implementing privacy policies and procedures

Privacy Rule: *See* **Health Insurance Portability and Accountability Act of 1996**

Private law: The branch of law concerned with the rules and principles that define rights and duties among people and among private businesses

Privilege: A concept that protects confidential communications between provider and patient related to diagnosis and treatment from disclosure during civil and some criminal misdemeanor litigation

Privileged communication: Communication shared between two parties—such as physician and patient, clergy and parishioner, husband and wife, and attorney and client—that is considered privileged; may be defined by state law

Privilege statutes: Laws that legally protect confidential communications between a provider (e.g., physician, psychologists, marital therapist) and a patient from disclosure during civil and some criminal misdemeanor litigation

Pro se: In a lawsuit, an individual who represents himself or herself in lieu of having an attorney

Procedural due process: Applies due process to the federal and state governments; provides that the government shall not take a person's life, liberty, or property without due process of law; procedural due process intends fair processes and procedures

Procedural law: The court's rules that guide a lawsuit from the time it begins through completion, whether it culminates in a trial or ends with a settlement or dismissal

Production of documents: A discovery method initiated by a subpoena duces tecum, which requests that an individual bring documents or other records to court

Protected health information (PHI):   A term defined in the HIPAA Privacy Rule as "individually identifiable health information that is transmitted by electronic media, maintained in electronic medium, or transmitted or maintained in any other form or medium" (45 CFR 160.103)

Psychotherapy notes: Behavioral health notes recorded by a mental health professional that document or analyze the content and impressions of conversations that are part of private counseling sessions; they are not part of the health record and do not contain information such as diagnosis, prescriptions, treatment modalities, and test results

Public key infrastructure (PKI):   A key system with two keys, a private key and a public key

Public law (PubL):   The branch of law concerned with the federal, state, or local government and its relationship to individuals and business organizations; the most familiar form of public law is criminal law

Public record laws: Laws that provide public disclosure upon request of any information of any public body in a state, except as otherwise exempt by state regulations

Punitive damages: Damages that exceed compensatory damages and serve to punish the defendant(s)

Q

QIO: *See* **Quality improvement organization**

Quality: "Doing the right thing, at the right time, in the right way, for the right person—and having the best possible results" (AHRQ)

Quality improvement: The overall processes a facility has in place to make sure healthcare is safe, effective, patient centered, timely, efficient, and equitable

Quality improvement organization (QIO):   Community-based organization selected by the Centers for Medicare and Medicaid Services to conduct quality-related activities

Qui tam: The "whistleblower" provisions of the False Claims Act, which provide that private persons, known as relators, may enforce the act by filing a complaint, under seal, alleging fraud committed against the government

R

RBAC: *See* **Role-based access control**

Recovery Audit Contractors (RACs):   Private organizations utilized by the Department of Health and Human Services to identify underpayments and overpayments associated with services paid under the Medicare program; RACs are paid a contingency fee based on the amount of overpayments and underpayments identified

Red Flag Rules: A provision under the Fair and Accurate Credit Transaction Act (FACTA) that requires financial institutions and creditors—including many healthcare organizations—to develop and implement written programs that identify, detect, and respond to red flags that may signal the presence of identity theft

Red flags: Suspicious documents, information, or behaviors that indicate the possibility of identity theft

Redisclosure: Disclosure by a healthcare organization of information that was created by and received from another entity

Regional Health Information Organization (RHIO):   A health information organization that brings together healthcare stakeholders within a defined geographic area and governs health information exchange among them for the purpose of improving health and care in that community

Registry: A database including information about a particular disease or condition; more information is obtained for registries than is required for communicable diseases

Relator: Private persons who may enforce the False Claims Act by filing a complaint, under seal, alleging fraud committed against the government

Release of information (ROI):   The act of making information known; the release of confidential health information about an identifiable person to another person or entity; release, transfer, provision of access to, or divulging in any other manner of information outside the entity holding the information (45 CFR 160.103) (*see also* **Disclosure**); the process of disclosing protected health information from the health record to another party

Relevant evidence: Evidence having a tendency to make the existence of any fact more probable or less probable

Report cards: Comparative data about healthcare providers reported on websites such as health-grades.com or by organizations such as the National Committee for Quality Assurance and Centers for Medicare and Medicaid Services

Request for admissions: A discovery method that asks the opposing party in litigation to admit to certain facts so the facts do not have to be proven

Request restrictions: Under the Privacy Rule, the right of an individual to request that a covered entity limit the uses and disclosures of protected health information to carry out treatment, payment, or healthcare operations

Requests: Ways in which access, use, and disclosure of patient information are made, which may include mail, telephone, physical presence of the requester, fax, or e-mail

Required standards: The implementation specifications of the HIPAA Security Rule that are designated "required" rather than "addressable"; required standards must be present for the covered entity to be in compliance

Res ipsa loquitur: Latin for "the thing speaks for itself"; an exception to the plaintiff having the burden of proof in which the facts or circumstances accompanying an injury may raise a presumption, or at least permit an inference, of negligence on the part of the defendant or some other individual who is charged with negligence and the burden of proof is shifted to the defendant

Res judicata: Latin for "a matter already judged"; a legal doctrine that bars litigation between the same parties on matters already determined in a former lawsuit

Rescue doctrine: Principle that if a tortfeasor creates a circumstance that places a victim in danger, the tortfeasor is liable not only for the harm caused to the victim but also for the harm caused to any person injured in an effort to rescue that victim

Respondeat superior: Latin for "let the master answer"; the doctrine under which a hospital holds itself responsible for the actions of its employees provided those individuals were acting within the scope of their employment or at the hospital's direction at the time of the activity in question

Respondent: The party against whom a petition is filed on appeal

Restraints and seclusion: Ways of managing behavior; the right of patients to be free from non–medically necessary restraints and seclusion is protected under the Medicare Conditions of Participation

Retaliation and waiver: Rights protected under the Privacy Rule. To ensure the integrity of individuals' right to complain about alleged Privacy Rule violations, covered entities are expressly prohibited from retaliating against anyone who exercises his or her rights under the Privacy Rule, assists in an investigation by the Department of Health and Human Services or other appropriate investigative authority, or opposes an act or practice that he or she believes is a violation of the Privacy Rule; individuals cannot be required to waive the rights that they hold under the Privacy Rule in order to obtain treatment, payment, or eligibility for enrollment or benefits

Retention: A mechanism for storing records, providing for timely retrieval, and establishing the length of time that various types of records will be retained by the healthcare organization

Retention schedule: A timeline for records retention based on factors such as federal and state laws, statutes of limitations, age of patient, competency of patient, accreditation standards, AHIMA recommendations, and operational needs

Revenue cycle: The supervision of all administrative and clinical functions that contribute to the capture, management, and collection of patient service revenues

Revisions: Corrections or alterations to the health record

RHIO: *See* **Regional Health Information Organization**

Risk analysis: The process of identifying which risks should be proactively addressed and which risks are lower in priority

Risk control techniques: Prevent or reduce the chances or effects of a loss occurrence

Risk evaluation: The final step in the risk management process, which involves evaluating each piece of the process to determine whether objectives are being met

Risk exposure or identification: A systematic means of identifying potential losses that requires an understanding of the facility's business, legal, organizational, and clinical components

Risk financing: Methods used to pay for the costs associated with claims and other expenses—most commonly, liability insurance

Risk management: The processes in place to identify, evaluate, and control risk; defined as the organization's risk of accidental financial liability

Risk treatment: The application of risk control and risk financing techniques to determine how a risk should be treated, often aimed at preventing or reducing the chances or effects of a loss occurrence

ROI: *See* **Release of information**

Role-based access control (RBAC): A control system in which access decisions are based on the roles of individual users as part of an organization

Root cause analysis: A tool designed to identify the basic underlying factors that contributed to a sentinel event

Rubber signature stamp: A type of authentication for paper records; stamp must be used only by the person identified by the stamp in accordance with laws, standards, and regulations

Rule of reason analysis: Court determination of whether an antitrust violation exists; includes analysis of affected geographic markets, product or service involved, nature of the industry, motivation of the alleged illegal activity, and impact of the activity on the industry

S

Safe harbor exception: Activities designated by the Office of Inspector General as not subject to prosecution and protect the organization from civil or criminal penalties

Safe Harbor method: The removal of eighteen specified identifiers about an individual or the individual's relatives, employers or household members to de-identify protected health information

Safe Medical Devices Act (SMDA): A federal program that requires reporting to the Food and Drug Administration (FDA) and the product manufacturer of the medical device any occurrences that have or may have contributed to serious illness, serious injury, or death

SAMHSA: *See* **Substance Abuse and Mental Health Services Administration**

Secondary data: When data from a record are used for purposes other than what was intended

Security: 1. The means to control access and protect information from accidental or intentional disclosure to unauthorized persons and from unauthorized alteration, destruction, or loss; 2. The physical protection of facilities and equipment from theft, damage, or unauthorized access; collectively, the policies, procedures, and safeguards designed to protect the confidentiality of information, maintain the integrity and availability of information systems, and control access to the content of these systems

Security incident: An event in which the security of a system was breached or threatened

Security officer or chief security officer: An individual responsible for overseeing privacy policies and procedures

Sentinel event: An unexpected occurrence involving death or serious physical or psychological injury, or the risk thereof (Joint Commission 2006)

Separation of powers: Among the three branches of federal and state governments, the authority of each is limited in order to inhibit the ability of any one branch of government to become autocratic

Service: The means by which a defendant is notified of a lawsuit

Settlement: Determining the outcome of a legal case between the parties without pursuing the matter through to trial

Shadow Record: A duplicate record kept for the convenience of the provider or facility; it usually is an exact duplicate of the original health record and should not contain documentation that is not in the original record

Sherman Anti-Trust Act: First passed in 1890, one of several antitrust laws that collectively make it illegal to restrain trade through contracts or conspiracies and prohibit price fixing and mergers that lessen competition, enforced by the Federal Trade Commission (FTC) and the Department of Justice (DOJ)

Short form consent: In the context of human subjects research, a written document stating that the elements of informed consent required by the Common Rule have been orally presented to and understood by the subject or the subject's legally authorized representative

Slander: Defamation in an oral form

SMDA: *See* **Safe Medical Devices Act**

Social media: A collection of online technologies and practices that people use to share opinions, insights, experiences, and perspectives; often used by healthcare organizations as marketing tools and mechanisms to communicate with consumers or patients

Social Security Administration (SSA): A division of the federal government that administers rehabilitation and disability services for people suffering from physical or mental disabilities that affect their ability to work or return to work in a timely manner

Sole proprietorship: A legal business entity in which a single owner elects not to insulate his or her personal assets through the use of a corporation or other legal form

Special damages: Arrive out of the special character, condition, or circumstances of the event or person injured

Special jurisdiction: A type of court in which particular areas of the law have been carved out for resolution (for example, small claims, domestic relations, juvenile, or probate courts)

Specific performance: A court order that requires the party that breached a contract to honor its contractual obligations

Spoliation: Intentional destruction, mutilation, alteration, or concealment of information relevant to a legal proceeding

SSA: *See* **Social Security Administration**

Stand-alone authorization: An authorization for the use or disclosure of one's protected health information that is separate from an informed consent for treatment or participation in a research study

Standard of care: What an individual is expected to do or not do in a particular situation, established by statute or ordinance, judicial decision, professional associations, or by practice; in healthcare professions, it is the exercise of reasonable care by healthcare professionals with similar training and experience in the same or similar communities

Stare decisis: Latin for "let the decision stand"; a legal doctrine stating that local courts within a court system are bound to follow (apply) the decisions of higher courts in the same court system in order to determine the outcome of a case, as long as the fact pattern of the case in the higher court is similar to that of the current case

Stark Law: *See* **Federal Physician Self-Referral Statute**

State action: When a private entity such as a hospital takes on the characteristics of a public organization; the private organization is then held to government standards such as due process

Statute of limitations: A statutory enactment that places time limits on certain claims

Statute of repose: Statute enacted to add new provisions, subject to certain exceptions, that provide a maximum amount of time within which to discover and file a claim; maximum or absolute limitations

Statutory law: Law based on statutes, which are created by the legislative branch of the government (the House of Representatives and the Senate)

Steward: The person responsible for ensuring the integrity and security of electronic information and records (*see also* **Custodian of health records**)

Stewardship: Refers to responsibility for ensuring the integrity (accuracy, completeness, timeliness) and security (protection of privacy as well as protection from tampering, loss, or destruction) within the context of electronic information and records management

Strict liability: A theory under which a person is responsible for the damage and loss caused by his or her acts and omissions regardless of fault

Structured settlement: An arrangement by which the claim is paid in installments rather than in one lump sum settlement

Subject matter jurisdiction: A form of jurisdiction based on the content or substantive area of the case being brought

Subpoena: Legal order that commands an individual to give testimony or commands the production, inspection, copying, testing, or sampling of books, documents, electronically stored information, or tangible items

Subpoena ad testificandum: A subpoena that primarily seeks an individual's testimony

Subpoena duces tecum: A subpoena instructing the recipient to bring documents and other records to a deposition or to court

Substance Abuse and Mental Health Services Administration (SAMHSA):   A division of the Department of Health and Human Services that, in 2004, published a document explaining the relationship between HIPAA and the Alcohol and Drug Abuse Regulations regarding confidentiality and release of information

Substantive due process: Guarantees that laws are fair, reasonable, and not arbitrary; allows for challenges to a law's content and substance

Substantive law: Law that defines the rights and obligations that arise between two or more parties, such as torts and contracts

Sudden emergency doctrine: Relieves a person of liability if, without prior negligence on his or her part, that person is confronted with a sudden emergency and acts as an ordinarily prudent person would act under the circumstances

Summons: A document that gives the defendant notice of the lawsuit and explains the defendant's procedural obligations

Sunshine laws: *See* **Open records laws, Public records laws**

Supremacy Clause: A clause of the US Constitution that states that federal law is supreme over any conflicting state law

Supreme Court: The highest court in the US legal system; hears cases from the US Courts of Appeals and the highest state courts when federal statutes, treaties, or the US Constitution is involved

Supreme courts: Courts of final decision making, which exist at both the federal and state levels; other courts must abide by decisions of the supreme courts

Syndromic surveillance: Refers to monitoring nonspecific clinical information that may indicate a bioterrorism-associated disease before a specific diagnosis is made

System security: Totality of safeguards including hardware, software, personnel policies, information practice policies, disaster preparedness, and oversight of these components; protects both the system and the information contained within from unauthorized access from without and from misuse from within; enables the entity or system to protect the confidential information it stores from unauthorized access, disclosure, or misuse, there by protecting the privacy of the individuals who are the subjects of the stored information

T

Technical safeguards: Security measures that are based on technology rather than on administration or physical security, including access control, unique user identification, automatic logoff, and encryption and decryption

Telephone callback procedures: A form of entity authentication in which a modem dials into the system and a special callback application asks for the telephone number from which the call was placed

Term of art: Word or phrase with a specific meaning in a defined subject, such as PHI (protected health information) in HIPAA

Termination of access: An administrative safeguard that is used when an employee changes job position, takes on new job roles or duties, or terminates employment with the organization

Therapeutic privilege: A doctrine that has historically allowed physicians to withhold information from patients in limited circumstances

Timeliness: The completion of a health record within timelines established by legal and accreditation standards and by organizational policy and medical staff bylaws

Title VII of the Civil Rights Act of 1964:   A law that, in combination with the Equal Employment Opportunity Act of 1972, prohibits discrimination based on age, race, color, sex, religion, or national origin

Tokens: Devices such as key cards that are inserted into doors or computers in order to gain entry

Tolled: Delay, suspend, or hold off effect of a statute

Tort: A civil wrong for which the law provides a remedy in the form of a lawsuit to recover damages

Tort law: Law that involves the right of an individual, corporation, or other legal entity to recover damages for a loss caused by the defendant (tortfeasor or wrongdoer)

Tort reform: The variety of measures intended by legislatures to overhaul the justice system; with regard to medical malpractice, such reforms are intended to diminish the number of lawsuits and large jury verdicts, stabilize the market, and ultimately reduce premiums for physicians

Tortfeasor: Wrongdoer, defendant

TPO: *See* **Treatment, payment, and healthcare operations**

Transfer of health records: The movement of a record from one medium to another (for example, from paper to microfilm or to an optical imaging system) or to another records custodian

Transplant registries: Database of patients who need organs as well as databases of potential donors

Trauma registry: A registry designed to identify the types of traumatic injuries incurred in the state, currently required by 37 states

Traumatic injury: A wound or injury included in a trauma registry

Treatment, payment, and healthcare operations (TPO):   Collectively, these three actions are functions of a covered entity that are necessary for the covered entity to successfully conduct business; thus, many of the Privacy Rule's requirements are relaxed or removed where protected health information is needed for purposes of treatment, payment, or healthcare operations

Trial: The stage in a lawsuit after the pretrial phase if the parties do not negotiate a settlement and the case is not dismissed

Trial courts: The first and lowest level of the US federal court system or of a state court system

Trier of fact: Judge or jury responsible for deciding factual issues

Trojan horse: A destructive piece of programming code that hides in another piece of programming code that looks harmless, such as a macro or an e-mail message

Types of requests: The ways in which requests for access, use, and disclosure of patient information are made, which may include mail, telephone, physical presence of the requester, fax, or e-mail

U

UHCDA: *See* **Uniform Health-Care Decisions Act**

Ultra vires act: A decision by a corporation's governing body or executives that goes beyond the express or implied powers of the corporation; such an act is usually void and can result in personal liability if financial loss results, if it was taken with the knowledge that the action was beyond the scope of power, or if it was made in bad faith

Unavoidable accident: An occurrence that could not have been foreseen or anticipated in the exercise of ordinary care and that results without the fault or negligence of either the defendant or the plaintiff

Unbundling: A billing practice in which providers use multiple procedure codes for a group of procedures instead of the appropriate comprehensive code in order to inappropriately maximize reimbursement

Unconditioned authorization: Authorization is not required in order to receive treatment or some other service or benefit

Uniform Anatomical Gift Act: An act that provides suggested standards for all aspects of organ donation, including who may make anatomical gifts and how intent to make anatomical gifts should be expressed—designed to create uniformity in this area across all 50 states

Uniform Durable Power of Attorney Act: Federal statute that provides a mechanism for individuals to deal with their property in the event of incapacity

Uniform Electronic Transactions Act: Federal statute that makes electronic transactions as enforceable as paper transactions, removing barriers to electronic commerce and increasing trust associated with electronic business transactions

Uniform Guidelines on Employee Selection Procedures: A set of guidelines published by the Equal Employment Opportunity Commission to guide selection of employees; the overriding principle is that selection of employees must be made on qualifications related to job performance

Uniform Health-Care Decisions Act (UHCDA): A model law created in 1993 that provides that an individual may give an oral or written instruction to a healthcare provider that remains in force even after the individual loses capacity, and suggests decision-making priority for that individual's surrogates

Uniform Photographic Copies of Business and Public Records as Evidence Act (UPA): Federal statute, with state versions, that makes admissible as evidence the reproduction of any record that has been retained in the regular course of business and kept by a process that accurately reproduces the original in any medium; supports the transition from paper to electronic storage of information

Union steward: A representative of the employee in a unionized environment

Unique identifier: A combination of characters and numbers assigned and maintained by the security system and used to track individual user activity; user ID

United States Code (USC): The compilation of all federal statutes

Unusual event: A type of event that often must be reported to the state; may include unexpected occurrences resulting in death or serious injury unrelated to the natural course of a patient's illness or underlying condition, an incident resulting in the abuse of a patient, medication errors, transfusion errors, transfusion reactions, falls resulting in fractures, wrong patient/wrong site surgical procedures, and operative complications

Upcoding: *See* **Overcoding**

USC: *See* **United States Code**

Use: HIPAA definition with respect to individually identifiable health information, the sharing, employment, application, utilization, examination, or analysis of such information within an entity that maintains such information (45 CFR 160.103)

User: An individual with rights to use a particular secured system or access a particular physical area

User-based access control (UBAC):   A security mechanism used to grant users of a system access based on the identity of the user (HHS n.d.)

Uses, disclosures, and requests: The three types of situations in which protected health information is handled and the Privacy Rule governs

Utilization review: The process of determining whether the medical care provided to a specific patient is necessary according to preestablished objective screening criteria at time frames specified in the organization's utilization management plan

V

Vendors: Outside companies such as consultants and those who sell equipment and supplies, perform release-of-information functions, provide laundry or food services, or repair equipment that have a presence in a healthcare facility and may or may not be business associates

Verdict: The decision rendered by the jury at the end of a trial; in criminal cases, in order to convict or acquit a defendant, a unanimous vote is required

Version management: The manner in which an organization handles the numerous versions that may exist of a document or collection of data

Vertical restraint of trade: Situation in which two or more entities at different levels in a distribution chain act together to restrain trade

Vital record: Records concerned with births, deaths, marriages, divorces, abortions, and late fetal deaths; each state requires that a certificate be completed that verifies the vital event

Voir dire: The process through which a jury is selected

W

Wagner Act: *See* **National Labor Relations Act of 1935**

Waiver of privilege: An exception to physician–patient privilege that occurs when a party claims damages for a mental or physical injury; the party thereby waives his or her right to confidentiality to the extent that it is necessary to determine whether the mental or physical injury is due to another cause

Warranties: Statements of fact in a contract that are made by one party to induce another party to enter into the contract

Weight of the evidence: The amount of consideration the judge or jury gives a particular record or piece of evidence when deciding the factual issues of the case

WEP: *See* **Wired equivalent privacy**

Whistleblower: An individual who discloses wrongdoing by an organization to the authorities or to the public

Wired equivalent privacy (WEP):   A form of encryption used to authenticate the sender and the receiver of messages over networks, particularly when the Internet is involved in the data transmission; should provide authentication (both sender and recipient are known to each other), data security (safe from interception), and data nonrepudiation (data sent have arrived unchanged)

Workers' compensation: Legislation that ensures that employees who are injured on the job or become ill as a result of a job are provided with some means of support while recovering from their illness or injuries

Workforce: Under the HIPAA Privacy Rule, employees, volunteers, trainees, and other persons, whether paid or not, who work for and are under the direct control of the covered entity

Workstation: A computer designed to accept data from multiple sources in order to assist in managing information for daily activities and to provide a convenient means of entering data as desired by the user at the point of care

Worm: A special type of computer virus that stores and then replicates itself

Writ of execution: A method of collecting judgment that directs the appropriate law enforcement official to seize the defendant's real or personal property to satisfy the debt owed to the plaintiff

List of Cases

Ace v. State of New York, 146 Misc.2d 954, 553 N.Y.S.2d 605 (1990)

Acuna v. Turkish, 384 NJ Super. 395 (App. Div. 2006)

Adams v. St. Francis Regional Medical Center, 264 KS 144, 955 P.2d 1169 (1998)

American Color Graphics v. Rayfield Foster, AL Civ. App., 838 So.2d 374 (2001)

Anderson v. Strong Memorial Hospital, 140 Misc.2d 770, 531 N.Y.S.2d 735 (1988)

Andrews v. Ohio Dept. of Transp, Court of Claims No. 2002-05336-AD (2002)

Batson v. Kentucky, 476 U.S. 79 (1986)

Berger v. Sonneland, 101 WN. App. 141, 1 P.3d 1187 (2000)

Biddle v. Warren General Hospital, 86 Ohio St. 3d 395 (1999)

Broek v. Park Nicollet Health Services, MN App. Unpub. (2003)

Coleman Parent Holding Inc. v. Morgan Stanley & Co., FL Dist. Ct. App. 892, So. 2d 496 (2004)

Connecticut v. Abney, 88 CT App. 495; 869 A.2d 1263 (2005)

Cruzan v. Director, Missouri Department of Health, 497 US 261; 110 Sect. 2841 (1990)

Darling v. Charleston Community Memorial Hospital, 33 IL 2d 326, 211 N.E.2d 253, 14 A.L.R. 3d 860 (IL Sept. 29, 1965)

Dillard v. Pittway Corp., 719 So.2d 188, 193 (Ala. 1998)

Duncan v. Scottsdale Medical Imaging, Ltd., 70 P.3d 435; 415 AZ Adv. Rep. 43 (2003)

Emergicare Systems Corporation v. Bourdon, 942 S.W. 2d 201 (Tex. App. 1997)

Erie Railroad Co. v. Tompkins, 304 U.S. 64 (1938)

Estate of Berhinger v. Medical Center at Princeton, 249 N.J. Super. 597, 592 A2d 1251 (N.J. Super. L. 1991)

Fabich v. Montana Rail Link, Inc., MT Daist., 2005 ML 135

Fairfax Hospital v. Curtis, 249 VA 531; 457 S.E.2d 66 (1997)

Fierstein v. DePaul Health Center, MO Ct. App. E.D., 24 S.W.3d 220 (2000)

Fletcher v. South Peninsula Hosp., 71 P.3d 833 (Alaska 2003)

Fred's Stores of Tennessee v. Brown, MS App., 829 So. 2d 1261 (2002)

Griswold v. Connecticut, 381 U.S. 479 (1965)

Hake v. George Wiedemann Brewing Co., 23 Ohio St. 2d 65(1970)

Hamilton v. Ashton, 846 N.E.2d 309 (IN Ct. App. 2006)

Hammonds v. Aetna Casualty & Surety Co., 243 F. Supp. 793 (N.D. Ohio 1965)

Herr v. Wheeler, 634 S.E.2d 317, 320 (Va. 2006)

Hospital Authority of City of St. Marys v. Eason, 222 Ga. 536 (1966)

In the Matter of J.B., 172 NC App. 1; 616 S.E.2d 264 (2005)

In the Matter of Robert Quackenbush, 156 NJ Super. 282; 382 A.2d 785 (1978)

In re Quinlan, 70 NJ 10. 355 A.2d 647 (1976)

In re Storar, 52 NY 2d 363; 420 N.E.2d 64; 52 NY 2d 382; 420 N.E.2d 73 (1981)

In re Search Warrant App. No. 125-4, 852 A.2d 408 (PA Super.2004)

Johnson PPA v. Atlantic Health Services, P.C., 2000 WL 1228275 (Conn. Super. Aug. 21, 2000)

Kadlec Medical Center v. Lakeview Anesthesia Associates, No. Civ.A. 04-0997 (E.D.La. May 19, 2005).

Kohl v. Tirado, 256 GA App. 681, 569 S.E.2d 576 (2002)

Lehman v. Haynam, 164 Ohio St. 595 (1956)

Lemuz By and Through Lemuz v. Fieser, 933 P.2d 134 (Kansas 1997)

Limbaugh v. Florida, 887 So.2d 387 (2004)

Lipschitz v. Stein, NY App. Div., 10 A.D.3d 634, 781 NYS.2d 773 (2004)

Mapes v. District Court, 250 MT 524; 822 P.2d 91 (1991)

Martin v. Baehler 1993 WL 258843 (Del. Super. 1993)

Nielsen v. Braland, 264 MN 481, 119 N.W.2d 737 (1963)

Order of Railroad Telegraphers v. Railway Express Agency, 321 U.S. 342 (1944)

The Pension Committee of the University of Montreal Pension Plan, et al., v. Banc of America Securities, LLC, et al., SDNY, 05 Civ. 9016 (2010)

Phillips v. Covenant Clinic, 625 N.W.2d 714, Iowa (2001)

Provena Covenant Medical Center v. Department of Revenue, 2010 WL 966858, 10 (2010)

Rea v. Pardo, 132 A.D.2d 442, 522 N.Y.S.2d 393 (1987)

Reese v. Bd. of Directors of Memorial Hosp. of Laramie Co., 955 P.2d 425 (Wyo. 1998)

Roe v. Wade, 410 U.S. 113 (1973)

Riverside Hosp., Inc. v. Johnson, 272 VA 518, 636 S.E.2d 416 (2006)

Sanders v. Spector, 673 So.2d 1176 (La. App. 1996)

Schloendorff v. Society of New York Hospital, 211 NY 125; 105 N.E. 92 (1914)

Silvestri v. General Motors, 4th Cir., 271 F.3d 583, 591 (2001)

Smith v. McVicker, 5th App. No. 2003AP120092, 2004- Ohio-4217 (2004)

Smith v. Rossi, 115 A.D. 2nd 899; NY App. Div. (1985)

Strickland v. Pinder, 899 A.2d 770 (D.C. Ct. App. 2006)

Swartz v. Cartwright, 15 MS L. Rep. (2002)

Tarasoff v. the Regents of the University of California, 17 Cal. 3d, 425, 551 P 2d 334, 132 Cal. Rptr. 14 (Cal. 1976)

Thompson v. Ulysses Cruises, Inc., 812 F. Supp. 900 (S.D. Ind. 1993)

Trujillo v. Trujillo, 71 CA App. 2nd 257, 162 P.2d 64 (1945)

Uncapher v. Baltimore & O.R. Co., 127 Ohio St. 351, at syllabus (1933)

Union Pacific R. Co. v. Botsford, 141 US 250; 11 Sect. 1000 (1891)

United States. v. Gibson, No. CR04-0374RSM, 2004 WL 2237585 (W.D. Wash. August 19, 2004)

United States v. Syme, 3rd Cir., 276 F.3d 131 (2002)

Wagner v. Int'l Railway, 232 N.Y. 176 (1921)

Wesley Medical Center v. Clark, 234 KS 13, 669 P.2d 209, 220–221 (1983)

Williams v. American Medical Systems, 248 Ga. App. 682, 684 (2001)

Williams v. Sprint/United Management Company, 230 F.R.D. 640 (D. Kan. 2005)

Wilson v. Merritt, 142 Cal. App. 4th 1125, 48 CA Rptr. 3d 630 (2006)

Zubulake v. UBS Warburg, SDNY, 217 FRD 309 (2003)

Zubulake v. UBS Warburg, 220 FRD 212 (2003)

Zubulake v. UBS Warburg, 229 FRD 422 (2004)

Index

Note: Page numbers with *f* indicate figures; those with *t* indicate tables.